H. KELIKIAN, M.D.
Associate Professor, Department of Orthopaedic Surgery
Northwestern University Medical School and Senior Attending Staff of Chicago
Wesley Memorial Hospital

HALLUX VALGUS, ALLIED DEFORMITIES OF THE FOREFOOT *and* METATARSALGIA

W. B. Saunders Company, Philadelphia & London

W. B. Saunders Company: West Washington Square
Philadelphia, Pa. 19105

12 Dyott Street
London WCIA IDB

833 Oxford Street
Toronto 18, Ontario

Hallux Valgus, Allied Deformities of the Forefoot and Metatarsalgia ISBN 0-7216-5355-3

 Press of W. B. Saunders Company. Library of Congress catalog card number 65–11549.

Print No.: 9 8 7 6 5 4

Preface

The extensive bibliographies in this book must be taken as testimony of the author's intellectual indebtedness to others—in particular to the great surgeons of the past. The historical asides in the text may help to place surgical concepts in proper perspective and perhaps counteract the curious notion that important observations were recorded only in recent decades.

The author wishes to express his gratitude to Irmgard Karolina Strassburger for the drawings which illustrate this book; to Miss Vicki Catalani, of the Chicago Wesley Memorial Hospital, for the photographic illustrations; to Miss Georgia Price, of the Northwestern University Medical School Library, and to Miss Kathleen Worst, of the American College of Surgeons Library, in tracking down for me little-known journals and rare books; and to Mrs. Rose Boyian, who made innumerable retypings of the manuscript. Without their help work often would have come to a full standstill.

No less a debt is owed to Miss Lena Ohannes Kupelian, who made faithful translations from many languages of source material whose reading enriched my own life as a surgeon and made possible my fuller understanding of the sustained attention thoughtful surgeons have everywhere given to the problems of deformity and discomfort with which we all must deal.

But the greatest obligation of all I owe to my own family, who quietly supported an endeavor which often seemed endless and who missed—I hope as much as I—the many hours of pleasant companionship I once enjoyed with them.

My publishers, too, had to know patience. Beyond this passive virtue they displayed also a sensitive appreciation of my purposes and a thorough technical knowledge of how to secure the results in engraving and printing which I wanted.

H. Kelikian

Contents

INTRODUCTION

More than a hundred years ago, Volkmann (1856) complained that the "affection" that "not only deforms the foot in a most clumsy way but also makes the gait uncertain and continuous walking painful" had not received from surgeons the attention it deserved. According to their social status, patients with what we now call hallux valgus were relegated to barbers to have their calluses trimmed, or to bootmakers to have their shoes adjusted. Hallux valgus was considered as belonging to "a low class surgery." Volkmann wrote: "The handbooks of surgery pass over it mostly in silence."

Not long ago the deformities of the toes, including hallux valgus, were classed with comparatively insignificant surgical problems. Blundell Bankart (1935) discussed hallux valgus, hallux rigidus, anterior metatarsalgia, and hammered toes under the general heading, *Minor Maladies of the Foot.* Ezra Jones (1940) felt "a bit embarrassed in presenting such a lowly subject as bunion operation" to the New England Surgical Society. Sixty-nine years earlier Jacques Reverdin (1881) betrayed no such squeamishness, nor offered an apologetic preamble, when he discussed the treatment of hallux valgus before the more austere International Medical Congress.

In the course of the discussion that followed Mayo's (1920) paper on hallux valgus, Calvin commented: "Some celebrated surgeon has said that there is no such thing as minor surgery, and the fact that Dr. Mayo undertakes to present a subject like this means that he considers the treatment of bunion as an important surgical procedure." It is tempting to give the expanded version of the cliché Calvin quoted: "There is no such thing as minor surgery, but there are minor surgeons,"—men with blunted perception who remain blind to the manifold problems of hallux valgus and allied forefoot deformities. To Mayo's name, Calvin might have added those of Broca, Volkmann, Hueter, Hamilton, Reverdin, Riedel, Hoffa, Schede, Fowler, Halstead, Robert Jones, and Hohmann, none of whom might be regarded as a minor surgeon. These men and many others we would classify as major surgeons have accorded serious attention to hallux valgus.

The question may be asked: "Why a long monograph on such a subject?" The answer is implicit in the title of this treatise: hallux valgus is not an isolated condition; it is related to the other deformities of the forefoot. The complexity of hallux valgus has been tacitly recognized for some time—Picqué (1902) considered it a complex lesion—but the concept received widespread expression around the third decade of the present century. Massart (1934) spoke of the deformities—not the deformity—of hallux valgus and insisted that the structural changes were not solely confined to the proximal joint of the great toe. The phrase *hallux valgus complex* simultaneously appeared in several languages. Mau (1938) entitled his article *Hallux-valgus Komplex*. Huc and Thyes (1938) referred to the pathological complexity of hallux valgus—"le complex pathologie de l'hallux valgus." Under the heading *Hallux Valgus Complex,* Creer (1938) included a multitude of deformities ranging from the spreading of the metatarsal arch to "swelling of the foot from oedema, not due to general conditions."

The extensive literature on hallux valgus and allied forefoot deformities supplies the second justification for the length of this monograph. Eighteenth century authors—Le Dran (1731), Rousselot (1769), Laforest (1782), and Camper (1781)—dwelt at some length on the deformities of the toes. Early in the nineteenth century both Brodie (1822) and Boyer (1826) specifically referred to the condition we now call hallux valgus. Since the publication of Froriep's (1834) *Commentatiuncula de Ossis Metatarsi Primi Exostosi,* a staggering number of articles has been written on this subject. To use a popular figure of speech, the grain lies hidden in the haystack; it must be sought, sifted, and brought to light. Diligent search takes time; adequate exposure requires space—not a few pages, but many. A critical appraisal of the vast literature should not be amiss. The least we hope to accomplish is to clarify some of the confusion.

A third justification for the length of this monograph lies in the fact that there is not a single work in English that deals in detail with this subject. In French, in addition to more than a dozen book size theses, there are the comprehensive surveys of Mauclaire (1896), Mouchet (1922), Verbrugge (1933), and Lelièvre (1952). In German, besides Cornils' (1890) dissertation, there are the detailed studies of Payr (1894), Heubach (1897), Simon (1918), Hohmann (1925), Timmer (1930), and Bade (1940). Offhand, one recalls Aievoli's (1895) essay in Italian, and Khoury's (1947) monograph in Spanish.

In wading through what has been written, one finds a number of stock statements that need reappraisal. The literature is cluttered with numerous conjectures concerning the causation of malformed toes; greater emphasis is being placed on evolutionary antecedents and on heredity, and less on civilized habits. It has become fashionable to overlook the obvious—shoes as one of the major causes of malformed toes—and indulge in conjectures. Theories that are not universally accepted by professional anthropologists and embryologists have been flaunted by clinicians as established facts. It is understandable that the sophomoric sibling who wanted to follow the footsteps of Darwin or Bardeen, but somehow got sidetracked into the unglamorous avocation of treating twisted toes should—out of sheer nostalgia or in response to the secret whisperings of his suppressed desire—attempt to relate his thoughts with those of his student-day idols. There is nothing wrong in trying to connect clinical observations with the general body of scientific knowledge, provided that he who attempts such correlation is well versed in both fields, or at least has studied the pros and cons of the controversial question. When the clinician starts with a fixed idea and seeks confirmation in the work of a scientist, and eschews contrary opinions, he is liable to be misled, and if influential, in his turn mislead others.

An influential orthopedic surgeon started the trend in the twenties; he surmised that hallux valgus—rather, metatarsus primus varus—might be a "reversion to the branch-grasping Simian type great toe, described by Morton." He did not seem aware that Morton's theory had been subjected to severe criticism by more than one professional anthropologist. He also suspected "a persistence of the embryo great toe, described by Lebloc" and did not appear to have taken sufficient pains to spell embryologist Leboucq's name correctly.

Leboucq's name was again conjured lately—this time with correct spelling. Since the earliest days of his orthopedic practice, another surgeon wrote, he had been aware of the frequent association of "metatarsus varus primus with bunions." At the time, however, he had not known that the same observation had been made by anthropologists long before orthopedic surgeons had thought of it. He mentioned Leboucq, who as early as 1882, had pointed out that the divergence of the first metatarsal was due to the extreme angle made by the plane of the distal articular facet of the cuneiform bone with the long axis of the foot. "This angle," the orthopedic surgeon attested, "approaches that found in prehensile arborial foot of the primates."

Leboucq (1882) studied the shape of the innermost cuneiform in embryos. He found that in 20 mm. specimens the tibial border of this bone was shorter than its fibular margin, which made its distal articular facet slope obliquely forward. This in turn induced the first metatarsal to diverge inward, away from its fellows. As development progressed, the tibial side of the cuneiform bone grew more rapidly than the fibular border, gradually straightening the plane of the distal articular facet until, in 40 mm. embryos it assumed the position it occupied in adults. Leboucq made no attempt to correlate "bunions" with the oblique setting of the innermost cuneometatarsal joint. Commenting on Leboucq's findings, no less an authority than Garrit S. Miller, Jr. (1920), of the United States National Museum said: "The course of the individual development in the embryo appears to be that which a divergent hallux without prehensile specification would pass through in assuming the human structure." Miller did not discern any "gorriloid taint" in the development of human hallux. It all appears to depend on which anthropologist or embryologist one chooses to quote from, and how one interprets and slants what one reads.

There are few reports in the literature of attempts to correlate local changes involving the toes with the general derangement of the forefoot. As for the treatment, the literature abounds with descriptions of innumerable appliances that were—and still are—prescribed for palliative as well as corrective purposes. There are far too many operative procedures on the record for the surgical correction of hallux valgus. Metcalf (1912) summarized 15 different operations; Timmer (1930) mentioned 25; Verbrugge (1933) outlined 51; Perrot (1946) counted 68; and McBride (1952) named 58. "Such variety of methods," McBride wrote, "can mean but one thing, namely that hallux valgus is a recalcitrant disorder."

This is a discreet understatement, not the whole truth. Most surgical procedures on record have scant, extremely tenuous, often untenable principles to support them. A number of operations are possible only on paper, in drawings or blueprints. Behind some of them lurks the desire of the progenitor to perpetuate his name by linking it to a supposedly new method. Lack of historical perspective might have led some of these authors to claim originality for a procedure that had been tried in the past and justly or unjustly relegated to limbo. Frequently one favored technique is applied to all grades of deformities: the cases are not objectively studied and surgically individualized.

Many methods have been indiscriminately ascribed to men who can hardly be said to have first devised or described them. Nor can it be said that these writers have canvassed the past records conscientiously, separated the sound from the slick, and assimilated the best. What is offered as new is often an amalgam of shopworn platitudes presented in streamlined verbiage. Even more disheartening is the complacent acceptance by the neophyte of what he reads. In most instances he merely sees the label and does not probe further. Concise, compact descriptions attract him. He shuns details. A diagram or two and a sketchy direction satisfy him; he remembers an operation by the name of the man who last described it.

It appears that all one has to do is to slip in the epithet "new" or prefix an operation with the possessive "my" or "author's." Those interested, including the author himself, can see and read the printed testimony and perhaps believe—which they usually do—that no one else had thought of it before. If the author had any qualms about the matter, he threw in a statement that began with the sentence, "At the time I first performed this operation I was not aware that it has been. . . ." Pretense of ignorance has been used to camouflage lack of intellectual integrity. It is possible that some writers resorted to such apologia inadvertently: they utilized a stock style of introducing a supposedly original method. In either case, by the indiscriminating reader, such an author is certain to be considered the co-originator if not the inventor of the supposedly new operation.

The author of these lines feels no compulsion to cavil or castigate. His is merely an attempt to rectify the record, or to put it tersely, organize the confusion. He may be in error about some points. If so, he would welcome the opportunity to be corrected. In criticizing others he feels the way Frank Hamilton (1884) must have felt when he wrote in the preface of his book: "From the beginning of his studies, the Author has found one of his most difficult labors in attempting to eliminate from the branch of science which he has undertaken to teach, the numerous 'false facts' or unreliable statements derived from these several sources; and this must be accepted as his apology for his repeated expressions of scepticism in reference to testimony, some of which has been accepted, as is believed without sufficient examination, by writers whose opinions might be regarded as of more value than his own."

In the present monograph the surgical treatment of forefoot deformities has been allotted considerable space and the discussion of the palliative management curtailed disproportionately. Some may take this as a token of the author's familiarity with the former, or conversely, of his limited experience in the latter. On his part the author concedes a measure of justification in such a verdict. He confesses he is prejudiced in favor of surgery. Unless he has to—because of the patient's unfavorable health or reluctance to submit to surgery—he does not pad shoes and prescribe plates in the hope of obtaining a lasting cure. He admits that external appliances sometimes allay the discomfort caused by forefoot deformities, but they do not correct them: they merely temporize.

REFERENCES

Aievoli, E.: Hallus valgus. *In* rapporto alla statica ed alla meccanica del piede. Arch. di. Ortop. *12*:225–254, 1895.

Bade, P.: *Der Hallux valgus.* F. Enke, Stuttgart, 1940.

Bankart, A. S. B.: The treatment of minor maladies of the foot. Lancet. *1*:249–252, Feb. 2, 1935.

Boyer, A.: *Traité des Maladies Chirurgicales.* 3rd Ed. Paris. *2*:73–76, 1826.

Brodie, B. C.: *Pathological and Surgical Observations on the Diseases of the Joints.* Longmans, London, 1822, pp. 350–362.

Camper, P.: *On the Best Form of Shoe.* Published with Dowie's treatise *The Foot and Its Covering.* R. Hardwicke, London, 1861, pp. 1–44. The French version, called *Dissertation sur le Meilleur Forme des Souliers,* appeared in Paris, 1781.

Cornils, P.: *Ueber Gelenkresectionen bei Arthritis Deformans und Hallux valgus.* Inaugural-Dissertation. G. Neuenhahn, Jena, 1890, pp. 5–43.

Creer, W. S.: The hallux valgus complex. Brit. Med. J. *2*:5–9, July 2, 1938.

Froriep, R.: *Commentatiuncula de Ossis Metatarsi Primi Exostosi.* Berolini: Joanni de Wiebel., 1834, pp. 1–8.

Hamilton, F. G.: *A Practical Treatise on Fractures and Dislocations.* 7th Ed., Philadelphia, H. C. Lea's Son & Co., pp. v–vii, 1884.

Heubach, F.: Ueber Hallux valgus und seine operative Behandlung nach Edm. Rose. Dtsch. Ztschr. Chir. *46*:210–275, 1897.

Hohmann, G.: *Der Hallux valgus und die übrigen Zehenverkruemmungen.* Ergeb. Chir. Orthop. *18*:308–376, 1925.

Huc, G., and Thyes: Tactique opératoire dans l'hallux valgus. Rev. d'Orthop. *25*:720–721, 1938.

Jones, E. A.: McBride operation for hallux valgus. Tr. New Eng. Surg. Soc. *23*:57–60, 1940.

Khoury, C.: *Hallux Valgus.* Lopex & Etchegoyen, Buenos Aires, 1947.

Laforest: *L'Art de Soigner les Pieds.* 3rd Ed., Lebigre, Paris, 1782, pp. 87–95.

Leboucq, H.: Le développement du premier métatarsien et de son articulation tarsienne chez l'homme. Arch. Biol. *3*:337–344, 1882.

Le Dran, H. F.: *Observations in Surgery* (Tr. by J. S. Surgeon). J. Hodges, London, 1739, pp. 359–368. The original French edition—*Observations de Chirurgie,* Chas. Osmond, Paris—appeared in 1731.

Lelièvre, J.: *Pathologie du Pied.* Masson et Cie, Paris, 1952, pp. 319–331 and 556–557.

McBride, E. D.: Hallux valgus bunion deformity. Am. Acad. Orthop. Surgeons *9:*334–346, 1952.

Massart, R.: Les résultats déplorables des opérations d'hallus valgus. Bull. Mem. Soc. Chir. *26:*669–674, 1934.

Mau, C.: Der Hallux valgus-Komplex. Med. Klin. *38:*1317–1321, 1938.

Mauclaire, P.: Clinodactylie externe et interne, déviations latérales des orteils. Presse Méd. *4:*205–210, 1896.

Mayo, C. H.: The surgical treatment of bunions. Minnesota Med. J. *3:*326–331, 1920.

Metcalf, C. R.: Acquired hallux valgus: Late results from operative and non-operative treatment. Boston Med. Surg. J. *167:*271–277, 1912.

Miller, G. S.: Conflicting views on the problem of man's ancestry. Am. J. Phys. Anthropol. *3:*232–245, 1920.

Mouchet, A.: Pathogénie et traitement des difformités du gros orteil. Rev. d'Orthop. *9:*583–613, 1922.

Payr, E.: *Pathologie und Therapie des Hallux Valgus.* W. Braumueller, Wien und Leipzig, 1894, pp. 1–77.

Perrot, A.: Pied plat transverse et hallux valgus, pathogénie et traitement. Schweiz. Med. Wchnschr. *76:*362–366, 1946.

Picqué, L.: Note sur une cas d'hallux valgus. Bull. Mem. Soc. Chir. *28:*518–525, 1902.

Reverdin, J.: De la déviation en dehors du gros orteil (hallux valgus, vulg. "oignon," "bunions," "Ballen.") et de son traitement chirurgical. Tr. Internat. Med. Congr. *2:*408–412, 1881.

Rousselot: *Toilette des Pieds.* Paris, 1769, pp. 93–99.

Simon, W. V.: Der Hallux valgus und seine chirurgische Behandlung, mit besonderer Berücksichtigung der Ludloff'schen Operation. Burns Beitr. Klin. Chir. *111:*467–537, 1918.

Timmer, H.: *Die Behandlung des Hallux valgus.* J. A. Barth, Leipzig, 1930, pp. 1–62.

Verbrugge, J.: *Pathogénie et Traitement de L'Hallux Valgus.* Mem. Bull. Soc. Belge d'Orthop. Lielons, Bruxelles-Ouest, 1933, pp. 3–40.

Volkmann, R.: Ueber die sogenannte Exostose der grossen Zehe. Virchow's Arch. Path. Anat Physiol. *10:*297–306, 1856.

Chapter One

CLARIFICATION OF TERMINOLOGY

In discussions about hallux valgus and allied forefoot deformities, the greatest source of confusion is the lack of agreement as to what constitutes the central axis to which side-to-side movements of the toes should be referred. Failure to distinguish between deformities produced by muscle activity, dynamically, and those caused by static forces, has led some authors to employ contradictory terms in describing the deviations of the great toe and its metatarsal. Another set of misleading terms can be related to the easy analogical deductions suggested by the structure and function of the hand. The popular designation *bunion* and its derivative *bunionectomy* are at present used too loosely and indiscriminately; they require redefinition. The term *exostosis,* as applied to the prominent medial eminence of the first metatarsal head, has not met with general approval and *exostectomy* has come to denote resection of more than the abnormal bony excrescence. The similes of the *anterior transverse arch* and of the *tripod of the foot* have been rejected repeatedly but continue to crop up in the literature time and again.

Axes of reference. The midline of the body, when extended, falls midway between the feet; the axis of the foot itself passes through the second toe. Continental authors prefer the midsagittal plane as basis of reference for both movements and deformities of the toes. With a few exceptions, English-speaking writers have adopted a dual standard: for movement, the axis of the foot is selected; for deformities, the midline of the body is chosen (Fig. 1–1).

It is universally agreed that the axis of the hand traverses the middle finger. By way of analogy the third toe was considered as the conveyor of the axis of the foot. It was argued that the body of the talus sustains the entire weight and serves as the distributor of superimposed stresses. When the line representing the long axis of this portion of the talus is extended anteriorly, it passes through the third toe. Another spurious argument pertains to the odd number of toes. Since there are five toes it was assumed that the middle one or the third constituted the conveyor of the longitudinal axis of the foot.

Careful anatomical studies have refuted the above contentions. Wood Jones (1920) pointed out that the primitive midline of the pentadactyle hand passes through the third finger, this being the most stable digit, since its metacarpal is solidly mortised into the carpus. In the

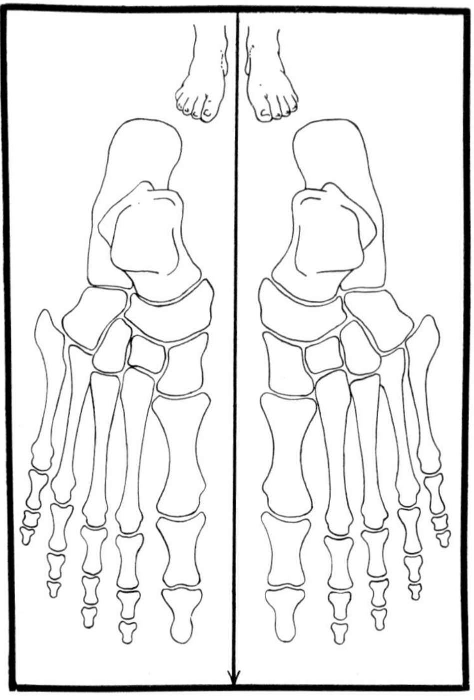

Figure 1–1. Midsagittal axis.

human foot the second metatarsal is slotted into the tarsus, which makes this bone the least movable, hence the most stable. "Our second toe," Wood Jones wrote, "has become the fixed point from which and to which the other toes are moved. The fixed midline of the foot has shifted toward the elongated first digit, and the evidence derived from the study of the bones is confirmed by the evidence derived from the study of the muscles." Studies of intrinsic muscles—especially dorsal (abducting) and plantar (adducting) interossei—have definitely consigned to the second digit the distinction of being the legitimate bearer of the longitudinal axis of the foot. In the hand the third finger is supplied by two dorsal interossei, and this digit possesses no volar interosseous muscle. In the foot the second toe gives anchorage to two dorsal interossei and no plantar interosseous inserts into it (Figs. 1–2 and 1–3).

Clinical observation also corroborates the view that the axis of the hand trav-

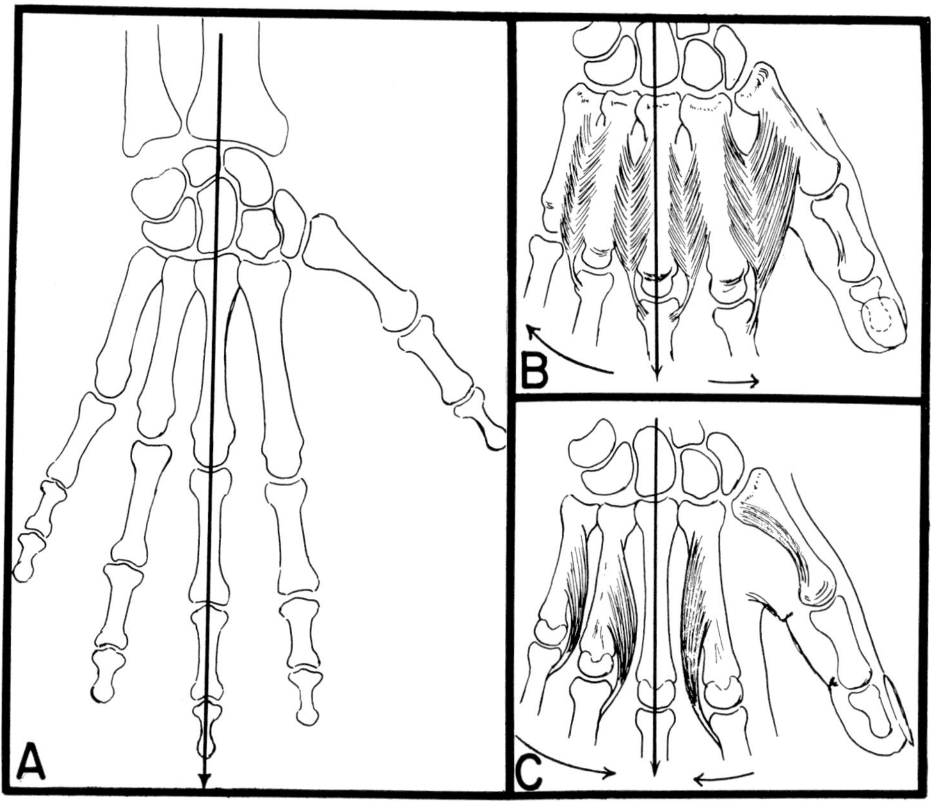

Figure 1–2. Axis of the hand.

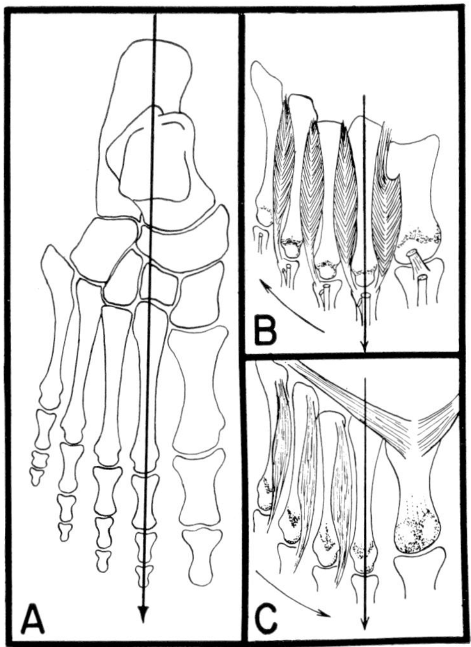

Figure 1–3. Axis of the foot.

erses the third finger while the axis of the foot passes through the second toe. For some reason congenital syndactylia involving only two digits seems to favor the web space on the postaxial—in the hand ulnar, in the foot fibular—side of the digit serving as the conveyor of the long axis. In the hand congenital syndactylia most often affects the third interdigital space; in the foot the second cleft is most commonly involved. Even in normal individuals the web between the second and third toes extends farthest forward, thus denoting a tendency toward confluence of these two—the axial and the first postaxial—digits. In the hand the third or the axial finger is the longest. This is not always the case in the foot. At one time it was thought that in what was called "ideal Greek type" the second toe was longer than the rest. More modern observers—including Wood Jones (1949)—claim that 1>2>3>4>5 "is the normal human formula." By "normal" is probably meant "the more common" (Fig. 1–4).

Lack of agreement about the axis of reference of the foot has induced authors in the past to variously describe side-to-side deviations of the hallux or its metatarsal. "Hallux valgus," Walsham (1896) wrote, "is the dislocation of the great toe inward at the metatarsophalangeal joint. It is frequently connected with an enlarged bunion over the inner side of the joint." Here "inward" is used in reference to the axis of the foot, and "inner" to the side of the foot nearer the midplane of the body. Keller (1904) called the tibial side of the first metatarsal "lateral." Whitman (1907) described hallux valgus as a "deformity in which the great toe is turned outward." Binnie (1913) defined it as an "inward deviation." In the footnote Binnie indicated that the word "inward" was "used in relation to the middle line of the foot." A page or two later, in assaying the steps of the then popular Weir operation,

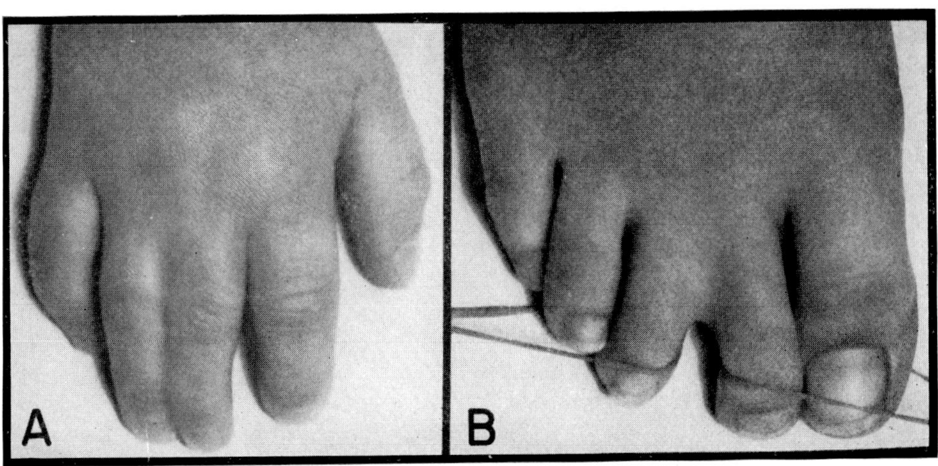

Figure 1–4. Syndactylia affecting the hand (*A*) and the foot (*B*).

Binnie wrote: ". . . divide the inner side of the joint capsule, i.e., the side next to the second toe. If the sesamoid bones are dislocated outward, remove them." In the footnote Binnie again saw fit to explain: "The words 'outer' and 'inner' are used in relation to the middle line of the foot and not of the body." Yet even as careful a writer as he fell prey to verbal confusion. He spoke of the "outward" displacement of sesamoids. If consistent, he should have said "inward," which in his language would have meant "the side next to the second toe." In hallux valgus, sesamoids are not displaced away from the second toe, but toward it.

Most authors now regard inner, internal, medial, tibial, and inward as relating to the side of the foot nearer to the midline of the body; their opposites —outer, external, lateral, fibular, and outward—refer to the border of the foot furthest away from the midsagittal plane of the body.

Abduction and adduction. These words are derived from the Latin verb *ducere,* which means to *lead.* From the same root came the French *duc,* Italian *duce,* and English *duke,* all of which mean leader. Adduction and abduction respectively signify being led *to* and away *from* an agreed axis. They imply dynamism or movement by muscle action.

Formerly, almost all Continental authors considered the midline of the body as the axis of reference for abduction and adduction of the great toe: the muscle that moves the hallux away from the midsagittal line was called abductor and the one that draws the hallux toward it was named adductor. This standard still persists in some parts of Europe. English-speaking authors regard the axis of the foot as the basis of reference: the muscle that moves the hallux toward the second toe is called adductor; the one that pulls it away, abductor. Obviously the two standards conflict: what one group calls adductor the other names abductor and vice versa. For the leg or the foot as a whole, it is universally agreed that the midline of the body should be taken as the basis of reference. The disagreement concerns the toes only, especially the hallux (Fig. 1–5).

Varus and valgus. The word "valgus" originally meant wry, bowlegged. At the beginning of the last century, the meaning of the word was reversed and valgus came to be used for knock-knees, and varus for bowlegs. By the turn of the century the converse use of these terms had become so deeply entrenched that Clarke (1900) finally conceded: "The fact that in Latin the terms 'valgus' and 'varus' were used inversely to the manner in which we use them need hardly be made the subject of discussion, since their misuse has become so well established that their meaning is never in doubt."

The term *hallux valgus* was first introduced into the literature by Carl Hueter (1871, 1877). He described this deformity as an *abduction contracture* in which the great toe is turned away from the median plane of the body. Most Continental and some English-speaking writers continued to use the word *abduction* in connection with hallux valgus. Others employed the axis of the foot for reference and described this deformity as an *adduction contracture.* Well aware of the dilemma, Clarke (1900) suggested that the Continental standard might be acceptable if a qualifying phrase is introduced in the definition. Clarke defined hallux valgus as a "deformity in which the great toe, when the foot is at rest, assumes a position of abduction from the median plane of the body."

Sir Robert Jones (1924) gave the following definition: "Hallux valgus is a deformity of the first metatarsophalangeal joint whereby the great toe is deflected outwards, or, in other words, adducted towards the center of the foot." Steindler (1943) had this to say about hallux valgus: "In this condition the big toe is abducted by the combined action of the extensor hallucis longus, the short extensors of the big toe and the adductor." It is conceivable that the phrase "short extensors" contains a misprint as the big toe has only one short extensor. The incongruity of the statement, "the big toe is abducted . . . by the adductor" becomes understandable if we remember that Steindler had Continental education and wrote in English. Straub (1951) said that in hallux valgus the great toe was "in abduction" and the "contracture of the adductor hallucis muscle" played a role in the production of this deformity. The opposite malformation, hallux varus, was described by Lewin (1959) as "adduction of the big toe."

In time, the Continental view dominated. Even by English-speaking writers, varus and valgus are now referred to the midsagittal axis: varus signifies inclination toward the midline of the body; valgus denotes divergence in opposite directions. Both adjectives imply static shift of position and not, as in the case of adduction and abduction, movement by muscle activity. Disregard of this point has led more than one author to use varus and valgus as though they were synonymous with adduction and abduction.

The lack of distinction between the two sets of terms, or the tendency to use them interchangeably, has been extended to descriptions of the exaggerated inward inclination of the first metatarsal. Here again what some authors call *adduction* the others consider *abduction*. Robinson (1918), Kleinberg (1932), McElvenny (1944), and Straub (1951) described the varus of the first metatarsal as *adduction,* while McMurray (1936) spoke of it as *abduction*. It is presumed that the first metatarsal is capable of independent movement and its positional shift is brought about by muscle activity.

Except for the comparatively weak first dorsal interosseous, no muscle gains discrete attachment into the first metatarsal to lever it, and it alone, into an independent position. The two muscles that insert into this bone—the anterior tibial and long peroneal—also connect with the innermost cuneiform. When the anterior tibial tightens, it lifts the inner border of the foot: the cuneiform and the metatarsal move together. Because of the obliquity of the anterior tibial muscle, in the initial stage of the movement known as dorsiflexion, the forefoot is drawn toward the midline of the body, which we may concede and call adduction; at the same time the forefoot is inverted. At the completion of the dorsiflexion, the forefoot is abducted and everted. Here the words *adducted* and *abducted, inverted* and *everted,* denote dynamic muscle activity and not fixed static stance. For established inward inclination of the first metatarsal we prefer the more legitimate and no less descriptive *metatarsus varus,* instead of *metatarsus adductus*. In the literature one also meets with *metatarsus adductovarus*—a needlessly cumbersome compounding.

Pronation and supination. It is often stated that adduction of the forefoot combined with inversion constitutes supination, and that abduction and

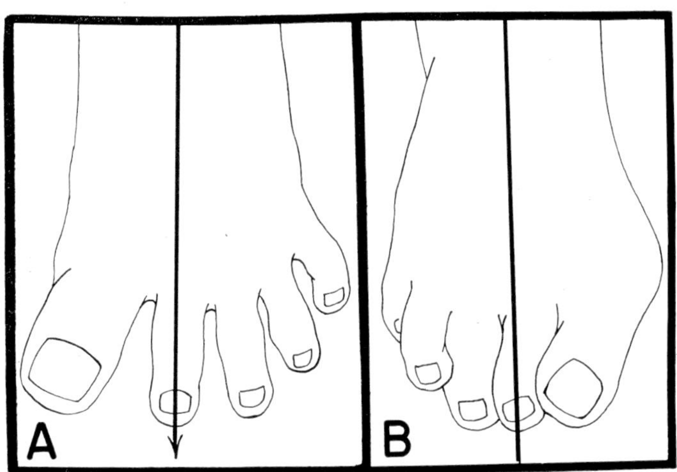

Figure 1–5. Abduction and adduction of the toes.

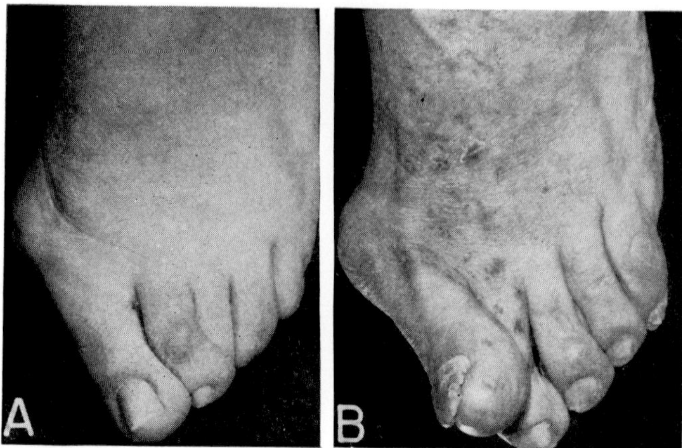

Figure 1–6. Hallux valgus with axial rotation of the great toe.

eversion evolve into pronation. More than one author of recent vintage has used the word pronation in connection with metatarsus varus. Lewin (1959) wrote: "Metatarsus varus or pigeon-toe is remnant of the prehensile function of the great toe. A moderate degree is favorable unless it is associated with pronation."

When the radius rotates around the ulna and the palm is turned up, the hand is said to be supinated; rotation in reverse direction, which brings the palm down, is called pronation. We may concede that the sole of the foot is in a position of permanent pronation when it rests on a flat surface. We may also say that it is more pronated when its tibial border is lowered and fibular side raised. But we cannot imagine the sole of the foot turning up until its dorsum comes to contact the said flat surface. The most we can say is that the foot is only partly supinated when its tibial border is elevated.

The rotation of the foot does not take place in the proximal segment of the limb as in the case of the hand, but around its own longitudinal axis. The forefoot rotates as a whole, not in parts: one cannot speak of independent pronation and supination of the first metatarsal or any metatarsal. The first metatarsal actively inverts or everts with the innermost cuneiform, since it shares with this bone the insertions of anterior tibial and the long peroneal tendons. Because of its firm connection with the other midtarsal bones, the medial cuneiform cannot rotate much without forcing its mates on the lateral side to follow suit. Outer metatarsals in turn invert or evert with the midtarsal bones. For the forefoot, it is perhaps best to use the terms inversion and eversion instead of supination and pronation. German authors prefer to use the last two.

Hiss (1937, 1949) introduced a confusing term, *pedevert*, meaning everted foot. He described eversion as "an outward curving of the foot upon itself, a condition in which the mesial side is not in alignment." Normally the medial border of the heel, the navicular bone, and the head of the first metatarsal are said to conform to a base line; in *pedevert* the forefoot is pictured as swinging away from this line. It is presumed that the forefoot has rotated around a dorsoplantar axis. Inversion and eversion of the forefoot takes place around the heel-to-toe or longitudinal axis.

In the more advanced stages of hallux valgus the great toe is rotated around its own long axis. Some authors describe this torsion as pronation, others call it eversion. According to Stein (1938), "The great toe is maintained in a position of eversion." Mikhail (1960) stated: "The big toe is rotated inward . . ." In the first statement the pulp of the toe is taken for reference; in the second, the nail. The great toe twists on its long axis in such a way as to make its nail slant inward and face the midsagittal plane while its pulp faces away from it. This rotary shift is legitimately described as eversion (Fig. 1–6).

Bunion and bunionectomy. Perhaps the most indiscriminately used term is the popular *bunion*. There are several possible sources for this word: the Italian *bugnone,* the old French *buigne,* and the old English *bunny*. They all mean swelling. According to the Encyclopaedia Britannica (1910), these words probably came from a common origin now lost. It is thought that the word *bunch* came from the same root; it was originally used to signify the hump, the swelling on a camel's back. Shipley (1945), thought old French *bugne* gave bunion. Skinner (1949) wrote after bunion: "Probably from Italian *bugnone,* a lump; from Greek *Bovvos,* a hill or eminence. The Italian bugnone is allied to the old French bugne or buigne, meaning swelling. This is probably the same as the old English bunny, a small swelling. All probably derive from the Greek Bovvos."

The term *bunion* ignores the misalignment of the great toe and relates merely to the swelling at its base. There is a bunion in every case of hallux valgus but the converse is not true. The prominence along the inner border of the forefoot may exist in the absence of outward deviation of the great toe. The swelling may consist of thickened soft tissue or bone, or of both; it may be caused by bursal, tendon sheath, or joint inflammation and there may be calcareous deposits around the region. Not infrequently the skin itself is thickened. It has become customary to qualify the term bunion according to the position of the swelling and call it medial, dorsal, or plantar (Figs. 1–7 to 1–12).

The analogous word for *bunion* in French is *oignon* and in German, *Ballen*. But neither of these popular terms has been dignified by the suffix *ectomy*. Whoever is responsible for advocating the mongrel *bunionectomy* knew, we surmise, "a little Latin and less Greek." Carelessly used to denote diverse surgical procedures for correction of hallux valgus, *bunionectomy* should be narrowed down to its original significance, namely, the effacement of the prominence at the base of the great or small toe. We would prefer to discard the term altogether and employ instead a more hybrid—and from an etymological point of view, legiti-

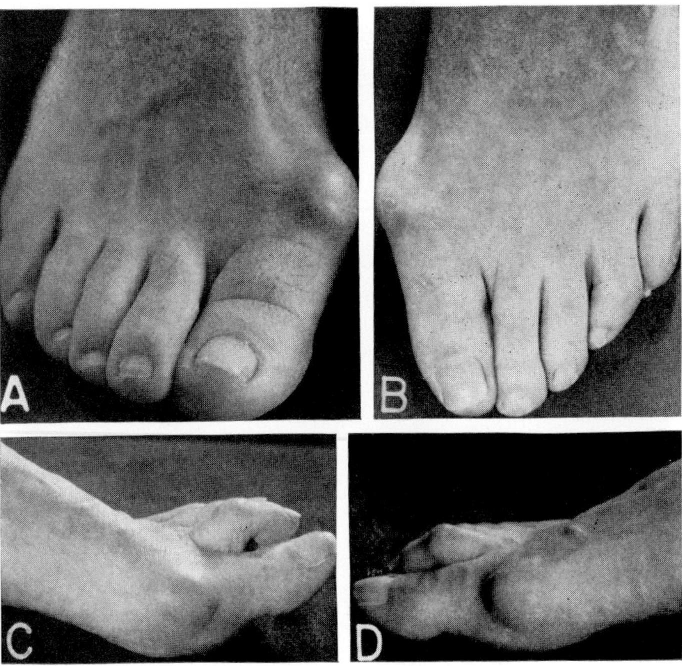

Figure 1–7. Cases of bunion due to prominent medial eminence and thickening of the overlying soft tissues.

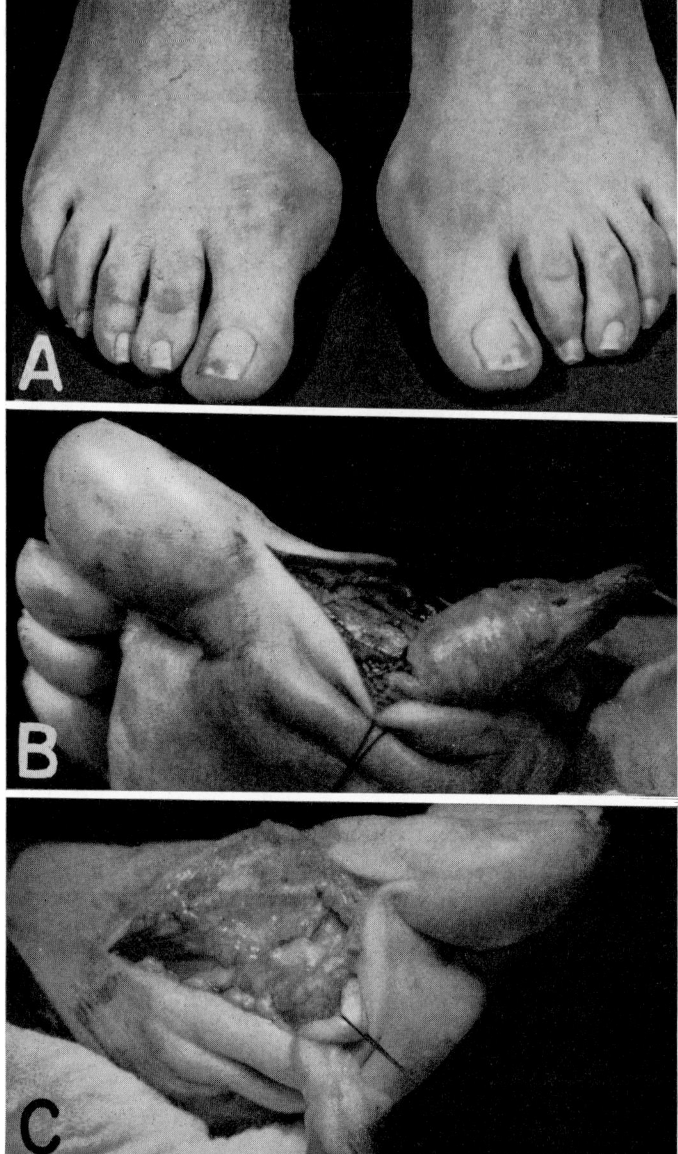

Figure 1–8. Bilateral bunion due to tumefied synovial sheath of the long flexor tendon.

mate–compounding such as *bursectomy* or *condylectomy*. Numerous authors use the term *exostectomy*.

Exostosis and exostectomy. Ever since Froriep (1834) commented on the exostosis of the first metatarsal, there have been recurrent controversies as to whether in hallux valgus the bony prominence over the medial aspect of the base of the great toe is due to new formation, or it merely represents the medially displaced portion of the metatarsal head. What we now know as hallux valgus, Froriep called *exostosis of the first metatarsal bone.* He thought that, at its point of attachment outside the articular cavity, the medial collateral ligament "drew the material of the bone" from behind the metatarsal head, "by the very action of strength," meaning by active tension. Volkmann (1856) placed the new deposit inside the joint proper. According to him bony and cartilaginous vegetations imparted to the first metatarsal head the appearance of possessing two condyles: one, true and lateral, still

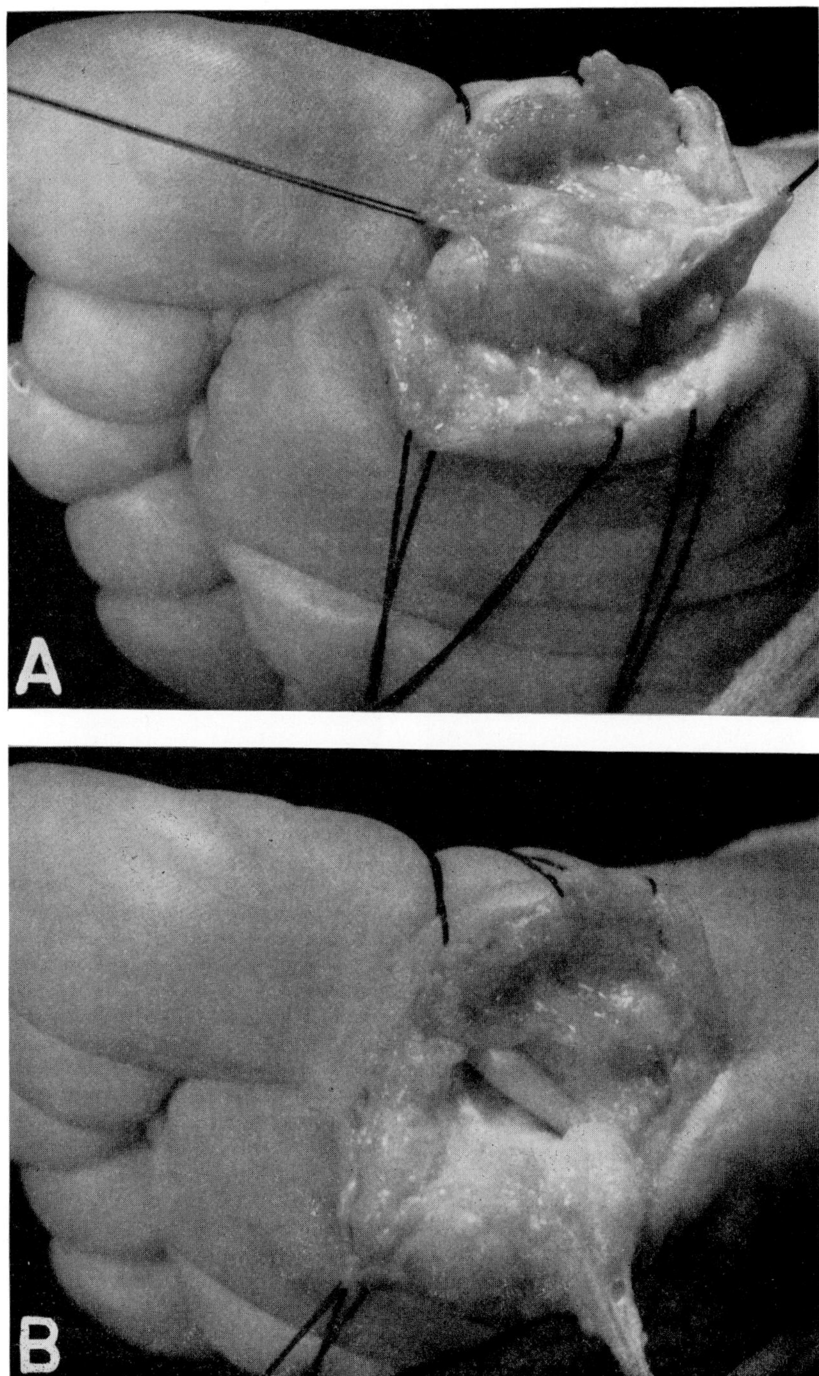

Figure 1–9. Unilateral bunion due to multilocular cyst emanating from the flexor sheath.

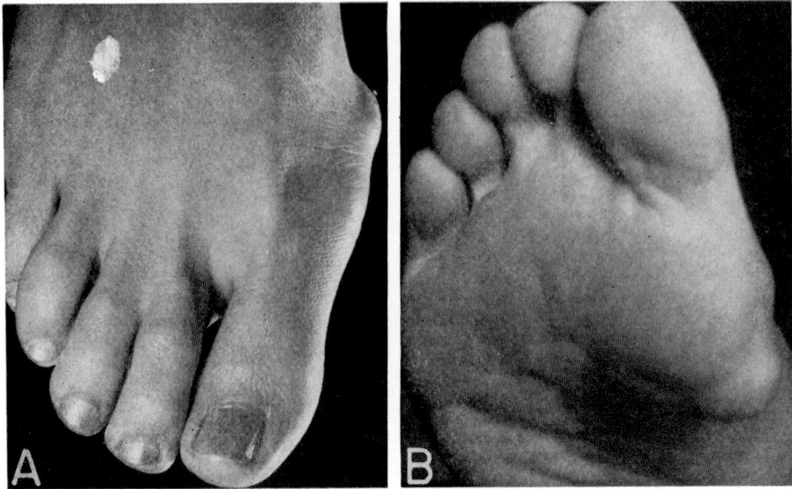

Figure 1–10. Plantar bunion as seen from the dorsal (*A*) and medial (*B*) aspects.

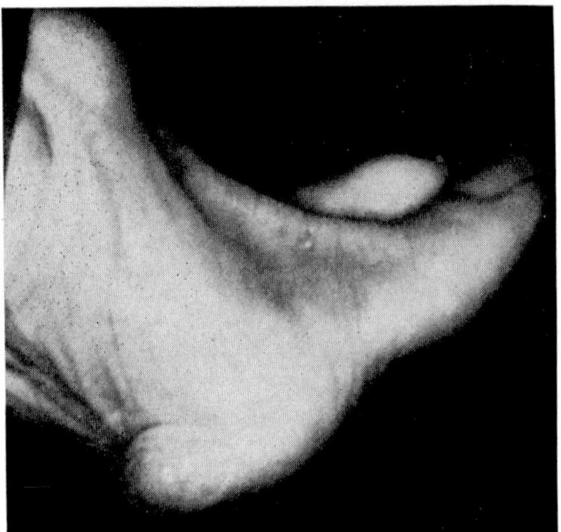

Figure 1–11. Plantar bunion.

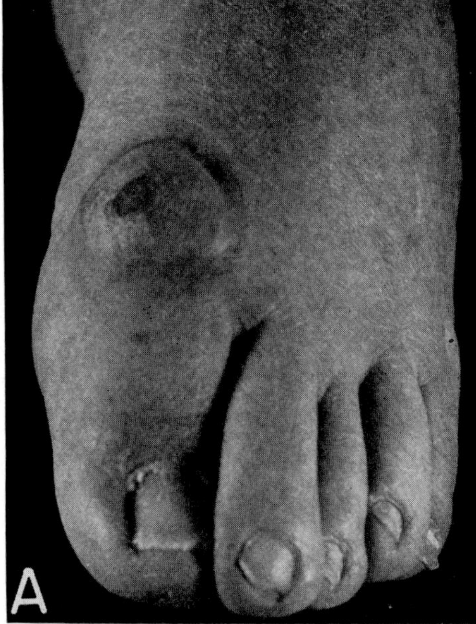

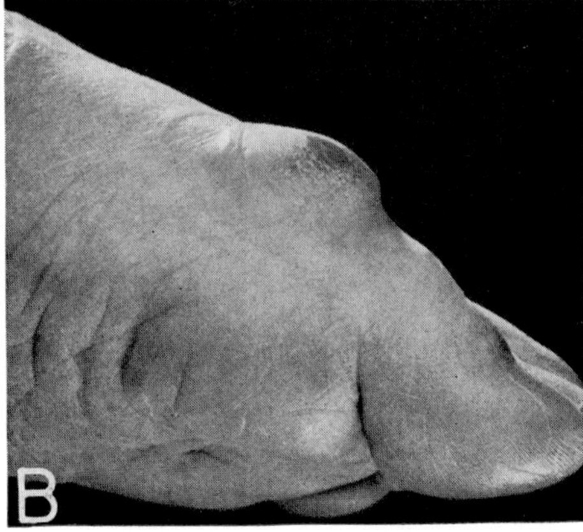

Figure 1–12. Dorsal bunion.

in line with the proximal phalanx; the other, medial, or pseudocondyle, consisting mainly of irregular accretion of cartilage and bone.

It is not generally known that Richard Volkmann of ischemic contracture fame was a poet besides being a surgeon: he wrote and published poetry under the pen name, Richard Leander. He did not write his surgical essays in Latin as had Froriep, nor in the stilted scientific jargon of the period; he composed them in a picturesque, effective prose. What he wrote was widely read and retained. Many of Volkmann's original observations about the structural changes in hallux valgus—the displacement of sesamoids, effacement of the ridge on the undersurface of the metatarsal head, the inward inclination of this bone, widening of the innermost intermetatarsal space—have now survived for over a century.

As with most conscientious literary craftsmen, Volkmann suggested more than he said. It was inferred by later writers that in hallux valgus, the deformity of the great toe was related to arthritis. Volkmann said that in what was then popularly called *Ballen* in Germany and *exostosis of the great toe* in more scientific circles the head of the first metatarsal, especially on its medial aspect, was definitely enlarged; it acquired "vegetative" accretion of bone and cartilage in a manner analogous to malum coxae senilis or almost identical with it.

In the ensuing decades the literature on hallux valgus became flooded with such phrases as a "hyperplastic process in the joint," "proliferation of the inner portion of the head," "expansion of the bone," and the "picture of arthritis deformans." Hueter (1871, 1877), who was perhaps the most influential authority on the subject in the seventies, spoke of "the picture of exostosis." Reverdin (1881) gave tacit sanction to this concept by recommending "ablation of exostosis" as a preliminary step to the subcapital cuneiform osteotomy we have come to connect with his name.

Haines and McDougall (1954) mentioned Froriep and Volkmann as the proponents of the contention that in hallux valgus "the medial eminence was a pathological neomorph, a true exostosis." They placed Lane on the top of dissenters with this theory. Thirteen years before Lane, Rose (1874) wrote: "The head of the metatarsal bone now forms a remarkable protuberance, which is still more enlarged by a bony proliferation of the bony tissue, caused or promoted by the continued pressure upon, the irritation of, the affected joint. Froriep described this affection as exostosis of the great toe, after proliferation of the bony tissue had taken place. In most cases, however, there exists only expansion of bone, and rarely exostosis."

Lane was born in 1856, the year Volkmann's article appeared. Three decades later, Lane (1887) wrote an essay on developmental deformiti that contained a section devoted to "abduction of the great toe." Lane referred to an article he had written during the preceding year and had shown "that what had been regarded as the cause of displacement was in reality the effect." He meant to say that arthritic change in hallux valgus was the result and not the cause of deviated toe. According to him the portion of the first metatarsal head no longer in contact with the base of the proximal phalanx generally wasted. In late stages of hallux valgus, Lane thought, the inner condyle of the metatarsal head actually shrank; by implication it did not hypertrophy or form new bone.

There ensued an army of dissenters. Heubach (1897) wrote: "In severe cases of hallux valgus, there is no exostosis; on the contrary, we find rather flattening of the joint to the extent that it became concave rather than convex." Silver (1923) thought that the medial prominence was due mainly to the subluxation of the head of the metatarsal and only to a lesser degree to hypertrophy. Stein (1938) was perhaps the most outspoken dissenter. "The so-called exostosis removed at operation," he wrote, "is usually a myth." Haines and McDougall (1954) arrived at the following conclusions: "Apart from osteophytic lipping which squares off the outline of the eminence as it is seen in radiographs and a small amount of lipping of the ridge of the metatarsal there is no evidence of new bone growth. In chronic cases the eminence may degenerate or disappear."

Most surgeons would now agree that in hallux valgus the bony prominence at the base of the great toe consists mainly of the medially displaced part of the head of the metatarsal. There may be a few osseous or cartilaginous excrescences on the inner margin of the articular surface of the head and along the medial aspect of the bone. Organized exostoses are seen more commonly on the dorsal and lateral side of the joint. Dorsal exostoses are seen most commonly in connection with hallux rigidus; lateral spurs

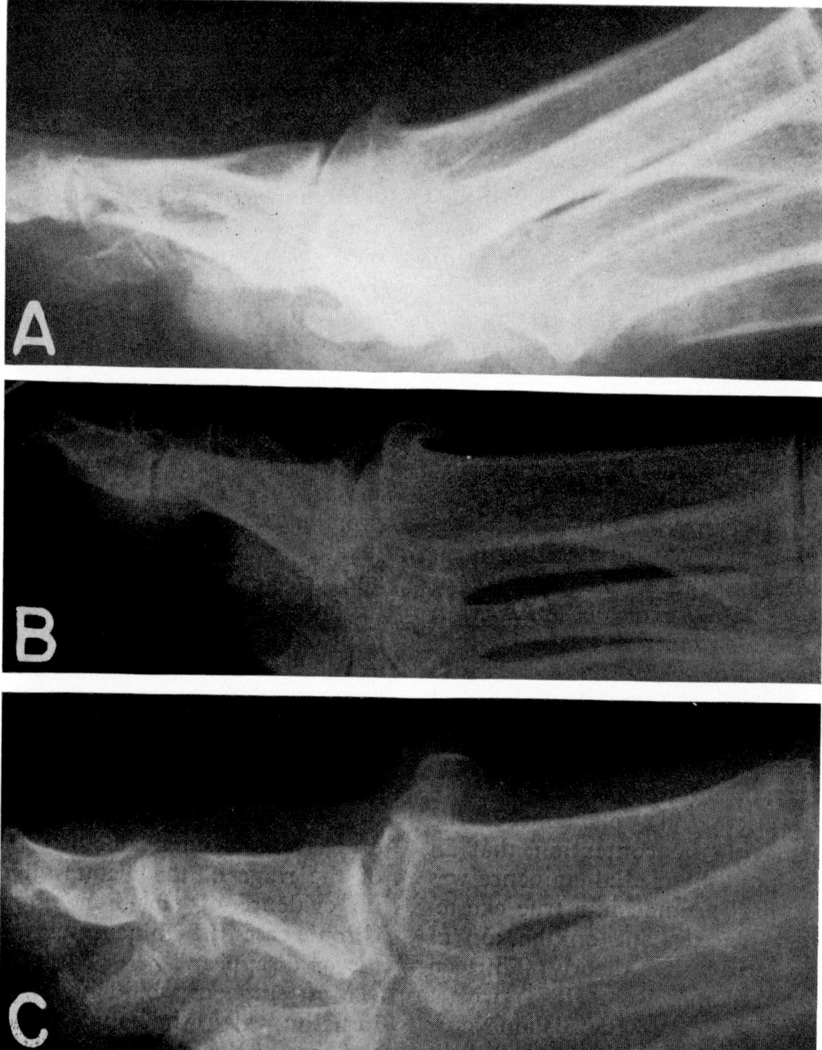

Figure 1–13. Dorsal osteophytes.

are usually associated with hallux valgus. Occasionally plantar exostoses emanate either from the metatarsal head or from the sesamoids. At times the base of the proximal phalanx gives rise to an exostosis (Figs. 1–13 to 1–15).

Exostosis as applied to the irregular deposits over the subluxated portion of the first metatarsal head is a misnomer and *exostectomy* hardly describes the operation for which it is often used—namely, resection of the medially displaced portion of the head. For this operation the author prefers a more specific appelation: *sagittal resection of the medial eminence.* Not infrequently the sesamoids are mushroomed and have developed peripheral osteophytes, in which instance the entire bone is resected—*ostectomy* or *sesamoidectomy* is performed.

The author must confess that it is not easy to dispose of such solidly transfixed terms as *exostosis* and *exostectomy* or divest them of the meaning assigned by convention. In the ensuing pages, when the author uses them, it should be understood that he is doing so out of historical necessity. Too many established and deserving contributors have employed them. Compared to *bunion* and *bunionectomy,* they have some redeeming features: they convey a scientific aura and their use is not confined to English-speaking countries, but is universal.

The anterior metatarsal arch and the tripod of the foot. Another pair of historically sanctioned terms that have caused considerable confusion pertains to the imaginary arch slung transversely across the heads of the metatarsal bones and to the supposed three weight-bearing points of the foot. These two designations—*anterior metatarsal arch* and the *tripod of the foot*—are interrelated since both are based on the supposed selective areas of contact of the foot with the ground. The foot is said to rest on three points: the medial tubercle of the os calcis posteriorly and the heads of the first and fifth metatarsal bones anteriorly.

In most cases of hallux valgus, and often independent of this deformity, the sole beneath the central metatarsal heads bulges in a plantar direction; compared to the domed depression proximally under the distal row of tarsal bones, this region conveys the impression that a veritable arch has collapsed or become reversed. It must have been such an impressionistic deduction that led orthopedic surgeons in the past, and some even now, to visualize an arch underneath the metatarsal heads. It is supposed that normally the heads of the second, third, and fourth metatarsals are lifted off the ground; the contact of these bones with the supporting surface is considered pathological. A multitude of epithets have been used to qualify this state

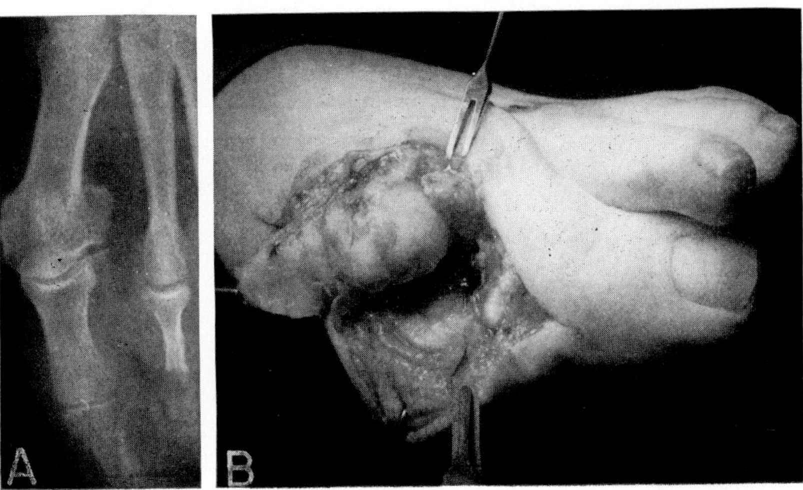

Figure 1–14. Lateral osteophytes as shown in roentgenograph (*A*) and during surgical exposure (*B*).

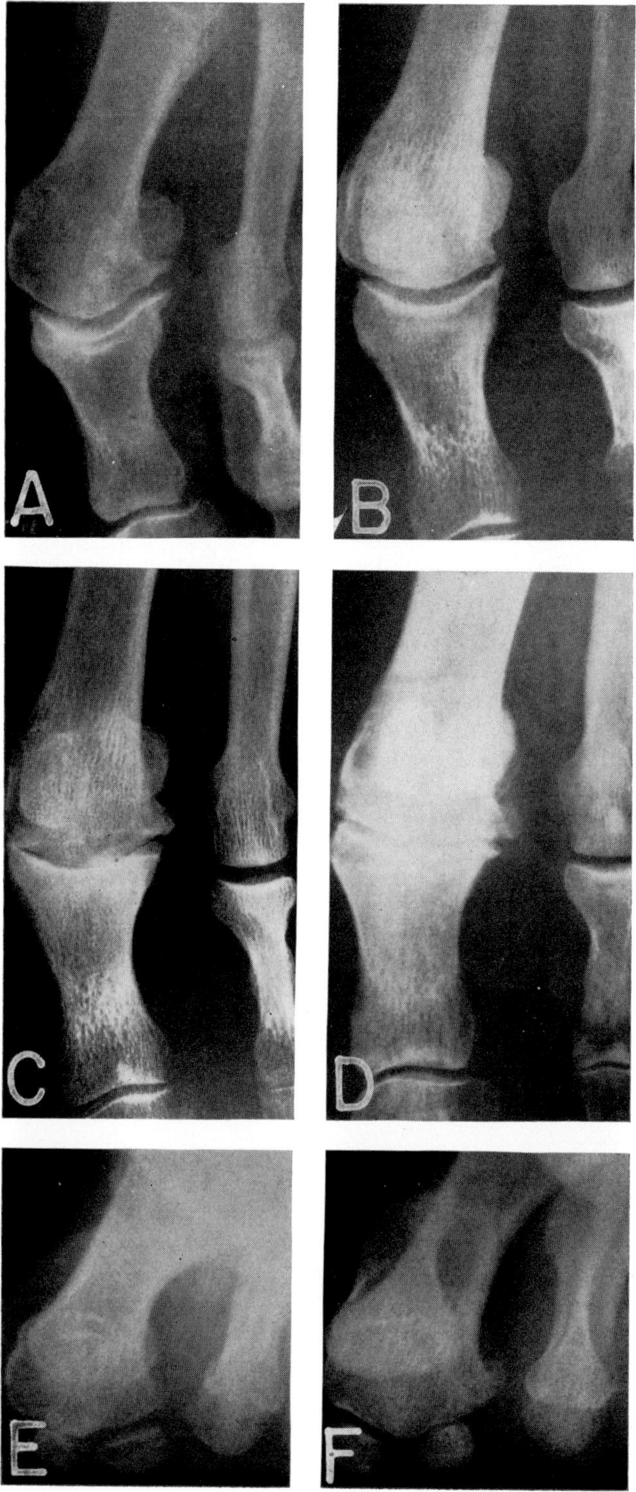

Figure 1–15. Assorted roentgenographs showing lateral osteophytes.

of imaginary arch: obliterated, effaced, flattened, weakened, broken down, dropped, depressed, decompensated, sunken, collapsed, and reversed. The adjective *anterior* is used to distinguish the supposed arcuate arrangement of the metatarsal heads from the *transverse arch* of the anatomists, which lies further posteriorly under the distal row of tarsal bones. Some clinicians call the latter *posterior* metatarsal arch. The transverse arch under the distal row of tarsal bones gradually diminishes anteriorly and is nonexistent at the level of the metatarsal heads. The anatomists categorically deny the existence of an arch under the metatarsal heads and also reject the subsidiary simile—*the tripod of the foot* (Figs. 1–16 and 1–17).

In criticism of the traditional concept of anterior metatarsal arch, formed by the heads of the metatarsal bones, D. J. Morton (1930) wrote: "There is no such arch or arch conformation in this particular region of the foot, for each bone has direct contact with the ground through the intervening tissues." Elftman (1934) conducted a cinematic study

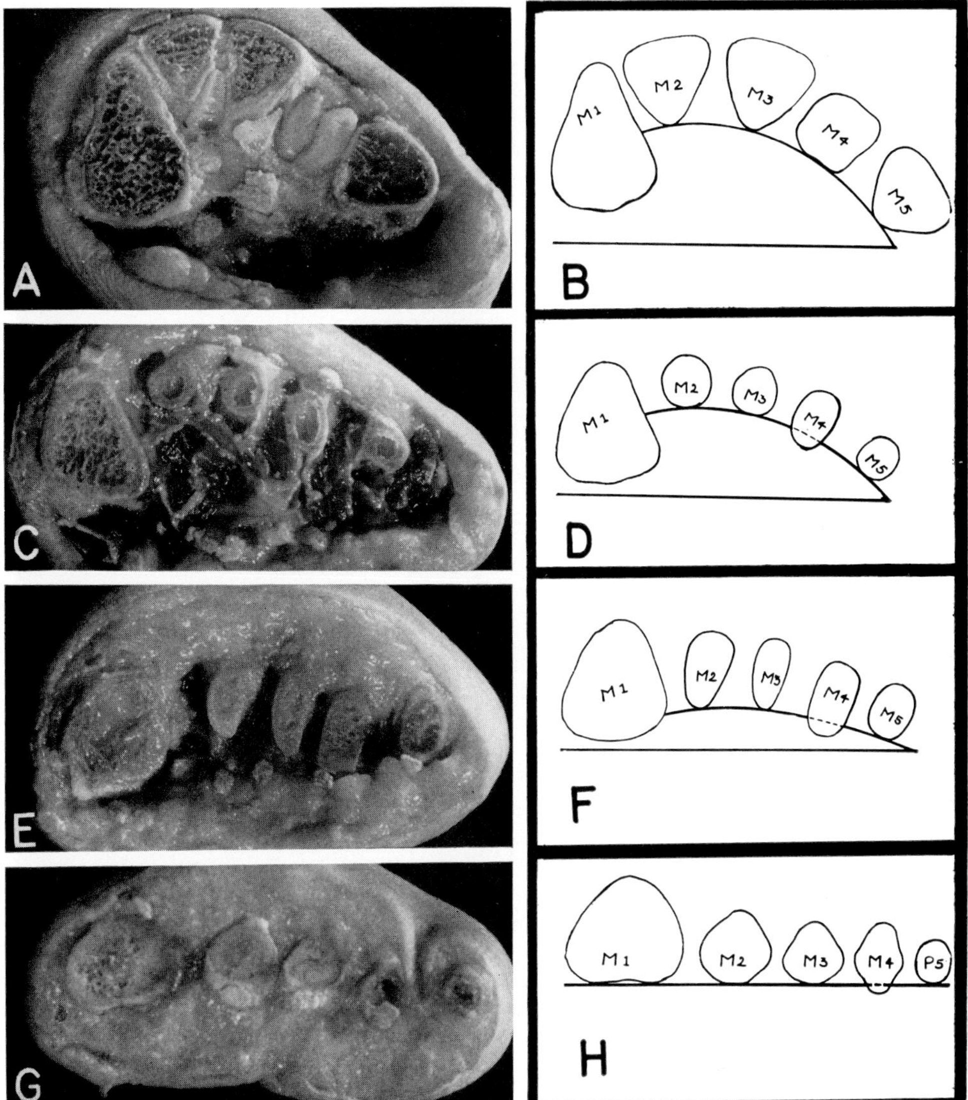

Figure 1–16. Cross sections of the forefoot through the base of the first metatarsal (*A* and *B*), through the proximal third (*C* and *D*), through the neck (*E* and *F*) and through the head (*G* and *H*).

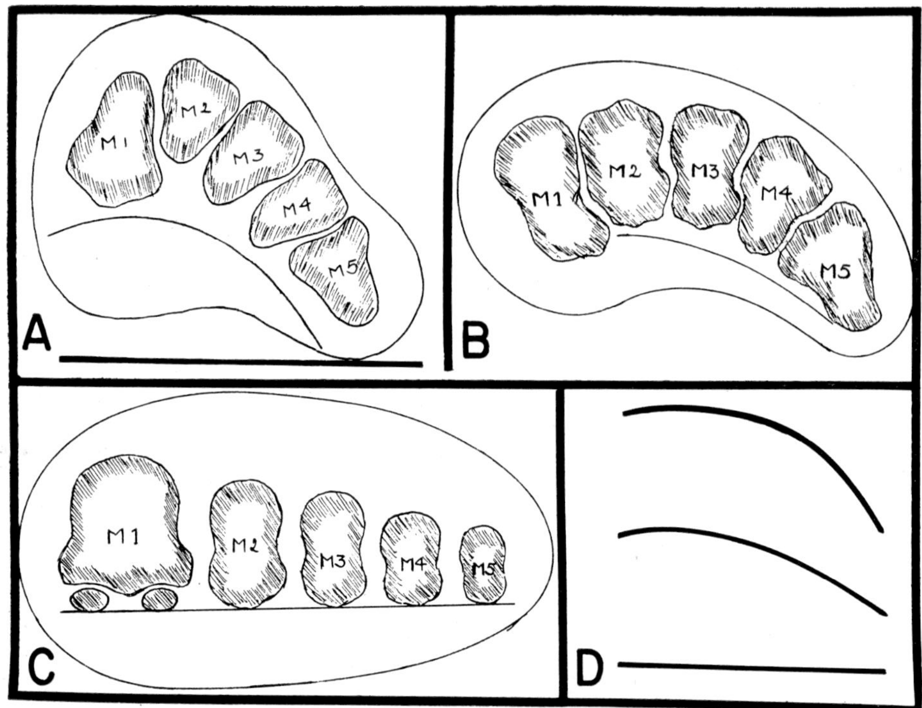

Figure 1–17. The transverse arch of the anatomists diminishes as it approaches the level of the metatarsal heads, where there is no arcuate arrangement.

of pressure distribution in the human foot and concluded that the whole area under the metatarsal heads sustained the body weight. Bruce and Walmsley (1938) studied cross sections of fetal and adult feet; their observations, they said were "in keeping with the experimental results of Morton." Russell Jones (1941) wrote: "If one will stand barefooted on five strips of paper about ⅝ inch wide placed parallel with the foot under the respective metatarsal heads, and have an assistant pull the strips from under the foot, one will discover that the foot is no tripod."

It may be asked: how should one designate the splaying of the marginal metatarsal bones if not by collapse of the anterior metatarsal arch? Truslow (1925) coined *metatarsus primus varus,* which relates to the exaggerated medial inclination of the first metatarsal. Silfverskiöld (1927) suggested the name *metatarsus latus.* This term was adopted by Hauser (1939), who described it as "spreading of the anterior part of the foot due to separation of the heads of the metatarsal bones from each other." He indicated that the chief deformity was varus of the first metatarsal and in a similar way the fifth metatarsal splayed away from the fourth. *Metatarsus latus* describes the widening of the transmetatarsal span from one border of the forefoot to the other; it bears no reference to the more troublesome plantar prominence of the central metatarsal heads. Perrot (1946) preferred the term *transverse flat foot—pes transversus planus. Triangular flatfoot* is another name. Lake (1952) used the term *splay foot.*

It is obvious that a comprehensive term to describe the plantar protrusion of the central metatarsal heads has not yet been given an adequately descriptive name. Until an appropriate one is found, we remain content with the less pretentious, perhaps least objectionable *splayfoot,* the analogue of German *Spreizfuss. Splaying of the forefoot* is perhaps preferable since it localizes the disturbance. One must make a distinction between the splaying of the metatarsal heads along a horizontal line and their positional shift in coronal plane. In the young, one often sees the heads of the marginal metatarsals fan out sideways on weight-bearing. To a degree this type of splaying is considered physiological. But when the forefoot overflows the limits set by the sole of the shoe and the vamp causes pressure and chafing on the side of the marginal metatarsal heads, one can no longer speak of physiological splaying. There is the question of pain and pain is not physiological. The term *metatarsus latus* may well be reserved for the side to side splaying of the marginal metatarsal heads on a horizontal plane. In the more complicated variety these bones not only seem to have spread sideways but they also tilt up in dorsal direction throwing the capitalia of the central metatarsals into greater plantar prominence. Some authors claim actual descent of the central metatarsal heads plantarward. It is a matter of relativity (Figs. 1–18 to 1–20).

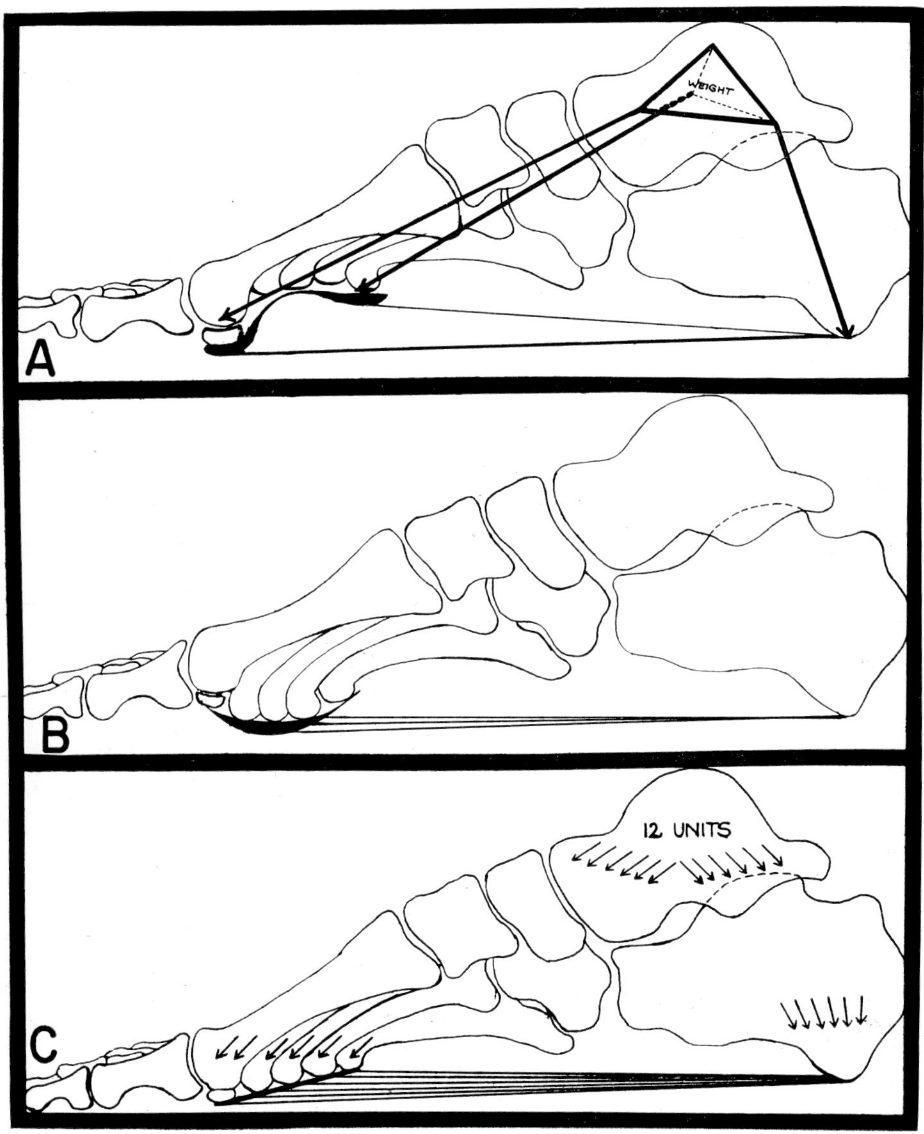

Figure 1–18. The tripod of the foot (*A*), the collapse of the anterior transverse arch of the clinicians (*B*) and the more modern concept of weight distribution in stance (*C*).

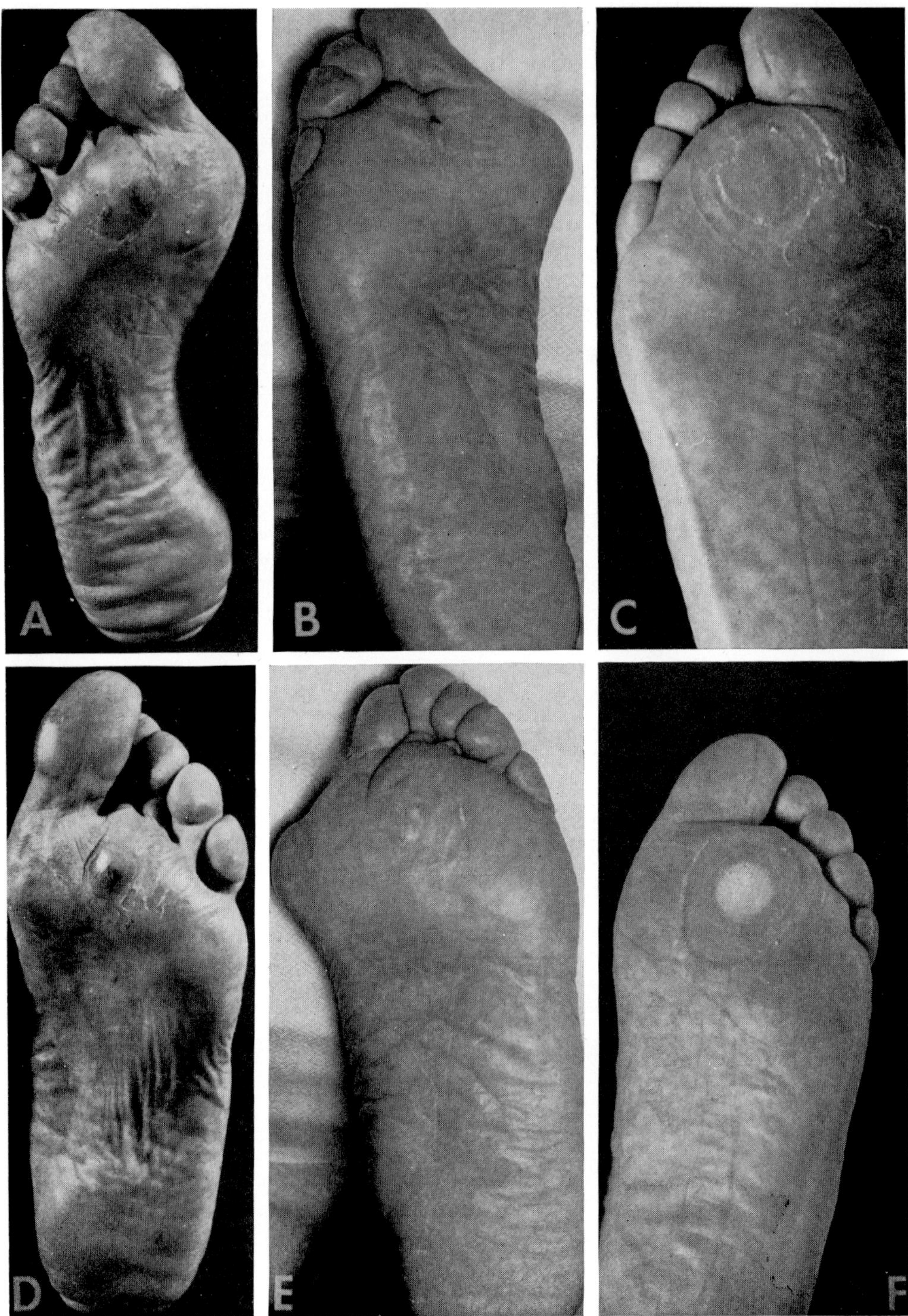

Figure 1–19. Unilateral cases with apparent plantar bulge of the area under the central metatarsal heads.

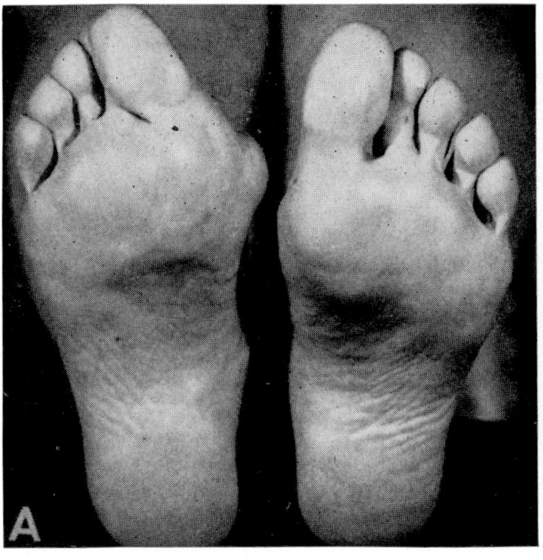

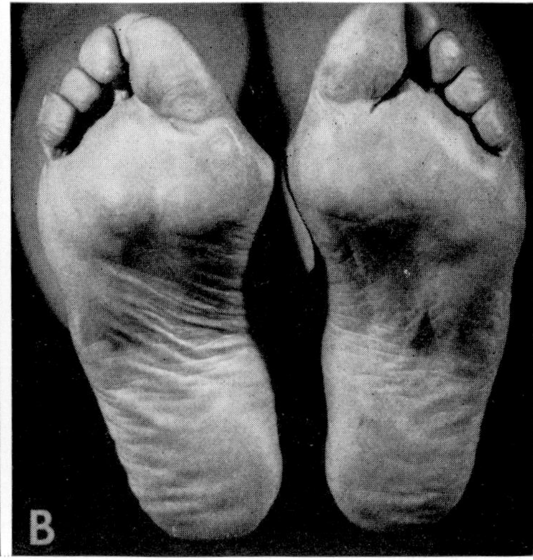

Figure 1–20. Bilateral cases with apparent plantar bulge of the area under the central metatarsal heads.

REFERENCES

Binnie, J. F.: *Manual of Operative Surgery.* 6th Ed., Philadelphia, Blakiston, 1913, pp. 1032–1036.

Bruce, J., and Walmsley, R.: Some observations on the arches of the foot and flatfoot. Lancet *2:*656–659, 1938.

Clarke, J. J.: Hallux valgus and hallux varus. Lancet *1:*609–611, 1900.

Elftman, H.: A cinematic study of the distribution of pressure in the human foot. Anat. Rec. *59:*481–491, 1934.

Encyclopaedia Britannica: Bunion. 11th Ed., Cambridge, England, University Press, *4:*798, 1910.

Froriep, R.: *Commentatiuncula de Ossis Metatarsi Primi Exostosi.* Berolini: Joanni de Wiebel, 1834, pp. 1–8.

Haines, R. W., and McDougall, A.: The anatomy of hallux valgus. J. Bone Joint Surg. *36:*272–293, 1954.

Hauser, E. D. W.: *Diseases of the Foot.* Philadelphia, W. B. Saunders Co., 1939, pp. 113–117.

Heubach, F.: Ueber Hallux valgus und seine operative Behandlung nach Edm. Rose. Dtsch. Ztschr. Chir. *46:*210–275, 1897.

Hiss, J. H.: *Functional Foot Disorders.* Los Angeles University Press, 1937, pp. 123–184.

Hiss, J. H.: *Functional Foot Disorders.* 3rd Ed., Los Angeles, The Oxford Press, 1949, pp. 323–387.

Hueter, C.: Klinik der Gelenkkrankheiten. 1st Ed., Leipzig, F. C. W. Vogel, 1871, pp. 339–351. 2nd Ed., 1877.

Jones, F. W.: *The Principles of Anatomy As Seen in the Hand.* London, J. & A. Churchill, 1920, pp. 42 and 219–220.

Jones, F. W. *Structure and Function As Seen in the Foot.* 2nd Ed., London, Baillière, Tindall & Cox, 1949, pp. 32–38.

Jones, R.: Discussion on the treatment of hallux valgus and rigidus. Brit. Med. J. *2:*651–656, 1924.

Jones, R. L.: The human foot. An experimental study of its mechanics, and the role of its muscles and ligaments in the support of the arch. Am. J. Anat. *68:*1–39, 1941.

Keller, W. L.: The surgical treatment of bunions and hallux valgus. New York Med. J. *80:*741–742, 1904.

Kleinberg, S.: Operative cure of hallux valgus and bunions. Am. J. Surg. *15:*75–81, 1932.

Lake, N. C.: *The Foot.* London, Baillière, Tindall & Cox, 1952, pp. 116 and 231.

Lane, W. A.: The causation, pathology and physiology of the deformities which develop during young life. Guy's Hosp. Rep. *44:*307–317, 1887.

Lewin, P.: *The Foot and Ankle.* Philadelphia, Lea & Febiger, 1959, pp. 124–156.

McElvenny, R. T.: A study of hallux valgus: its cause and operative management. Quart. Bull., Northw. Univ. Med. Sch. *18:*286–297, 1944.

McMurray, T. P.: Treatment of hallux valgus and rigidus. Brit. Med. J. *2:*218–221, 1936.

Mikhail, I. K.: Bunion, hallux valgus and metatarsus primus varus. Surg. Gyn. Obst. *111:*637–646, 1960.

Morton, D. J.: Structural factors in static disorders of the foot. Am. J. Surg. *9:*315–328, 1930.

Perrot, A.: Pied plat transverse et hallux valgus, pathogénie et traitement. Schweiz. Med. Wchnschr. *76:*362–366, 1946.

Reverdin, J.: De la déviation en dehors du gros orteil (hallux valgus, vulg. "oignon," "bunions," "Ballen.") et de son traitement chirurgical. Trans. Internat. Med. Congr. *2:*408–412, 1881.

Robinson, H. A.: Bunion, its causes and cure. Surg. Gyn. Obst. *27:*343–345, 1918.

Rose, A.: Resection considered as a remedy for abduction of the great toe—hallux valgus—and bunion. Med. Rec. *9:*200–201, 1874.

Shipley, J. T.: Bunion. In *Dictonary of Word Origins.* 2nd Ed., New York, The Philosophical Library, 1945, p. 61.

Silfverskiöld, N.: Metatarsus latus und Hallux valgus. Acta. Chir. Scand. *61:*443–560, 1927.

Silver, D.: The operative treatment of hallux valgus. J. Bone Joint Surg. *5:*225–232, 1923.

Skinner, H. A.: Bunion. In *The Origin of Medical Terms.* Baltimore, Williams & Wilkins Co., 1949, p. 68.

Stein, H. C.: Hallux valgus. Surg. Gyn. Obst. *66:*889–898, 1938.

Steindler, A.: *Orthopedic Operations.* Springfield, Ill., Chas. C Thomas Co., 1943, pp. 547–550.

Straub, L. R.: Affections of the feet. In *The Specialties in General Practice* (R. L. Cecil, ed). Philadelphia, W. B. Saunders Co., 1951, pp. 125–134.

Truslow, W.: Metatarsus primus varus or hallux valgus? J. Bone Joint Surg. *7:*98–108, 1925.

Volkmann, R.: Ueber die sogenannte Exostose der grossen Zehe. Virchow's Arch. Path. Anat. Physiol. *10:*297–306, 1856.

Walsham, W. J.: *Surgery: Its Theory and Practice.* Philadelphia, Blakiston, 1896, p. 784.

Whitman, R.: *A Treatise on Orthopedic Surgery.* Philadelphia, Lea Brothers & Co., 1907, pp. 717–751.

Chapter Two

THE FUNCTIONAL ANATOMY OF THE FOREFOOT

Flexors and extensors of the toes. It is not definitely known who initially promulgated the concept of *pes altera manus.* Blandin (1833) mentioned it. Duchenne (1867) perpetuated it: he was responsible for the remark that muscles moving the toes functioned like the muscles acting on fingers. This statement was carried by book after book and surgeons reading them subjected the foot to operations that may have proved beneficial when carried out on the hand but were useless when tried on the foot. Too often it was—and still is—forgotten that in the foot, stability takes precedence over movement, and attempts to restore *muscle balance* are futile without establishing *bone balance.*

There is some justification to the seemingly absurd but pertinent point made by Wood Jones (1949) that it would be better for the surgeon dealing with the disabilities of the foot had he never learned the structure and function of the hand. "To liken the action of the muscles of the foot to that of the hand," Wood Jones wrote, "is to abandon all hope of understanding the ordinary mechanics of standing and walking." Wood Jones defined the hand as "a tactile, testing, grasping organ," designed for fine movements of isolated parts; the foot, he said, subserved "the function of . . . support and propulsion of the body in bipedal orthograde progression," and it effected "gross movements of parts acting as a whole."

The primary function of the finger is movement, and for this it needs to be free, to act, as it were, in midair. The finger owes its fine movements to the intricate arrangement of intrinsic muscles, in particular, the interossei and the lumbricals. In the hand these small muscles flex the proximal phalanges of the second to fifth fingers and extend the middle and the terminal segments.

"When the electrodes are placed over one of the interossei, with the foot off the ground and held at right angles to the leg," Duchenne wrote, "it is observed that three different movements take place: (1) abduction or adduction according to the position of the interosseous; (2) flexion of the proximal phalanx; (3) extension of the distal two phalanges." Duchenne deduced: "physiologically the extensor digitorum longus is only the extensor of the proximal phalanges and . . . the interossei are the real extensors of the middle and distal phalanges."

The phrase that betrays the fallacy of Duchenne's deduction is *the foot off the ground.* Levick (1921, 1932) electrically stimulated the dorsal interossei when the foot was planted on the ground. He found that the simultaneous action of four dorsal interossei, with the toes fixed, was "to bunch up" the metatarsal bones in such a way as to raise "the transverse arch." Levick thus corroborated what had been said before by Ellis—namely, that acting from their fixed points of insertion distally, the muscles of the foot moved the proximal segments from where their fleshy fibers originate. Wood Jones (1949) formulated this concept as follows: "The moving end of the muscles of the leg and foot is often the opposite end from that of the homologous muscle in the forearm and hand."

Obviously the foot functions principally when it is on the ground, at which time the muscles attached to the toes do not flex, extend, abduct, or adduct them, but fix them firmly to establish a point from which the body can be propelled forward. Unlike the fingers, the toes are designed for leverage and stability, and they require a solid surface to press on.

Pressors and tractors. Practically all important ideas about the function of the forefoot—for that matter of the foot as a whole—were formulated by Ellis of Gloucester. With the exception of Little (1839), who was afflicted with clubfoot and described that deformity in great detail, we can think of no one whose intense interest in his chosen subject could match that of Ellis, who himself suffered from a lame foot caused by injury. It was this accident, Ellis confessed, that had directed his attention to "foot-physiology."

Ellis (1874–1899) devoted something like 30 years to this subject. He pointed out that the weight of the body fell on two abutments—the heel, and the expanded front part of the sole, or *the tread.* The two parts did not serve the same purpose: one rested on the heel but rose on the tread to move forward. Man had been classed as plantigrade but in every step he took he alternately became digitigrade; in running he remained so. A man's hand, Ellis said, was admirably designed for grasping but his foot was intended to merely press on the ground, and it could best exert such pressure if the great toe remained extended in all its length.

Ellis took issue with the view—expressed in the anatomy books of the period, notably Quain's (1892)—that the *flexor and extensor muscles* of the toes, including the *lumbricals* and the *interossei,* acted like the corresponding muscles of the hand. Ellis demurred: while this was true if the toes were used as fingers, it was altogether untrue when the toes were used as toes. Then the *flexors* did not flex; they were *pressors* of the toes against the ground. The extensors did not extend; they were tractors: they acted from the toes as fixed points and drew the movable body forward. In the hand the two sets of muscles were antagonistic; in the foot they cooperated. The pressing-down action of the flexors was necessary to give a fixed point from which the extensors could act. "When in action as toes," Ellis wrote, "the toes serve as pressing, and not like fingers, as grasping organs."

Ellis considered the terms *origin* and *insertion* as applied to muscles misleading. They suggested that muscles always acted from their fleshy origins as fixed points and on their tendinous insertions as movable ones. In the foot the converse was true. The long extensors acted from the fixed point of the toes and pulled the movable leg forward; the long flexors of the toes similarly aided in the propulsion of the body, and as they contracted, their taut tendons lifted the overlying metatarsal heads and relieved them of the excessive stress.

According to Ellis, the principal action of the toes is to give a good foothold by active pressure on the ground, so as to supplement the passive pressure of the body weight. The toes are necessary if only to provide their corresponding metatarsal bones protection from pressure on the ground. To the lack of this influence Ellis ascribed the callosities on the sole. He mentioned Pollosson's (1889) *anterior metatarsalgia* and added: "Show me the condition of the toes in any foot, let me see how their functions are exercised, and I will predict the condition of the plantar arch." It was implied that if the toes did not firmly press down and broaden the tread, metatarsalgia would inevitably ensue.

Ellis distinguished the posture of the great toe during pressing-down action from that of the lesser digits: the hallux lay flat and straight and offered a larger area of contact to the ground; in the same act the smaller toes became bent, humped-up in the middle, allowing only the pulp of the terminal phalanx to press down. The bending of the lesser digits, Ellis stated, was proportional to the vigor with which they pressed on the proffered surface. But however vigorously the hallux bore down, it did not bend; it remained straight in all its length. Both in function and structure the great toe differed from the lesser digits; it served as a solid base from which the body could be propelled onward while the lesser toes merely gripped the ground. This last action had been erroneously interpreted as prehension or grasping: there was nothing to grasp; the toe nails were not turned into the ground; the sole of the foot was never used as a palm; the smaller toes merely turned their distal phalanges toward the ground and pressed on it.

The great toe, Ellis explained, has two phalanges and two flexor muscles, one for each phalanx. The two muscles cooperated in keeping the hallux straight in all its length. But in order to keep the great toe straight, from which, as a fixed point, the long flexor could effectively act, the short flexor had to hold the proximal phalanx down, to stabilize it. Ellis made it clear that if the short flexor failed in this function, the long flexor would cause knuckling at the interphalangeal joint and only the tip of the great toe would touch the ground. The area of surface contact would be curtailed and the pressing-down action of the great toe would weaken (Fig. 2–1).

Recent interpretations. Without mentioning Duchenne and Ellis, Lambrinudi (1927–1942) revived their ideas and in his zeal for oversimplification—of which he was a master—he left out some important points and authored several misleading statements. Lambrinudi considered the foot as a *second class lever* with the head of each metatarsal serving as a *fulcrum*. He assigned two duties to the toes: *prehensile and ambulatory*. When walking without shoes on soft crumbling soil, he said, the toes gripped the ground in order to stabilize the fulcrum, but on firm smooth surface the necessity of stabilizing the fulcrum no longer existed. The toes then lay straight and firm against the ground to enlarge the fulcrum and relieve the metatarsal heads of constant pressure.

Ellis would have approved of the phrase *straight and firm* as applied to the great toe but not to the lesser digits. Lambrinudi appears to have transposed what Ellis said about the great toe to the smaller digits. Curiously, in the drawing Lambrinudi used to illustrate the function of long extensors and flexors, the interossei and lumbricals, the lesser digit was shown with two phalanges instead of three. Ellis would have frowned on the word *prehensile,* which Lambrinudi used lavishly in connection with the pressing-down action of the toes. Ellis could also have told Lambrinudi that *grip* and *grasp* are not synonymous.

Wood Jones (1949) acknowledged Ellis' authority and paraphrased his ideas with some fidelity. "The business of bending the free toes and straightening them back again," Wood Jones wrote, "is an occupation that is neither important nor often indulged in . . . digital flexors act in permitting the toes to grip the ground at the moment of take-off . . . in the two-jointed big toe, the flexors . . . pull it flat against the ground for leverage, while the flexors of the other toes bend them actively so as to permit them to dig themselves in . . . In this action the function of the digital flexors is to stabilize the toes against the supporting surface. Nothing more is required of them."

Boileau Grant (1958) did not mention Ellis but echoed his views: "In man the toes are not used for prehensile pur-

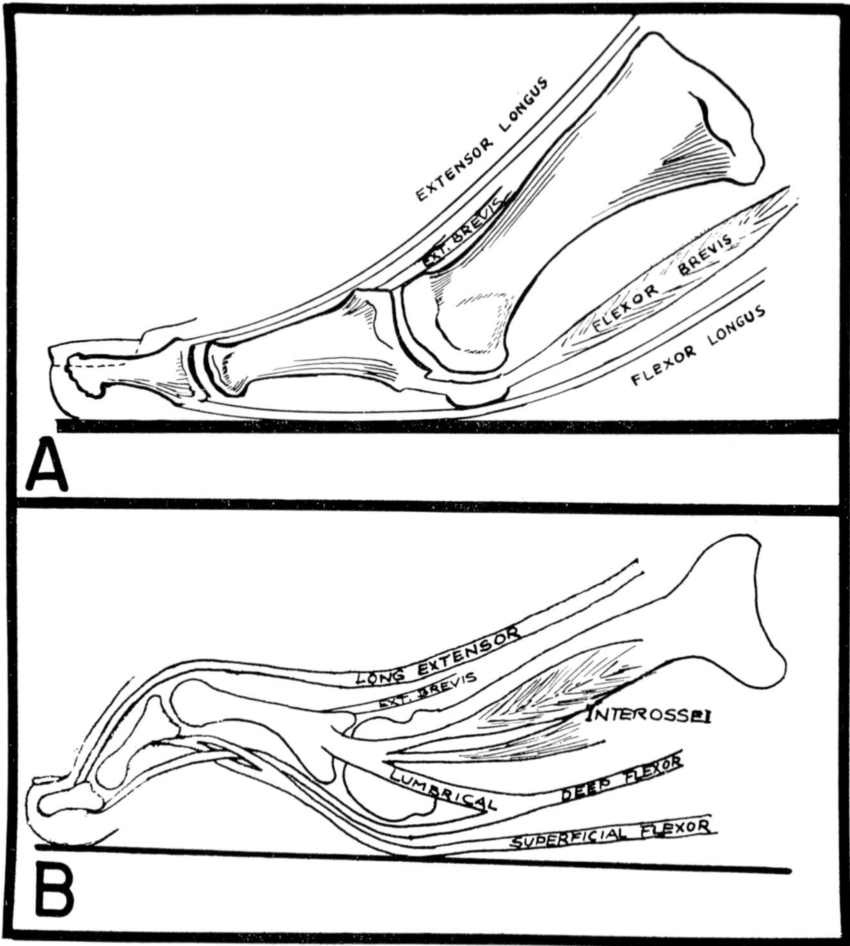

Figure 2–1. The positions of the great toe (*A*) and one of the smaller toes (*B*) during their pressing down action.

poses; their function is to press into the ground and there to form a friction surface during the act of walking. They afford a purchase for the forward thrust of the body at each step. If there were no toes, when the heel left the ground one would rise on the uneven heads of the metatarsals."

Somehow all three—Lambrinudi, Wood Jones and Grant—who borrowed extensively from Ellis also subscribed to Duchenne's view; namely that, as in the hand, pedal interossei flexed the proximal phalanges of the lesser toes and extended the distal two segments. This concept presupposes that by way of the dorsal expansion of the extensor tendons, the interossei and lumbricals of the foot reach the middle and terminal phalanges beside being inserted into the base of the proximal bone.

The destiny and the function of pedal interossei and lumbricals. John Hilton (1877), the author of the classic *Rest and Pain,* was perhaps the first to cast doubt on the orthodox view of disposition of intrinsic muscles in the foot. His criticism was couched in the law he formulated: *The nerve-trunk supplying a joint supplies also the muscles moving the joint, and the skin over the insertions of these muscles.* Hilton singled out the second toe to demonstrate the difference in nerve distribution as compared to the corresponding finger of the hand. "But here," Hilton wrote, "is a marked difference, apparently, in distribution of the plantar nerve from the median or ulnar nerves in the hand, this plantar nerve (analogous to the branch of the median nerve) does not pass towards the dorsum of the toes, but confines itself to its under surface; and it seems upon careful examination, that the interossei and lumbricals do not extend themselves so completely along the dorsum of the toe as the corresponding muscles do upon the dorsum of the finger. Again we have, on a small scale, the same thing expressed with equal precision—that the same nerve that supplies the muscles supplies also the skin over the insertion of these muscles."

Spalteholz (1923) was one of the few anatomists to stress the fact that pedal interossei and lumbricals only flex the proximal phalanges of the lesser toes without extending the second and third phalanges as in the hand. Forster (1927) could not find anything resembling the "classic and regular image of fingers" in the general arrangement of the extensor expansion in the back of each small toe. According to him, interossei are attached exclusively to the sides of the bases of the proximal phalanges. Manter (1945) noted a number of variations of the interosseous muscles of the human foot. Pertinent to the point under discussion, he wrote: "The tendons of the interosseous muscles insert into the proximal phalanges at the tubercles which are present on each side of the bases of these bones. A part of each tendon is firmly attached to the capsule of the metatarsophalangeal joint blending with the thickened plantar portion of the capsule. Continuation of the tendons dorsally into the extensor aponeurosis, as described in some current gross anatomy textbooks, could not be found, though it was searched in several feet . . ."

In walking, pedal interossei merely stabilize proximal phalanges. They do not—as was surmised by Lambrinudi, Wood Jones, and Grant—keep the two terminal phalanges extended, thus preventing the toes from "curling under at each step." This function is in part performed by the long extensors of the toes. Also, the surface one steps on resists such curling action.

The range of toe flexion and extension. Wright (1928) stated that the metatarsophalangeal joints allowed "fully 90 degrees of hyperextension . . ." The age at which this range is possible was not given. Obviously flexion and extension at the metatarsophalangeal joint diminish with advancing age and the number of years shoes are worn. These movements reach wider range in toe dancers. In women who have been wearing high heels the toes can be passively extended to a greater degree. Another factor that comes into play is the position of the foot in relation to the leg. Passive flexion of the toes is augmented when the foot is dorsiflexed at the ankle; the toes can be pushed further dorsally when the foot is plantarflexed. In general, active extension is more free at the metatarsophalangeal joint than flexion; at the interphalangeal joint flexion is freer.

Speaking of flexion and extension permitted at the metatarsophalangeal articulation of the great toe, Hiss (1937) said: "This joint motion may normally run to one hundred and thirty degrees. In the average type of normal foot it will be around ninety. Then division is made between plantar flexion and dorsal extension. These ordinarily are divided equally, forty five degrees each." This "division" appears arbitrary; at the metatarsophalangeal joint of the hallux greater range of motion is permitted in dorsal than in plantar direction. Out of the total range only a small fraction consists of flexion (Figs. 2–2 and 2–3).

Watson-Jones (1941) stated that normally the metatarsophalangeal joints of the toes were "level" and the whole row might be regarded as one articulation at which movement occurred with each step as weight was transmitted to the toes. The metatarsophalangeal joints do not lie on the same dorsoplantar plane; the second and third and sometimes the first metatarsal heads may reach the same line anteriorly, but the fourth does not extend as far forward as its fellow on the tibial side, and the head of the fifth is far behind the fourth. Watson-Jones is correct in regarding all five metatarsophalangeal joints as one in permitting passive yield in the dorsal direction. Very

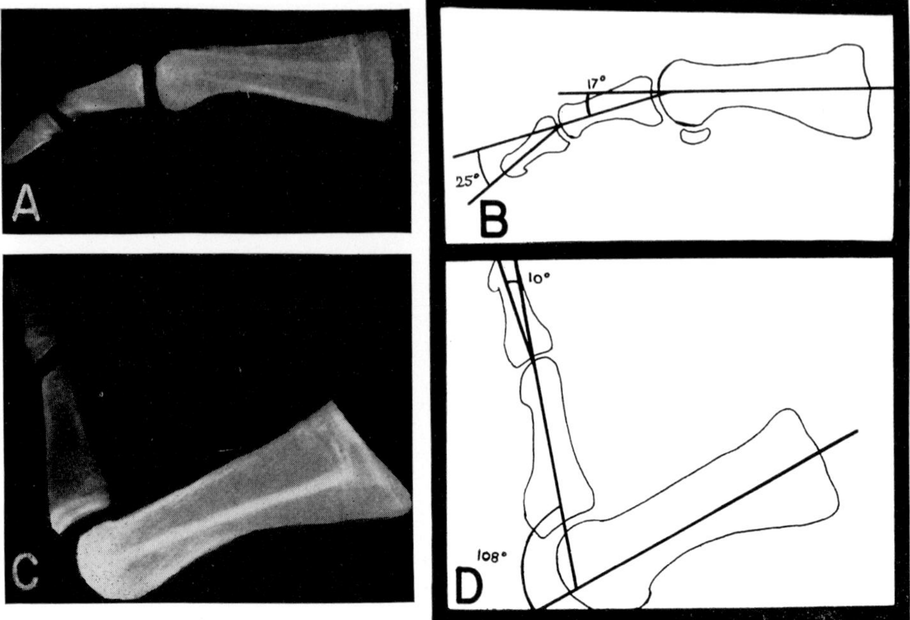

Figure 2–2. Flexion (*A* and *B*) and extension (*C* and *D*) of the hallux in a boy.

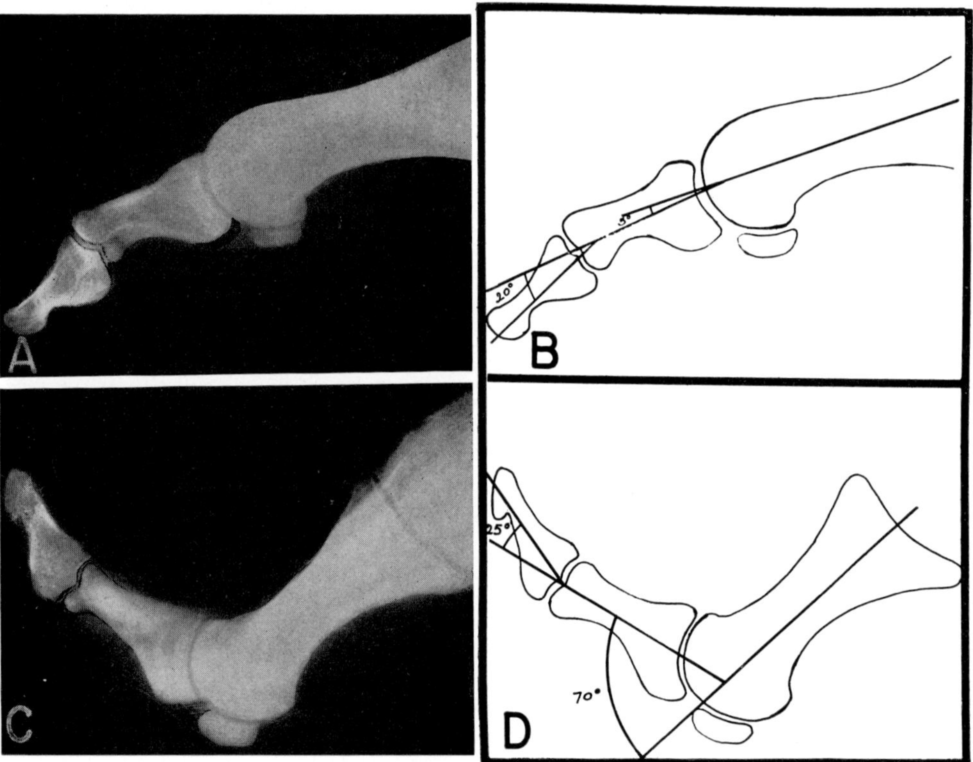

Figure 2–3. Flexion and extension of the hallux in an adult.

few individuals can actively flex or extend their toes independent of one another (Figs. 2–4 to 2–8).

Joseph (1954) studied 50 male subjects with the aid of radiographs and found a wide variation between individuals in the range of movement allowed at the joints of the great toe. "At the metatarsophalangeal joint," he wrote, "dorsiflexion is much more free than plantar flexion. The opposite is the case at the interphalangeal joint. . . . There is an inverse ratio between active and passive dorsiflexion: the greater the range of active dorsiflexion, the less the range of additional passive dorsiflexion."

After operations on the toes, especially on the hallux, passive yield in dorsal direction is more important than active extension. Some degree of active flexion, sufficient to stabilize the toes on the proffered surface, is desirable.

Opposability of the hallux. A recurrent theme in the literature relates to the prehensile propensity of the great toe in infants, in unshod natives, and in armless people. It all started with Camper (1781). "I remember seeing at Amsterdam, twenty-five years ago," Camper wrote, "a man who had, in place of arms, merely short immovable appendages, and who executed with his feet all

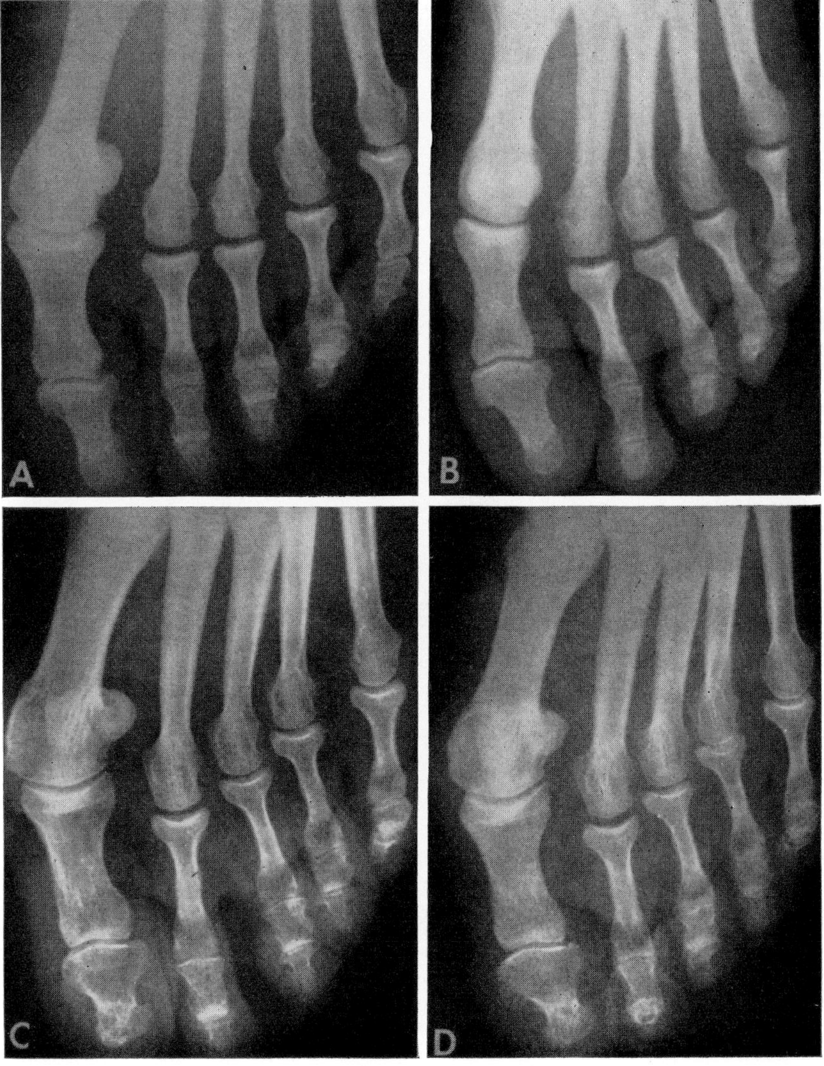

Figure 2–4. The line of metatarsophalangeal joint in various roentgenographs.

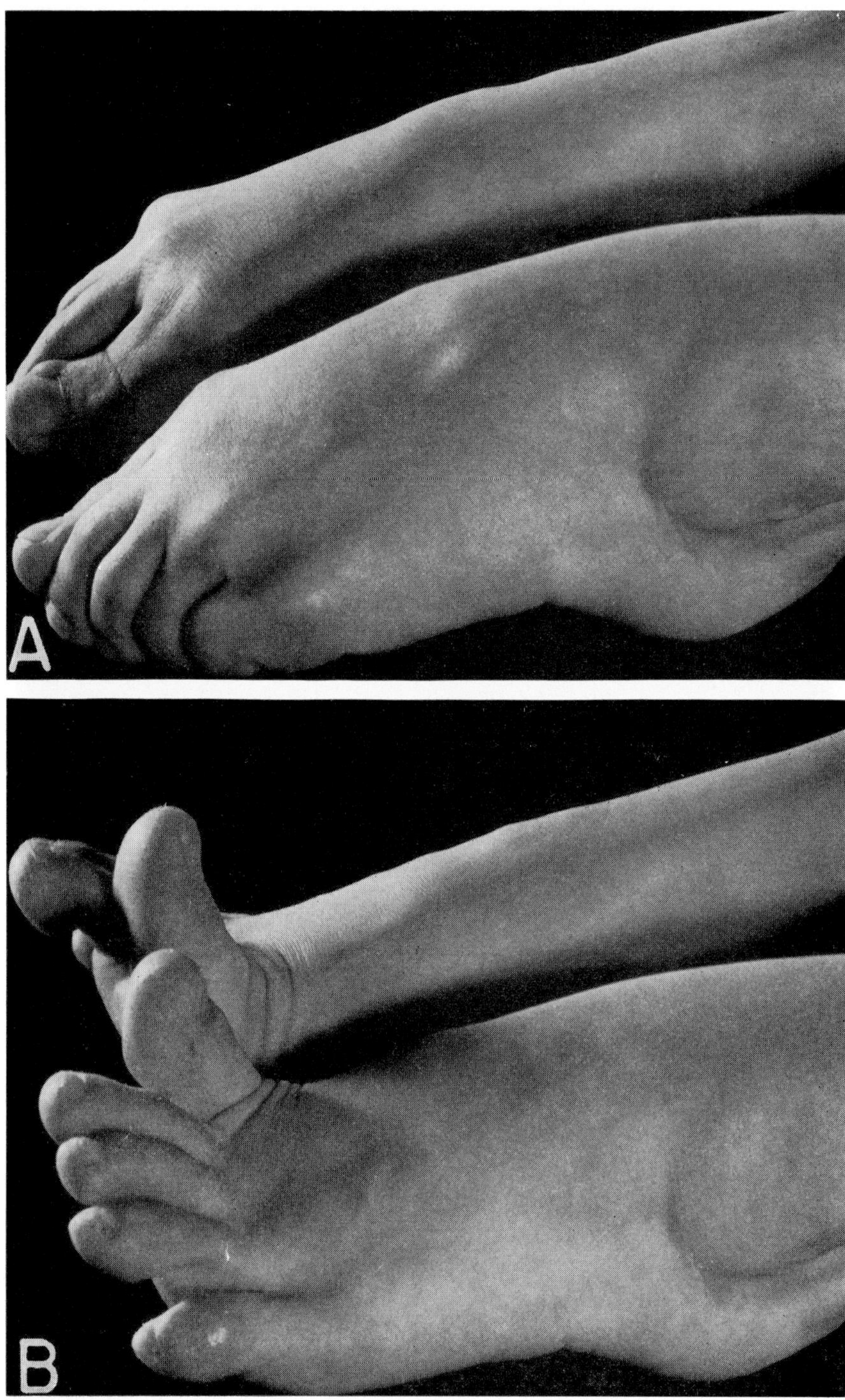

Figure 2–5. Flexion (*A*) and extension (*B*) of the toes. The great toe does not bend as far down but tilts up more than smaller digits.

those actions for which we employ our fingers. He could write, cut his own pens, fire a pistol, etc." Huxley (1863) spoke of "the great amount of mobility, and even some sort of opposability" of the hallux in barefooted natives. Hoffmann (1905) extolled the accomplishments of another young man born without hands illustrating "to what extensive intricate uses the commonly cramped and abused foot may be put."

Wood Jones (1929) took issue with Huxley on the question of opposability of the great toe. In the hand, Wood Jones argued, the movement culminating in opposition took place at the carpometacarpal joint. In the foot of arboreal primates prehension depended on motion permitted at the innermost cuneometatarsal joint. In armless human beings the movement that produced pulp-to-pulp contact between the great toe and lesser digits took place at the metatarsophalangeal articulation. Wood Jones (1949) conceded that there was some embryological evidence of divergent great toe in man. "As for adult human hallux," Wood Jones wrote, "the alignment of its metatarsal with that of the second and its inclusion in the common bond of the deep transverse ligament render any suggestion of opposability . . . absurd. . . . *Movements of human big toe are metatarsophalangeal move-*

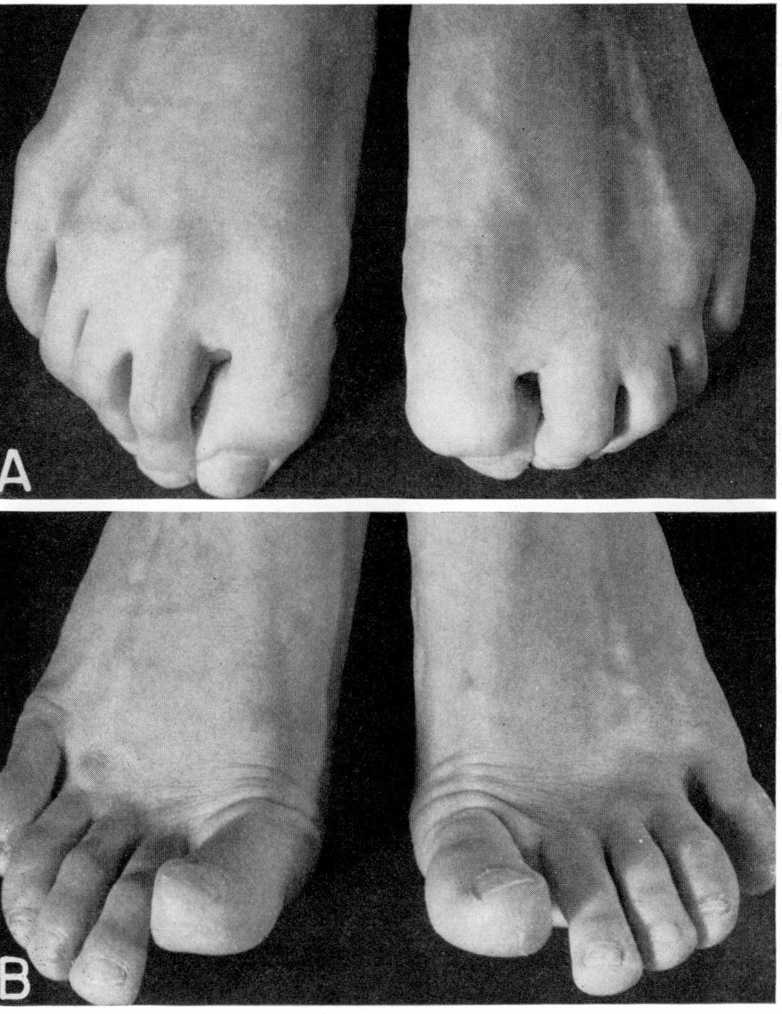

Figure 2–6. Flexion (*A*) and extension (*B*) of the toes as seen from the dorsal aspect.

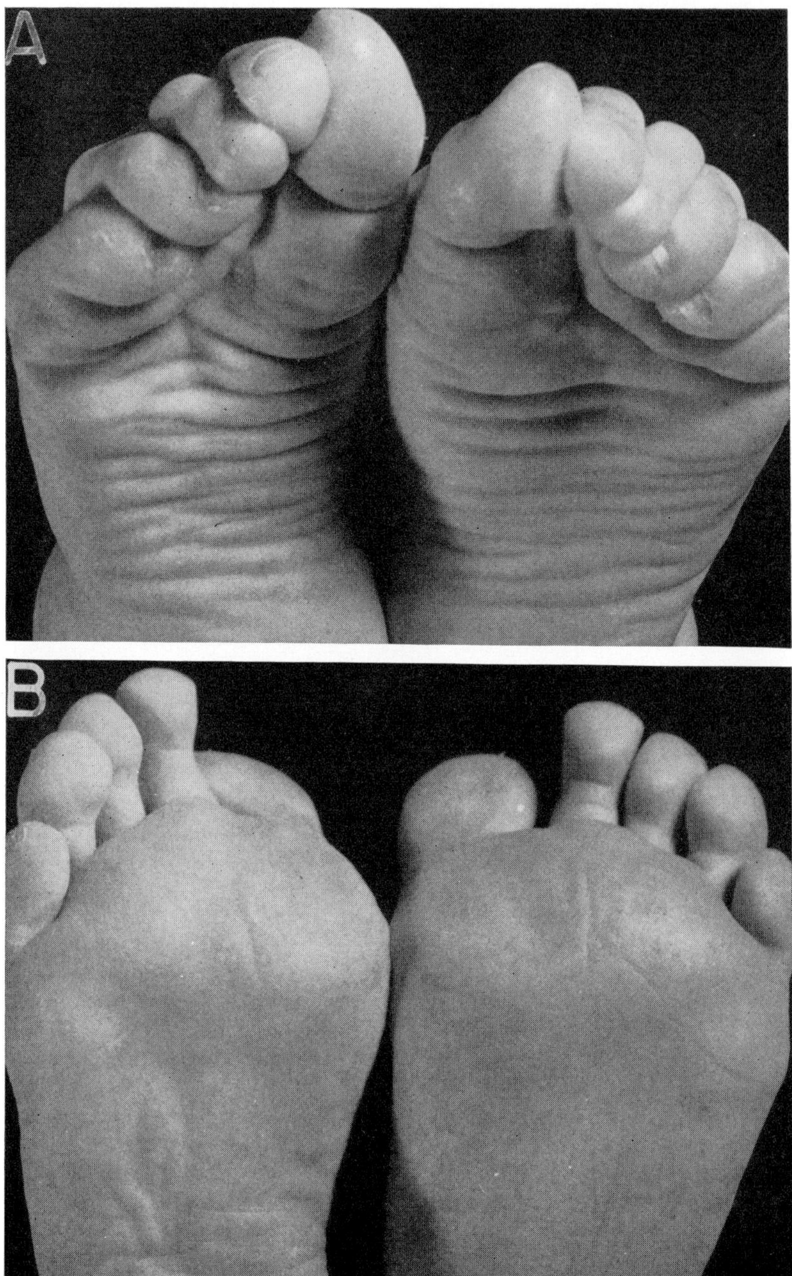

Figure 2–7. When the toes are flexed, a dimple (*A*) forms under the second metatarsal head. In extension (*B*) of the toes the depression disappears.

ments and it can not be too strongly emphasized that opposition is a movement carried out at the tarsometatarsal and not metatarsophalangeal joint."

Movement permitted at the first cuneometatarsal joint. The distal articular facet of the first cuneiform is mildly convex; that of the base of the metatarsal is correspondingly concave. The dorsoplantar diameter of the joint is twice as long as its transverse measurement. The plane of the joint slants medially and inclines plantarward. The curve of the articular facets is a measure of the mobility of this joint; the tibial slant and the forward tilt of its plane, respectively, determine the degree of medial and plantar inclination of the first metatarsal. Normally the innermost cuneometatarsal joint allows 10 to 15

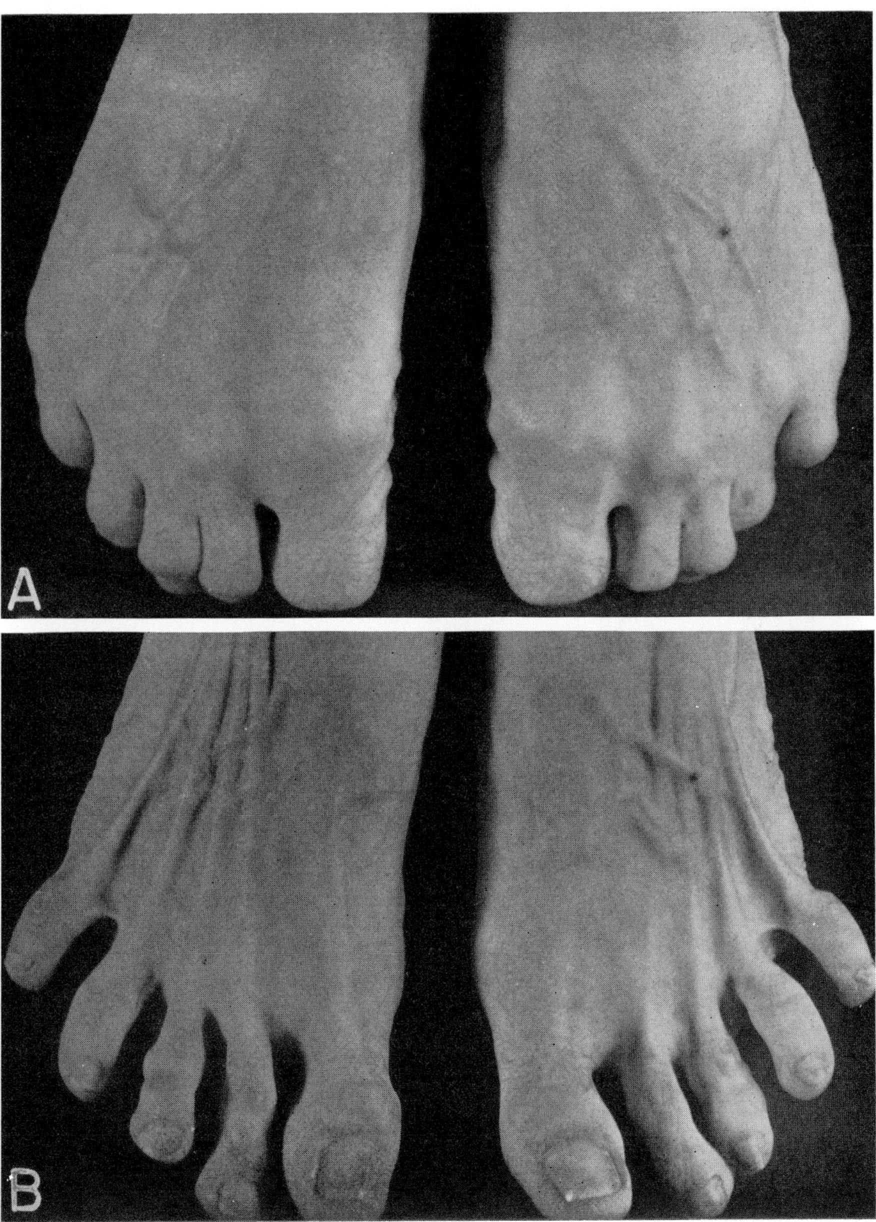

Figure 2–8. During flexion (*A*) of the toes the second metatarsal head bulges dorsally and the central digits converge. In extension (*B*) the toes diverge.

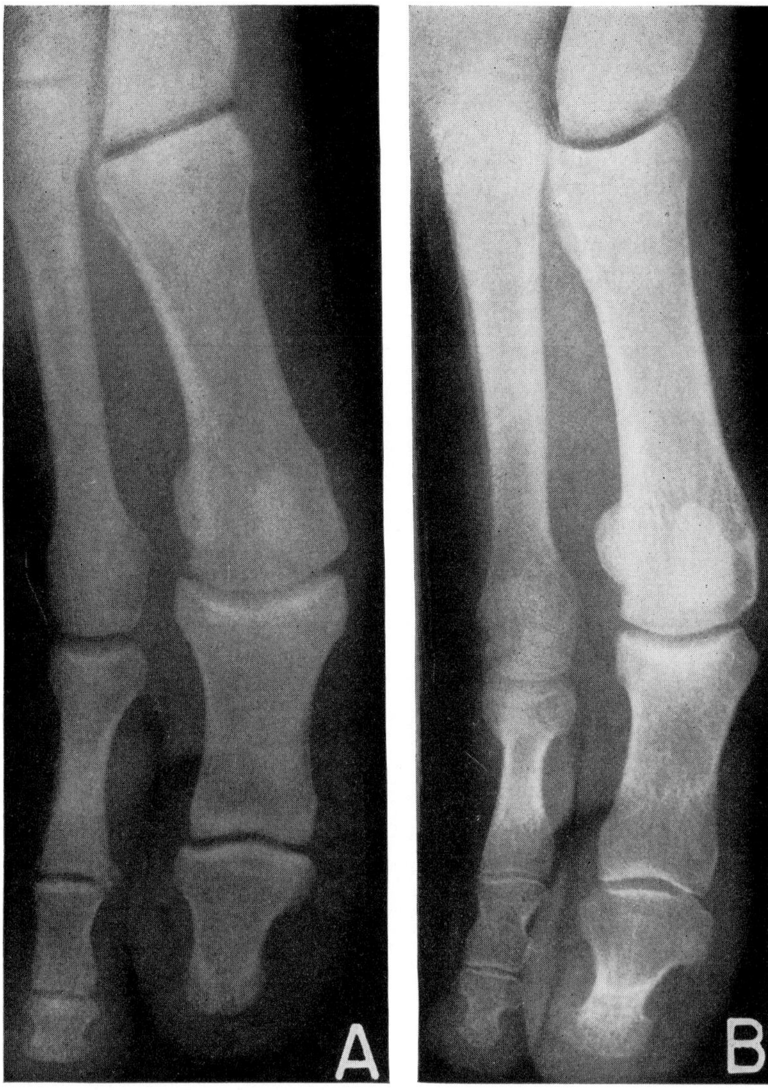

Figure 2–9. The innermost cuneometatarsal joint: oblique setting (*A*), and curved configuration (*B*).

degrees of passive up-and-down movement. Side-to-side motion is about half of that range. The limited mobility permitted at this joint contributes to the resilience of the longitudinal arch—or what some prefer to call bow or spring—without weakening its stability. With accentuated curve of the facets there is greater range of mobility—even hypermobility, which is not desirable (Fig. 2–9).

Moderate medial slant of the articular plane of the innermost cuneometatarsal joint is considered normal. It gives the first metatarsal slight varus inclination —about 5 to 8 degrees—as measured by the angle formed between its own longitudinal axis and that of the second metatarsal. This small degree of inward inclination enhances the weight-sustaining power of the first metatarsal. With greater obliquity of the articular plane, the first metatarsal would go into more varus, which is not desirable. Diminished plantar inclination of the articular plane is accompanied by dorsal tilt of the first metatarsal head and consequent failure of this bone to sustain its share of the body weight.

Distribution of body weight in the forefoot. In numerous articles, but especially in two books—*The Human Foot,* and *Human Locomotion and Body Form* —D. J. Morton (1935, 1952) tried to establish a norm concerning the amount of weight sustained by the heads of the five metatarsal bones: "In the function of weight-bearing, the foremost physiological feature consists of the relative equality of the supporting contact of each metatarsal bone: Recognition of such a contact as normal condition and as part of the foot mechanics refutes the widely held concept of an anterior transverse arch. It is obvious that these bones cannot support weight unless they have contact with the ground; and if they have contact, then there can be no arch conformation."—Morton meant distally under the metatarsal heads—"Each metatarsal bone transmits approximately an equal amount of weight with the exception of metatarsal I, which carries a double load."

In the foot, Morton distinguished two axes: (1) *axis of balance,* running between second and third metatarsals; and (2) *axis of leverage,* located between first and second metatarsals. He said that in standing, out of twenty-four units of body weight, twelve were supported by each foot, and out of twelve, six units were carried by the heel and six by the forefoot. "In the passive act of standing," Morton wrote, "four medial units of weight are transmitted through the talar neck by metatarsal I, II and III, and two lateral units pass to metatarsal IV and V through the anterior process of the calcaneous and cuboid bone." In other words, there are three units on either side of *axis of balance.* Of the three medial units, the first metatarsal carries two and the second metatarsal, one. The three lateral units are equally distributed on the third, fourth, and fifth metatarsal. Thus, the ratio of weight distribution is 2:1:1:1:1. In walking, when one shifts from one foot to the other and the heel of the latter is lifted off the ground, 24 units of body weight are carried by the five metatarsals. The axis of leverage serves as the dividing line: twelve units are carried by the first metatarsal head; the heads of the lateral four bones sustain three units each: the ratio of weight distribution is 4:1:1:1:1 (Fig. 2–10).

Subdivision of the foot into separate functional units. Ellis (1889) said that, in relation to its fellow, each foot "is the complement as well as the counterpart"; taken singly the two sides of the foot "differ materially in structure and in function as well as in form: the inner side serves as a springy lever from which the body is propelled onward; the outer half acts as a buttress to give additional area of support where such support is not afforded by the foot on the other side."

Lambrinudi (1938) considered the outer part of the foot essentially a balancing organ and the inner segment "a lever and a spring to absorb shock." Wood Jones (1949) quoted both Ellis and Lambrinudi and found it difficult to determine "when and by whom this fundamental truth, so commonly and completely ignored in textbook teaching, was first enunciated." He himself wrote: "The human foot is designed with an outer part functionally specialized as a static, stabilized, supporting organ and an inner part destined as the elastic, mobile, dynamic organ of propulsion." Du Vries (1959) said the outer border of the foot formed a buttress for stability and balance; he considered the inner portion "essentially a lever."

Manter (1946) sounded a note of dissent but his findings appear to have passed unnoticed. He carried out an experiment with loaded cadaver feet and measured the degree of compression in the joints of the foot. "The results," Manter wrote, "contradict the suggestion that the lateral subdivision of the foot is the primary weight-bearing element. Furthermore, there is no indication that the foot should be divided into two functional units."

The question remains unsettled. It is perhaps safe to say that the medial tier of bones of the foot are joined to one another with curved surfaces; these joints allow greater resilience. The bones of the lateral portion have mainly plane articular facets; the outer midtarsal joints yield to the pressure from above only slightly (Fig. 2–11).

Speaking of the forefoot as a unit, Wiles (1934) restated a well known principle as follows: "The bones of the fore-

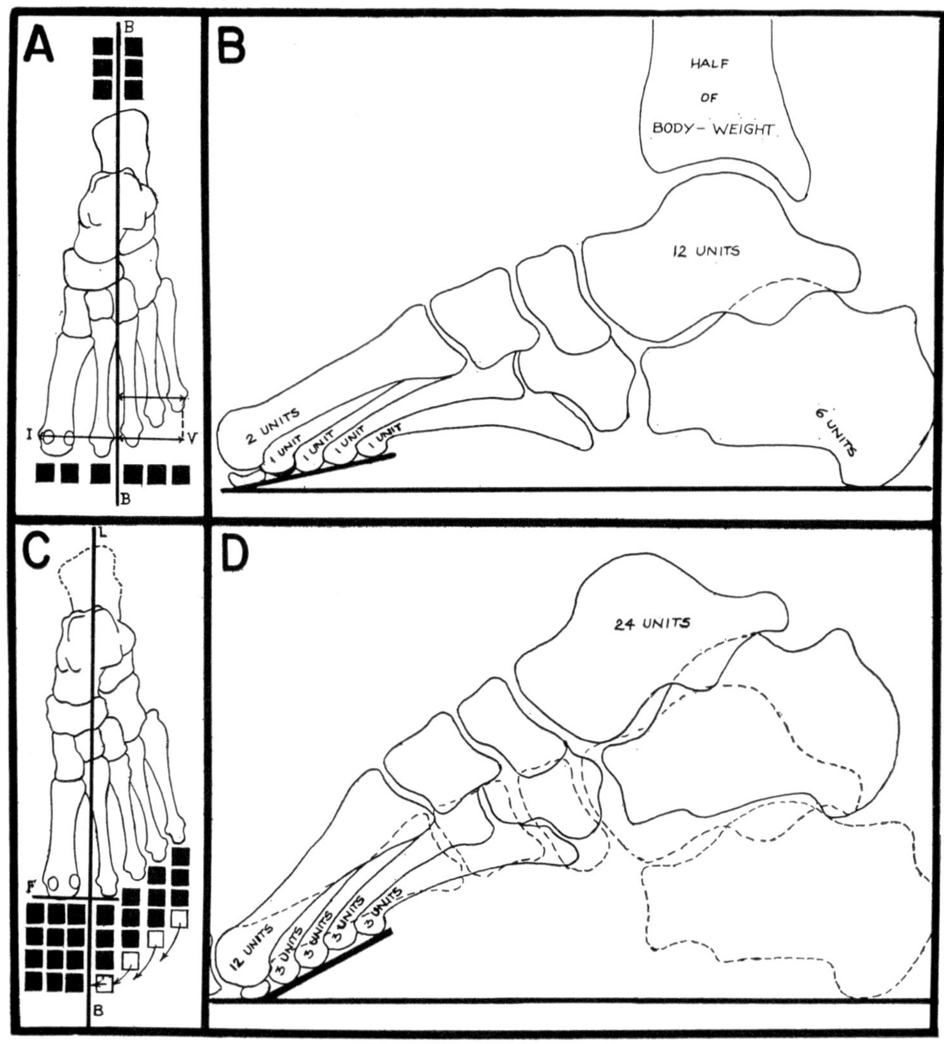

Figure 2–10. Axis of balance (*A*), weight distribution in stance (*B*), axis of leverage (*C*), and weight distribution during take-off (*D*). (*A* and *C*, redrawn from D. J. Morton's books and articles.)

foot, all those in the front of the midtarsal joints, are connected closely together by interosseous ligaments which limit but the slightest movement between them. Consequently, the whole forefoot must move as one piece (only the first metatarsal showing any considerable independent movement). Moreover, the forefoot is very closely attached to the os calcis by the long and short plantar ligaments. On the other hand, there is no close union between the forefoot and the astragalus. The forefoot and the os calcis must therefore move as one piece around the axis of the astragalus so that the main movement of the foot occurs at the subastragaloid and astragaloscaphoid joint."

When the forefoot inverts and everts, or as some would have it, supinates and pronates, the movements take place mainly in talocalcaneal, talonavicular, and calcaneocuboid joints and the forefoot follows as an end point, its own articulations contribute very little to the sum total of rotary movement. The same is true of plantarflexion and dorsoflexion, which are permitted primarily at the ankle; the distal joints add their increment with diminishing range until the metatarsophalangeal junction is reached.

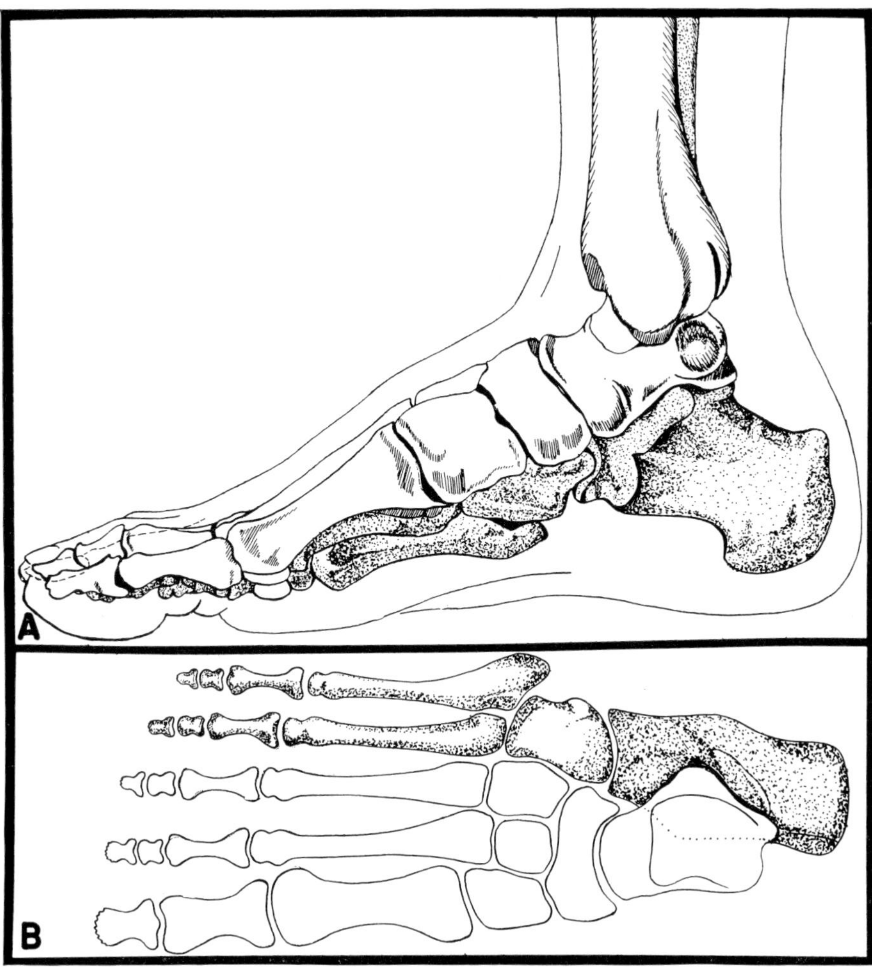

Figure 2–11. The medial springy "lever" and the lateral *(dotted)* supporting buttress of the foot.

REFERENCES

Blandın, P. F.: *A Treatise on Topographical Anatomy* (Tr. from French by A. Sidney Doane). New York, Moore & Payne, 1833, pp. 354–367.

Camper, P.: *On the Best Form of Shoe,* published with Dowie's treatise, *The Foot and Its Covering.* London, R. Hardwicke, 1861, pp. 1–44. The French version, called *Dissertation sur le Meilleur Forme des Souliers,* appeared in Paris, 1781.

Duchenne, G. B.: *Physiology of Motion* (Tr. by E. B. Kalpan). Philadelphia, J. B. Lippincott Co., 1949, pp. 370–439. The original French edition appeared in 1867.

DuVries, H. L.: *Surgery of the Foot.* St. Louis, C. V. Mosby Co., 1959, pp. 21–56.

Ellis, T. S.: The influence of muscular action in prevention and cure of flat-foot. Paper read before the Gloucester branch of British Medical Association in 1874.

Ellis, T. S.: *On the Arch of the Foot.* Gloucester, J. Bellow, 1877, pp. 1–22.

Ellis, T. S.: Position of rest in fatigue and in pain, 1878, pp. 1–8. (Octavo)

Ellis, T. S.: The physiology of the feet. Lancet *1:*1113–1115, 1884.

Ellis, T. S.: The physiology of the feet. Popular Science Monthly *28:*395–400, 1886.

Ellis, T. S.: Deformities of the great toe. Brit. Med. J. *1:*1157–1158, May 27, 1887.

Ellis, T. S.: *The Human Foot: Its Form and Structure, Functions and Clothing.* London, J. & A. Churchill, 1889.

Ellis, T. S.: *The Human Foot: Its Form and Structure, Functions and Clothing.* In Wood's Medical and Surgical Monograph, Vol. 6, 1890.

Ellis, T. S.: On some points in the physiology of the foot. Trans. Roy. Med. Chir. Soc. *80:*171–190, 1897.

Ellis, T. S.: Hallux valgus and hammer toe. Lancet *1:*1155–1156, 1899.

Forster, A.: Considération sur l'attitude des orteils chez l'homme. Arch. d'Anat. d'Histol. d'Embryol. *7*:247–261, 1927.

Grant, J. C. B.: *A Method of Anatomy.* Baltimore, Williams & Wilkins Co., 1958, pp. 462 and 502.

Hilton, J.: *Rest and Pain.* London, G. Bell & Sons, 1877, pp. 175–176.

Hiss, J. M.: *Functional Foot Disorders.* Los Angles University Press, 1937, pp. 73–78.

Hoffmann, P.: Conclusions drawn from comparative study of the feet of barefooted and shoe-wearing peoples. Am. J. Orthop. Surg. *3*:105–136, 1905.

Huxley, T. H.: *Man's Place in Nature and other anthropological essays.* New York, D. Appleton & Co., 1894, p. 119. The title essay originally appeared in 1863.

Jones, F. W.: The distinctions of the human hallux. J Anat. *63*:408–411, 1929.

Jones, F. W.: *Structure and Function As Seen in the Foot.* 2nd Ed., London, Baillière, Tindall & Cox, 1949, pp. 1–4 and 200–214.

Joseph, J.: Range of movement of the great toe in men. J. Bone Joint Surg. *36*:450–457, 1954.

Lambrinudi, C.: An operation for claw-toes. Proc. Roy. Soc. Med. *21*:239, 1927.

Lambrinudi, C.: Use and abuse of toes. Postgrad. M. J. *8*:459-464, 1932.

Lambrinudi, C.: Functional aspect: action of foot muscles. Lancet *2*:1480–1482, 1938.

Lambrinudi, C.: Discussion on painful feet. Proc. Roy. Soc. Med. *36*:47–51, 1942.

Lambrinudi, C., and Stamm, T. T.: A report on the work in the orthopaedic department of Guy's Hospital. Guy's Hosp. Rep. *89*:184-225, 1939.

Levick, G. M.: The action of the intrinsic muscles of the foot and their treatment by electricity. Brit. Med. J. *1*:381–382, 1921.

Levick, G. M.: On arch-raising rôle of certain intrinsic muscles of the foot. J. Anat. *67*:196–197, 1932.

Little, W. J.: *A Treatise on the Nature of Club-Foot and Analogous Distortions.* London, W. Jeffs, 1839.

Manter, J. T.: Variations of the interosseous muscles of the human foot. Anat. Rec. *93*:117–124, 1945.

Manter, J. T.: Distribution of compression forces in joints of the foot. Anat. Rec. *96*:313–321, 1946.

Morton, D. J.: *The Human Foot.* New York, Columbia University Press, 1935, pp. 105–149 and 187–195.

Morton, D. J.: *Human Locomotion and Body Form.* Baltimore, Williams & Wilkins Co., 1952, pp. 70–75.

Pollosson, A.: De la métatarsalgie antérieure. Province Méd. *6*:1–3, Feb. 9, 1889. See Lancet, *1*:436, 1889 and *1*:553, 1889.

Quain, J.: *Quain's Elements of Anatomy.* London, Longmans, Green & Co., 1876. Vol. 1, p. 260. The same statement appeared on page 274, Vol. II, Part 2, 1892.

Spalteholz, W.: *Hand Atlas of Human Anatomy.* Edited and translated from the 7th German edition by L. F. Barker. Philadelphia, J. B. Lippincott Co., 1923, Vol II, pp. 372–377.

Watson-Jones, R.: *Fractures and Other Bone and Joint Injuries.* Baltimore, Williams & Wilkins Co., 1941, p. 163.

Wiles, P.: Flat-feet Lancet *2*:1089, 1934.

Wright, W. G.: *Muscle Function.* New York, P. B. Hoeber, 1928, pp. 83–95.

Chapter Three

CLINICAL FEATURES

HALLUX VALGUS COMPLEX

It is seldom that hallux valgus is an isolated entity. More often it is associated with other deformities of the forefoot, sometimes the entire foot. What appears to be simply a deviation of the great toe toward the fibular border of the foot is due to the unseen shift of position of at least two bones. From its base forward the first metatarsal inclines medially and the proximal phalanx is deflected in the opposite direction. The joint between these two bones knuckles toward the midline of the body and presents a prominence along the tibial margin of the forefoot. The outward deviation of the great toe is usually accompanied by rotation around its own longitudinal axis, the nail of the hallux slants medially, and the pulp turns toward the second toe. The great toe may ride over the second digit or slip under it (Figs. 3–1 to 3–4).

The outward deviation, axial rotation, and overriding are merely some of the features—the most striking but not necessarily the most troublesome—of the interrelated deformities. Ingrown toenail, with or without infection, is not an uncommon accompaniment of hallux valgus and the discomfort caused by it may overshadow that due to knuckling of the joint. The lesser toes—especially the second and third—are pushed toward the outer border of the foot. They are crowded together, hammered, and clawed. The central toes—the second more than the others—are retracted and deviated, and their basal phalanges are displaced at the metatarsophalangeal joint both in dorsal and lateral direction. The heads of corresponding metatarsals appear to have taken a relatively more plantar position.

The small toe may be in exaggerated varus. The fifth metatarsal inclines fibularward to a marked degree until its head is partly out of contact with the base of the proximal phalanx. It presents a deformity along the outer border of the forefoot that has become known as *bunionette.* The space between the fourth and fifth metatarsals is widened. The first metatarsal assumes a greater varus inclination and the distance between it and the second metatarsal is also widened. In short, the forefoot is splayed. Each of these entities presents its own set of symptoms and physical findings. On the one hand there is the apparent or occult deformity; on the other there is pain. There is discomfort associated with wearing shoes and interference with proper functioning of the foot both in standing or walking.

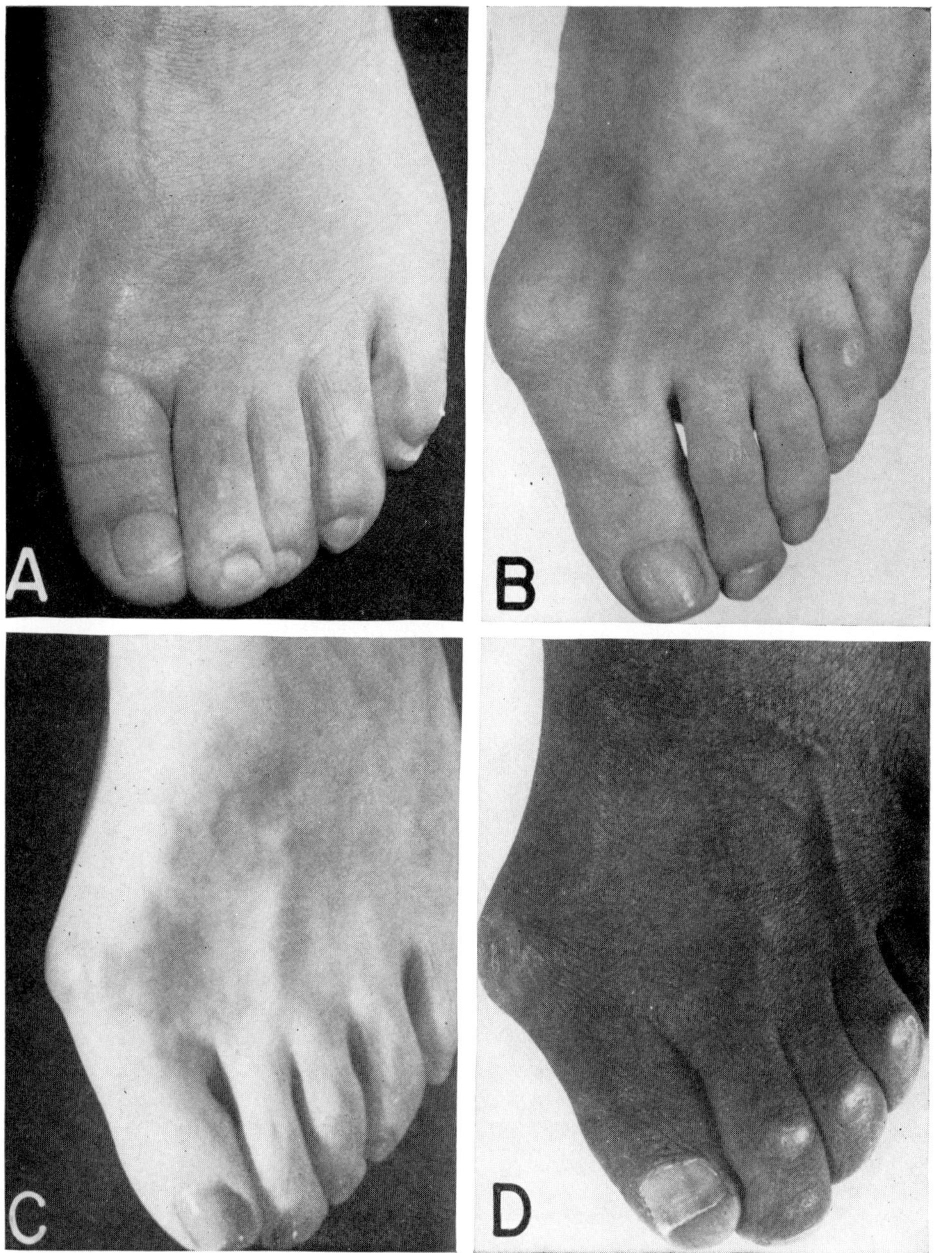

Figure 3–1. Grades of outward deviation of the great toe.

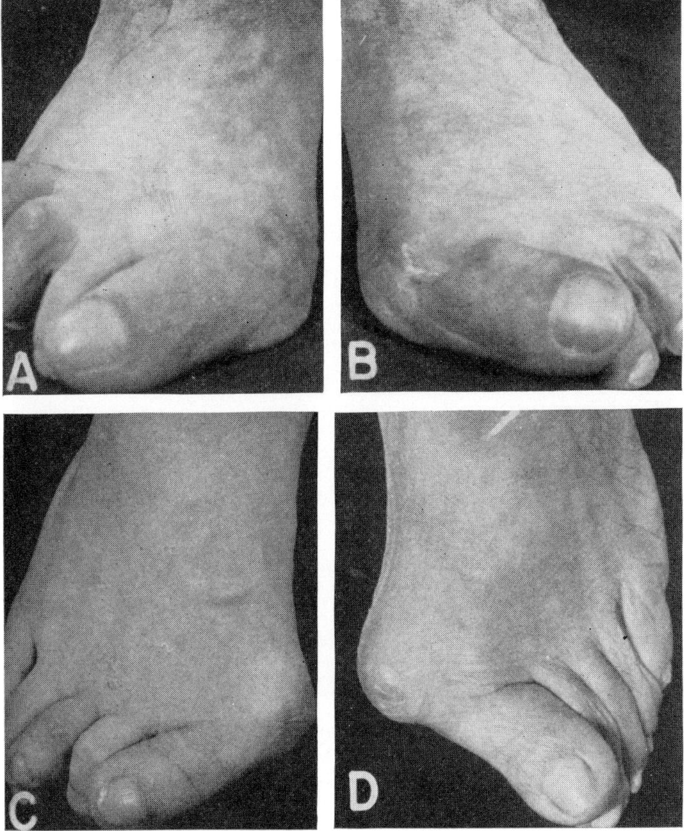

Figure 3–2. Outward deviation with axial rotation.

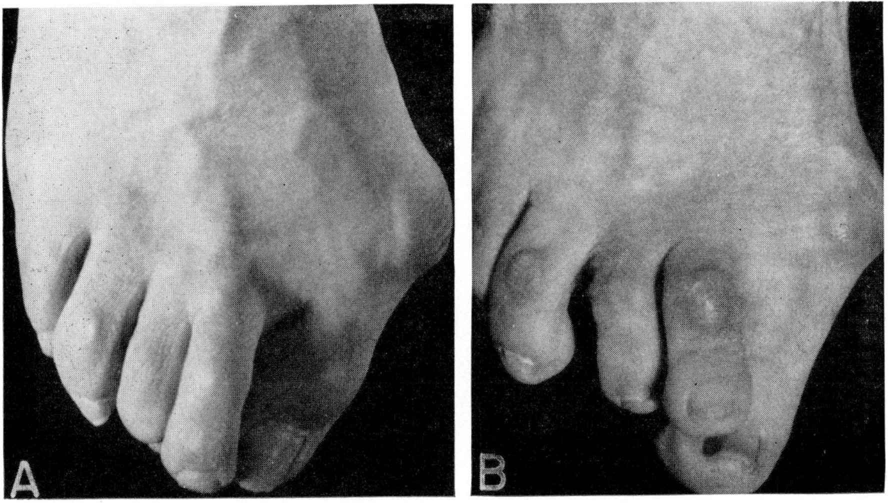

Figure 3–3. Mild (*A*) and more advanced (*B*) overriding second toe.

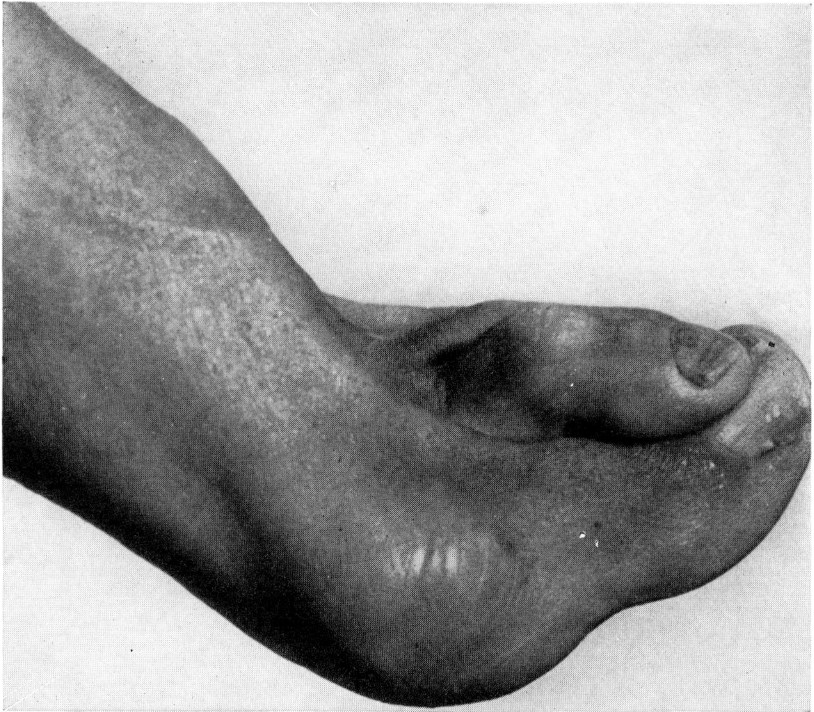

Figure 3–4. Overriding second toe as seen from the medial aspect.

Bunion pain. The degree of deformity of the great toe is not a measure of the severity of the symptoms. Even the most severely twisted hallux may be asymptomatic. What makes the patient come for consultation is pain, difficulty in being fitted with shoes, corns, and keratoses. Many merely seek cosmetic improvement.

A classic example of extreme discomfort caused by hallux valgus was recorded by Camper (1781). "One of my friends, residing in Amsterdam, suffered from a bunion," Camper (1781) wrote, "all attempts to cure which were in vain tried for more than a year. The sufferer was forced to keep to the house and neglect his business, in consequence of the insupportable pain he suffered in walking." Another example was provided by Pitha. Rose (1874) quoted him as follows: "An old surgeon having suffered greatly from abduction of the great toes finally, in his 75th year, cured it radically by placing first one foot on a block of wood and chopping the toe off with a chisel and hammer, and subsequently repeating the same on the other foot. In spite of his old age both wounds healed promptly." Here the word "abduction" is used in reference to midsagittal line. Rose deleted the following sentence from the original statement by Pitha and Billroth (1868): "This case gives at least a good illustration of the torment that a case of bunion can cause."

Bursitis. In hallux valgus the prominence along the inner border of the forefoot consists mainly of the medially displaced portion of the first metatarsal head. Between this bone and the overlying skin a synovial sac is formed that may distend with fluid, become inflamed, result in regional cellulitis, rupture, and discharge pus through a sinus. During the fulminant phase of inflammation the skin over the bursal tumefaction is red and tense; it is parchment-thin in the center and thick around the periphery; there may be lymphangitic lines streaking up the leg. When the inflammation abates and the swelling subsides, the skin becomes puckered and corrugated; in chronic cases the integument is indurated and calloused.

Besides aggravating the local pain at

the inner base of the great toe, the inflamed or infected bursa may cause fever and leukocytosis: it may evolve into a bursal abscess, cellulitis, or lymphangitis. In the aftermath of local infection the skin sometimes becomes painfully adherent to the underlying bone. Years after the resolution of noninfectious bursitis, one may see on roentgenographs shadows along the medial aspect of the first metatarsal head suggesting calcareous deposits. Pain caused by corns on hammered and clawed toes must be included in this group because there is often a bursa underneath the hardened skin.

Arthritic pain. Often it is difficult to dissociate the discomfort due to the knuckling of the joint and distended bursa from the pain caused by arthritis of the first metatarsophalangeal articulation. Support and immobilization afforded by the shoe should alleviate arthritic pain; walking and weight-bearing aggravate it. In arthritis, movements of the toe are limited; passive motion may elicit crepitation; forced extension is painful. One may palpate marginal spurs.

Metatarsalgia. Undoubtedly the most disabling deformity of the forefoot—usually associated with hallux valgus but also occurring independently—is the one characterized with the word *splaying.* In the preceding chapter we suggested that splaying failed to adequately describe the plantar bulge of the central metatarsal heads—also called obliteration, collapse, and reversal—of the anterior metatarsal arch. Viewed from the plantar aspect, the area just proximal to the bases of the toes presents a convexity both from side to side and from front to back. This appearance is accentuated by the dorsal retraction of the lesser toes that usually accompanies the more severe grades of hallux valgus. On deep palpation one may elicit tender points and also feel the heads of the second, third, fourth, and sometimes fifth metatarsals.

The integument under the plantarly prominent metatarsal heads is often keratotic. It may even ulcerate as in diabetics and patients afflicted with spina bifida. Plantar ulcers of neuropathic origin have been explained on the basis of dulled or absent sensibility. Perhaps equally important is the factor of diminished motor power. Toes that cannot effectively bear down on the proffered surface fail to disperse the stress thrown on the metatarsal heads. The skin under these bones responds to excessive pressure by becoming thick. The blood supply of the central portion of the pressure keratosis is cut off by excessive peripheral scarring; this area sloughs and results in an ulcer (Figs. 3–5 and 3–6).

Metatarsalgia, with or without plantar keratosis, is the most distressing symptom of hallux valgus complex. Most commonly it is chronic and diffuse. Occasionally it simulates T. G. Morton's (1876) "affection" with paroxysmal pain confined to the third interdigital area. In long-standing fixed incarcerations of the central metatarsal heads, degenerative changes also involve the corresponding joints, causing persistent pain and limitation of motion. One cannot overstress the point that toes that fail to flex at the metatarsophalangeal articulations, fail to contact the proffered surface, and fail to bear down on it with sufficient

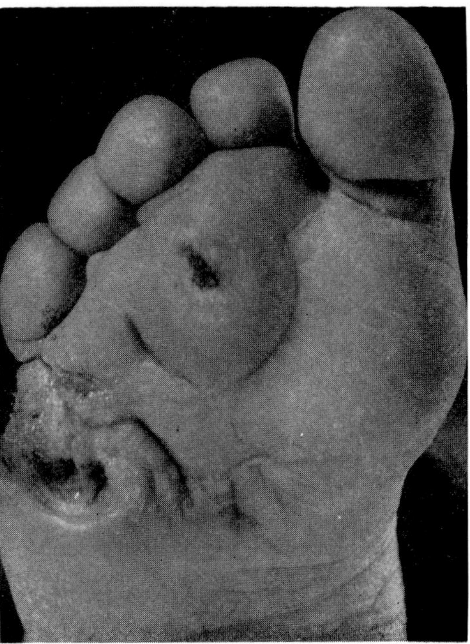

Figure 3–5. Fungating plantar ulcer due to diminished sensation caused by spina bifida.

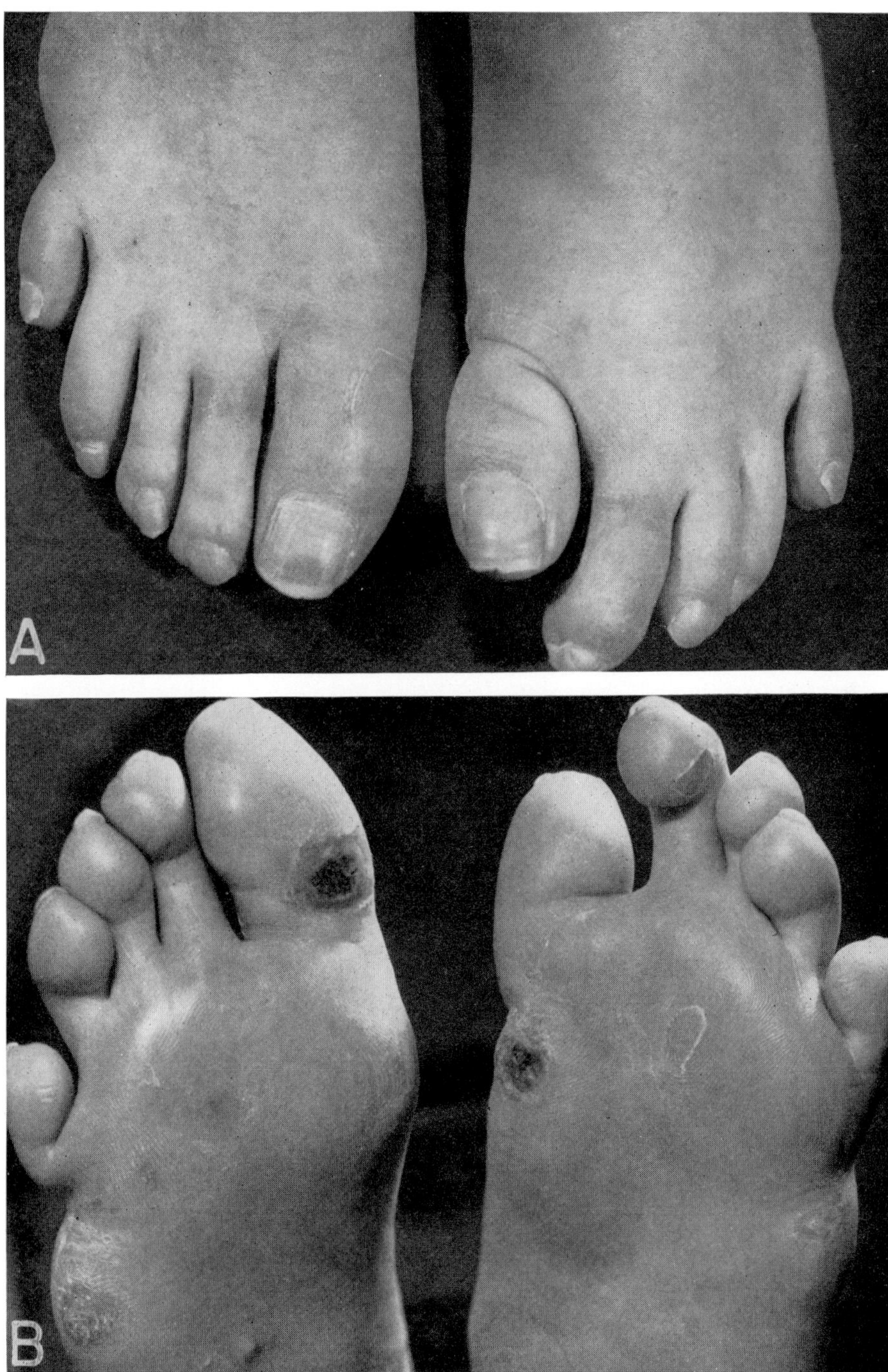

Figure 3–6. Spina bifida causing bilateral plantar keratoses mainly owing to the diminished motor power of the toes.

force are perhaps the most common cause of metatarsalgia. When the hallux rides over the second toe, it cannot obviously contact the proffered surface, broaden the tread, and relieve its metatarsal of the excessive load. The resulting metatarsalgia is usually confined to the area of the foot under the sesamoids. When the second toe has mounted over the hallux, it too cannot touch the ground and fails to relieve its own metatarsal of some of the stress. Hammered, clawed, overriding, and deviated third, fourth, and fifth toes are likewise accompanied by pain under their respective metatarsal heads. Quite frequently more than one toe is involved and the resulting metatarsalgia is diffuse. Pressure keratoses on the plantar aspect of the forefoot provide objective evidence of the location and extent of metatarsalgia (Figs. 3–7 to 3–12).

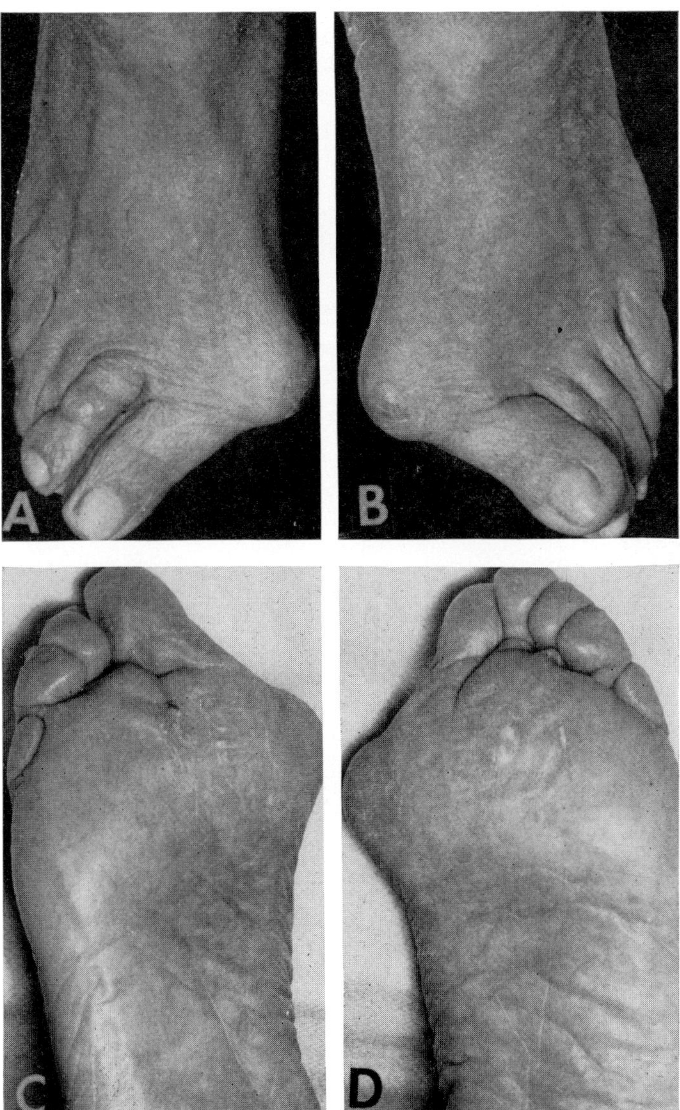

Figure 3–7. Bilateral hallux valgus with apparent plantar bulge of the area under the central metatarsal heads.

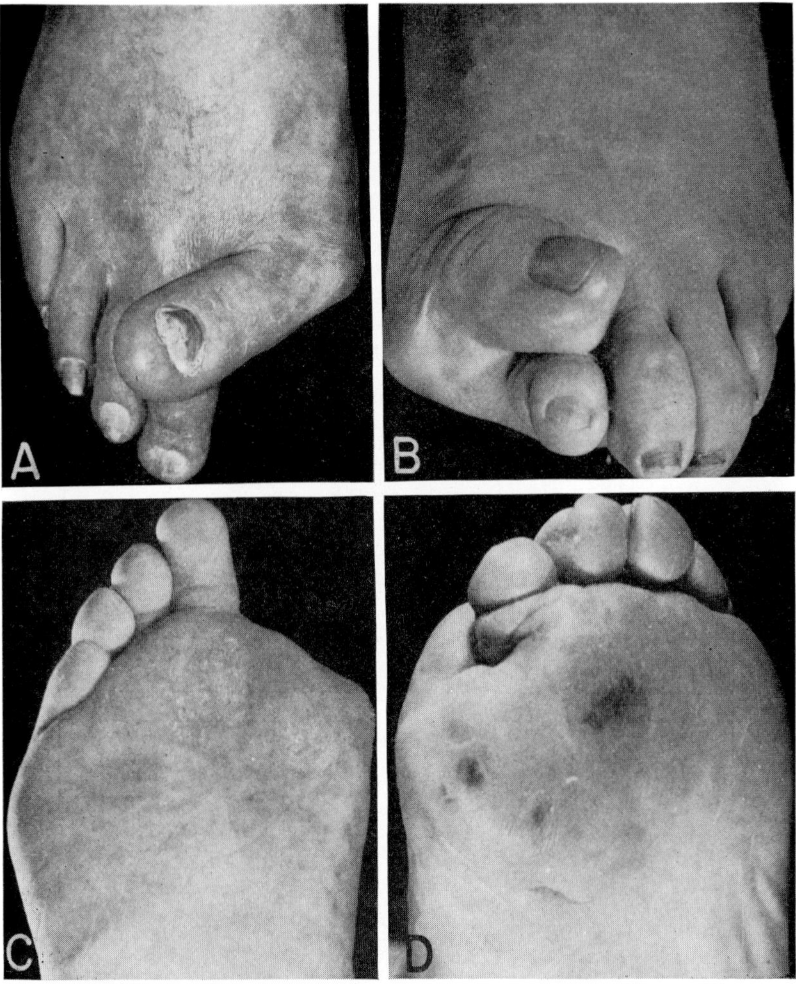

Figure 3–8. Two cases of overriding hallux: dorsal and plantar views of one foot (*A* and *C*), and of the other foot (*B* and *D*). Note the plantar keratosis (*D*).

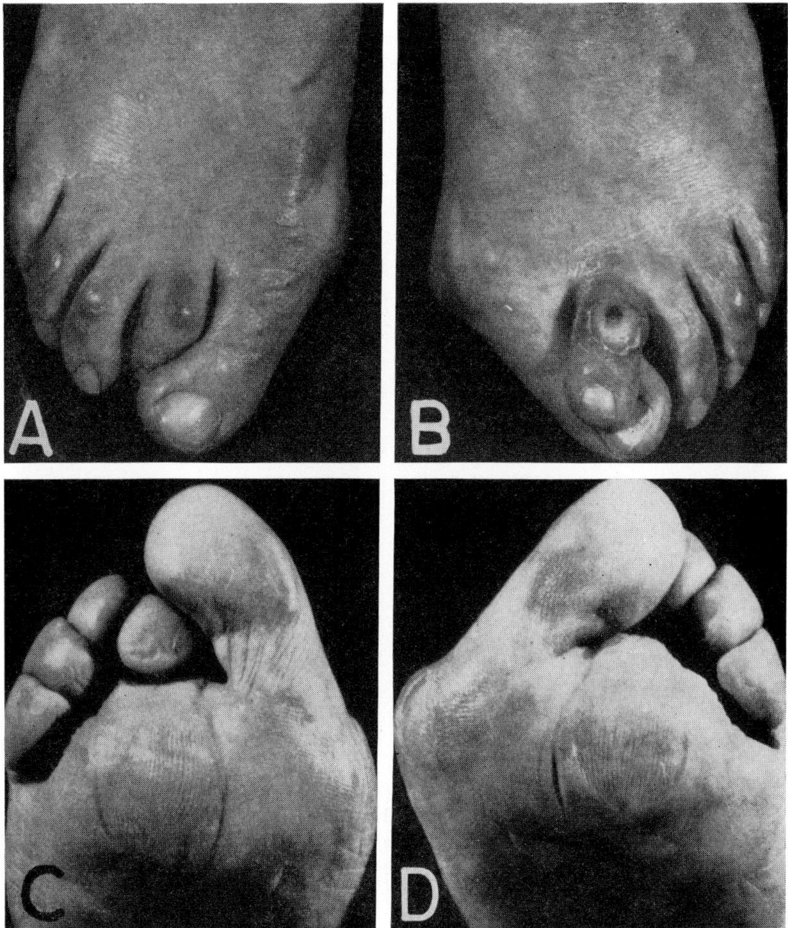

Figure 3–9. Bilateral hallux valgus with hammered second toe on the right side (*A* and *C*) and overriding second digit on the left (*B* and *D*). Metatarsalgia was more severe on the left side just behind the toe that failed to touch the ground.

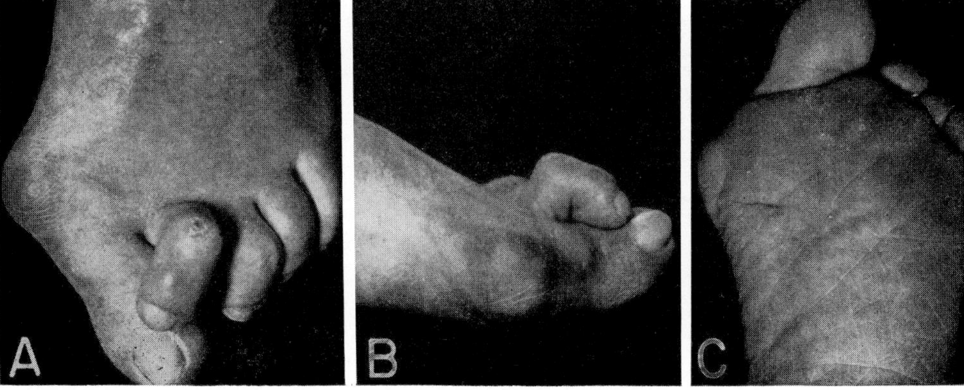

Figure 3–10. Unilateral hallux valgus and overriding second toe with metatarsalgia and small keratosis under the second metatarsal head.

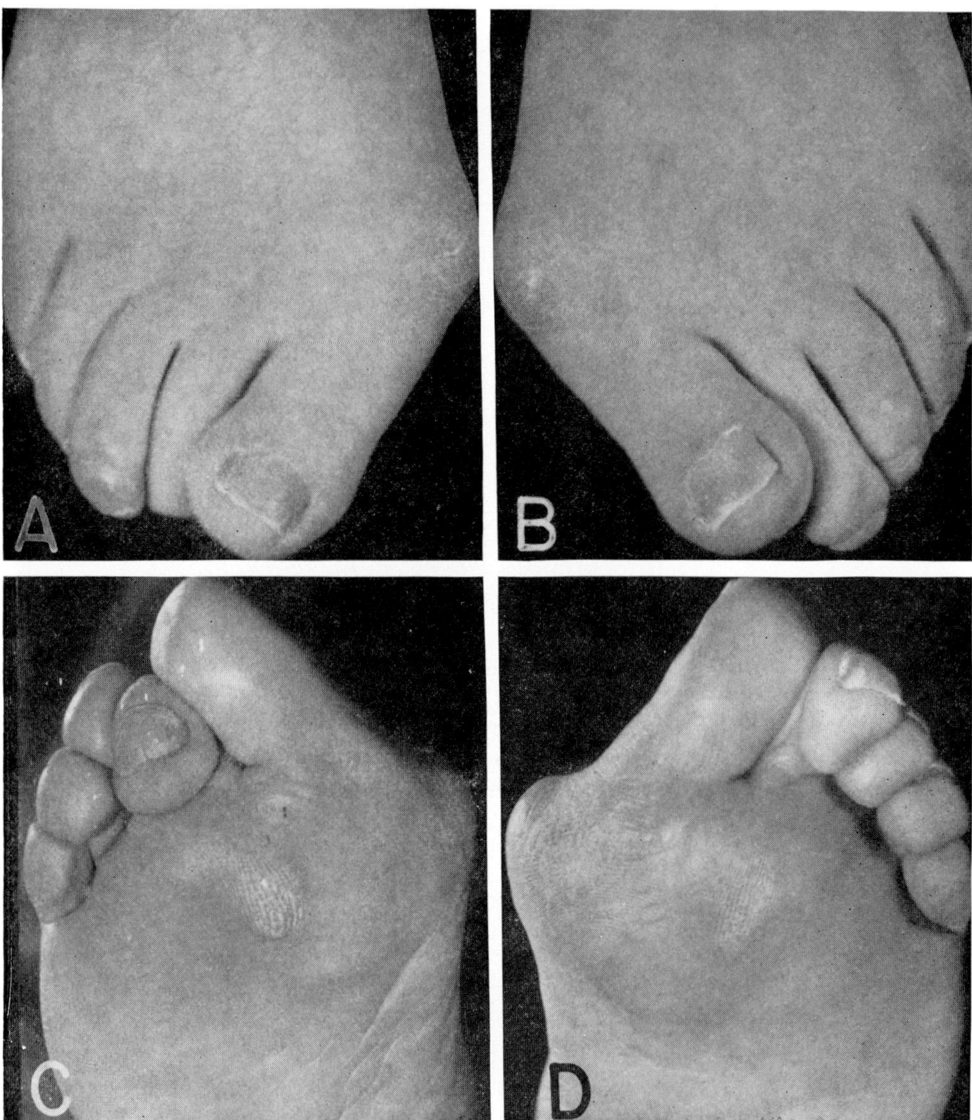

Figure 3–11. Bilateral hallux valgus. The hammered second toe on the right side touched the ground, but it was stiff and could not press down effectively to relieve the stress on its metatarsal. The patient complained of pain under the second metatarsal head.

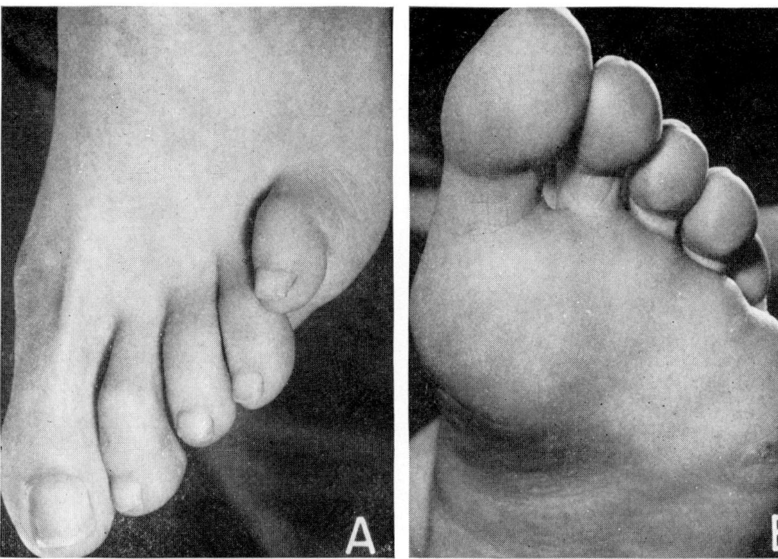

Figure 3—12. Clawed fifth toe with keratosis and pain under its metatarsal head.

REFERENCES

Camper, P.: *On the Best Form of Shoe,* published with Dowie's treatise, *The Foot and Its Covering.* London, R. Hardwicke, 1861, p. 39. The French version, called *Dissertation sur le Meilleur Forme des Souliers,* appeared in Paris, 1781.

Morton, T. G.: A peculiar and painful affection of the fourth metatarsophalangeal articulation. Am. J. Med. Sci. *71:*35–45, Jan. 1876.

Pitha, V., and Billroth: *Handbuch der Allgemeinen und Speziellen Chirurgie.* Stuttgart, F. Enke, 1868, Vol. 4, pp. 371–378.

Rose, A.: Resection considered as a remedy for abduction of the great toe—hallux valgus—and bunion. Med. Rec. New York *9:* 200–201, 1874.

Chapter Four

CAUSAL RELATIONS

In his monograph on hallux valgus, Quevedo (1894) enumerated 19 authorities with varying views as to the cause. Boniface (1895) grouped the divergent concepts under four classes: mechanical, muscular, "diathesique," and anatomical. Walsham and Hughes (1895) spoke of ligamentous and arthritic causes. Mauclaire (1896) added osseous and neurogenic factors to this list and distinguished between congenital and acquired hallux valgus. Kirmisson (1899) related hallux valgus to rheumatism, hemiplegia, infantile paralysis, and other systemic affections. Metcalf (1912) mentioned the following causes: "softening of the internal lateral ligament"—Malgaigne's (1852) view; "loss of muscular equation" —Nélaton's (1859) concept; flatfoot—Goldthwait's (1893) contention; and "trauma to the metatarsophalangeal joint"—Payr's (1894) proposition. Mouchet (1922) mentioned heredity and trophic disturbances. Frejka (1924) considered rickets as a cause. Hamsa (1937) offered an extensive etiological classification of hallux valgus.

Congenital hallux valgus. Sporadic cases of congenital hallux valgus have been reported by Mauclaire (1896), Clarke (1899), Blumenthal and Hirsch (1905), Klar (1905), Zesas (1906), Joachimsthal (1907), Mouchet (1919), Heller (1928), Hoffmann (1936), Meyerding and Upshaw (1947), and McCormick and Blount (1949). Keizer (1950, 1952) gave a detailed account of a newborn boy, the first child of a father in whose family hallux valgus formed a heredity trait. The mother had rubella during the first months of pregnancy; the baby had bilateral hallux valgus. Gutzeit (1914) reported a case in which the outward deviation of the great toe occurred at the interphalangeal joint. He called it *hallux valgus interphalangeus.* Daw (1935) added two similar cases. Rutt (1961) interpolated the photograph of another case of bilateral *phalanx hallucis valga* (his terminology). In a single period of 3 months, we saw two such cases (Figs. 4–1, 4–2).

Hallux valgus appearing at birth as a fixed deformity is rare. But there are those who consider the outward deviation of the great toe secondary to the exaggerated inward inclination of the first metatarsal, which they insist, is congenital and predetermined and represents an "arrest of ontogeny." Metatarsus primus varus is common at birth. Con-

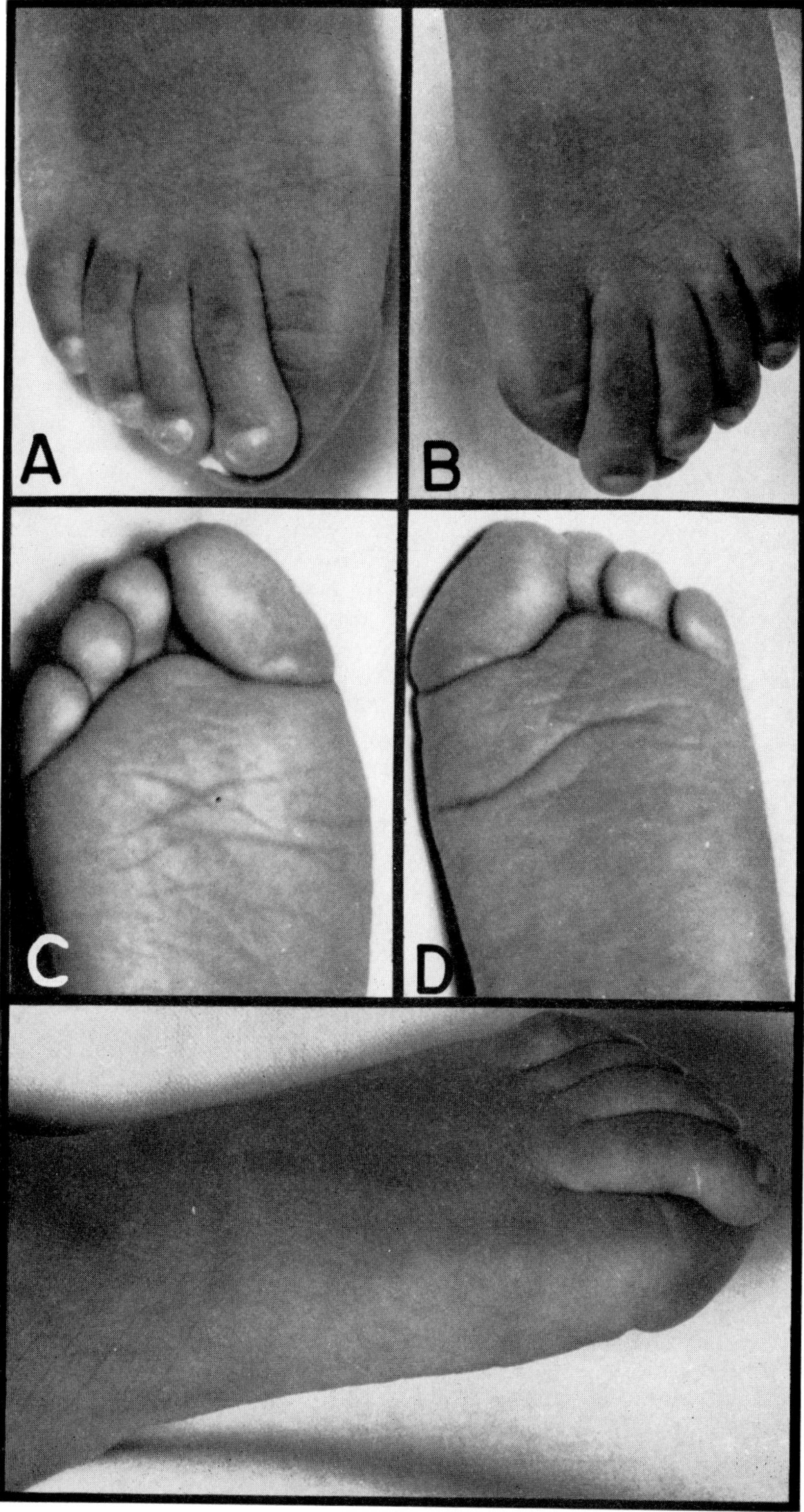

Figure 4–1. Congenital hallux valgus interphalangeus in a boy 18 months old.

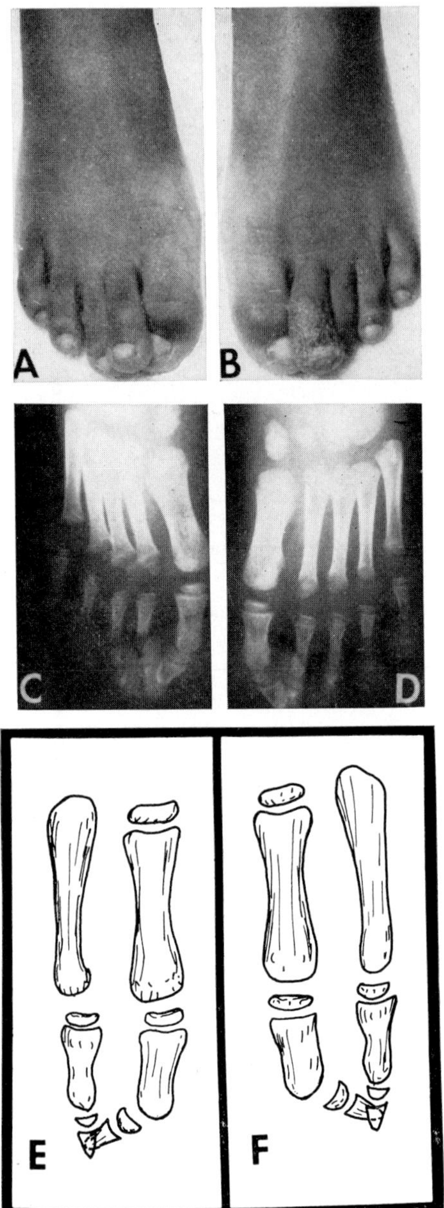

Figure 4–2. Hallux valgus interphalangeus in another child.

cealed supernumerary phalanx may be the cause of outward deviation of the great toe (Fig. 4–3).

Heredity. Durlacher (1845) spoke of hereditary predisposition in the occurrence of deformed toes and indicated that the first digit was principally affected. Digital distortion, he added, was peculiar to some families. "I saw, some time since," he wrote, "a remarkable illustration of the hereditary nature of the distorted toe in the person of a gentleman of the name of O'Caghan or Caen. While in attendance on him, I observed that he had a singularly-formed toe, and remarked that the distortion was peculiar to different families. He smiled at my observation, and told me that medical men were not alone aware of that fact, for that when travelling near the Giant's Causeway, he stopped at an inn kept by a man named Dick Caen, and claimed his hospitality on the score of relationship. The man stared at him, and said, 'Then by my shoul, sir, if you are an O'Caghan, you must have Prince O'Caghan's crooked toe.' "

Kirmisson (1902) spoke of a girl, aged 12½ years, with bilateral hallux valgus. Her mother had an identical deformity. Sandelin (1922) surveyed 536 cases of hallux valgus and noted hereditary influence in 54 per cent. McElvenny (1944) cited the case of a woman whose grandfather and father had a "bunion" on the right foot but not on the left. "This woman," McElvenny wrote, "has a bunion on her right foot but not on her left." Johnston (1956) studied the seven-generation pedigree of a family showing hallux valgus. He arrived at the following conclusion: "The anomaly appears to be transmitted as an autosomal dominant with incomplete penetrance."

It is now generally agreed that there is such an entity as hereditary familial hallux valgus (Fig. 4–4).

Age. Hallux valgus may be present early in life without causing discomfort. Payr (1894) placed its inception between the ages of 14 and 16 in girls and a little later in boys. In their survey of school children, Hardy and Clapham (1952) noted progressive increase of the lateral deviation of the great toe with advancing age. Symptomatic hallux valgus is more common after 40 years.

Sex. More women than men suffer from hallux valgus complex. Payr (1894) placed the ratio between male and female at 3:2. Lake (1952) considered the disproportion to "equal at least ten to one." If one is to judge by the number of those who seek advice, 50 females to one male would come closer to a more correct ratio. This preponderance in

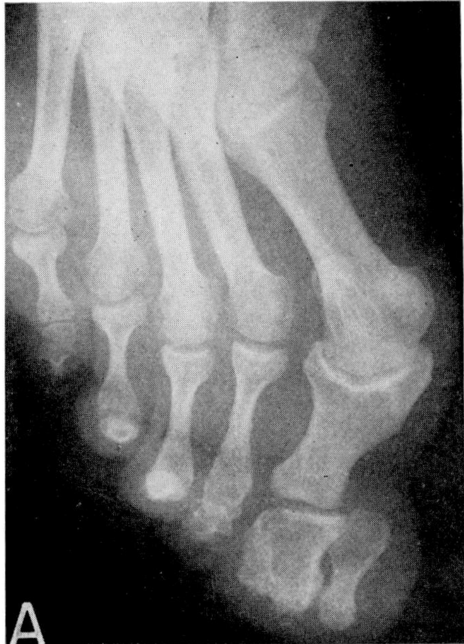

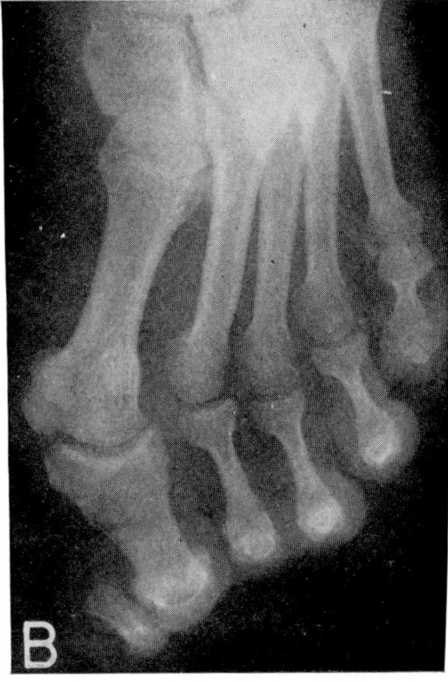

Figure 4–3. Congenital hallux valgus due to reduplication of the distal phalanx of the great toe.

women has been ascribed to their pointed, compressive, high-heeled shoes. After almost half a century of intensive practice of orthopedic surgery, Sir Robert Jones (1924) said: "I have never seen a normal foot in women who have worn fashionable boots. . . ."

Shoes. "From our infancy," Camper (1781) wrote, "shoes, as at present worn, serve but to deform the toes and cover the feet with corns. . . . It is evident that all the world did not imitate Socrates, who went barefoot. . . ." Durlacher (1845) wrote: "One of the most frequent and certain causes of a bunion is the wearing of shoes made too short, and with a narrow sole." Broca (1852) thought shoes exerted their deforming influence mostly on the toes. Meyer (1858) protested against "the arrogant absurdity of which fashion is guilty in forcing the foot into shoes which, instead of merely protecting it, disfigured it." From among the many detrimental effects of tapered, cramping footwear, Meyer singled out "the evils arising at the root of the great toe." Meyer started the trend for professional anatomists to crusade against fashion—"that most inexorable tyrant, to which the greater part of mankind are willing slaves." Flower (1880) blamed civilized footwear for

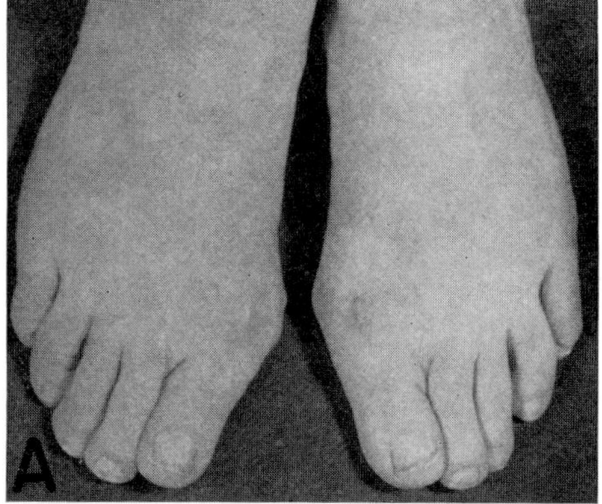

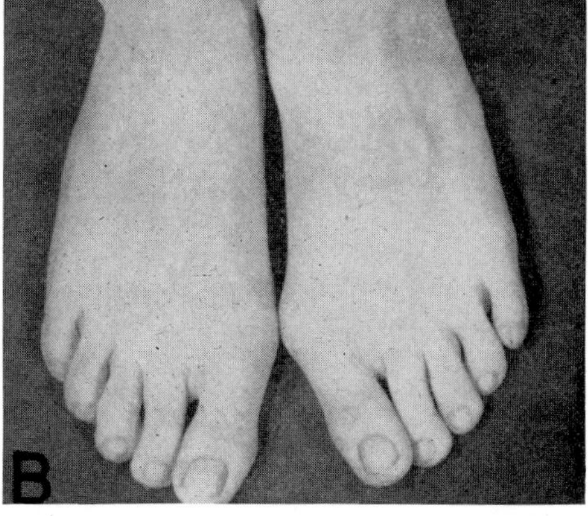

Figure 4–4. Bilateral hallux valgus of a middle aged woman (*A*) and her adolescent daughter (*B*).

"corns, bunions, ingrowing nails, and all their attendant miseries." After a lengthy vituperation along this line, he betrayed a note of defeatism by quoting Dr. Johnson as follows: "Few enterprises are as hopeless as a contest with fashion."

The very rare occurrence of hallux valgus in infants is often offered as an argument against the shoe as a cause. Then there is the contention that unshod natives sometimes manifest this deformity. Engle and Morton (1931) studied foot disorders among the natives of Belgian Congo and found them "free from the ordinary static foot trouble." Wells (1931) stated that the big toe of the Bantu was normally in valgus position, but it was not associated with any symptoms. Following his study of the feet of natives in Solomon Islands, James (1939) said that shoes compressed the feet and interfered with the blood supply of the muscles; structures became shortened; the foot lost its pliability, became less resilient and could not adapt itself to varying strains and positions. Barnicot and Hardy (1955) studied the position of the hallux in West Africans and recorded many instances of definite outward deviation, but the deformity was not attended with any discomfort. Lam Sim-Fook and Hodgson (1958) found that hallux valgus was more common among Chinese who wore shoes, while metatarsus primus varus prevailed among the unshod; in the latter, complaints referable to the forepart of the foot were nonexistent. It was implied that the occasional hallux valgus in the unshod was asymptomatic. Metatarsus primus varus as well as metatarsus "atavicus," "latus" and hypermobile first ray—all occurring in greater percentage in the unshod—were not accompanied by any subjective symptoms.

If one has to draw a conclusion from these reports, it would be that asymptomatic hallux valgus occurring among the unshod may be of hereditary origin but it is more likely an acquired deformity. Long ago Froriep (1834) was aware of the occurrence of hallux valgus—which he called *exostosis of the first metatarsal bone*—in people who had never worn shoes. The condition, he argued, was "especially common in those who walk with quick movements and vehemence throwing the full weight of the body towards the toes, which was the customary manner, dictated by necessity, among mountaineers and those who walked on rough roads or carried heavy weights." The unshod native has to tread on craggy, uneven terrain; he has to dig his toes into the ground for a more secure grip; he has to climb trees and curl his forefoot around bark and branches. Beside its deforming effect and the discomfort it causes, civilized footwear disposes of the necessity for developing muscle power: intrinsic muscles acting on the toes waste away and the joints stiffen.

Intrinsic factors. Fashionable footwear is classed as an extrinsic factor causing hallux valgus. The main intrinsic agents mentioned in the literature are: pes planus, advanced position of the great toe and its metatarsal, and metatarsus primus varus.

Pes planus. Riedel (1886), Goldthwait (1893), and many others who followed them connected flatfoot with hallux valgus. Silver (1923), F. Schede (1927), Anderson (1929), Hiss (1931), Verbrugge (1933), and Rogers and Joplin (1947) all noted the association of hallux valgus and *pronated foot.* Jordan and Brodsky (1951) wrote: "We regard the majority of cases of hallux valgus and hallux rigidus as acquired deformities resulting from foot pronation. The role of footwear is secondary, serving to aggravate an existing mild deformity or to produce manifest deformity where only potential hallux valgus previously existed as a result of foot pronation."

Hohmann (1951) contended that in flatfoot, owing to eversion of the os calcis from which it originates, the abductor hallucis shifts toward the outer border of the foot; the plantarly depressed tarsal bones bear down on this muscle and cause it to stretch and lose tone. The weakened abductor can no longer brace the medial capsule of the first metatarsophalangeal joint, nor can it counterbalance the adductors and maintain "forward position of the great toe." By implication Hohmann suggested that pes planus caused the abductor to be nonfunctional. Left without an opposing force, the adductors pulled the great toe toward the outer border of the foot.

Lake (1952) brought out a point that would seem to refute the concept of pes planus as a cause of hallux valgus. According to him, flatfoot is more likely to develop "in those whose employment demands prolonged standing and weight bearing," while hallux valgus occurred "in those whose feet are constantly active." Froriep (1834), we may remember, subscribed to a similar view. One of the main arguments against the concept of flatfoot as a cause of hallux valgus is that patients with pes planus alone outnumber those with the combined deformity. This is not saying that when hallux valgus and pes planus coexist, there may not be a causal connection between the two.

It is perhaps fair to say that in a limited number of cases pronated foot may be a predisposing factor. It may be reasoned that with the sinking of the inner border of the midfoot, the base of the first metatarsal is depressed downward, while its head tilts up. The medial capsule of the first metatarsophalangeal joint offers less resistance than the base of the proximal phalanx. The metatarsal head subluxates inward. The toebox of the shoe presses the tip of the hallux toward the outer edge of the foot. Less apparent is the impact of the ground or the sole of the shoe on the first metatarsal. In pes valgus, as the foot rolls outward, the counterpressure of the ground causes the first metatarsal to invert—or *supinate,* as German authors prefer to call it. Another approach to the problem is to consider that hallux valgus and pes planus stem from the same anatomical variety of foot—tapered in the heel, long and narrow in midportion, broad in the forepart, with hypermobile marginal metatarsals.

Advanced position of the hallux and its metatarsal. The presence of a comparatively long great toe or first metatarsal as a cause of hallux valgus has had a number of contenders: Mayo (1908, 1920), Simon (1918), Hardy and Clapham (1952) and Haines and McDougall (1954). Lake (1952) wrote: "No special form of foot, i.e., long, short, has been shown to be a factor nor is there any unequivocal proof that the relative lengths of the metatarsal bones have an etiological significance, although it may affect the secondary deformities."

Metatarsus primus varus. When William Anderson (1891) surmised "an irregularity of development, and unconnected with any vice in the foot covering" as a cause of hallux valgus, "especially those of very aggravated type," he could not have anticipated the controversy that has lasted now almost three-quarters of a century. Anderson could not be more definite; roentgenography had not yet come into practice. Seven years later, commenting on a paper by Steele (1898), Sayre said he had been resecting the medial eminence on the supposition that it was due to bony overgrowth. Sayre had changed his views since the advent of "skiagraphs." Recent study by the newer method had shown that the prominence at the base of the great toe was due to "a dislocation of the phalanx with marked separation of the first and second metatarsals . . ."

Loison (1901) studied cases of hallux valgus with the newer diagnostic method. He presented roentgenographs of patients who had been subjected to corrective surgery at the metatarsophalangeal joint but in whom the deformity had recurred. On the x-ray films he traced lines representing the longitudinal axes of the metatarsal and the phalanges of the great toe. When extended these lines formed an obtuse angle that opened outward. Loison said the formation of this angle was not only due to the outward deviation of the proximal phalanx but also depended on the inclination of the first metatarsal in the opposite direction. In surgical endeavors for correction of hallux valgus, closer attention should be paid to the base of the first metatarsal from where this bone begins to incline inward, Loison advised. Picqué (1902) was the first clinician to note the oblique setting of the innermost cuneometatarsal joint in a case of hallux valgus that he reported.

Loison and Picqué had a number of followers in Europe: Balacescu (1903) in

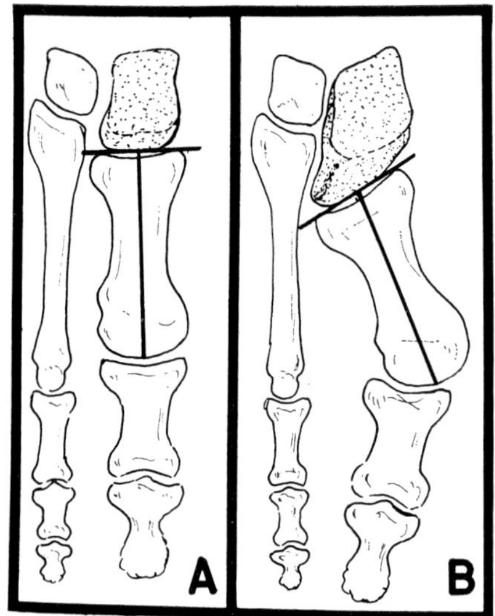

Figure 4–5. Transverse (*A*) and oblique (*B*) setting of the innermost cuneometatarsal joint.

Rumania, Riedl (1909) in Germany, and Albrecht (1911) in Russia. The first American to draw attention to "the approximal (sic) extremity of the metatarsal bone or its articulation with the cuneiform bone" was Young (1909) of Philadelphia. "In examining some x-ray plates within the past year," Young wrote, "I was impressed with the deformity of the tarso-metatarsal joint of the great toe in cases of hallux valgus; upon more careful investigation of these plates it seemed as if there were present a supernumerary bone, wedge-shaped in form, which by its shape and position produced this deformity." He was referring to the extremely rare os intermetatarseum. Young may be likened to a hunter who became infatuated with a decoy and forgot the real prey.

It remained for Ewald (1912) to set the matter straight. He discussed the shape of the innermost cuneiform bone. In hallux valgus this bone has a longer lateral than medial border. As a result the articular facet it presents to the base of the first metatarsal slants medially. The joint these two bones form is set obliquely, which in turn induces the first metatarsal to incline inward. In most cases of hallux valgus, Ewald stated, the varus of the first metatarsal is accompanied with trapezoid innermost cuneiform and oblique setting of its distal articular facet. Only in an occasional case is the innermost cuneiform rectangular and the plane of its distal articular facet transverse. In such a case Ewald supposed that the first metatarsal twists inward somewhere along its shaft (Fig. 4–5).

"In the medical literature," Mensor (1928) wrote, "ideas frequently are presented, forgotten and presented again. Within the past year a prominent orthopedic surgeon called attention to the varus deformity of the first metatarsal and suggested an operation similar to the one advocated thirteen years previously by Ewald. . . ." The reference is to Truslow (1925), whose article appeared exactly 13 years after Ewald's. Truslow proposed a new name, *metatarsus primus varus,* to replace hallux valgus. He thought the condition was due to an anatomical variation inherent in the individual's growth and development and was not an acquired deformity.

This was a revolutionary concept, something new—this theory of an innate factor causing hallux valgus instead of the shopworn alibi, shoes. Many—as Ely (1926) and Mensor (1928)—subscribed to it wholeheartedly; others, cautiously. Peabody (1931) wrote: "While it may be assumed that in some instances hallux valgus develops secondarily and inevitably from a congenital primus varus, we believe that in the majority of cases the deformity of the big toe joint is important."

Kleinberg (1932) considered "the adduction" of the first metatarsal bone and the obliquity of the cuneometatarsal joint primary—and hallux valgus secondary. Lapidus shifted the words of Truslow and coined *metatarsus varus primus.* "I believe that," Lapidus (1934) wrote, "congenital varus primus in the majority of cases is the primary deformity leading to secondary formation of hallux valgus. In other words, the medially opened angulation between the first cuneiform and the first metatarsal causes the compensatory angulation open laterally between the big toe and the first metatarsal."

The concept of metatarsus primus varus as a cause of hallux valgus has found numerous adherents—Dreesmann (1928), Durman (1957), and many others. There were also some dissenters. The same year that Ewald published his paper Metcalf (1912) wrote: "It is not uncommon . . . to have the internal cuneiform exuberant at its outer border, so that it forms an oblique base for the diverging metatarsal." Toward the end of his article Metcalf asked: "Is it not quite plausible to suppose that the inward displacement of the first metatarsal is due to the pressure transmitted from the tip of the outwardly displaced phalanx?" McMurray (1936) ascribed the exaggerated inward inclination of the first metatarsal to the pressure exerted by the base of the outwardly deviated proximal phalanx. Piggott (1960) likened the question of the priority of hallux valgus and metatarsus primus varus to the controversy surrounding "the-chicken-and-the-egg" sequence. He was inclined to believe that the valgus of the great toe is primary.

From the literature we have culled four distinct theories as to the cause of metatarsus primus varus: (1) It is due to the oblique setting of the innermost cuneometatarsal joint; (2) the curve at this joint enhances the mobility, and hence, the tendency of the first metatarsal to be pushed medially; (3) wedged between the first and second metatarsal heads, the lateral sesamoid pushes the former inward; and (4) the base of the outwardly deviated proximal phalanx of the great toe forces the first metatarsal medially (Fig. 4–6).

Whatever its future, the concept of metatarsus primus varus has stimulated considerable interest and has fostered a number of ingenious surgical procedures. It should be noted that even the most adamant advocates of metatarsus primus varsus as a cause of hallux valgus concede that ill fitting shoes initiate or at least aggravate the outward deviation of the great toe. Truslow (1925) believed that faulty shoes may be a causative factor. Ely (1926) considered the shoe as a contributing cause. Lapidus (1934) wrote: "An excellent example of this atavistic type of foot, with metatarsus varus primus presenting predisposition toward hallux valgus formation, was observed by the author in a case of middle-aged brother and sister. The sister developed 'bunions' in young age, as a result of wearing the usual distorting ladies' shoes, while the brother's feet remained normal, because of the straight last shoes, which checked this potential tendency. . . ."

It is perhaps safe to say that metatarsus primus varus predisposes and shoes provoke symptomatic hallux valgus. At the innermost cuneometatarsal joint the articular facets are reciprocally convex and concave, and the plane of articulation slants at an oblique angle medially. The oblique setting of the joint has had its share of emphasis as a determining factor in the causation of metatarsus primus varus. Not enough is said about the greater convexity of the distal articular facet of the medial cuneiform or the concavity of the corresponding surface of the first metatarsal. Greater curve at this joint denotes greater mobility. A hypermobile first metatarsal may cause its head to tilt up dorsally, throwing the heads of the lateral bones into relative plantar prominence. A hypermobile first metatarsal is more likely to incline inward and cause widening of the space between it and the second metatarsal. As the varus deflection of the first metatarsal increases, the valgus of the great toe becomes aggravated. There comes a time when arthritis intervenes and limits movements at the cuneometatarsal joint. Stabilized metatarsus primus varus is spoken of as being *fixed.*

Miscellaneous causes. *Arthritis.* In discussions of the causes of hallux valgus, arthritis was featured prominently until Lane (1886, 1887) insisted that arthritic change was the "effect" rather than the cause of the outward deviation of the great toe. Notwithstanding, influential authorities, such as Anderson (1891), Walsham and Hughes (1895), and Clarke (1900), considered arthritis as a cause. Anderson thought the direction of the great toe deviation was dependent on the position of osteophytes in the joint. Walsham and Hughes regarded "osteoarthritis . . . as the cause of the deformity." Clarke publicized Verneuil's con-

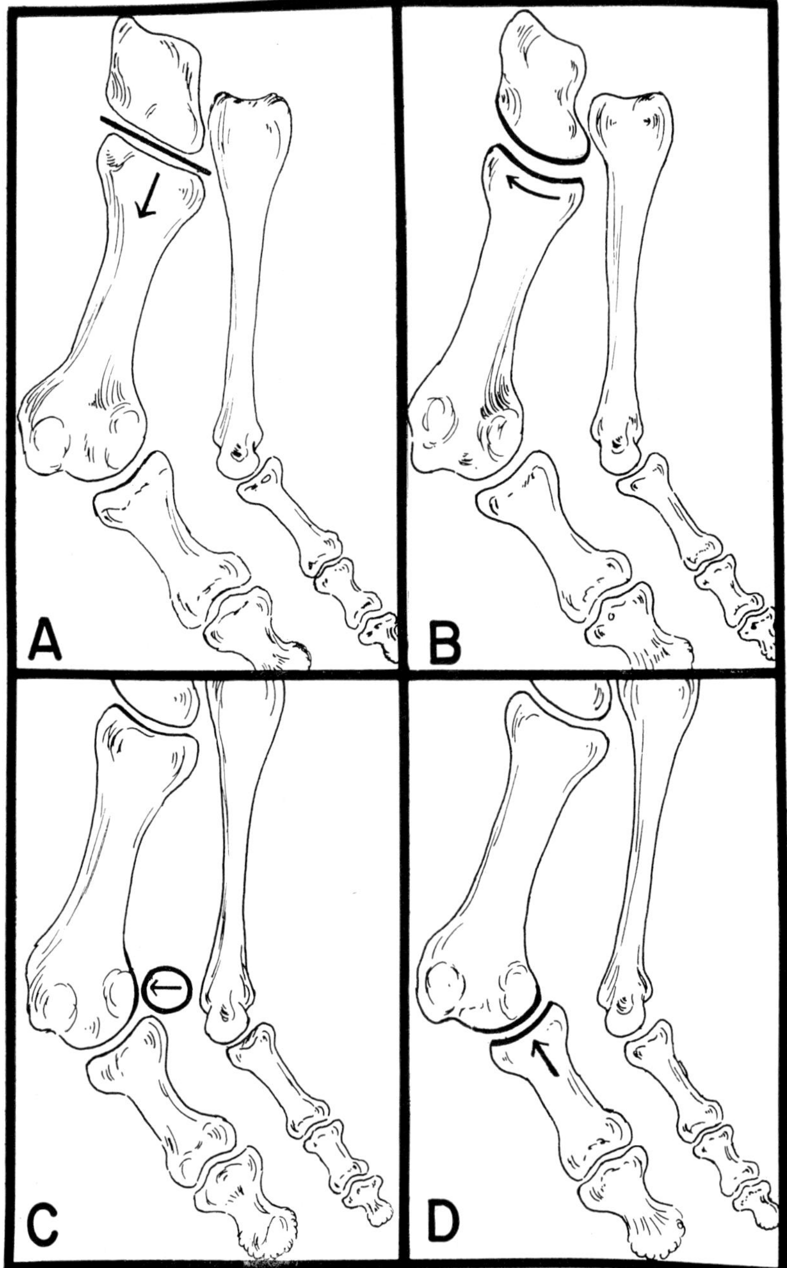

Figure 4–6. Diagrams illustrating theories concerning the causes of metatarsus primus varus: oblique setting of the cuneometatarsal joint (*A*), curved configuration of the cuneometatarsal joint (*B*), lateral sesamoid wedged between the first and second metatarsal heads (*C*), thrust by the base of the deviated proximal phalanx (*D*).

tention that every patient with hallus valgus belonged, *"ipso facto,* to the arthritic class." More recent authors writing on the subject go along with Lane and consider osteoarthritis the result and not the cause of hallux valgus. Rheumatoid arthritis is another matter; it is known to cause bizarre deformities of the toes, including hallux valgus (Fig. 4–7).

Muscular imbalance, contracture, or predominance. These have been considered in the etiology of hallux valgus. Dubrueil (1870) ascribed the outward deviation of the great toe to the predominance of the muscles that pull the toe away from the midsagittal plane over the muscle that draws it in opposite direction. Wyeth (1887) wrote: "The action of the muscles inserted into the base of the great toe must not be altogether overlooked in the etiology of the deformity. Of the five muscles which arise from the tarsus and the metatarsus and are inserted into this toe all but one tend to carry it toward the fibular side of the foot." Hagen-Torn (1925) placed the onus on the contracture of the adductor hallucis. McBride (1928) and many others have put the blame on the predominance of this muscle over the abductor hallucis. Kaplan (1955) found that in normal feet traction on the posterior tibial tendon produced no action on the great toe; in those with hallux valgus it enhanced outward deviation of the hallux. Dissection of the foot with hallux valgus revealed a sizable band connecting the tibialis posticus tendon with the origin of flexor hallucis brevis and the adductor obliquus. Kaplan considered this extension of the tibi-

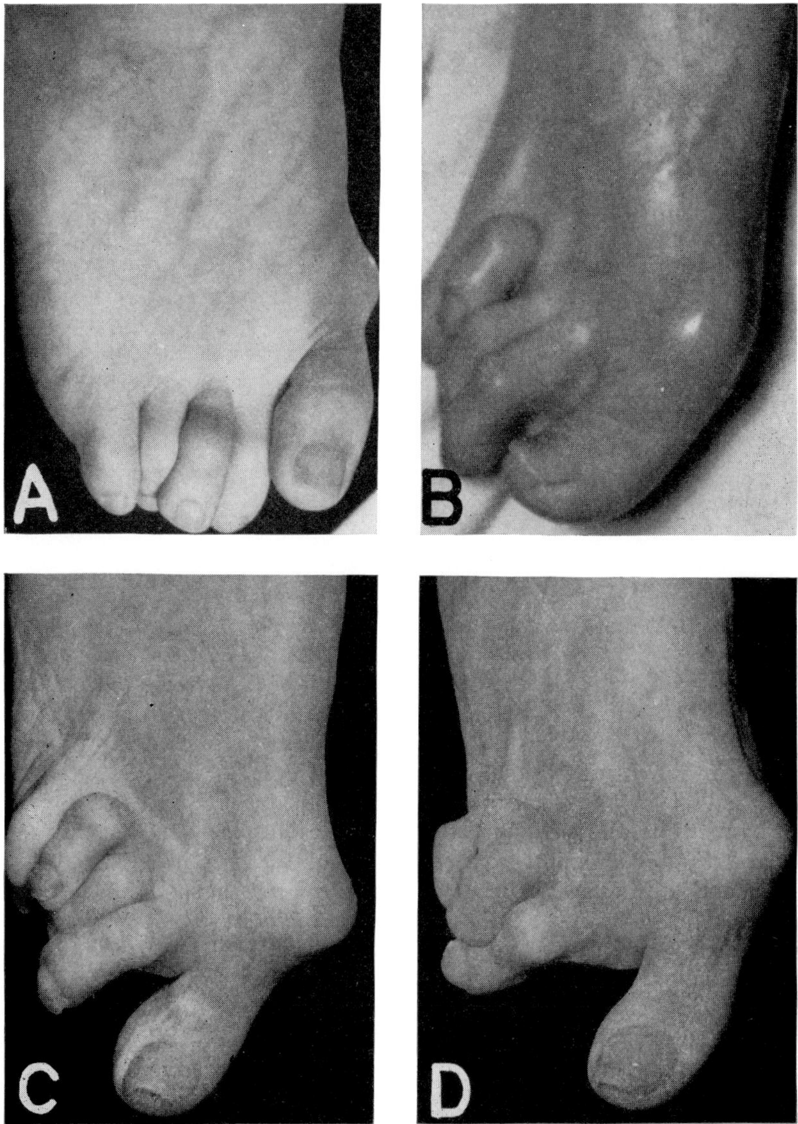

Figure 4–7. Rheumatoid arthritis with bizarre deformities of the toes, including hallus valgus.

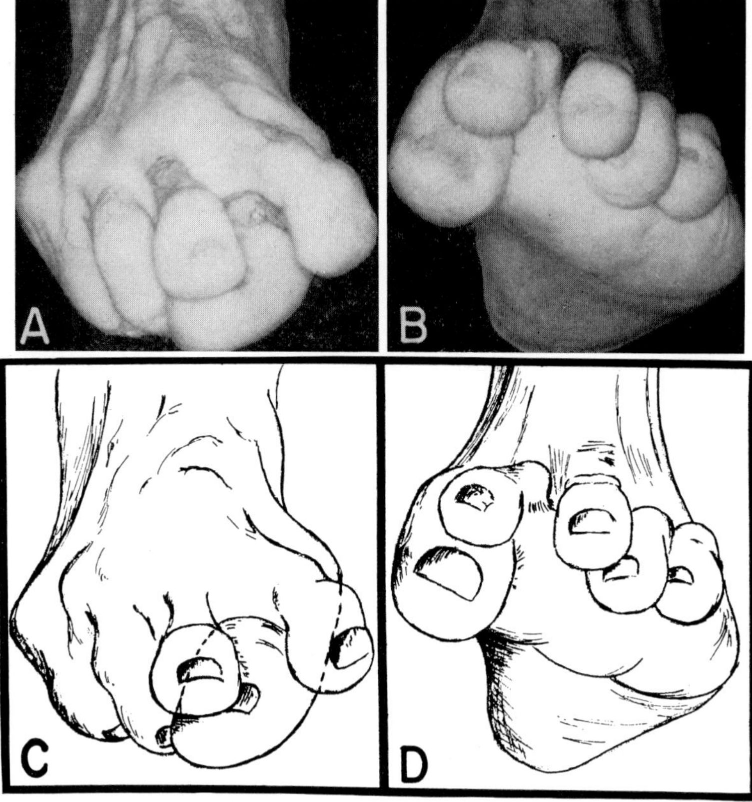

Figure 4–8. Bilateral hallux valgus and flexus in a case of spastic paralysis.

alis posticus insertion a contributing factor in the causation of hallux valgus. In ordinary cases of hallux valgus most writers regard muscular contracture, imbalance, or predominance as incidental to the deformity rather than the cause of it. After hallux valgus has become established, the contracted muscles and displaced tendons may aggravate the malposition of the great toe. It is unlikely that they play an active role initially. Occasionally in poliomyelitis, the flail hallux is pushed toward the outer border of the foot by the shoe. In cases of spastic paralysis the hallux is sometimes pulled under the second toe because of muscular imbalance (Figs. 4–8 and 4–9).

Sesamoid bones. As a cause of hallux valgus, sesamoid bones attracted considerable attention in the first two decades of the present century. Robinson (1918, 1928) wrote: "Bunion is a dislocation of the metatarsophalangeal articulation of the great toe . . . it is produced by the action of the sesamoid bones which are situated underneath the head of the first metatarsal bone." Robinson convinced a few of his contemporaries–Mayo (1920), among others. This view has long since been abandoned.

Os intermetatarseum. As a factor in hallux valgus, os intermetatarseum had only one advocate–Young (1909, 1910). Wheeler (1932) reviewed the roentgenographs of the feet in approximately 500 persons and concluded: "There is little evidence for the os intermetatarseum's contributing to either the presence or degree of severity of hallux valgus . . ." (Fig. 4–10).

Weak medial collateral ligament of the first metatarsophalangeal joint. This was considered as a cause of hallux valgus by Malgaigne (1852). Clarke (1900) suggested that the "softening of the internal ligament may also be due to traumatism or extension of inflamation from the superficial tissues"–meaning from the bursa. Mygind (1953) suspected a rupture of the fascia surrounding the

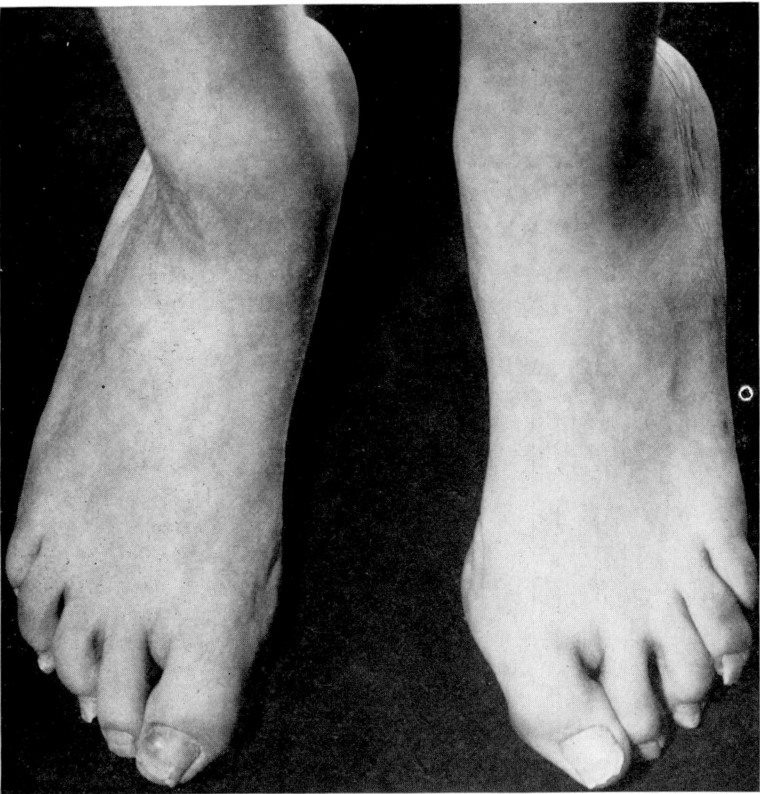

Figure 4–9. Unilateral hallux valgus in a girl, aged 12, afflicted with flaccid paralysis of the left leg and foot.

head of the first metatarsal. There are those who consider the contracture of the lateral collateral ligament as a cause. It is known that in hallux valgus the medial capsule and collateral ligament are elongated and the corresponding structures on the lateral side are contracted. These changes also belong to the category of effect and not of cause.

Trauma. Also considered as a factor is trauma. One could exaggerate the point and regard repeated impingement by the shoe on the great toe as chronic trauma. Payr (1894) suscribed to this view. He thought occupations that necessitated long hours of standing and walking were predisposing factors and mentioned the preponderance of hallux valgus among waiters, waitresses, messengers, and maids. Payr also recorded the occurrence of hallux valgus after the fall of a heavy object on the foot. He stated that binding the feet of young people was injurious. Needless to say, in rare instances of malunited fracture of the first metatarsal head or the base of the proxi-

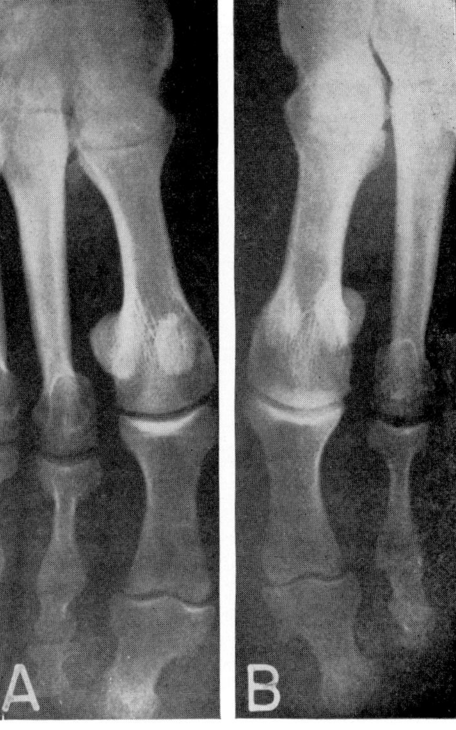

Figure 4–10. Bilateral os intermetatarseum.

mal phalanx, hallux valgus may result as a secondary deformity.

Congenitally absent, amputated, or hammered second toe. As a cause of hallux valgus this was mentioned by several authors—Bankart (1935) and Rutt (1961), among others. The second toe serves as a lateral buttress to the hallux. It is supposed that congenital hammering of the second toe paves the way for eventual development of hallux valgus.

Trophic disturbances. We have encountered a case of Charcot's arthropathy of the metatarsophalangeal joint of the great toe. In this instance the hallux deviated in the direction that the shoe pushed it—outward. In cases of trophic ulcers due to spina bifida or diabetes, the metatarsophalangeal joint is secondarily infected. The resulting pyogenic arthritis causes destruction of articular surfaces, and the toe may become deflected toward the fibular border of the foot.

Multiple factors. These were considered by Clarke (1900) and more recently by Hiss (1937) and Stein (1938). Clarke spoke of congenital and acquired causes. Hiss numerated the following agents: "(1) Phylogenetically developed stronger adduction than abduction; (2) tendon imbalance from lost abduction; (3) joint buckling from medial thrust of shoes; (4) Excess weight bearing on the great toe joint from eversion of the whole foot." Stein commented: "Any factors, extrinsic, or intrinsic, tending to shift this load more medially on the big toe, favor the development of hallux valgus. . . . The deformity primarily is merely a functional postural adaptation; later it becomes structural in character."

REFERENCES

Albrecht, G. H.: The pathology and treatment of hallux valgus (in Russian). Russk. Vrach. *10:*14–19, 1911.

Anderson, R. L.: Hallux valgus: report of end results. South. Med. Surg. *91:*74–78, 1929.

Anderson, W.: Contractions of the fingers and toes; their varieties, pathology and treatment. Lancet *2:*1–5, 1891; 56–57, 1891; 107–111, 1891; 161–163, 1891; Lancet *78:*279–282, 1891.

Balacescu, J.: Un caz de hallux valgus simetric. (in Rumanian). Rev. Chir. *7:*128–135, 1903.

Bankart, A. S. B.: The treatment of minor maladies of the foot. Lancet *1:*249–252, 1935.

Barnicot, N. A., and Hardy, R. H.: The position of the hallux in West Africans. J. Anat. *89:* 355–361, 1955.

Blumenthal, M., and Hirsch, K.: Ein Fall angeborener Missbildung der vier Extremitaten. Ztschr. Orthop. Chir. *14:*11–33, 1905.

Boniface, C.: *De L'Hallux Valgus,* (orteil en équerre). Thesis. Paris, G. Steinheil, 1895, pp. 17–40.

Broca, P.: Des difformités de la partie antérieure du pied produite par l'action de la chaussure. Bull. Soc. Anat. *27:*60–67, 1852.

Camper, P.: *On the Best Form of Shoe,* published with Dowie's treatise, *The Foot and Its Covering.* London, R. Hardwicke, 1861, pp. 1–44. The French version called *Dissertation sur le Meilleur Forme des Souliers* appeared in Paris, 1781.

Clarke, J. J.: *Orthopedic Surgery.* London, Cassell & Co., 1899, pp. 117–127.

Clarke, J. J.: Hallux valgus and hallux varus. Lancet *1:*609–611, 1900.

Daw, S. W.: An unusual type of hallux valgus (two cases). Brit. Med. J. *2:*580, 1935.

Dreesmann, K.: Hallux valgus und Metatarsus varus. Med. Klin. *24:*1740–1743, 1928.

Dubrueil, A.: De quelques difformités du gros orteil. Gaz. Hôpitaux *43:*50–51 and 54, 1870.

Durlacher, L.: *A Theatise on Corns, Bunions, the Diseases of Nails and the General Management of the Feet.* London, Simkin, Marshall & Co., Introduction, 1845, pp. 22–23.

Durman, D. C.: Metatarsus primus varus and hallux valgus. A.M.A. Arch. Surg. *74:*128–135, 1957.

Ely, L. W.: Hallux valgus. Surg. Clin. N. Amer. *6:*425–431, 1926.

Engle, E. T., and Morton, D. J.: Notes on the foot disorders among natives of the Belgian Congo. J. Bone Joint Surg. *13:*311-318, 1931.

Ewald, P.: Die Aetiologie des Hallux valgus. Dtsch. Ztschr. Chir. *114:*90–103, 1912.

Flower, W. H.: Fashion in deformity. Popular Science Monthly *17:*722–742, 1880.

Frejka, B.: Concerning the etiology of hallux valgus (in Czech). Bratisl. Lek. Listy *3:*310–327, 1924.

Froriep, R.: *Commentatiuncula de Ossis Metatarsi Primi Exostosi.* Berolini: Joanni de Wiebel, 1834, pp. 1–8.

Goldthwait, J. E.: The treatment of hallux valgus. Boston Med. Surg. J. *129:*533–535, 1893.

Gutzeit, R.: Über Hallux valgus interphalangeus. Verhandl. Dtsch. Ges. Chir. *43:*62–65, 1914.

Hagen-Torn, O.: Hallux valgus—eine transformatorische Folge und Ausdruck der Schaedigung der Fussagewoelbe. Arch. Klin. Chir. *135:*490–492, 1925.

Haines, R. W., and McDougall, A.: The anatomy of hallux valugus. J. Bone Joint Surg. *36:* 272–293, 1954.

Hamsa, W. R.: Hallux valgus: A study of end results of 339 bunionectomies. Nebraska Med. J. *22:*225–229, 1937.

Hardy, R. H., and Clapham, J.C.R.: Hallux valgus predisposing anatomical causes. Lancet *1:*1180–1183, 1952.

Heller, E. P.: Congenital bilateral hallux valgus. Ann. Surg. *88*:798–800, 1928.

Hiss, J. M.: Hallux valgus: its causes and simplified treatment. Am. J. Surg. *11*:50–57, 1931.

Hiss, J. M.: *Functional Foot Disorders.* Los Angeles University Press, 1937, pp. 263–294.

Hoffmann, H.: Die Phalanx Hallucis valga congenita. Ztschr. Orthop. Grenzgb. *65*:353–360, 1936.

Hohmann, G.: *Fuss und Bein.* Munich, J. G. Bergmann, 1951, pp. 145–192.

James, C. S.: Footprints and feet of natives of the Solomon Islands. Lancet *2*:1391–1392, 1939.

Joachimsthal, G.: *Handbuch der Orthopaedischen Chirurgie.* Jena, G. Fischer, 1907, pp. 710–720.

Johnston, O.: Further studies of the inheritance of hand and foot anomalies. Clin. Orthop. *8*:146–160, 1956.

Jones, R.: Discussion on the treatment of hallux valgus and rigidus. Brit. Med. J. *2*:651–656, 1924.

Jordan, H. H., and Brodsky, A. E.: Keller operation for hallux valgus and hallux rigidus. A.M.A. Arch. Surg. *62*(4):586–596, 1951.

Kaplan, E. B.: The tibialis posterior muscle in relation to hallux valgus. Bull. Hosp. Joint Dis. *16*:88–93, 1955.

Keizer, D. P. R.: Hallux valgus duplex congenitus avec hypospadias penis. Paris Méd. *40*:566, 1950.

Keizer, D. P. R.: Hallux valgus. Lancet *1*:1305, 1952.

Kirmisson, E.: Les difformités acquises des orteils envisagées au point de vue de leur étiologie. Rev. d'Orthop. *10*:133–138, 1899.

Kirmisson, E.: *Les Difformités Acquises, de l'Appareil Locomoteur, Pendant l'Enfance et l'Adolescence.* Paris, Masson et Cie., 1902, pp. 506–517.

Klar, M. M.: Ueber angeboronen Hallux valgus. Ztschr. Orthop. Chir. *14*:304–311, 1905.

Kleinberg, S.: The operative cure of hallux valgus and bunions. Am. J. Surg. *15*:75–81, 1932.

Lake, N. C.: *The Foot.* London, Baillière, Tindall and Cox, 1952, pp. 222–260.

Lane, W. A.: The causation and pathology of the so-called disease rheumatoid arthritis, and of senile changes. Tr. Path. Soc. London *37*: 387–447, 1886.

Lane, W. A.: The causation, pathology, and physiology of several of the deformities which develop during young life. Guy's Hosp. Rep. *44*:307–317, 1887.

Lapidus, P. W.: The operative correction of the metatarsus varus primus in hallux valgus. Surg. Gyn. Obst. *58*:183–191, 1934.

Loison, M.: Note sur le traitement chirurgicale de hallux valgus d'après l'étude radiographique de la déformation. Bull. Mem. Soc. Chir. *27*:528–531, 1901.

McBride, E. D.: A conservative operation for bunion. J. Bone Joint Surg. *10*:735–739, 1928.

McCormick, D. W., and Blount, W. P.: Metatarsus adductovarus, "skewfoot." J.A.M.A. *141*:449–459, 1949.

McElvenny, R. T.: A study of hallux valgus: its cause and operative management. Quart. Bull., Northw. Univ. Med. Sch. *18*:286–297, 1944.

McMurray, T. P.: Treatment of hallux valgus and rigidus. Brit. Med. J. *2*:218–221, 1936.

Malgaigne, J. G.: Mémoire sur la déviation latérale du gros orteil. Rev. Méd. Chir. *11*:212–224, 1852.

Mauclaire, P.: Clinodactyle externe et interne, déviations latérales des orteils. Presse Méd. *4*:205–210, 1896.

Mayo, C. H.: The surgical treatment of bunions. Ann. Surg. *48*:300–302, 1908.

Mayo, C. H.: The surgical treatment of bunions. Minnesota Med. J. *3*:326–331, 1920.

Mensor, M. C.: Hallux valgus; report of cases. Calif. West. Med. *28*:341–345, 1928.

Metcalf, C. R.: Acquired hallux valgus. Late results from operative and non-operative treatment. Boston Med. Surg. J. *167*:271-277, 1912.

Meyer, G.: *Why the Shoe Pinches* (Tr. by J. S. Craig). New York, R. T. Trall & Co., 1863, pp. 5–35. The German pamphlet was called *Die rightige Gestalt der Schuhe,* Zurich, Myer & Zeller, 1858.

Meyerding, W. H., and Upshaw, J. E.: Heredofamilial cleft foot deformity (lobster-claw foot or split-foot). Am. J. Surg. *74*:889–892, 1947.

Mouchet, A.: Hallux valgus, congénital bilatéral. Bull. Soc. Pédiat. *17*:298, 1919.

Mouchet, A.: Pathogénie et traitement des difformités du gros orteil. Rev. d'Orthop. *9*:583–613, 1922.

Mygind, H. B.: Some views on the surgical treatment of hallux valgus. Acta. Orthop. Scand. *23*:152–158, 1953.

Nélaton, A.: Élémens de Pathologie Chirurgicale. Paris, G. Baillière, 1859, Vol. 5, pp. 969–971.

Payr, E.: *Pathologie und Therapie des Hallux valgus.* Wien und Leipzig, Wilhelm Braumuller, 1894, pp. 1-77.

Peabody, C. W.: The surgical cure of hallux valgus. J. Bone Joint Surg. *13*:273–282, 1931.

Peck, J. L.: *Dress and Care of The Feet.* New York, S. R. Wells, 1871, pp. 1–85.

Picqué, L.: Note sur une cas d'hallux valgus. Bull. Mem. Soc. Chir. *28*:518–525, 1902.

Piggott, H.: The natural history of hallux valgus in adolescence and early adult life. J. Bone Joint Surg. *42*:749–760, 1960.

Quevedo, S.: De l'hallux valgus (orteil en équerre, en croix ou clinodactyle) et de son traitement chirurgicale. Thesis. Paris, G. Steinheil, 1894, pp. 47–52.

Riedel: Zur operativen Behandlung des Hallux valgus. Cbl. Chir. *44*:753–755, 1886.

Riedl, H.: Osteotomie des Keilbeines bei Hallux valgus. Arch. Klin. Chir. *88*:565–575, 1909.

Robinson, H. A.: Bunion: its cause and cure. Surg. Gyn. Obst. *27*:343–345, 1918.

Robinson, H. A.: Bunion: its cause and cure. Internat. Clin. *2*:64–76, 1927.

Robinson, H. A.: The etiology of bunion. Milit. Surg. *62*:807–813, 1928.

Rogers, W. A., and Joplin, R. J.: Hallux valgus, weak foot and the Keller operation: an end-result study. Surg. Clin. N. Amer. *27*:1295–1302, 1947.

Rutt, A.: Phalanx Hallux valga congenital. In *Spezielle Orthopaedie: Untere Extremitat* (edited by Hohmann, Hackenbrock, etc.): Stuttgart, George Thieme, 1961, pp. 1129–1130.

Sandelin, T.: Operative treatment of hallux valgus. Abstract in J.A.M.A. *80:*736, 1923. The original article appeared in Finska Läkaresällskapets Handlingar, Hesingfors, *64:*543, 1922.

Schede, F.: Hallux valgus, Hallux flexus und Fussenkung. Ztschr. Orthop. Chir. *48:*564–571, 1927.

Silver, D.: The operative treatment of hallux valgus. J. Bone Joint Surg. *5:*225–238, 1923.

Sim-Fook, L., and Hodgson, A. R.: A comparison of foot forms among the non-shoe and shoe-wearing Chinese population. J. Bone Joint Surg. *40:*1058–1062, 1958.

Simon, W. V.: Der Hallux valgus und seine chirurgische Behandlung, mit besonderer Berücksichtigung der Ludloff'schen Operation. Bruns Beitr. Klin. Chir. *111:*467–537, 1918.

Steele, A. J.: Hallux valgus extremis. Med. Rec. *54:*246–247, 1898.

Stein, H. C.: Hallux valgus. Surg. Gyn. Obst. *66:*889–898, 1938.

Truslow, W.: Metatarsus primus varus or hallux valgus? J. Bone Joint Surg. *7:*98–108, 1925.

Verbrugge, J.: *Pathogénie et Traitement de l'Hallux Valgus.* Mem. Bull. Soc. Belge d'Orthop., pp. 3–40, 1933.

Walsham, W. J., and Hughes, W. K.: *The Deformities of the Human Foot.* London, Baillière, Tindall & Cox, 1895, pp. 496–514.

Wells, L. H.: The foot of the South African native. Am. J. Phys. Anthrop. *15:*186–289, 1931.

Wheeler, P. H.: Os intermetatarseum and hallux valgus. Am. J. Surg. *18:*341–342, 1932.

Wyeth, J. A.: *A Text-Book on Surgery.* New York, D. Appleton & Co., 1887, pp. 735–736.

Young, J. K.: The etiology of hallux valgus or os intermetatarseum. Am. J. Orthop. Surg. *7:*336–341, 1909.

Young, J. K.: A new operation for adolescent hallux valgus. Univ. Penn. Med. Bull. *23:*459–468, 1910.

Zesas, D. G.: Zum angeboren Hallux valgus. Ztschr. Orthop. Chir. *15:*36–39, 1906.

Chapter Five

STRUCTURAL ALTERATIONS

Hohmann (1951) defined hallux valgus as a "static deformity, a concomitant symptom of splayfoot." Lake (1952) considered it a part of the widespread splaying of the foot. Both authors confined the basic disturbance to the forefoot since this is the part that bears the brunt of maximum stress during the take-off stage of walking. The underlying skeletal misalignment is usually three dimensional: there is deviation sideways, displacement in dorsoplantar direction, and axial rotation. The metatarsal bones fan out while the toes are crowded together. At the metatarsophalangeal joints there is a variable degree of deviation and displacement of the proximal phalanges. The first metatarsal bone rotates around its long axis allowing its under aspect to turn tibialward, while the plantar surface of the great toe faces toward the fibular border of the foot. At times the first metatarsal head tilts up while the base of the proximal phalanx of the great toe appears to have descended plantarward. Occasionally the reverse may take place: the first metatarsal head faces toward the ground while the base of the proximal phalanx of the great toe assumes a dorsal position. The proximal phalanges of the central toes usually incline toward the outer border of the foot and may have become subluxated at the metatarsal phalangeal joint both in lateral and dorsal directions. The fifth toe is usually in a varus position while its metatarsal has assumed a valgus position. In other words, the forefoot is splayed (Fig. 5–1).

The question may well be asked: Does hallux valgus ever occur without occult or manifest splaying of the forefoot? In congenital hallux valgus the great toe is seen to deviate in lateral direction before the child has borne weight on its feet and forced the metatarsal bones to spread out. Occasionally—because of a localized destructive disease of the first metatarsophalangeal joint or malunited fracture of one of the bones—the hallux inclines toward the outer border of the foot without an appreciable increase in the measurement of the transmetatarsal span. In hallux valgus interphalangeus the first intermetatarsal space is not widened: there is no metatarsus primus varus. More commonly, hallux valgus and splaying of the forefoot coexist (Fig. 5–2).

Skeletal foundation of splaying. The three cuneiform bones of the foot form a deep socket that opens toward the toes. The base of the second metatarsal is solidly slotted into this. The bases of

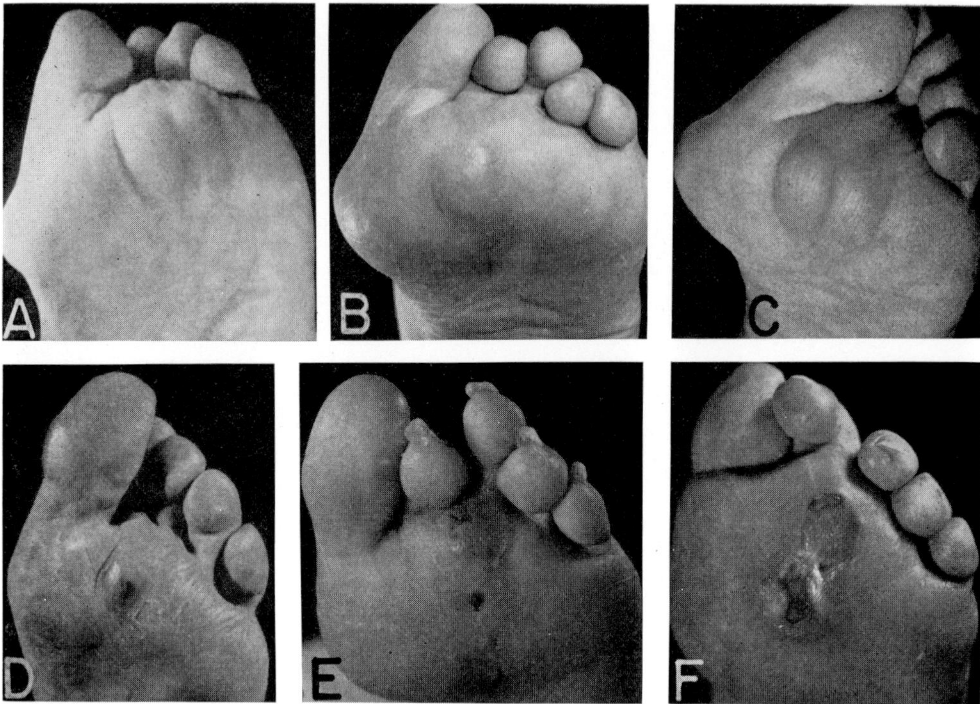

Figure 5–1. Splayed forefeet seen from the plantar aspect.

the three central metatarsals form a shallower notch, which receives the third cuneiform. The zigzag line of tarsometatarsal joints and the reciprocal interlocking of the bones at this junction enhance the stability of what anatomists consider the only transverse arch of the foot (Fig. 5–3).

Joints with flat articular facets permit only minimal motion and are therefore more stable. The second and third tarsometatarsal joints allow almost no movement. Grant (1958) stated that the fifth metatarsal could be plantarflexed and dorsiflexed freely, the fourth less freely, the third, second and first, very slightly, if at all. The reference is to passive motion. No metatarsal bone can be made to move alone actively. The comparative mobility of the fifth and fourth metatarsals is due to the oblique setting, the shallowness, and the mildly concave articular facet that the two together present to the cuboid bone. The base of the fifth metatarsal enters only partly into the formation of this joint. On its fibular aspect it is not flanked by another bone, as is the fourth metatarsal; hence, it enjoys greater mobility. Each of the three middle metatarsals is flanked on either side by another bone. The contiguous sides of the bases of all four lateral metatarsals articulate with one another. The intervening joint contains a synovial cavity on the dorsal aspect only. The plantar portion of the joint is spanned by interosseous ligaments, which are reinforced inferiorly by thick fibrous bands that resist splaying.

The first metatarsal is free on its tibial aspect. The articular facet the first metatarsal presents to the cuneiform proximally is extensive; it is mildly concave from side to side and in the dorsoplantar direction. The joint the first metatarsal forms with the innermost cuneiform lies about a centimeter distal from the second tarsometatarsal articulation, and it dips closer to the ground. Ordinarily, only the head of the first metatarsal rests on the ground, and this it does through the intermediary of two slippery ossicles—the sesamoid bones. The fifth metatarsal contacts the proffered surface most of its length; its tendency to splay is checked by the counterfriction of the

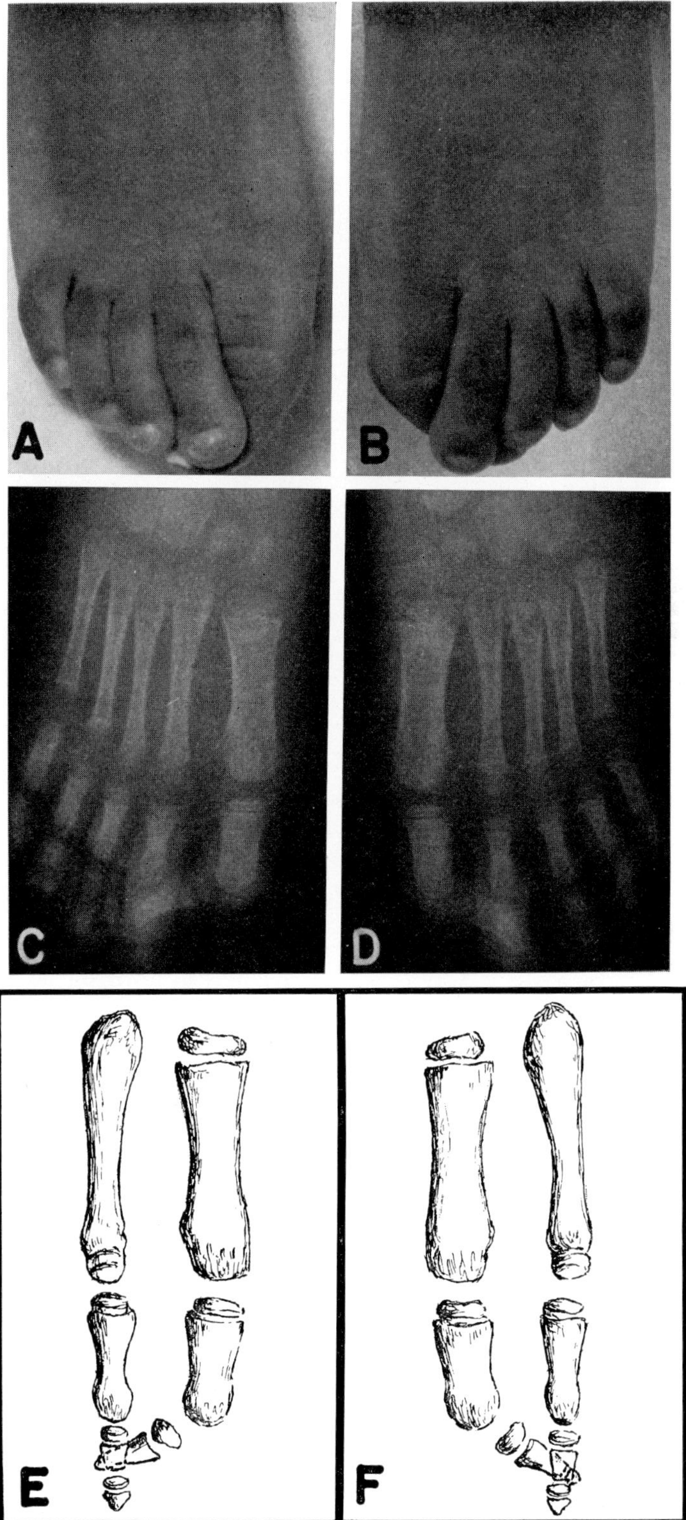

Figure 5–2. Bilateral congenital hallux valgus interphalangeus with no splaying of the forefoot nor any widening of the first intermetatarsal space.

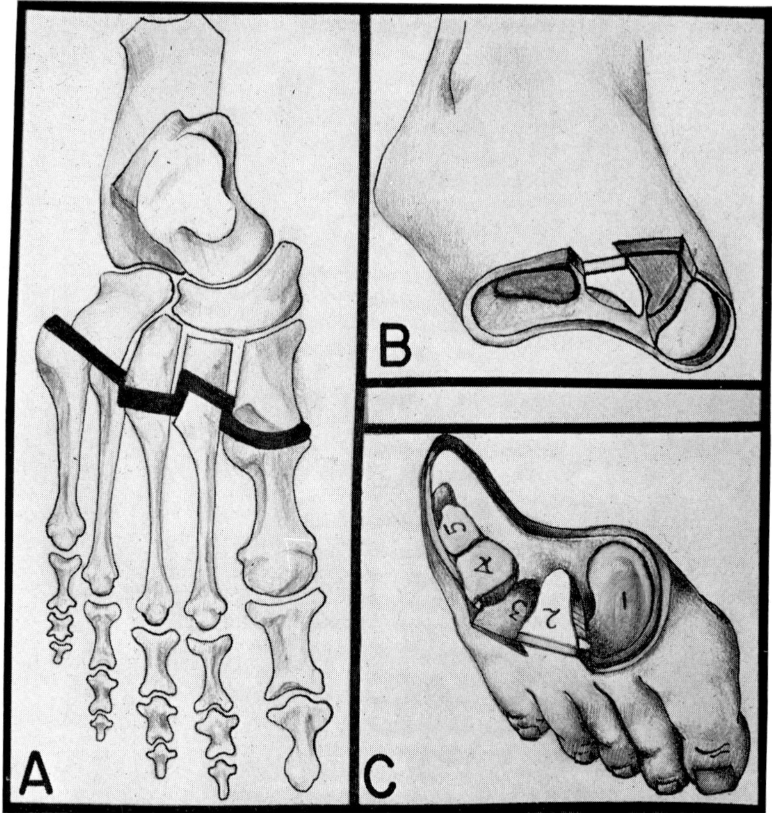

Figure 5–3. Interlocking of bones at the tarsometatarsal junction.

ground. Even though it yields less to compression from the side than the fifth metatarsal, the first metatarsal manifests greater tendency to splaying; it diverges from its neighbor more than the fifth, which means it does so more than any other metatarsal. It is not surprising that the exaggerated varus inclination of the first metatarsal is considered a cardinal sign of forefoot splaying.

Broca (1852) stated that, in what we now call hallux valgus, the first metatarsal underwent two positional changes: one in the direction of its long axis, the other around it. Broca was not clear about the last shift. From his writing one gets the impression that the first metatarsal and the innermost cuneiform turned their inferior aspects laterally and their superior borders medially. It was not stated whether the axis of the foot or the midline of the body is used for reference. German authors almost unanimously insist that in hallux valgus the first metatarsal is "supinated" and at the same time its head becomes tilted in a dorsal direction.

Cotton (1935) contended that "the collapse of the anterior metatarsal arch," which often accompanied hallux valgus, was due to "the ascent of the first member," rather than "descent" of the central metatarsal heads. Lambrinudi (1938) coined a new name, *metatarsus primus elevatus.* In hallux valgus, Stein (1938) thought, the metatarsal head was "inverted" in relation to the toe and the proximal phalanx was subluxated plantarward. Hauser (1950) stated that in response to the valgus position of the heel, or "pronation," the medial section of the anterior part of the foot went into "relative supination"; the counterpressure of the floor pushed the first metatarsal up and inward and its head was twisted in such a way as to turn its plantar surface medially.

Soft tissue safeguards against splaying. In the final analysis, muscles procure active dynamic protection against splaying as they do against other types of skeletal displacement; ligaments play a passive role. "The maintenance of the normal plastic form of the foot," Wood Jones (1949) wrote, "is due to the dual control exerted by the passive elasticity of the ligaments and the active contractibility of the muscles."

The ligaments bracing the anatomical transverse arch receive adequate aid from two powerful muscles—the *posterior tibial* and the *long peroneal*. Both these muscles are extrinsic to the foot. Their fleshy bellies are located in the leg; they send only their tendons to the foot. The posterior tibial tendon enters the sole of the midfoot from the inner border; the long peroneal penetrates it from the lateral side. Under the distal row of tarsal bones these tendons cross one another. Running close to the bone, the terminal digitations of the posterior tibial tendon capture all the bony components of the anatomical transverse arch except the bases of the first and the fifth metatarsals. The tendon of the long peroneal is slung underneath the midtarsus like a tie beam in bias—from its lateral point of entrance it passes forward and inward and connects with the innermost cuneiform and base of the first metatarsal. The only bone entering into the formation of the anatomical transverse arch that escapes being caught by the tendons of posterior tibial and long peroneal muscles is the base of the fifth metatarsal. This bone is secured by the short peroneal muscle, which lends a measure of lateral bracing. In the take-off, when greater strain is thrown on the forefoot, these extrinsic muscles contract and prevent the bony components of the anatomical transverse arch from spreading apart—splaying.

Distally the transverse span of the metatarsal heads—the "anterior metatarsal or transverse arch" of clinicians—receives no support from the muscles of the leg. This duty is assigned to weak, vestigial, intrinsic muscles. One thinks of the transverse head of the adductor of the great toe—*adductor transversus*. The origin of this muscle from the lateral metatarsal region, the transverse disposition of its fibers, and the insertion of its tendon medially into the great toe makes one think that it is ideally designed and situated to actively prevent splaying. Contrary to the impression conveyed by anatomical illustrations presented by various authors—McBride (1928), Hiss (1937), Stein (1938), McElvenny (1944), among others—adductor transversus does not originate from the metatarsal bones, but from the deep transverse ligament and the adjacent available margins of the intervening plantar pads. Its tendon inserts into the lateral sesamoid and the base of the proximal phalanx of the great toe and not into the first metatarsal, which most needs to be moored. Moreover, the muscle consists of slender fasciculi that lie below the middle metatarsals. They must get pinned down and cannot contract during take-off when such contraction is most needed. It is difficult to imagine how they can tighten under the body weight, lift the central metatarsal heads off the ground, and pull the marginal bones together (Fig. 5–4).

Of the remaining intrinsic muscles only the abductor hallucis can be said to lend the first metatarsal a measure of medial support—provided it has not slipped from the inner aspect of its head down under it, as it usually does in hallux valgus. The analogous muscle on the fibular side of the forefoot—the abductor of the small toe—inserts into the undersurface of the phalanx. It affords no lateral bracing to the fifth metatarsal. The experiments conducted by Levick (1921, 1932) indicate that when the toes are fixed, the interossei hold the metatarsal bones together and counteract the tendency of splaying. Pedal interossei insert mainly into the bases of the proximal phalanges. In hammered toe—which often accompanies hallux valgus—there is a variable degree of dorsal dislocation of the proximal phalanx at the metatarsophalangeal joint. With the dorsal shift of its point of insertion the interosseous tendon comes to lie on a higher plane in relation to the metatarsal head. It no longer acts as flexor of the metatarsophalangeal joint and may even serve as an extensor. Moreover, these retracted toes fail to touch the

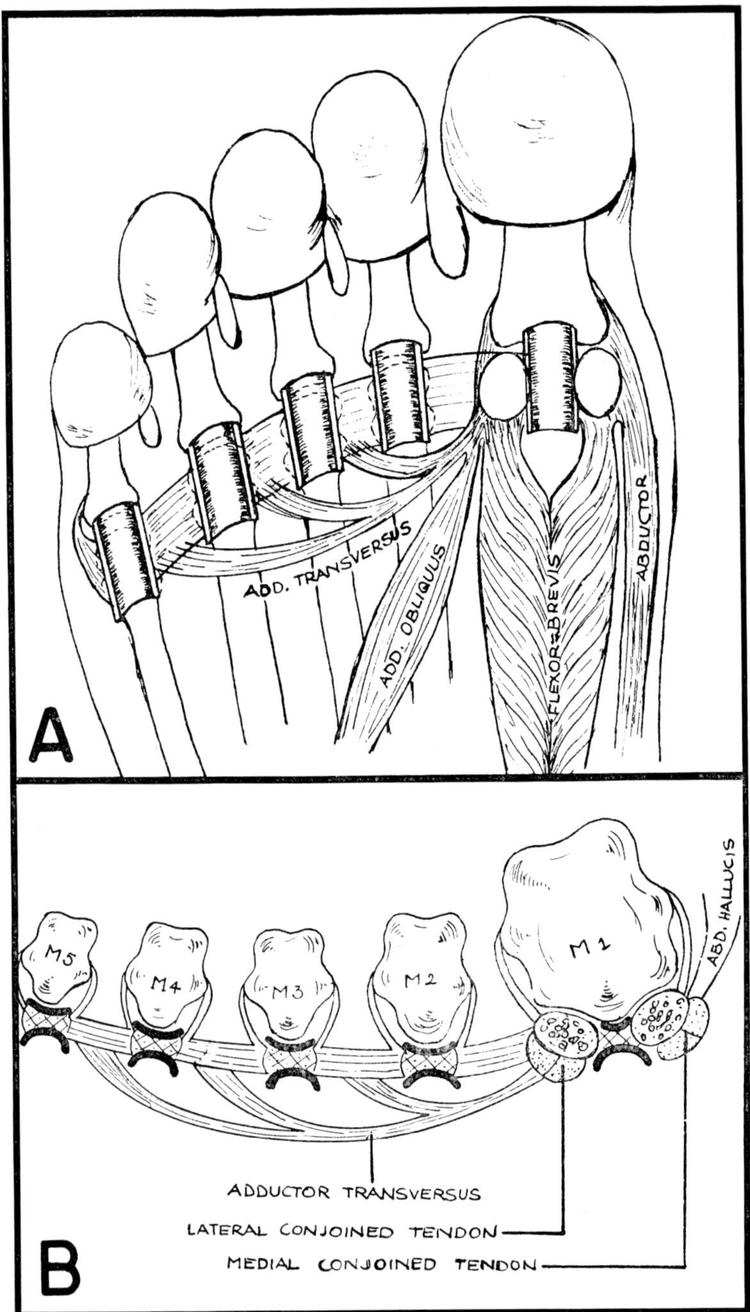

Figure 5–4. Adductor transversus.

proffered surface and press on it with sufficient force to establish fixed points from where the interossei can draw the metatarsal heads together—"bunch them up," as Levick said they would.

The responsibility of holding the metatarsal heads together falls to passive structures: *fascial encasement* of the forefoot but mainly on the deeper binding elements—the *plantar pads* and the bands of the deep *transverse ligament.* The latter consist of four separate bands, each of which bridges the gap between two flanking plantar pads. There are five plantar pads, one for each metatarsophalangeal joint. The pad belonging to the basal joint of the great toe is the largest. It contains a pair of sesamoid bones and has incorporated within its bulk two sizable conjoined tendons. The plantar pads of the four lateral joints consist of small, thin fibrocartilaginous plates; they receive no tendinous insertions and only rarely possess an osseous core. Medially and laterally each pad is suspended by the joint capsule and the collateral ligaments, which in turn bind the metatarsal head to the base of the proximal phalanx. Each pad receives two septal slips from the deeper surface of the plantar aponeurosis. Inferiorly the plantar pad is grooved and forms the roof of the flexor tunnel; superiorly it serves as the floor of the corresponding metatarsophalangeal joint. The metatarsal head rests on the plantar pad and is connected with it indirectly—by way of the capsule and the collateral ligaments of the joint and through loose areolar tissue proximally. The plantar pad procures more direct and firmer attachment distally with the proximal phalanx of the toe and moves with it. Because there are five plantar pads to be connected and four transverse bands, only three central pads blend with a band on either side. The free border of the sesamoid pad is suspended by the medial collateral ligament of the first metatarsophalangeal joint. The free border of the fifth pad connects with the lateral collateral ligament of the metatarsophalangeal joint of the small toe.

Superficial transverse plantar ligament is the name given by B.N.A. revision to the interlacing fibers of the distal portion of the plantar aponeurosis. Over the ball of the forefoot the aponeurosis thickens into a transverse strap. From the deep surface of this strap spring five pairs of septal slips; these run dorsally to connect with the margins of each plantar pad. Along their course, the septal slips provide fibrous encasement to the closely packed cells of fat. The adipose cushions lie between the plantar aponeurosis and the flexor tendons. Septal slips also contribute to the construction of the fascial tunnels of the flexor tendons. At the free borders of the great and small toes, the plantar aponeurosis curves around and splits into two layers. One of these continues to the dorsum of the foot and connects with the deep fascia of the region; the other, the deeper one, blends with the periosteum of the proximal phalanges of the first and fifth toes. On the dorsum of the foot the fascia thickens into fibrous expansions that hold the extensor tendons close to the bone. The best defined retinacular strap is the one slung over the extensors of the great toe—the *medial hood ligament*. This ligament curves inward along the tibial border of the great toe and blends with the periosteum of the proximal phalanx. It, too, does not connect with the metatarsal head. In hallux valgus the *hood ligament* moves with the phalanx and leaves the inner aspect of the joint unprotected. The superficial plantar ligament and deep fascia of the dorsum of the foot together provide the metatarsophalangeal region with a fibrous encasement—a belt.

Two separate, yet interconnected, binding systems thus hold the structures of the metatarsophalangeal junction together. On a deeper plane, four bands of the deep transverse ligament link together five plantar pads and thus provide a strap that extends from one side of the forefoot to the other. The medial margin of the strap is moored to the tibial side of the base of the proximal phalanx of the great toe; the lateral margin is anchored to the fibular border of the first phalanx of the small toe. On a plane closer to the skin, the plantar aponeurosis and the deep fascia of the dorsum of the forefoot provide this region with a circumferential strap. The two straps—one deep and transverse, the other circumferential and superficial—are linked together by septal slips that run in a dorsoplantar direction. The important point is that both straps are far more firmly connected with the proximal phalanges than with the metatarsal bones (Fig. 5–5).

The question arises: In splaying of the forefoot what is it that gives way? Stein (1938) surmised that, with exagger-

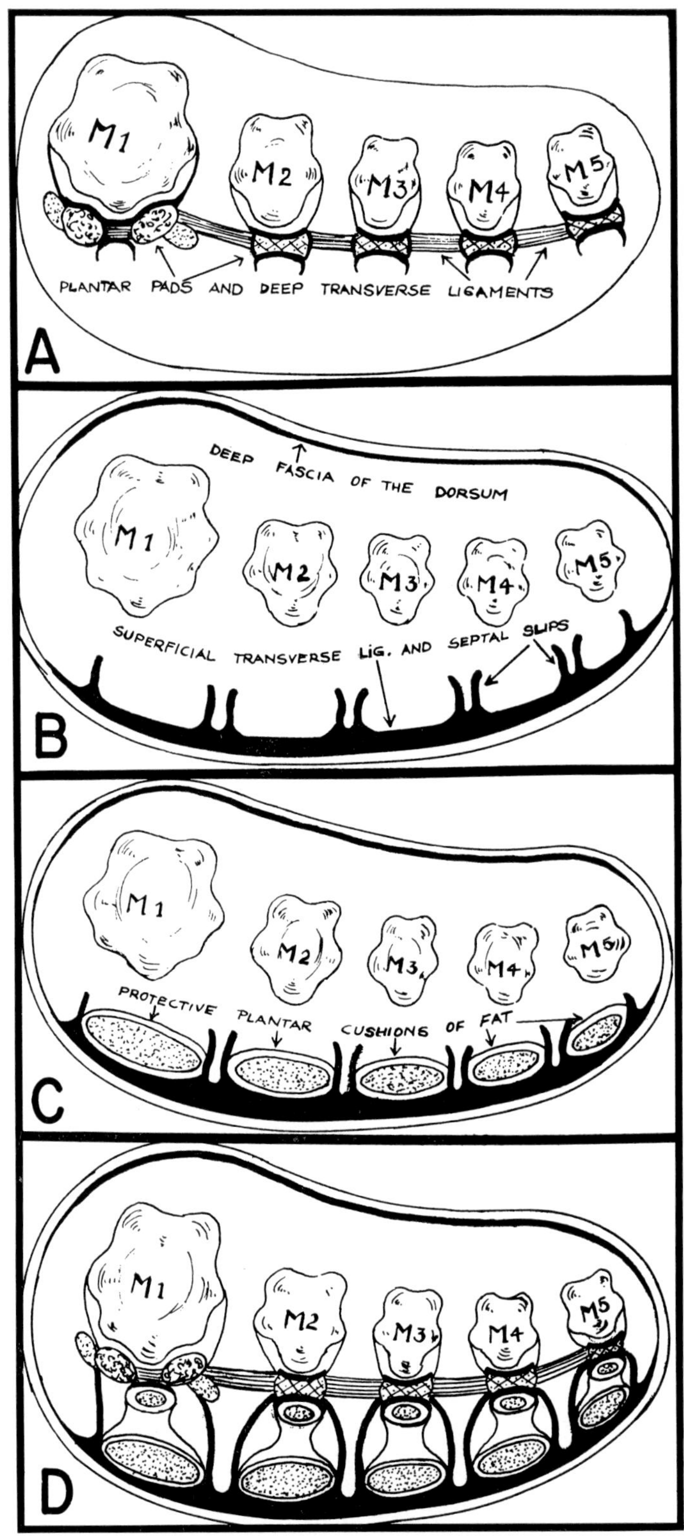

Figure 5–5. Soft tissue safeguards against splaying. Plantar pads and interlacing segments of the deep transverse ligaments (*A*). Superficial transverse ligaments and its septal slips (*B*). Protective cushions of fat between the septal slips (*C*). Interconnection of superficial and deep fascial straps (*D*).

ated varus of the first metatarsal, there is "a corresponding spreading and elongation of the transverse intermetatarsal ligament between it and the adjacent head." If this were true, the sesamoid pad would not shift toward the first intermetatarsal space. It has been erroneously supposed that the intermetatarsal segments of the deep transverse ligament firmly bind the adjacent metatarsal heads together and in splaying they "give way," "stretch," or "elongate." From what has been said it should be clear that the individual bands of the deep transverse ligament chain the flanking plantar pads. The metatarsal heads rest on these pads and therefore lie above the level of the deep transverse ligament.

According to Haines (1947), "In spread foot the deep transverse ligaments are intact, but the ligament which attaches the medial sesamoid to the first metatarsal bone is stretched." Haines and McDougall (1954) wrote: "The four deep transverse ligaments that bind together the five plantar pads of the metatarsophalangeal joints are not unduly stretched, so that as the metatarsals spread it is the ligaments that bind the pads to the heads of the metatarsals that give way." The reference is to the collateral ligaments of the first metatarsophalangeal joint, since their article dealt with the anatomical changes accompanying hallux valgus. It is the medial collateral ligament of this joint that stretches, allowing the first metatarsal to go into exaggerated varus and the sesamoid pad to migrate toward the fibular border of the foot.

Changes affecting the more closely related structures of the great toe. In full-blown hallux valgus several changes take place in and around the first metatarsophalangeal joint. They involve: the articular bones, the capsular and ligamentous structures, the muscles and the tendons, the bursa, and the skin.

The articular bones. The articular ends of the two main bones entering into the formation of the first metatarsophalangeal joint shift position in relation to one another. In mild cases of hallux valgus, outward deviation of the proximal phalanx is the sole feature. In severe deformities, axial rotation and subluxation enter into the picture. As the phalanx inclines outward and becomes displaced in a lateral direction, it leaves the medial articular surface of the metatarsal head unopposed and, hence, subject to unwonted friction by fibrous tissue instead of cartilage. The strip of erosion of the hyaline surface separating the displaced medial portion from the part of the head still in contact with the base of the phalanx was recorded by Riedel (1886), and given the name *sagittal groove* by Clarke (1900). Normally the underaspect of the first metatarsal head is marked with a median ridge, called the *crista*. This ridge is flanked on either side by two hyaline coated grooves, one for each sesamoid. In hallux valgus, because of the migration of the sesamoids, the median ridge is filed smooth, effaced. The undersurface of the first metatarsal head may also present patches of erosion, some of which communicate with the sagittal groove of Clarke. In more advanced cases of articular erosion, the interior of the metatarsal head is cystic due to the proliferation of marrow connective tissue in response to the denuded hyaline surface (Figs.5–6 to 5–9).

The *proximal phalanx* of the great toe presents a moderately concave articular facet to the globular head of the first metatarsal. The barrel shaped base of the phalanx gives insertion to the sesamoid pad, the joint capsule, the collateral ligaments, and the following muscles: abductor hallucis, both heads of the flexor brevis, the adductors, and the extensor brevis. The base of the proximal phalanx may be likened to the controlling post of a hammock. The joint capsule, the collateral ligaments, and the sesamoid pad form a shallow hammock that is reinforced laterally by the adductor obliquus and medially by the abductor hallucis. When the proximal phalanx deviates toward the outer border of the foot, subluxates, and everts, the hammock moves from under the metatarsal head. The fibular rim of the hammock, fenced by the adductor obliquus, rises up in a dorsal direction; the shallower tibial rim consisting of the abductor is lowered, allowing the head

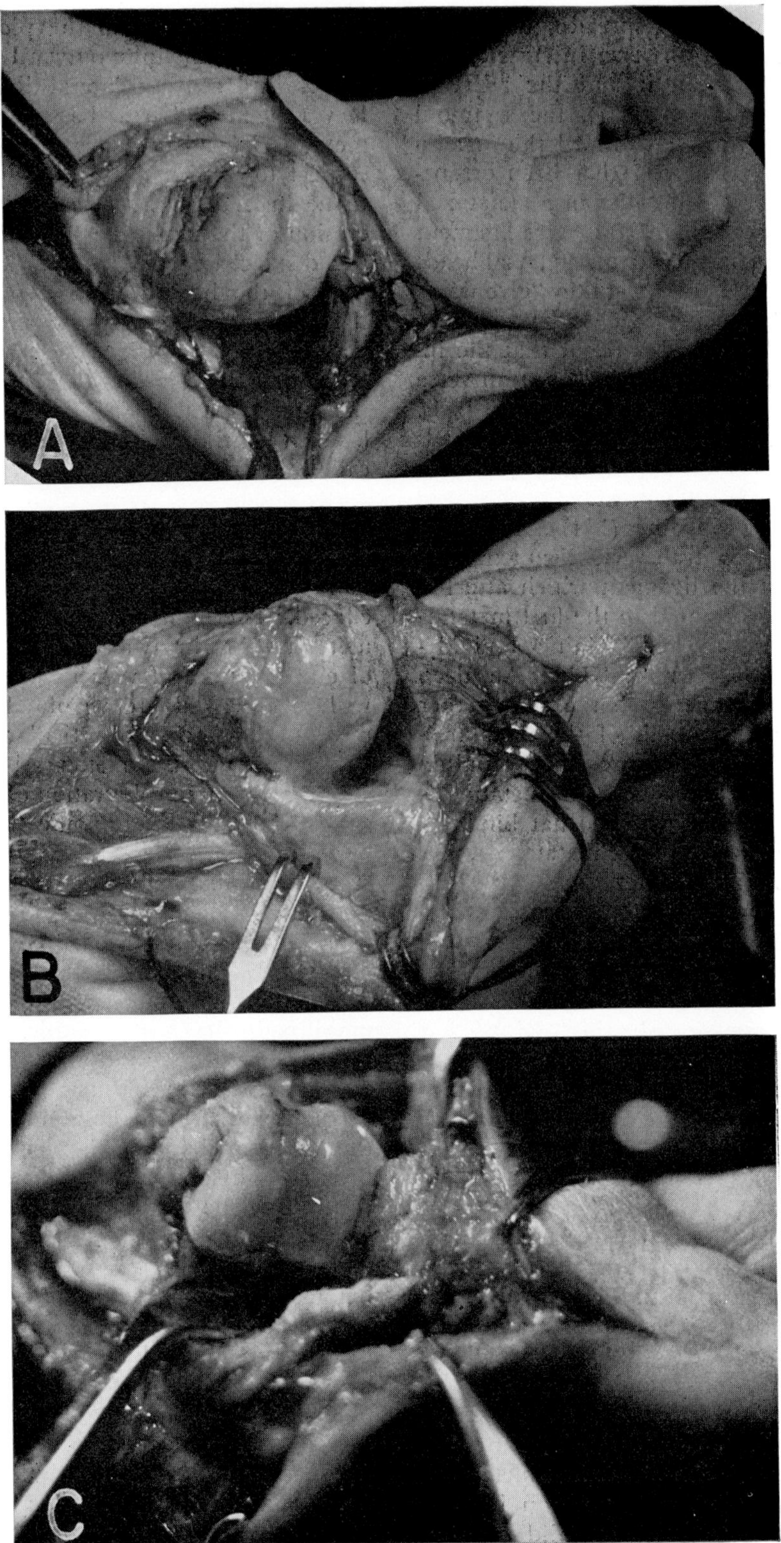

Figure 5–6. Sagittal groove as seen from the medial exposure of the first metatarsal head in three different cases.

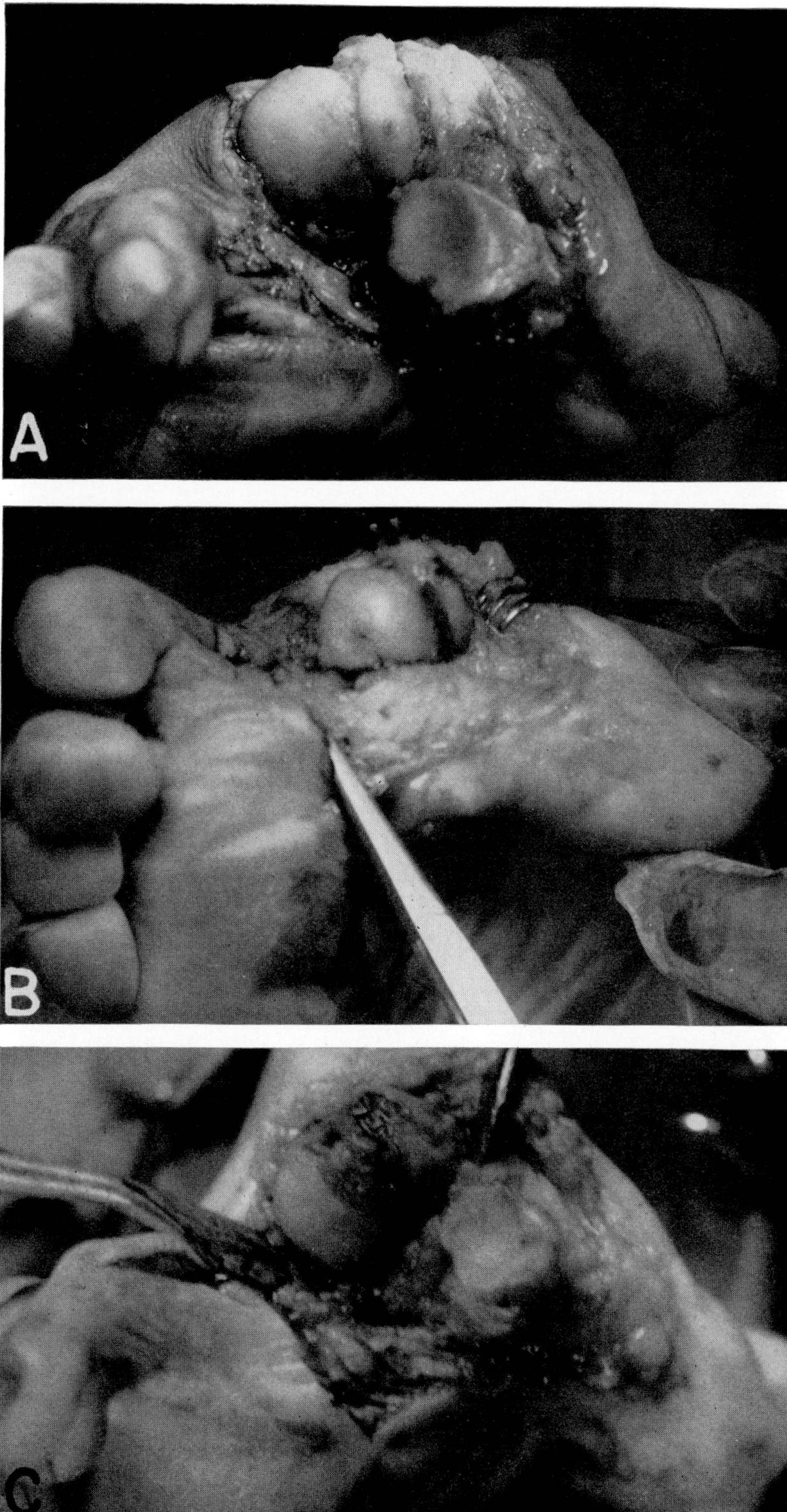

Fig. 5–7. Sagittal groove as seen when the first metatarsal head is exposed by interdigital incision in three other patients.

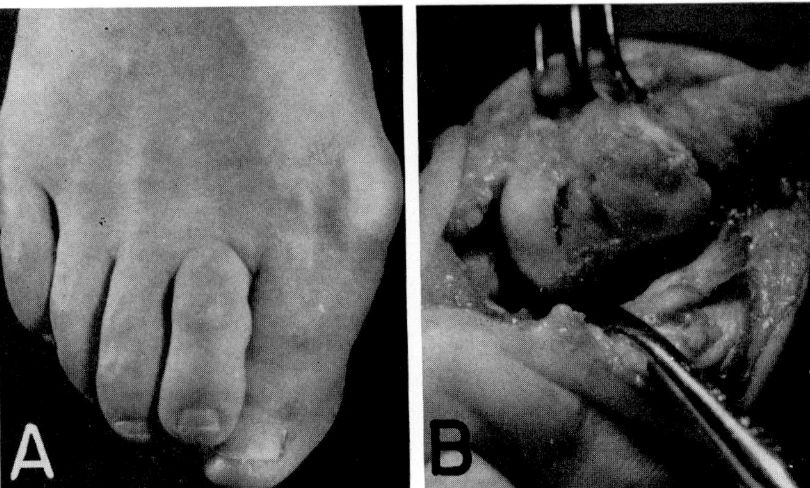

Figure 5–8. Hallux valgus (*A*) complicated with deep central ulcers (*B*) of the metatarsal head seen after surgical exposure.

of the metatarsal to go into varus (Figs. 5–10 and 5–11).

The *sesamoids* under the first metatarsal head are bound together by fibrocartilage; they are ringed by tendons, ligaments, and capsular tissue. The two ossicles move as one. All soft tissue structures that connect with the sesamoids insert into the base of the proximal phalanx of the great toe. The sesamoids move with the toe. In extension of the toe they shift forward; in flexion they glide backward. Side-to-side displacement of the sesamoids also depends on the position of the hallux. Shoe-wearing adults cannot actively abduct or adduct their great toes. Lateral migration of the sesamoids is to be regarded as evidence of outward deviation of the hallux. In some cases of hallux valgus the medial ossicle comes to lie under the ridge of the metatarsal head or in the groove originally occupied by the lateral sesamoid; the lateral sesamoid rides up along the fibular aspect of the head. In their new, mechanically incongruous location, the sesamoids wear out; they lose their hyaline coating, become mushroomed, form spurs and fragment. Incarcerated in the first intermetatarsal space, the fibular sesamoid may serve as a wedge and push the first metatarsal into greater varus. Adhesion between the sesamoids and the metatarsal head is not uncommon. Rarely, there is bony union between the displaced sesamoid and the metatarsal head (Figs. 5–12 to 5–14).

Capsular and ligamentous structures. The capsule of the first metatarsophalangeal joint is extensive. On either side it is reinforced with collateral ligaments—a medial and a lateral. Each ligament originates from the tubercles on the sides of the metatarsal head; the ligament then fans out to be inserted into the sesamoid pad below, and the proximal phalanx in front. With the outward deviation and eversion of the phalanx, the capsular structures on the fibular aspect of the metatarsophalangeal joint undergo shortening; those on the tibial side elongate. With outward deviation of the great toe, only the fibers of the medial collateral ligament connecting the two main bones are elongated. When there is also axial rotation, the fibers attached to the sesamoid pad are also stretched. The capsule and collateral ligament on the fibular side of the joint are contracted. The extent of this contraction depends on the degree of deviation of the hallux and the displacement of the sesamoids.

Muscles and tendons. A shift in position and structural changes may take place in muscles and tendons related to the great toe. With the axial rotation of the proximal phalanx—eversion--the tendon of the abductor hallucis slips from the medial side of the metatarsal head down under it. The adductor ob-

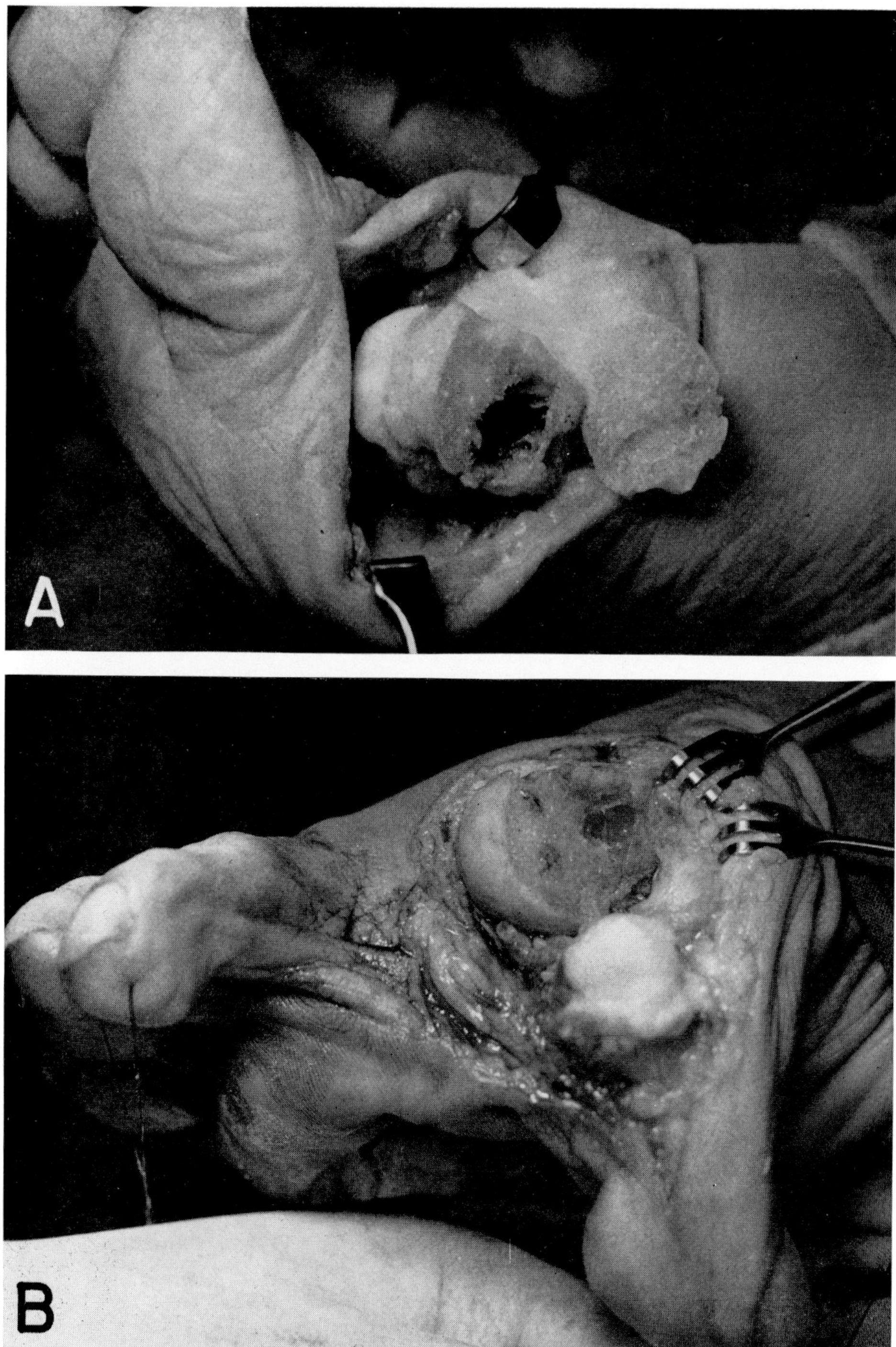

Figure 5–9. Cystic changes in the first metatarsal head as seen after sagittal resection of the medial eminence through medial (*A*) and interdigital approaches (*B*).

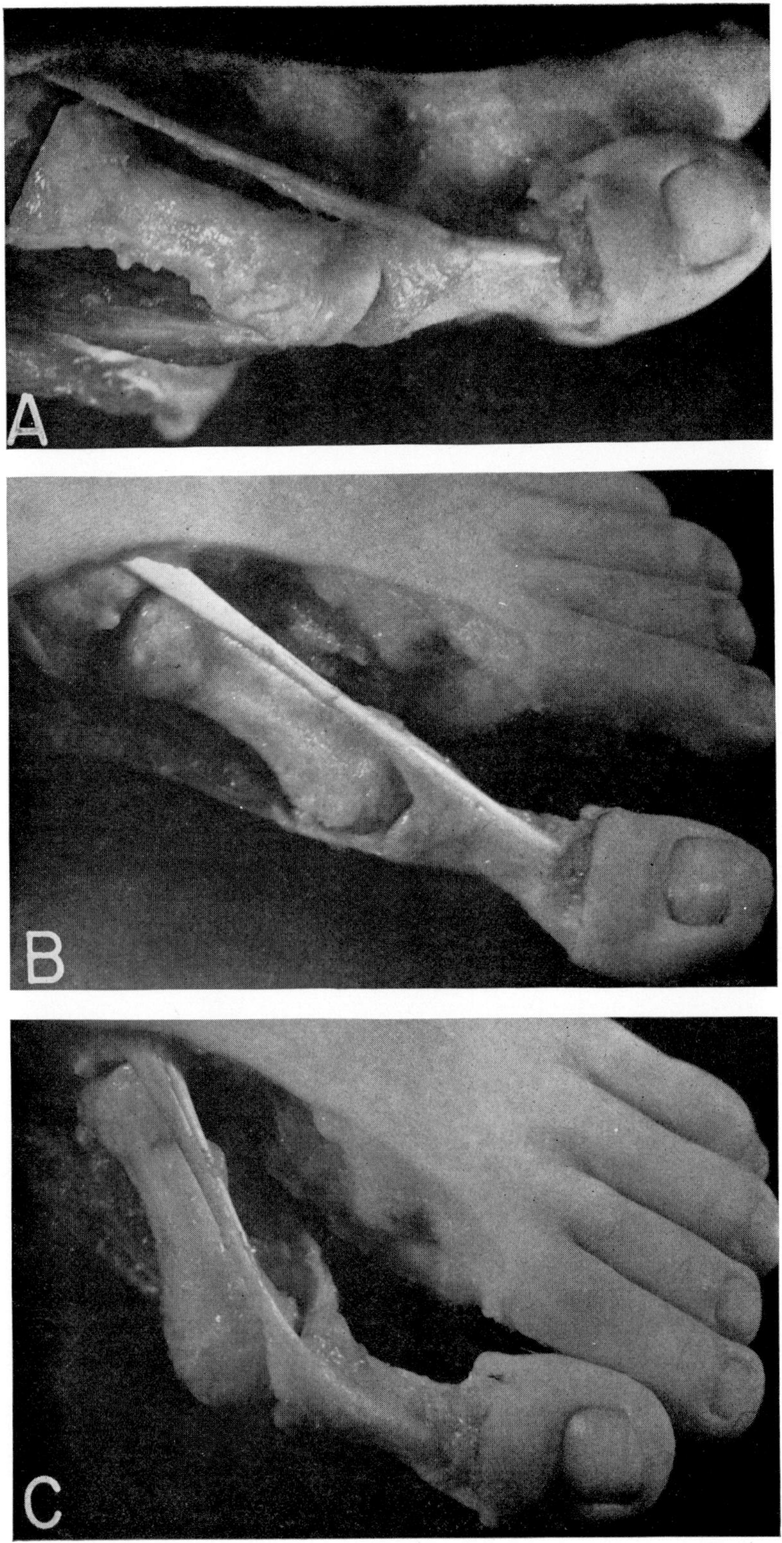

Figure 5–10. Dissected specimens. The hallux has been pushed laterally exposing the medial portion of the first metatarsal head (*A*). The hallux has been straightened (*B*). The great toe has been twisted until its nail slants medially (*C*): note the lateral sesamoid in the first interdigital space.

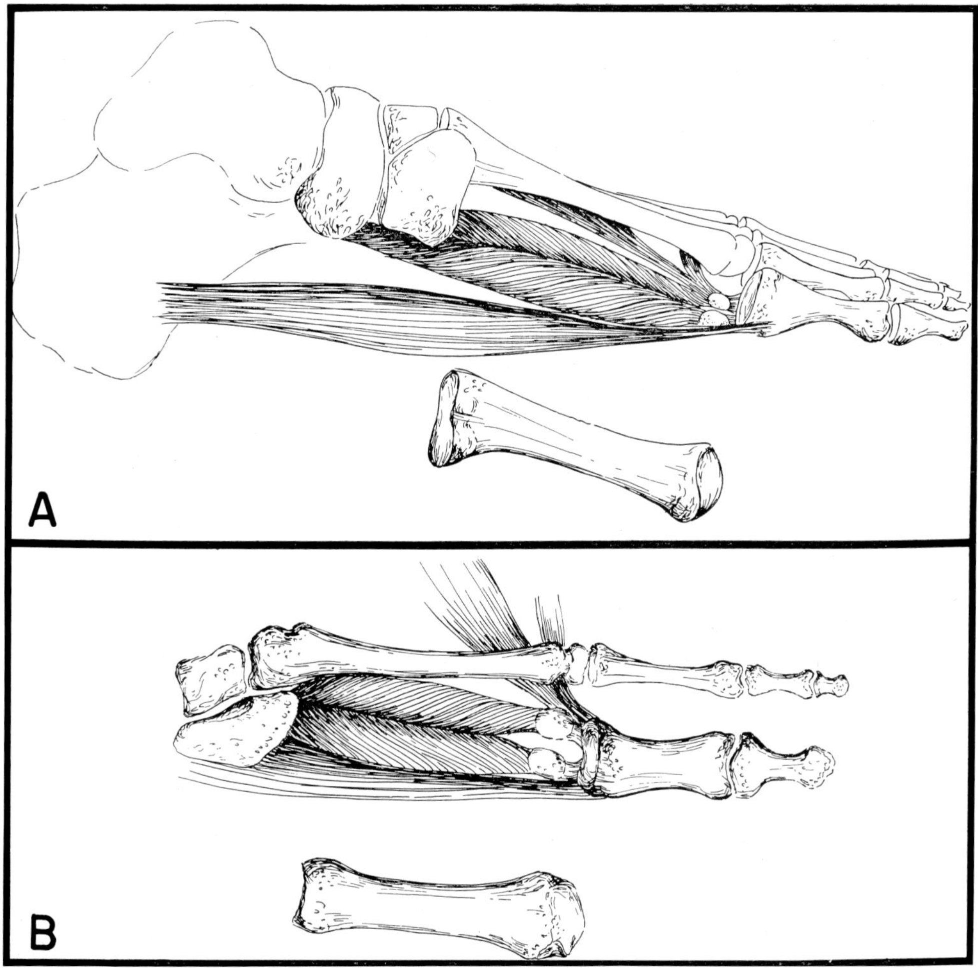

Figure 5–11. The "hammock" cradling the first metatarsal, seen from medial (*A*) and dorsal (*B*) aspects.

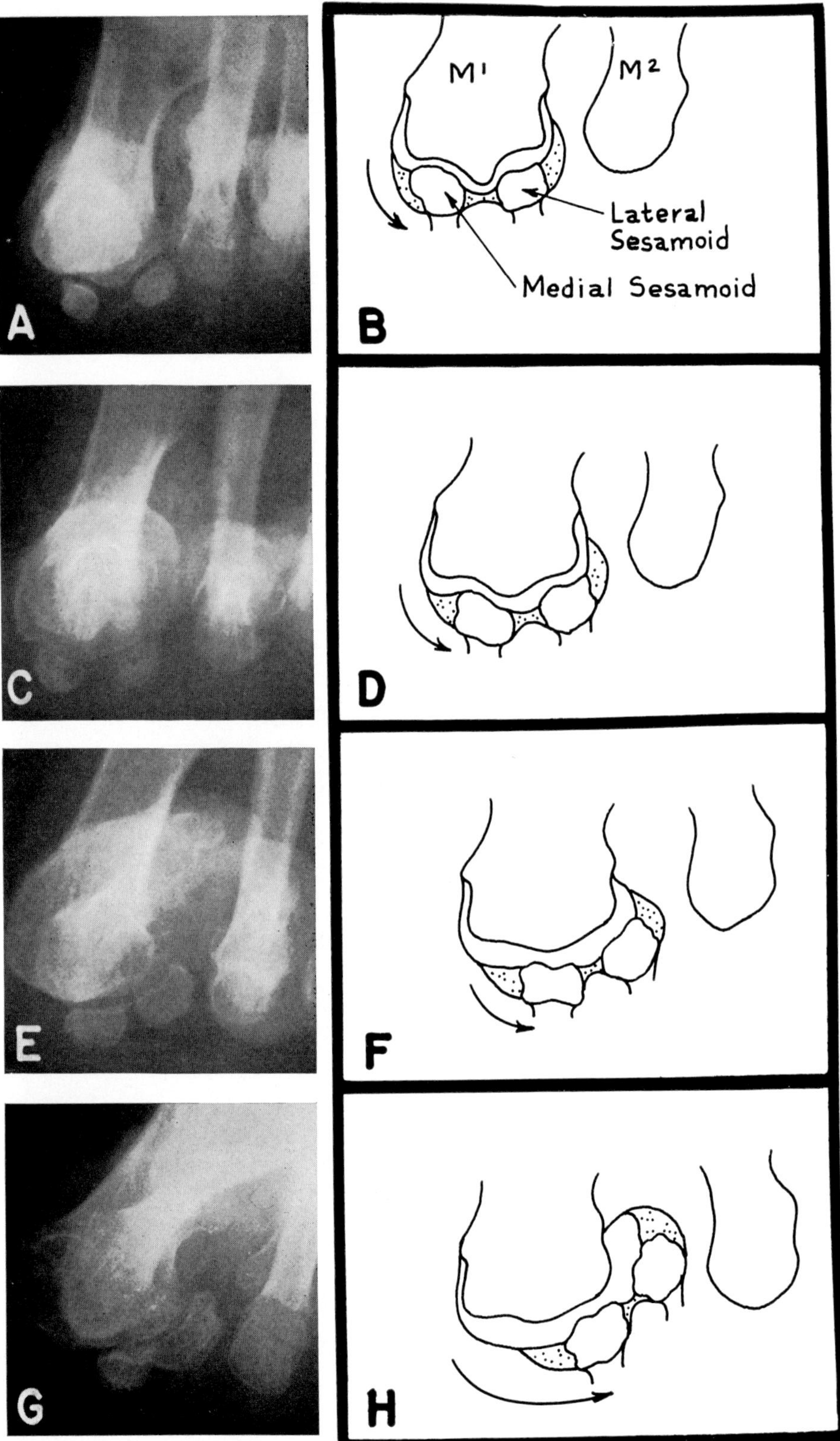

Figure 5–12. Migration of the sesamoid pad. Normal relation of the sesamoids and the first metatarsal head (*A* and *B*). Blunting of the crista and mild outward migration of the sesamoids (*C* and *D*). Effacement of the crista and more lateral shift of the sesamoids (*E* and *F*). Marked migration of the sesamoids and mushrooming of the lateral ossicle (*G* and *H*).

liquus on the other side of the joint moves to a dorsal position. The short flexors migrate outward. The tendon of the long flexor moves in a lateral direction with the overlying sesamoid pad, which forms the roof of its tunnel. Lying under the more loosely constructed *hood ligament,* the long extensor tendon becomes bowstrung. It may even present spindle shaped tumefaction where it is rubbed by the lip of the shoe vamp or toe box. The bowstringing of this tendon does not necessarily mean that it has undergone shortening in an absolute sense. In women who wear high heels and maintain a plantarflexed position of the foot at the ankle, there is compensatory lengthening of the long extensor. The short extensor of the great toe originates below the ankle. In hallux valgus it is contracted; its shortening is absolute. "The insertion of the innermost tendon of the extensor brevis digitorum into the base of the first phalanx of the big toe diagonally would cooperate in a valgus deviation," Collins (1899) wrote (Fig. 5–15)

Collins may have started the controversy concerning the functional perversion of muscles in hallux valgus. It is claimed that, with the axial rotation of the great toe, when it leaves the medial side of the first metatarsal head and comes to lie under it, the abductor hallucis ceases to serve as an abductor and acts as a flexor. The short flexor that has moved toward the first intermetatarsal space aids the adductor to pull the hallux into a greater valgus position. The bowstrung extensors and laterally displaced long flexor also augment the action of adduction and aggravate the valgus deformity of the great toe. It is conceivable that some measure of perverted muscle activity takes place in the earlier stages of hallux valgus—before marked arthritic changes have caused stiffening of the joint. After interlocking of the bones at the joint, the intrinsic muscles stop acting as muscles and serve as ligaments. In shoe-wearing adults the abductor hallucis merely serves as a medial brace to the first metatarsophalangeal joint, buttressing its capsule (Figs. 5–16 and 5–17).

Bursa. The bursa on the inner aspect of the first metatarsal head has been the subject of considerable discussion. Camper (1781) thought a bursa "naturally" existed in this area. Annandale (1866) spoke of synovial sacs that "normally occur in this situation." When inflamed and enlarged, they were called bunions, Annandale said. "But occasionally a bunion may be due to the formation of an adventitious bursa," he conceded. The adjective "adventitious" stuck in the literature; it now appears to have cast doubt on the existence of a true bursa in this region. Annandale also discussed bursitis occurring on the dorsal and plantar aspects of the first metatarsophalangeal joint as well as on its medial side. Most recent authors have overlooked the very troublesome thickening of the skin below the first metatarsophalangeal joint and the inflammation of the intervening bursa.

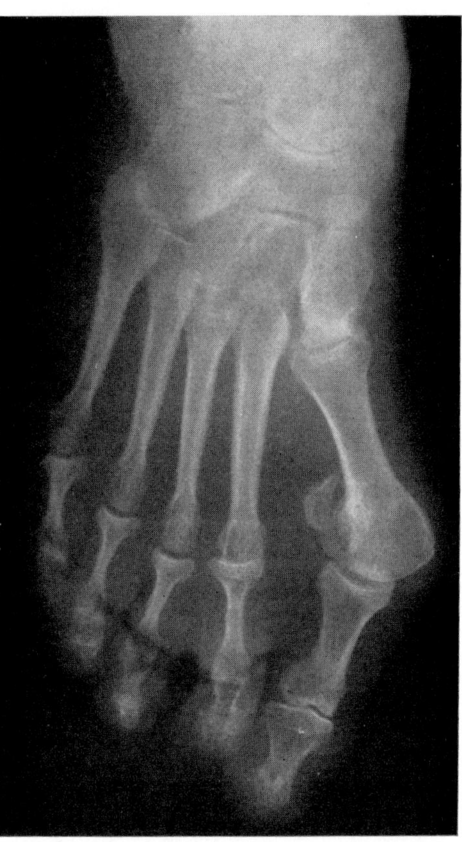

Figure 5–13. Spur arising from the proximal pole of the displaced, mushroomed lateral sesamoid.

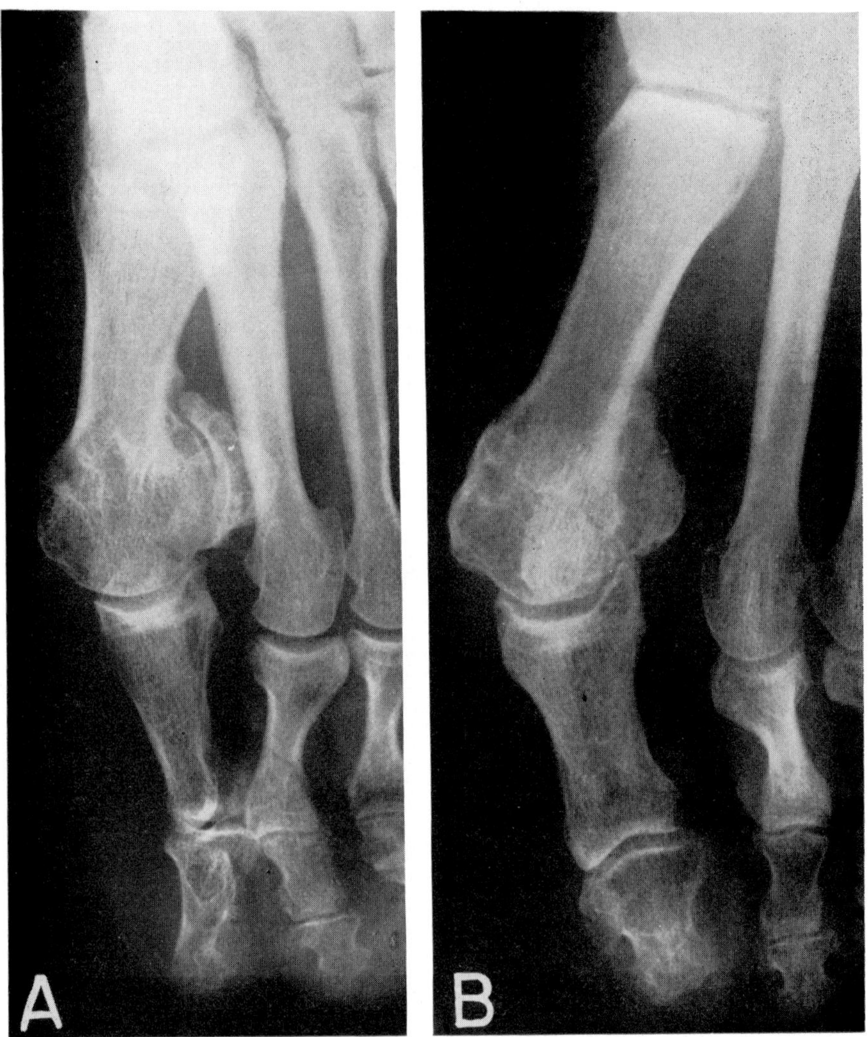

Figure 5–14. Fixation of the lateral sesamoid due to fibrous (*A*) and bony (*B*) ankylosis.

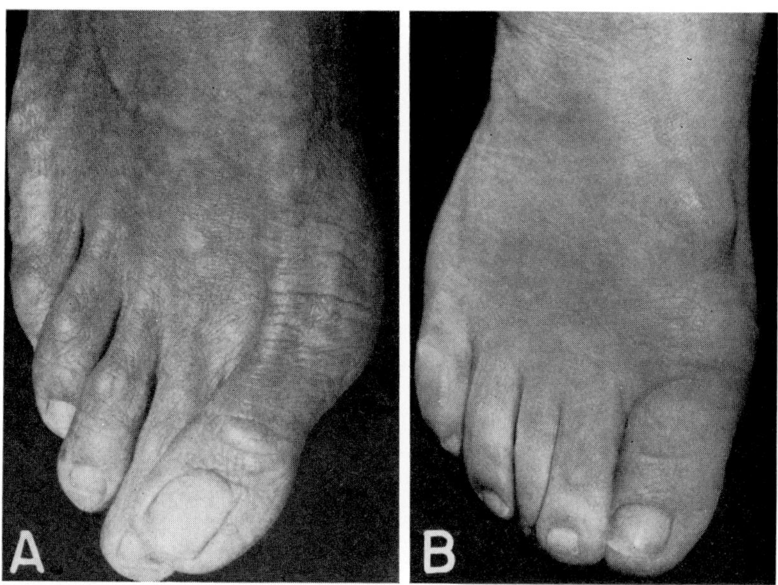

Figure 5–15. Bowstringing (*A*) of the long extensor tendon of the great toe. Thickening (*B*) of a segment caused by the vamp of the shoe.

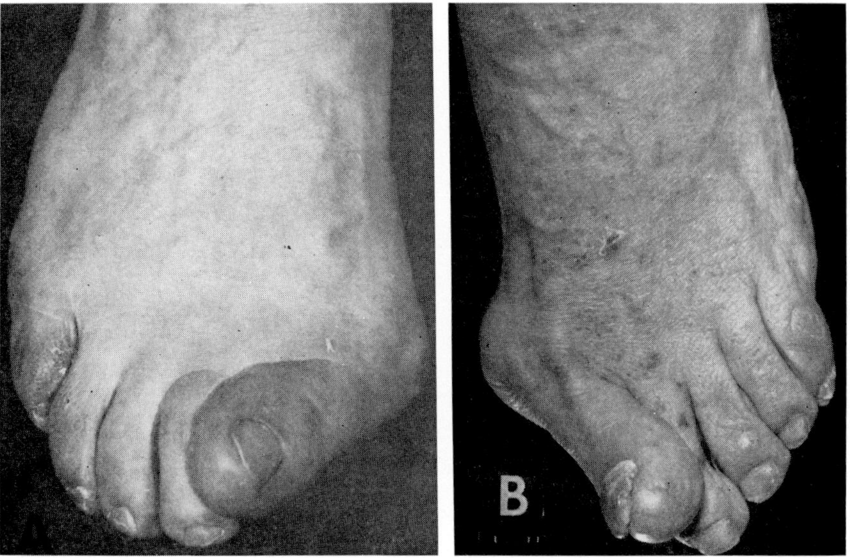

Figure 5–16. Axial rotation of the great toe in two different cases.

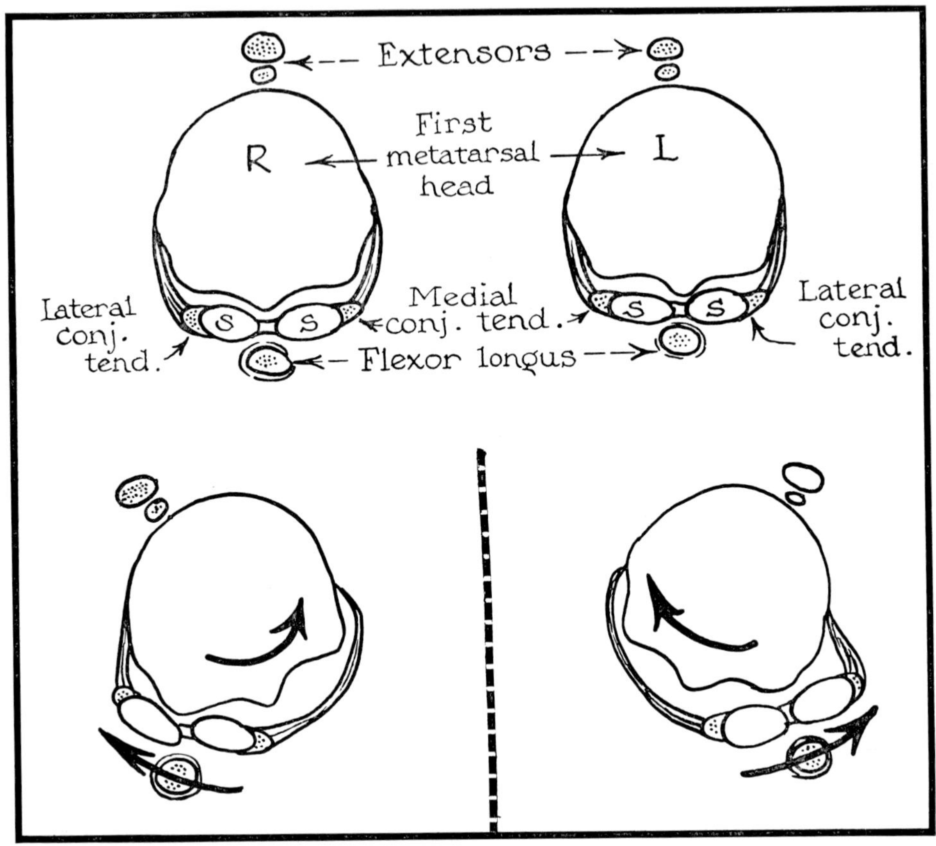

Figure 5–17. Axial rotation of the first metatarsal and outward migration of the sesamoid pad.

Chaput (1901) reported the largest hygroma on record. It bulged out from the medial aspect of the first metatarsophalangeal joint. It was polycystic and hemorrhagic, and measured 12 cm. long, 8 cm. wide, and 5 to 6 cm. deep. Poirier, who discussed Chaput's paper, said he had seen one the size of an egg. Multilocular bursae were also reported by Payr (1894). He dissected 128 cases of hallux valgus in cadavers and found that in about 10 per cent the mucous bag communicated with the joint cavity. Suppurative bursitis with regional cellulitis, sinus formation, or lymphangitis have been recorded in the past but seem to be rare now. In chronic nonsuppurative bursitis the wall of the sac becomes thick and its lining may be studded with villi; radiopaque deposits are at times visualized in the region of the bursa (Fig. 5–18).

Skin. The skin on the inner and plantar aspect of the great toe often undergoes cornification. Payr (1894) spoke about the constant pressure and chafing of the skin on the side of the prominent first metatarsal head. "This irritation," he wrote, "causes the skin to thicken and form a callus. . . ." Payr also mentioned the bluish frostbitten appearance of the skin. In old people with marked knuckling of the joint, the integument on the medial side is often parchment-thin and adherent to the underlying bone.

Changes affecting the lesser toes. With relative or real plantar descent of the central metatarsal heads, the proximal phalanges of the corresponding toes subluxate in a dorsal, and at times in a lateral, direction. The proximal phalanx assumes an extended position; the middle bone bends plantarward. The skin overlying the knuckled interphalangeal joint is chafed by the vamp of the shoe; it thickens into a hard callus. There are those who insist that in hammered toe a dorsally displaced proximal phalanx pushes the metatarsal head down toward the sole.

In splaying of the forefoot the most commonly affected smaller toes are the second and the fifth. The second toe is usually hammered. It may have slipped under the hallux or ride over it. As a result of widening of the first and fourth intermetatarsal spaces, the side-to-side span of the forefoot is increased. The fifth metatarsal inclines fibularward; its head presents a lateral eminence behind the base of the small toe. The bursa over this bony prominence may become irritated and inflamed. The bursa and bony prominence in this region have come to be known as a *bunionette*. The fifth toe responds to the valgus position of its metatarsal by going into a varus position (Fig. 5-19).

Correlation. In an established case of splaying, the first metatarsal inclines more than usually toward the midline of the body, and the fifth diverges away from it. The first metatarsal may also invert and allow its head to tilt up, while the hallux moves plantarward and turns to face the second toe. Because of the exaggerated inward inclination, inversion, and dorsal tilt of its head, the first metatarsal fails to carry its share of body weight. Greater stress is thrown on the outer bones—on the second, third, fourth, and sometimes the fifth metatarsal heads. Viewed from the plantar aspect the ball of the forefoot presents a convexity. This appearance is partly accounted for by the dorsal tilt of the first metatarsal head and the relative plantar prominence of the central capitalia. Because of the excessive stress to which they are subjected during the take-off phase of walking, or the permanent stress from high heels, the heads of the middle metatarsal dig their way plantarward and present palpable prominences under the skin of the sole.

It is to be remembered that four bands of the deep transverse ligament bind together five plantar pads, one for each metatarsophalangeal joint. Each plantar pad is connected moie directly and

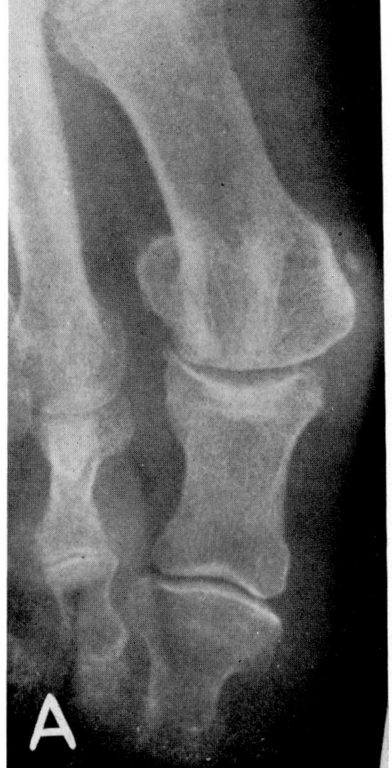

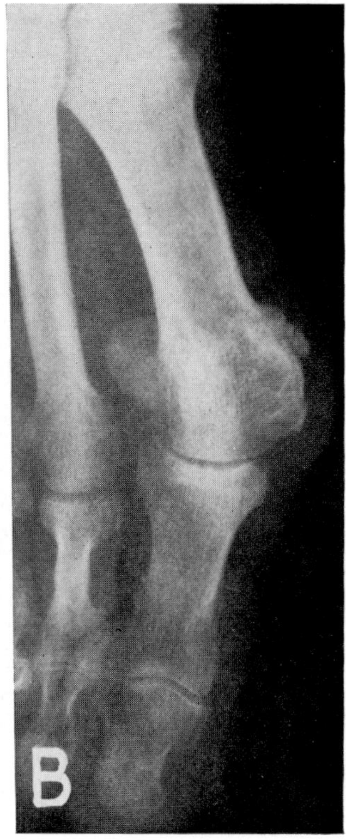

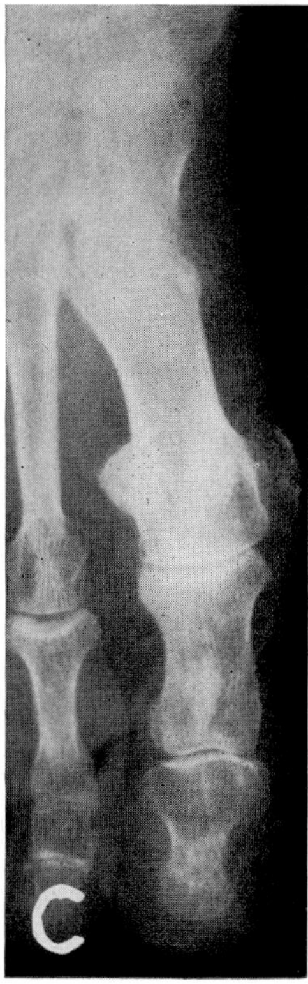

Figure 5—18. Calcarious deposits in the bursa.

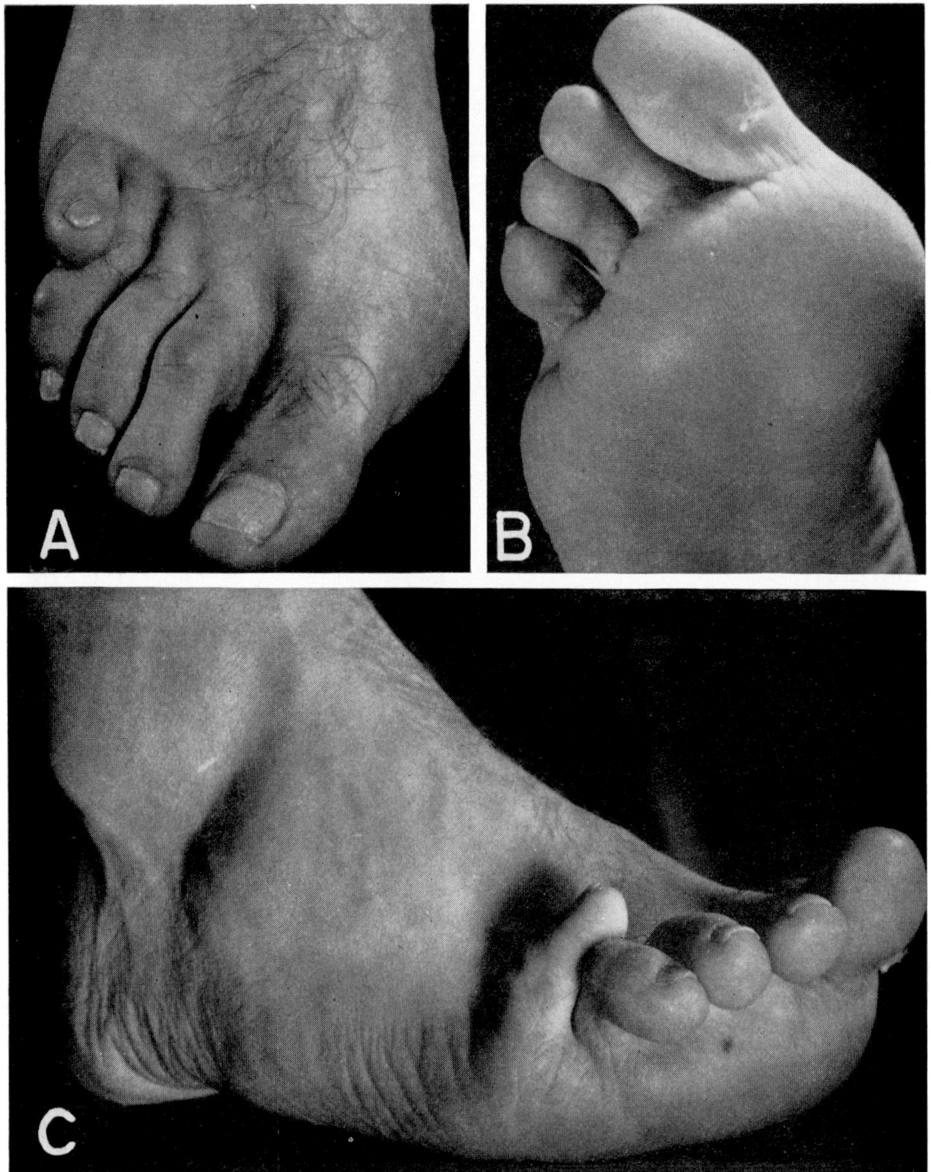

Figure 5–19. Hallux valgus, retracted central toes, and varus deformity of the fifth toe.

firmly with the base of the proximal phalanx than with the metatarsal head it lies under: the pad moves with the phalanx. The pad, moreover, forms the roof of the flexor tunnel, which is reinforced on the sides by septal slips emanating from the deep surface of the superficial transverse ligament. Before they reach the flexor tunnel and then pass dorsally to connect with the margins of the particular plantar pad, the septal slips encapsulate tightly packed clusters of fat cells, which absorb shock and save the metatarsal heads from wear. The most medial plantar pad, the one under the first metatarsal, gives anchorage to three sets of muscles—abductor hallucis, adductor hallucis, and flexor brevis—which restrain its forward excursion. No muscle inserts into any of the lateral plantar pads.

In hammered or clawed toe, the hyperextended proximal phalanx pulls the plantar pads—and with them the protective cushion of fat—from under the metatarsal head: the plantar pad and the cushion of fat now come to lie distal to the metatarsal head. The metatarsal head rests on loose areolar tissue, which becomes attenuated in time, leaving only the flexor tendons for support. In some instances the proximal phalanx is also subluxated sideways. It carries the plantar pad—and with it the flexor tunnel, the enclosed tendons, and the protective cushions of fat below them—to one side. In this case, the metatarsal head rests on the unpadded skin of the sole, where it can be palpated. The skin responds to the pressure from bone above and the

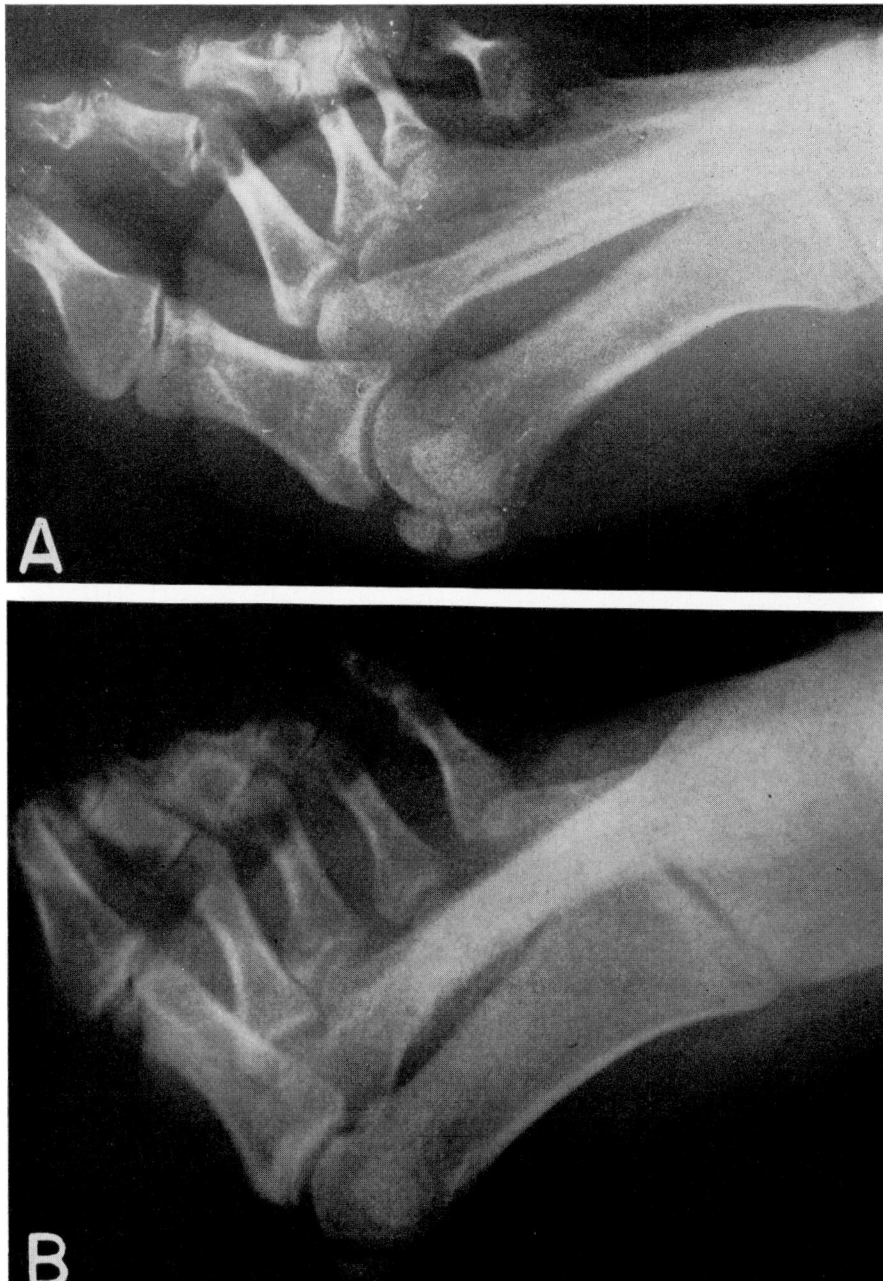

Figure 5–20. Clawed, retracted toes.

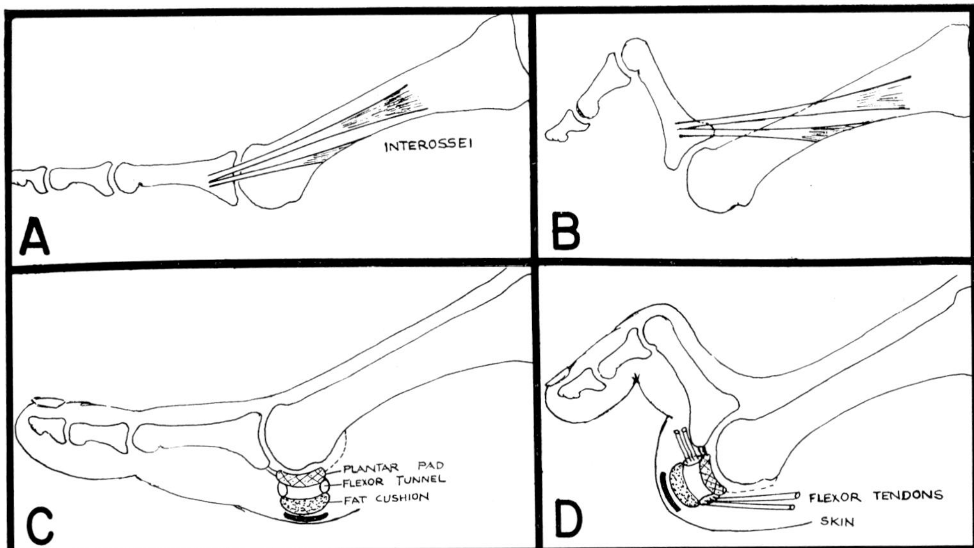

Figure 5–21. Structural changes associated with retracted toes. Normal relation of the pedal interossei and the metatarsal head (*A*). Dorsal shift of interossei in retracted toe (*B*). Soft tissue cushion under the metatarsal head (*C*). Forward shift of the cushion is a retracted, clawed smaller toe (*D*).

sole of the shoe below by becoming calloused and keratotic. Occasionally the central point of cornified integument ulcerates owing to insulation by scar and the cutting off of its blood supply. Unseen to the naked eye are the deep structural changes. In long-standing splaying, when the patient has walked on the metatarsal heads and not used the toes, the phalangeal bones atrophy (Figs. 5–20 to 5–24).

(*Text continued on page 95.*)

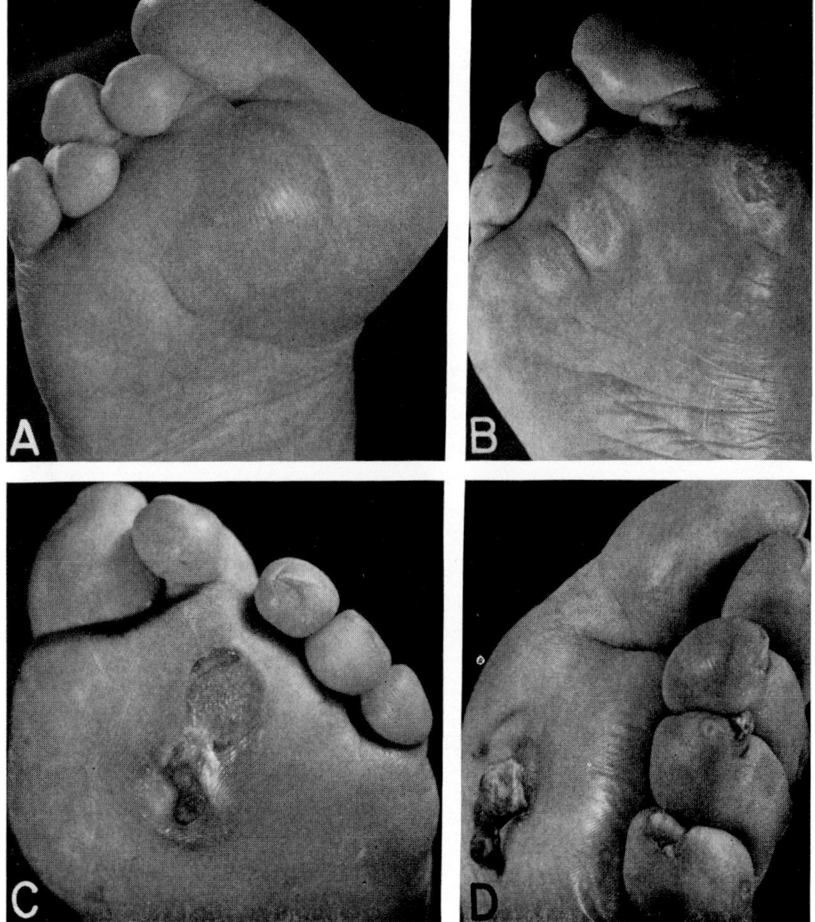

Figure 5–22. Plantar prominence of the area under the central metatarsal heads, keratoses, and ulcers.

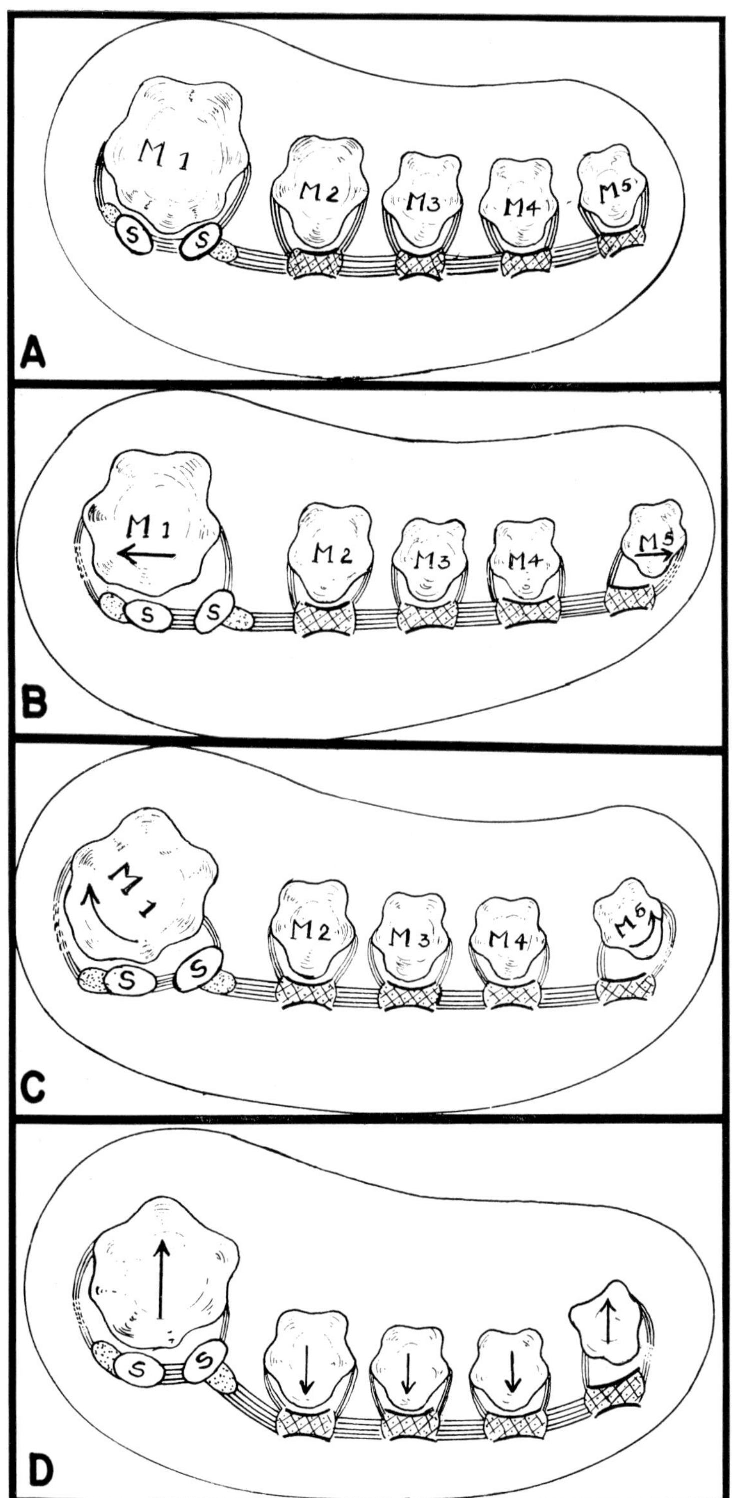

Figure 5–23. Relative shift of position of marginal metatarsal heads and the central capitalia. Deep transverse ligament and planter pads in relation to the overlying metatarsal heads (*A*). Marginal metatarsal heads have moved away from their immediate neighbors (*B*). Marginal metatarsals have rotated, the first medially, the fifth laterally (*C*). Marginal metatarsal heads have moved in a dorsal direction or what amounts to the same, the central capitalia have shifted plantarward (*D*); the medial collateral ligament of the first metatarsophalangeal joint and lateral collateral ligament of the fifth are shown stretched.

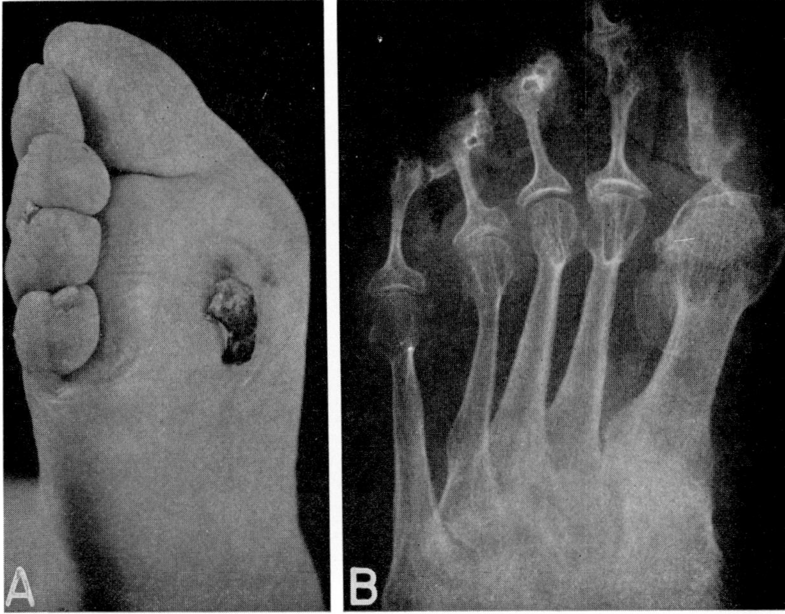

Figure 5–24. Long-standing plantar keratosis and retracted toes. Note the atrophy of the phalangeal bones.

REFERENCES

Annandale, T.: *The Malformations, Diseases and Injuries of the Fingers and Toes.* Philadelphia, J. B. Lippincott Co., 1866, pp. 110–127.

Broca, P.: Des difformités de la partie antérieure du pied produite par l'action de la chaussure. Bull. Soc. Anat. *27*:60–67, 1852.

Camper, P.: *On the Best Form of Shoe,* published with Dowie's treatise, *The Foot and Its Covering.* London, R. Hardwicke, 1861, pp. 1–44. The French version, called *Dissertation sur le Meilleur Forme des Souliers,* appeared in Paris, 1781.

Chaput, M.: Enorme bourse séreuse polykystique, hémorragique, développée sur un hallux valgus. Ablation. Résection de la tête métatarsienne. Ténopexie. Bull. Mem. Soc. Chir. *27*:769–770, 1901.

Clarke, J. J.: Hallux valgus and hallux varus. Lancet *1*:609–611, 1900.

Collins, W. J.: Hallux valgus and hammer toe. Lancet *2*:1028, 1899.

Cotton, F. J.: Foot statics and surgery. Tr. New Eng. Surg. Soc. *18*:181–208, 1935.

Grant, J. C. B.: *A Method of Anatomy.* Baltimore, Williams & Wilkins, 1958, p. 499.

Haines, R. W.: The mechanism of the metatarsals of spread foot. Chiropodist *2*:197–209, 1947.

Haines, R. W., and McDougall, A.: The anatomy of hallux valgus. J. Bone Joint Surg. *36*: 272–293, 1954.

Hauser, E.: *Diseases of the Foot.* 2nd Ed., Philadelphia, W. B. Saunders Co., 1950, pp. 92–125.

Hiss, J. M.: *Functional Foot Disorders.* Los Angeles University Press, 1937, pp. 263–294.

Hohmann, G.: *Fuss und Bein.* Munich, J. F. Bergmann, 1951, pp. 145–192.

Jones, F. W.: *Structure and Function as Seen in The Foot.* London, Baillière, Tindall & Cox, 1949, pp. 246–265.

Lake, N. C.: *The Foot.* London, Ballière, Tindall & Cox, 1952, pp. 233–256.

Lambrinudi, C.: Metatarsus primus elevatus. Proc. Roy. Soc. Med. *31*:1273, 1938.

Levick, G. M.: The action of the intrinsic muscles of the foot and their treatment by electricity. Brit. Med. J. *1*:381–382, 1921.

Levick, G. M.: On arch-raising rôle of certain intrinsic muscles of the foot. J. Anat. *67*:196–197, 1932.

McBride, E. D.: A conservative operation for bunion. J. Bone Joint Surg. *10*:735–739, 1928.

McElvenny, R. T.: A study of hallux valgus: its cause and operative management. Quart. Bull. Northw. Univ. Med. Sch. *18*:286–297, 1944.

Payr, E.: *Pathologie und Therapie des Hallux valgus.* Vienna Leipzig, Wilhelm Braumueller, 1894, pp. 1–77.

Riedel: Zur operativen Behandlung des Hallux valgus. Cbl. Chir. *44*:753–755, 1886.

Stein, H. C.: Hallux valgus. Surg. Gyn. Obst. *66*:889–898, 1938.

Chapter Six

EXAMINATION AND APPRAISAL

"The foot," said Lenox Baker (1953), "should have a thorough study and the operation should be directed to all correcting factors." He might have added: not only the foot, but the patient as a whole—the patient before the foot. There should be a clear understanding concerning the aim of surgery for hallux valgus. Is it to correct deformity or relieve pain? Is there metatarsalgia? Does the patient realize that correction of deviated great toe does not subdue plantar pain? What about hammered toes and pressure keratoses? Is the patient aware that on the average it takes 8 to 10 weeks to recover from most types of hallux valgus or hammertoe operations?

Some patients lack the stamina to go through a procedure that can be very painful the first few days. Patients often compare their slow recovery from foot surgery to relatively faster recuperation after other operations, especially abdominal. They may have to be reminded that postoperatively they did not walk on their bellies, and that weight-bearing in stance and ambulation add to the surgical trauma and retard the recovery. In addition there is the factor of relatively poor circulation of the toes as compared to the more central parts of the body.

Any surgeon who has operated on several hundred cases of hallux valgus will concede a percentage of failures. Patients should be warned of the possibility. They may also be given a hint of such common sequelae as swelling of the ankle and the leg, which follow any foot surgery, especially in elderly patients, more commonly in women than in men. At the same time, patients should not be unnecessarily alarmed; they must be assured that such complications are only temporary.

Beside emotional stability or lack of it, the surgeon ought to take into account the patient's age, occupation, and his general state of health. Advanced age by itself—without mental deterioration, cardiovascular disease, and other accompaniments of senility—does not contraindicate surgery. Perhaps because of mature ratiocination, stoicism, or limited activity, older patients tolerate radical surgical procedures better than young ones. A patient whose occupation necessitates long hours of standing or walking should not be subjected to resection of the main weight-bearing bones. Obese patients must be advised to reduce before surgery.

Naturally we would not resort to surgical correction of hallux valgus and related deformities of the forefoot in the presence of cardiovascular insufficiency, generalized arteriosclerosis, and severe diabetes. In the absence of circulatory disturbance of the foot itself, with adequate metabolic control, we do not, on the other hand, hesitate to correct deformed toes in moderate diabetics. In gouty patients we limit the surgery to such expedient procedures as evacuation of tophi, resection of calluses, bursectomy, and at most, excision of the medial eminence of the first metatarsal head.

The circulation of the foot. The most important preoperative examination of the foot is that directed toward ascertaining its circulatory state. Beside diabetes and generalized arteriosclerosis, one also thinks of thromboangitis obliterans. Varicose veins do not contraindicate surgery, but are better taken care of beforehand. Chronic thrombophlebitic states become aggravated after any foot operation.

Assessment of the arterial circulation of the foot is paramount. The toenails are tested for blanching and resumption of color. A more reliable blanching test is that of the pulp of the great toe. The base of the toe is pinched until its pulp becomes partly congested. The examiner then presses the tip of the top, releases the pressure, and watches the rate of return of pink hue. Tardy resumption of color suggests poor capillary circulation.

The two main arterial trunks—the dorsalis pedis and the tibialis posterior —are palpated. On the back of the foot the dorsalis pedis runs close to bone; it crosses the talonavicular and the naviculocuneiform joints. The best place to palpate the dorsalis pedis is over the second cuneiform just outside the long extensor tendon of the great toe. The foot should be placed at right angles to the leg. The examiner steadies his own hand by curling the thumb around the instep. The tips of his middle fingers seek the artery and gently compress it against the underlying bone. For palpation of the tibialis posterior, the examiner pivots his hand on the thumb. The fingers are placed proximal to the line joining the medial malleolus and the midpoint of the dome of the heel. The terminal segment of the posterior tibial artery lies about a finger's breadth behind the medial malleolus. It is best palpated by the third digit; being longer, this finger can locate the artery before it passes under the flexor retinaculum or the lancinate ligament. The foot should be inverted to relax the deep fascia of the leg, which covers the artery. An oscillometer, if available, may yield additional information (Figs. 6–1 and 6–2).

The hallux. Offhand, one observes the degree of outward deviation of the great toe and whether the hallux rides over or has slipped under the second digit. The plane of its nail is noted. If the nail slopes medially, valgus deformity is complicated with the axial rotation of the great toe, which means that the abductor hallucis has slipped under the first metatarsal head and the sesamoid pad has shifted fibularward. The quality of skin over the medial aspect of the first metatarsophalangeal joint is noted. When there has been previous cellulitis and parchment-like attenuation of the integument on the medial side, the joint is better approached through a dorsal or interdigital incision.

It is important to ascertain the range of motion at the first metatarsophalangeal joint. The hallux must possess a measure of pressing-down power and there must at least be 30 degrees of extension. Limited mobility of the first metatarsophalangeal joint and crepitation suggest erosion of the articulating surfaces. Dorsal spurs overlying the first metatarsal head may at times be palpated. Pain in the region of the sesamoids and tenderness on pressure suggest arthritic involvement of these small bones. The full extent of degenerative joint changes is often not revealed even after roentgenographic study and sometimes not until the time of surgical exploration (Fig. 6–3).

Associated deformities. One should note the presence of pronation of the foot as a whole, widening of the transmetatarsal span, retraction and overriding of lesser digits, and pressure kera-

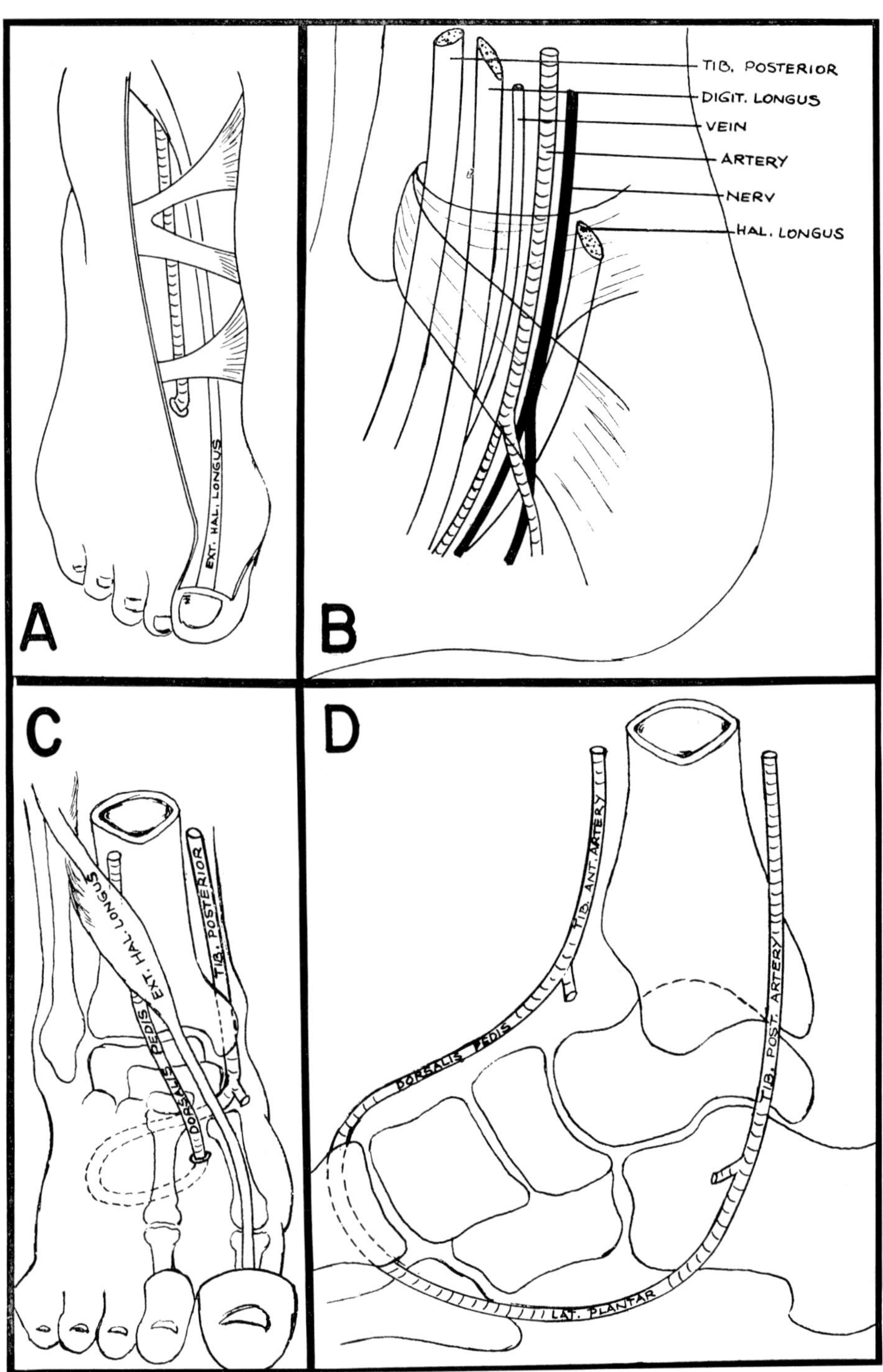

Figure 6–1. Dorsalis pedis and tibialis posterior arteries. These two vessels directly communicate with one another in the forefoot. Since their main trunks stem from the same vessel proximally, the leg and foot are provided with an arterial loop.

toses. Ingrown toenails and active fungus infections must be taken care of several months before surgery on bones. The same holds true of an infected draining bursa. The patient is asked to flex and extend his lesser toes. Active flexion is important, and there must again be something like 30 degrees of passive extension. Upward thrust against the plantarly prominent central metatarsal head should bring the corresponding toes down. If the toes do not yield, one must suspect fixed incarceration of the metatarsal heads. Side-to-side compression of the forefoot reveals if the splaying of the first and fifth metatarsals is functional or fixed. The patient is asked to bear weight on one foot; the spreading of the forefoot is noted (Fig. 6–4).

Roentgenographic study. Calcification of the walls of the main arterial trunks may sometimes be demonstrated in ordinary roentgenographs, but sclerotic vessels are better shown by soft tissue technique. Occasionally, in films taken after dorsoplantar exposure, the profunda branch of the dorsalis pedis will stand out as a "bull's eye" between the bases of the first and second metatarsals. Demonstrable sclerosis of the arteries of the foot contraindicates surgery (Fig. 6–5).

For adequate evaluation of the skeletal changes, three sets of x-ray films are taken: dorsoplantar and oblique views of the forefoot and axial exposure of the sesamoids. It may also be necessary to take similar exposures of the opposite foot for comparison. Two sets of dorsoplantar roentgenographs are taken: one with weight-bearing and another without. The two films are compared; when dry, they are superimposed. On the weight-bearing film widening of the first and fourth intermetatarsal spaces denotes dynamic splaying of the forefoot or hypermobile first and fifth metatarsal bones. One also looks for signs of arthritis involving the metatarsophalangeal joints. Indentation of the first metatarsal head suggests the presence of a sagittal groove. A comparatively short, undersized first metatarsal makes one suspect that this bone may not have been sustaining its share of body weight. Perhaps more significant is the thickening of the second metatarsal bone. In roentgenographs after dorsoplantar exposure one also notes rarefaction of the medial, non-

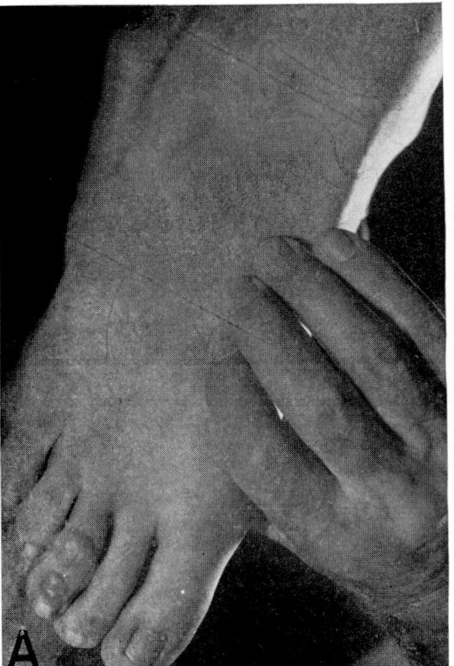

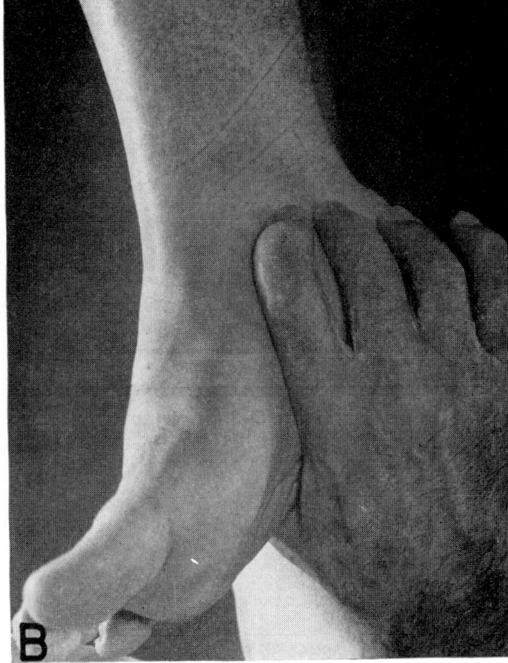

Figure 6–2. Palpation of dorsalis pedis and tibialis posterior arteries.

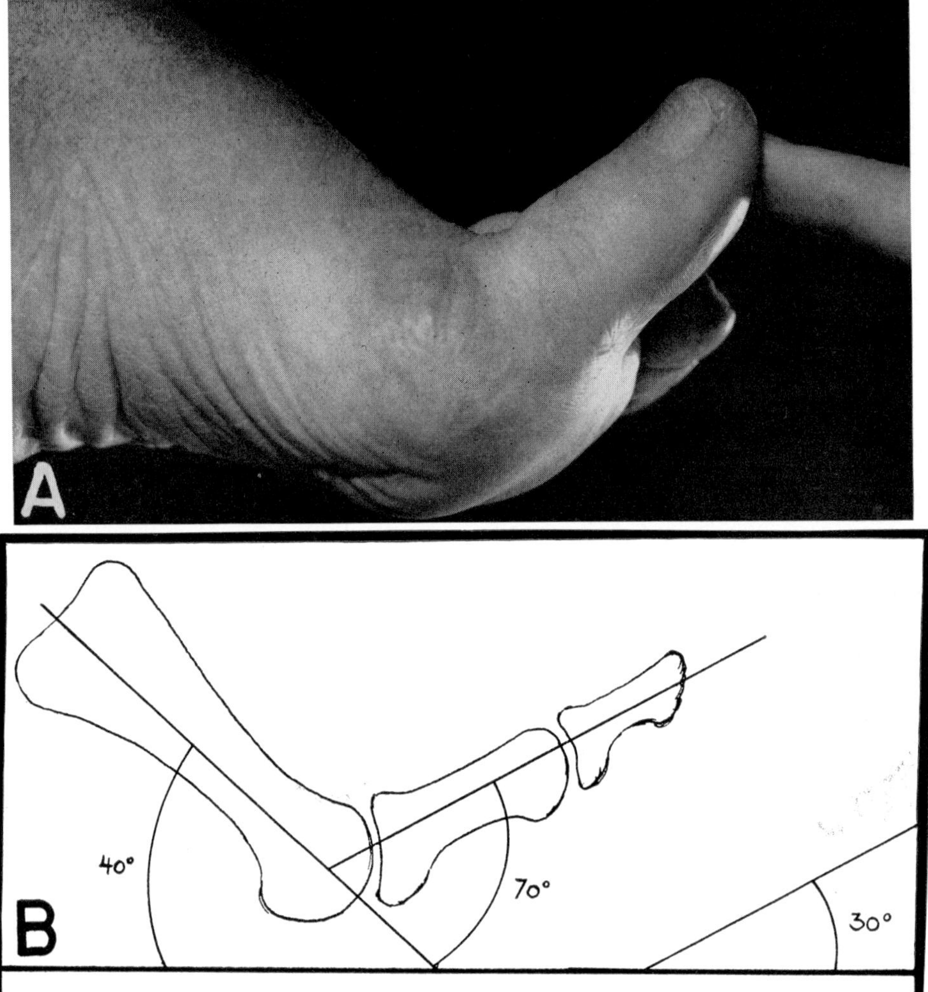

Figure 6–3. Accepted range of passive extension of the great toe.

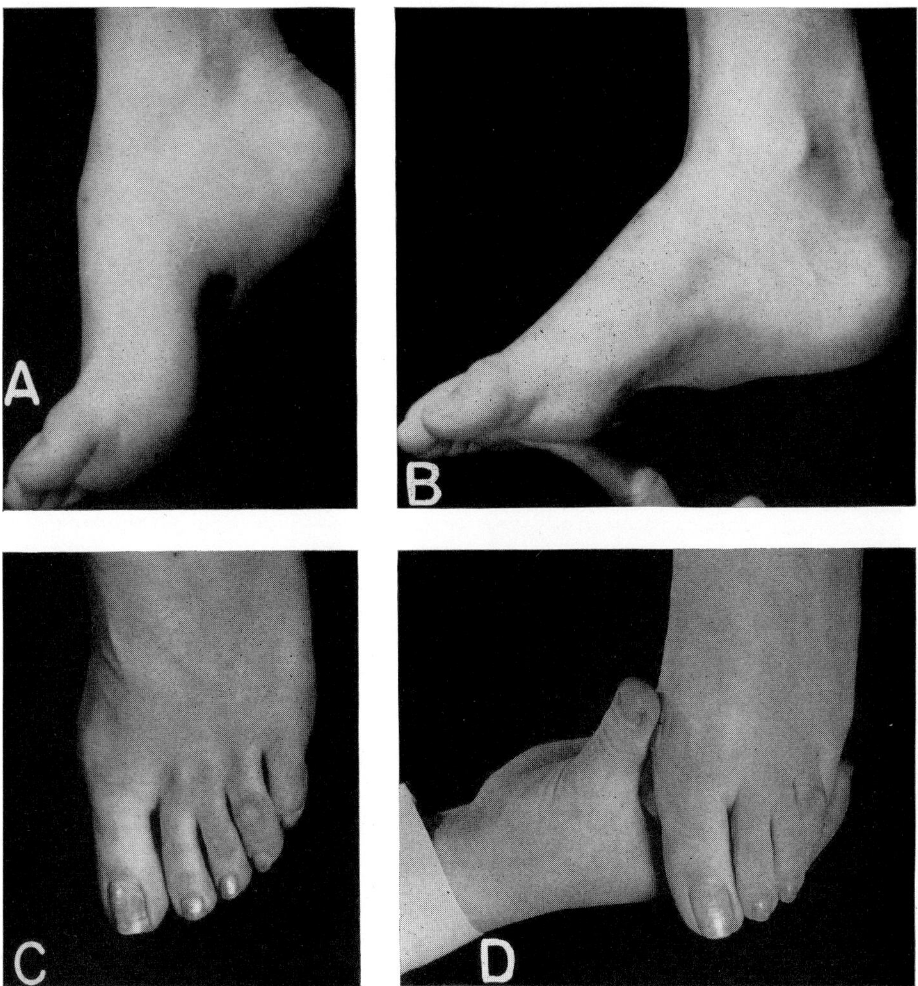

Figure 6–4. Tests to ascertain the resilience of the forefoot (*A* and *B*), and its compressibility (*C* and *D*).

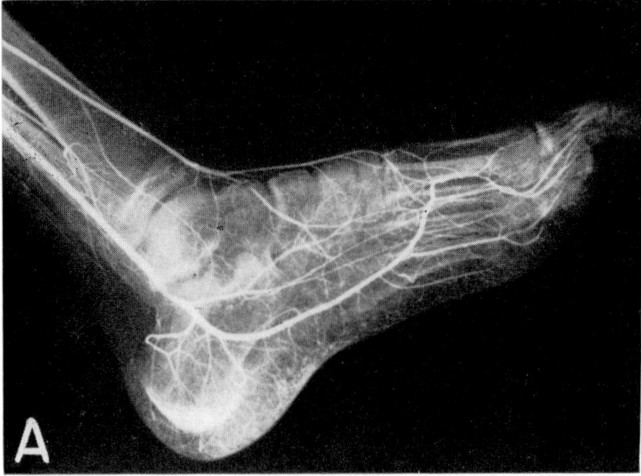

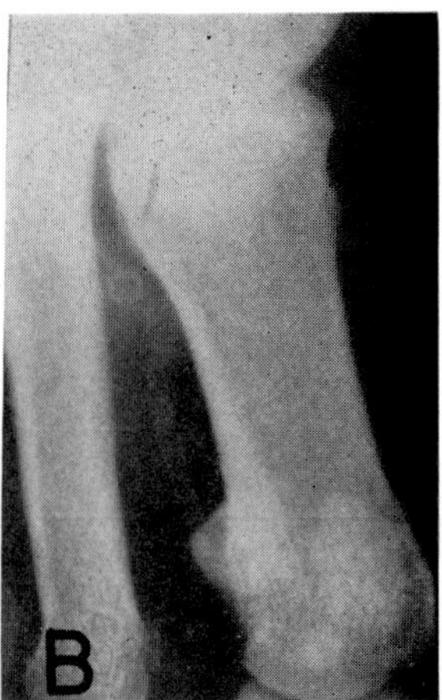

Figure 6–5. Circulatory disturbances. Arteriogram showing narrowing of the dorsalis pedis (*A*). Sclerosis of the artery connecting the dorsalis pedis with the lateral plantar branch of tibialis posterior (*B*).

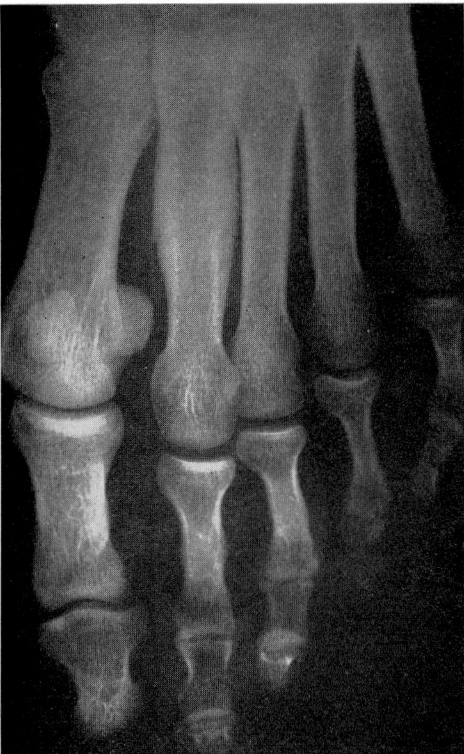

Figure 6–6. Stress hypertrophy of the second metatarsal in a case with short first metatarsal.

functioning part of the first metatarsal head. The translucence in this part of the bone may be diffuse or circumscribed; in the latter instance it is usually described as "cystic degeneration." One also observes fragmentation of the sesamoids: deviations of the lesser toes and dislocations of the metatarsophalangeal articulations (Figs. 6–6 to 6–15).

In oblique view roentgenographs, one particularly notes the relative plantar inclination of the metatarsal bones and the dorsal tilt of the proximal phalanges. The sesamoid bones are best visualized in films taken after axial or tangential exposure. Beside the outward displacement of the sesamoids and the effacement of the ridge (crista) on the undersurface of the first metatarsal head, the axial view gives added information about the fibular migration of the first plantar pad, osteochondritic changes involving the enclosed ossicles, and whether they are fragmented, mushroomed, or bipartite (Figs. 6–16 and 6–17).

Numerous attempts have been made to establish a norm and classify cases of hallux valgus according to the degree of deformity. From its base at the cuneometatarsal junction, the first metatarsal inclines slightly inward even in normal individuals. Between the first and second metatarsals there is always a measurable space. On dorsoplantar view roentgenographs, lines are traced through the long axes of the first and second metatarsals. When extended backward, these lines intersect and form an angle. Normally, in adults, this angle does not measure more than 8 degrees. Any measurement in excess of 10 degrees is considered indicative of varus

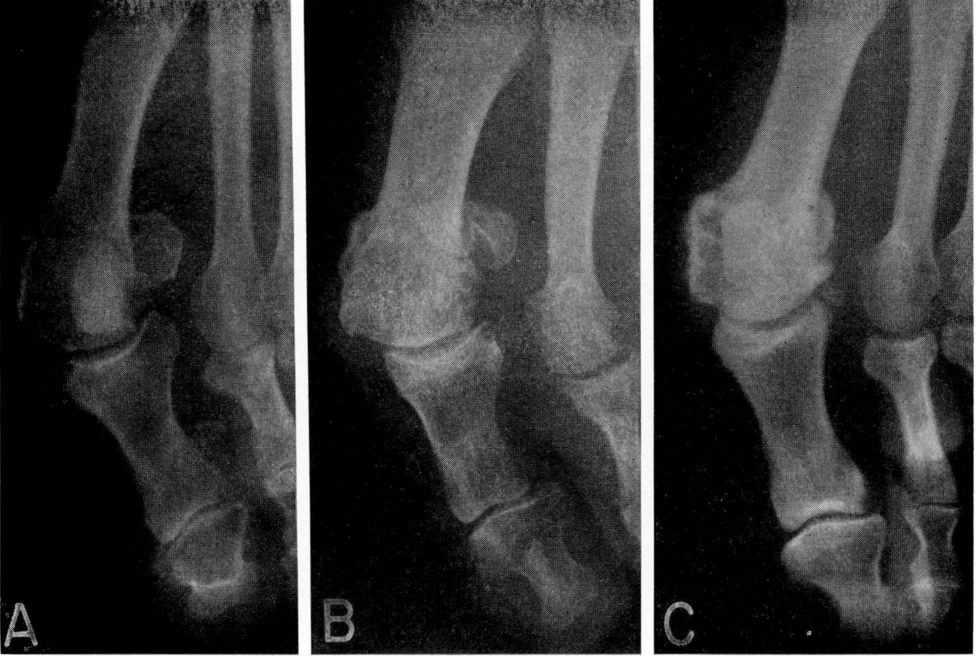

Figure 6–7. Squaring and sagittal groove of the metatarsal head. Note the ossicle in (*C*).

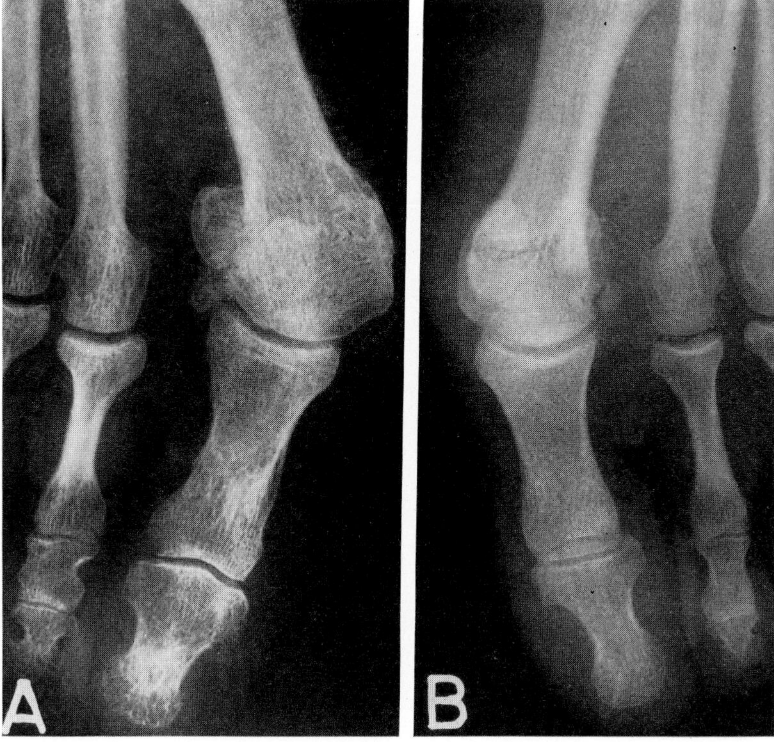

Figure 6–8. Seemingly detached ossicles in the lateral recess of the first metatarsophalangeal joint. Actually these pieces retain fibrous connections with either the metatarsal head or the lateral sesamoid.

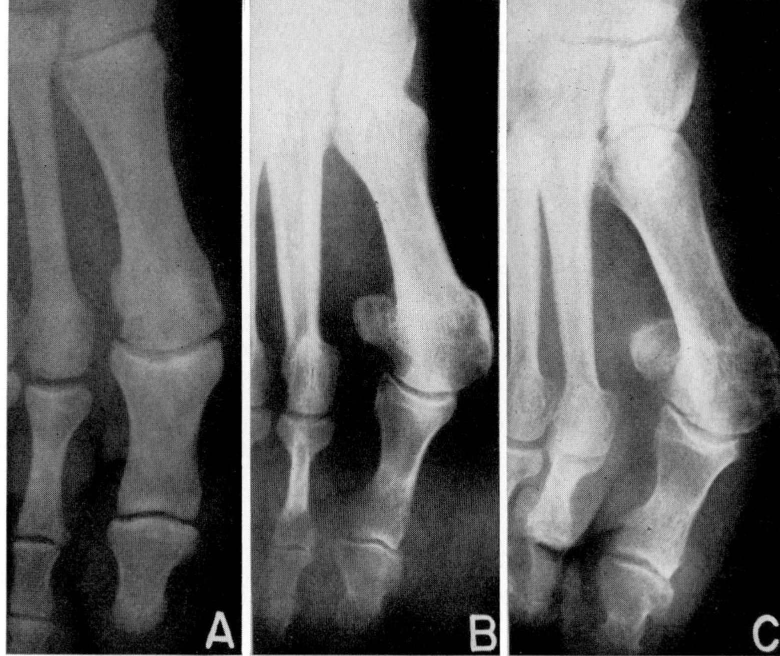

Figure 6–9. The articular cortex of the first metatarsal head. Normal configuration (*A*). Undulation (*B*). Notching (*C*).

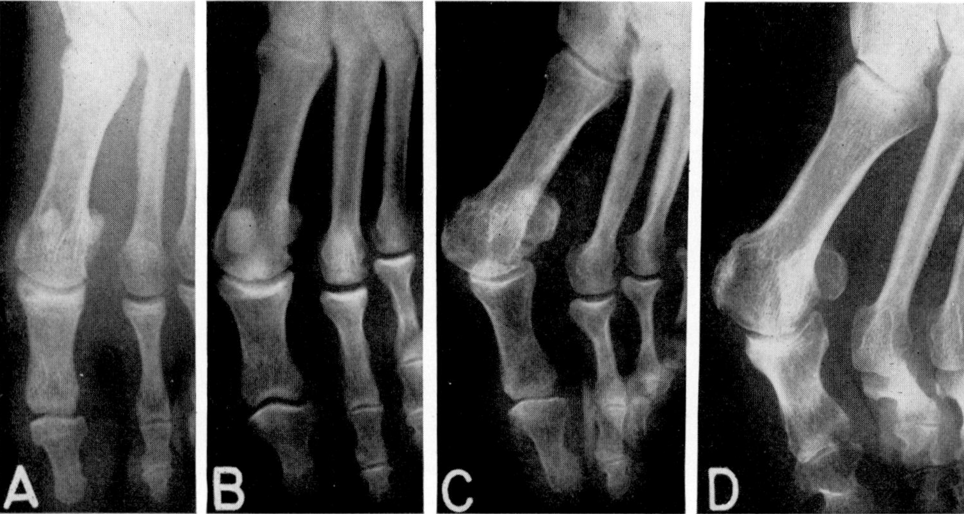

Figure 6–10. The first intermetatarsal space. In connection with metatarsus primus varus, this space would be wider were it not for the fact that in most cases the second metatarsal is also in varus position (*C* and *D*).

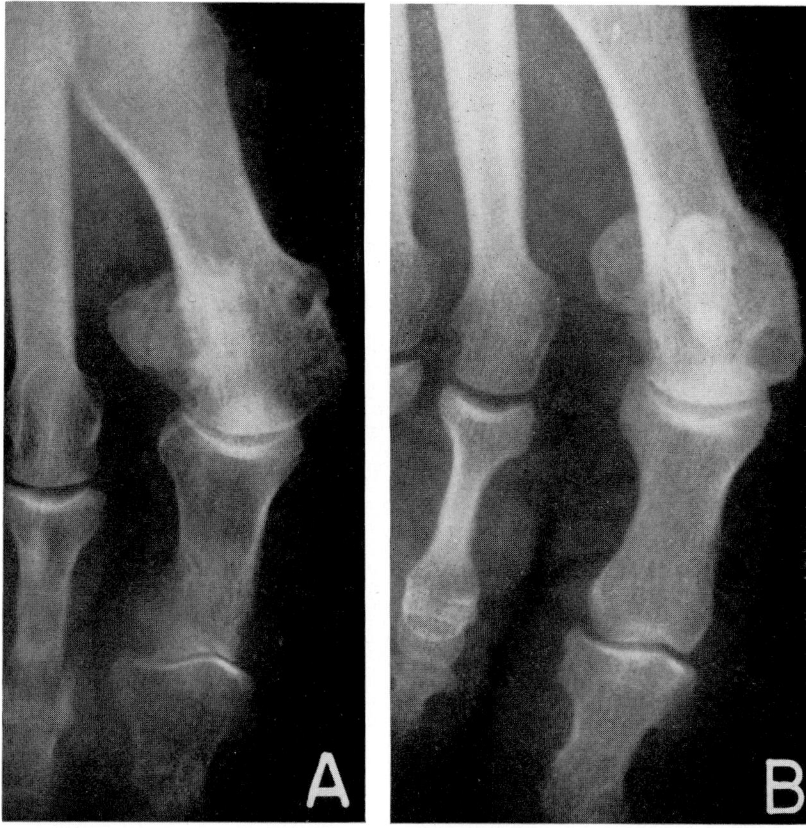

Figure 6–11. Radiolucent areas in the metatarsal head indicative of "cystic degeneration."

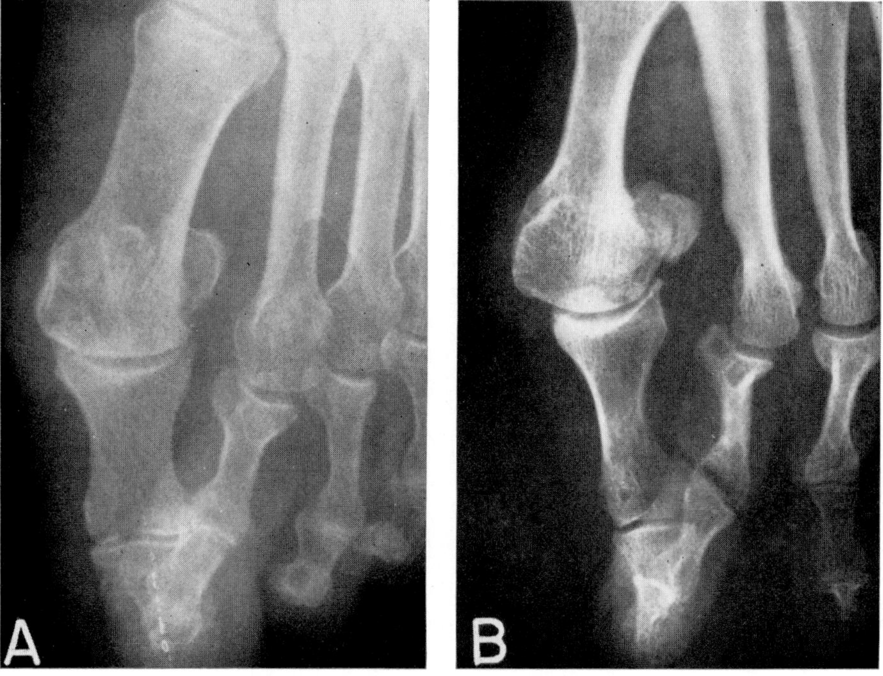

Figure 6–12. Medial subluxation of the second toe.

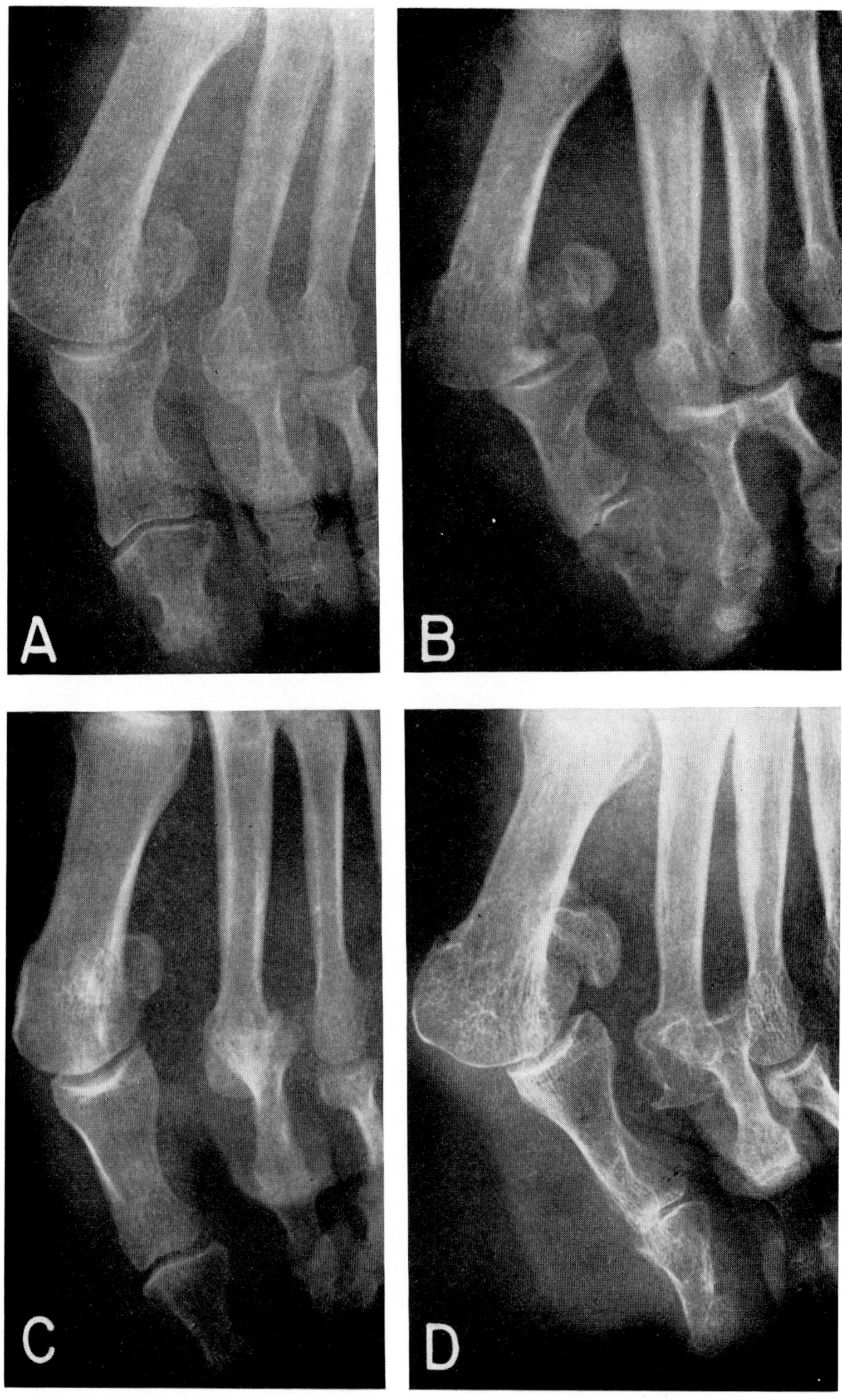

Figure 6–13. Lateral subluxation and dislocation of the second toe.

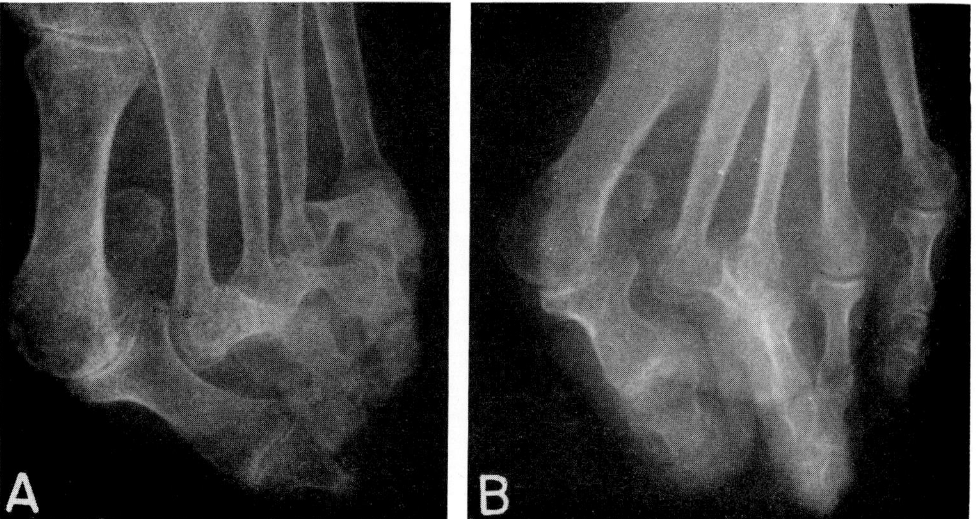

Figure 6–14. Multiple subluxations and deviations of the proximal phalanges.

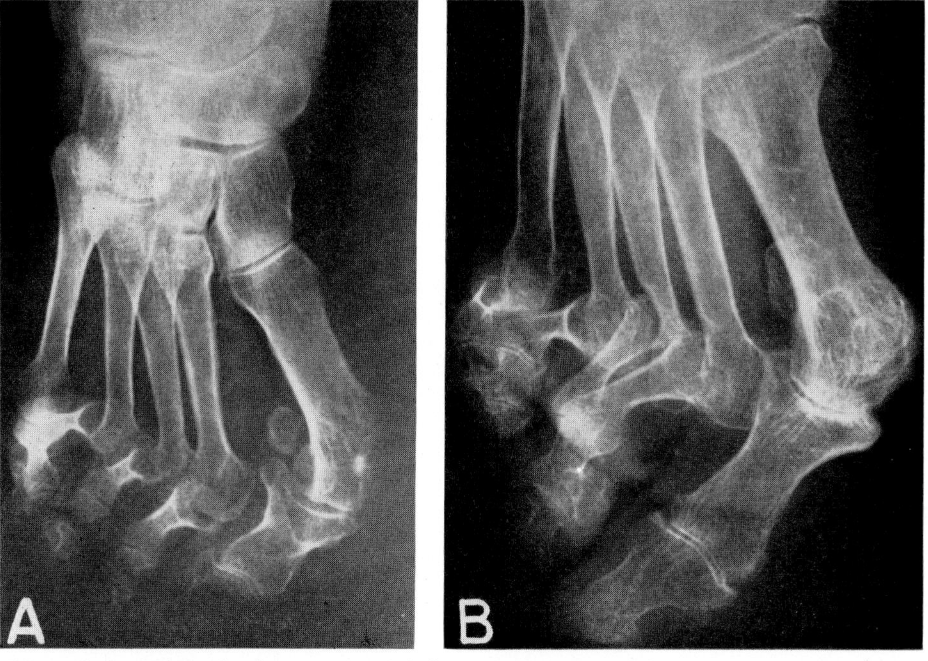

Figure 6–15. When the first metatarsal is in marked varus position and its head has not been subjected to intermittent pressure, the medial eminence will sometimes disappear (*A*). With use, in spite of marked varus, the head retains its globular shape and may even appear enlarged (*B*).

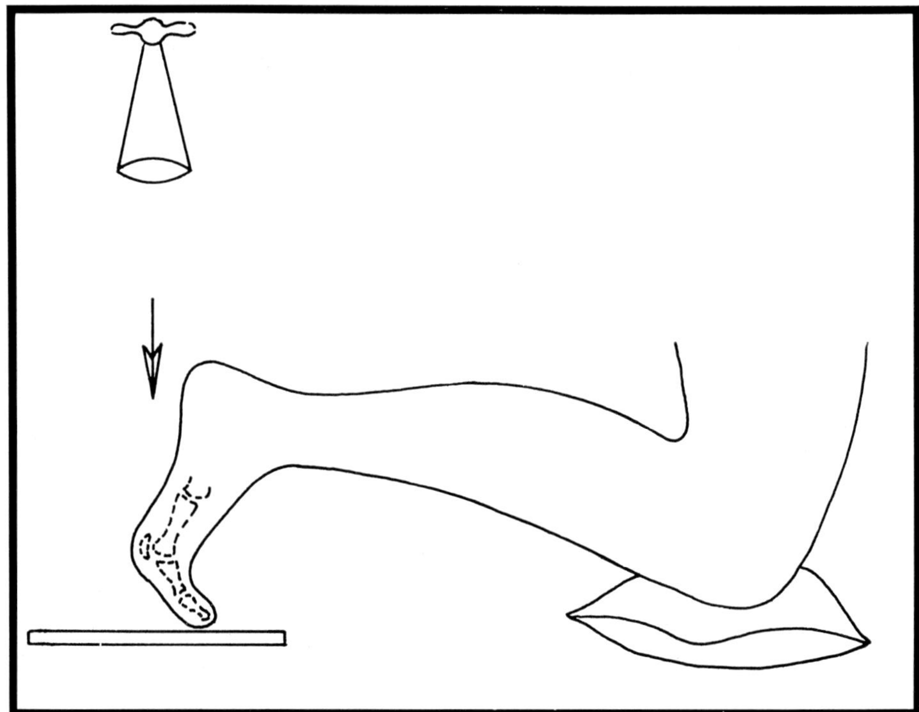

Figure 6–16. Roentgenographic technique for axial view of the sesamoids.

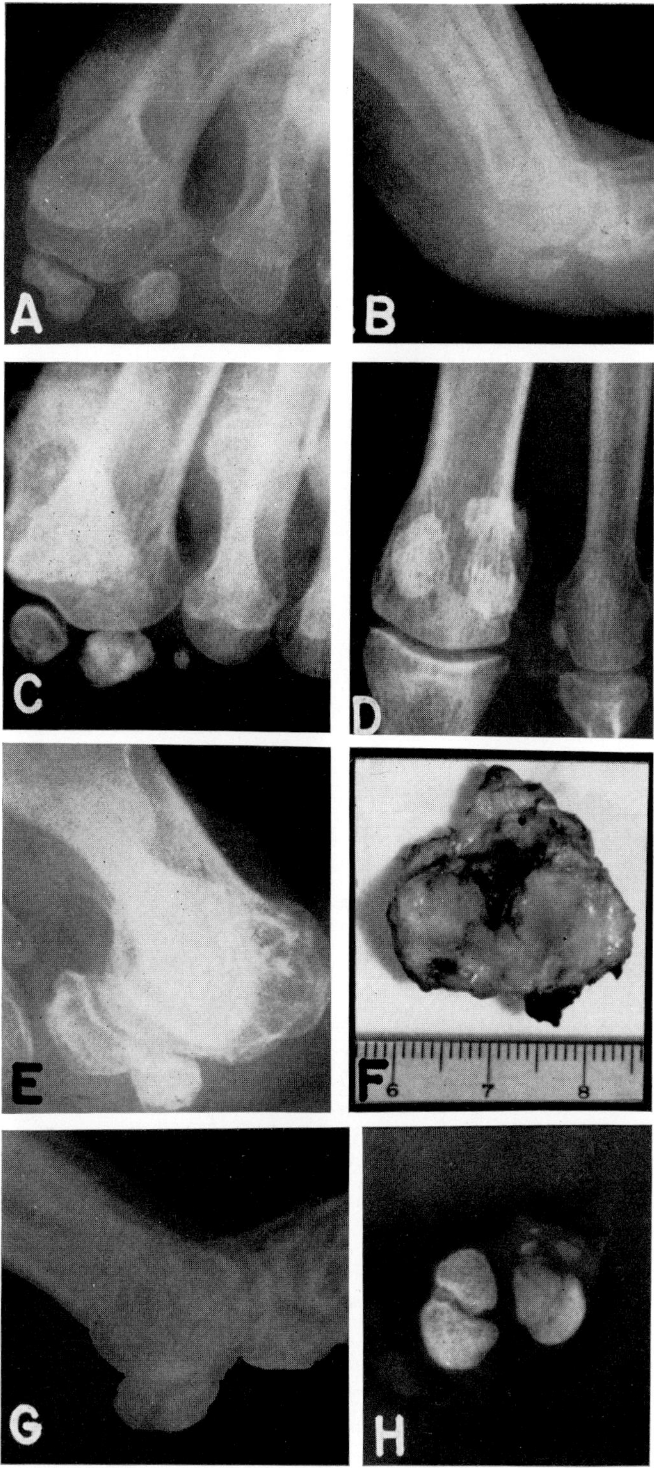

Figure 6–17. The sesamoid bones. Double medial sesamoid (*A* and *B*). Bipartite lateral sesamoid (*C* and *D*). Mushrooming (*E* and *F*). Split medial sesamoid (*G*). Sesamoid pad removed surgically (*H*).

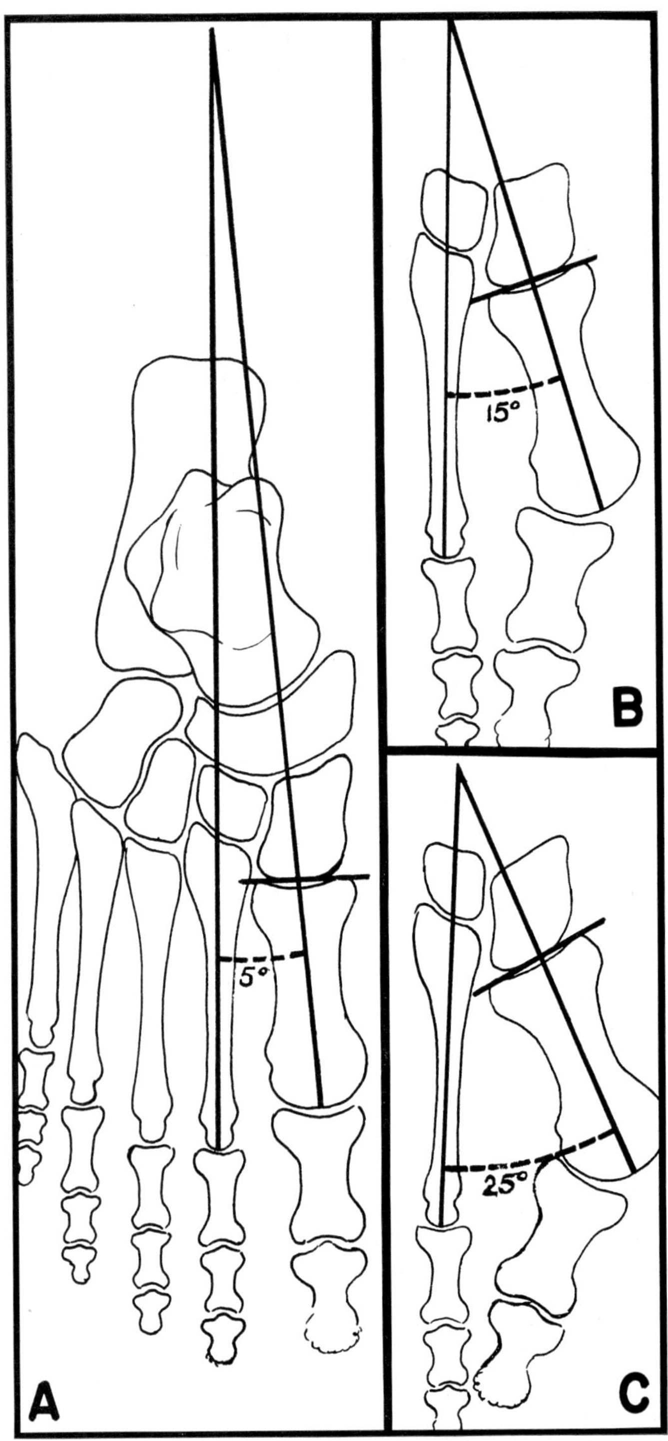

Figure 6–18. Measurements to ascertain the degree of varus of the first metatarsal.

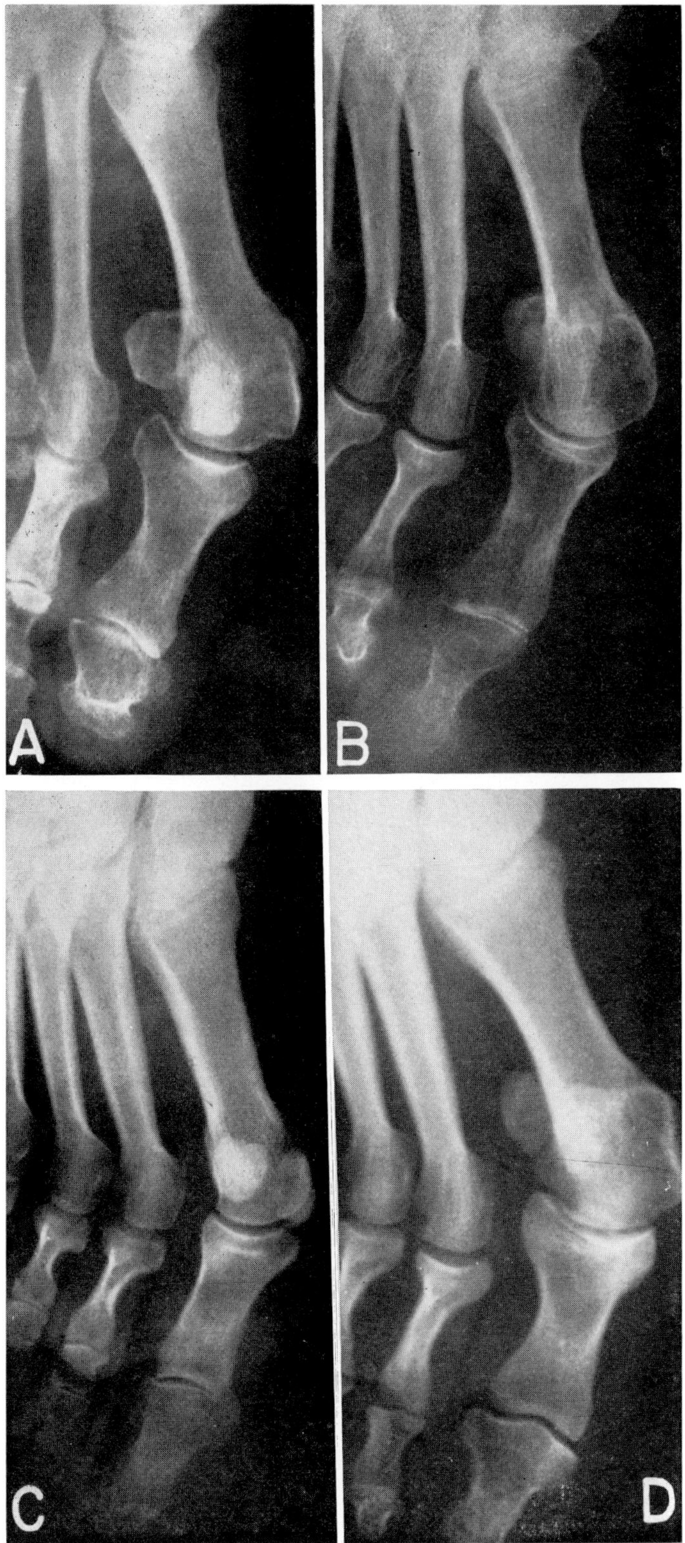

Figure 6–19. The orthodox method of determining the degree of varus of the first metatarsal cannot be considered valid in cases where the second metatarsal also inclines medially.

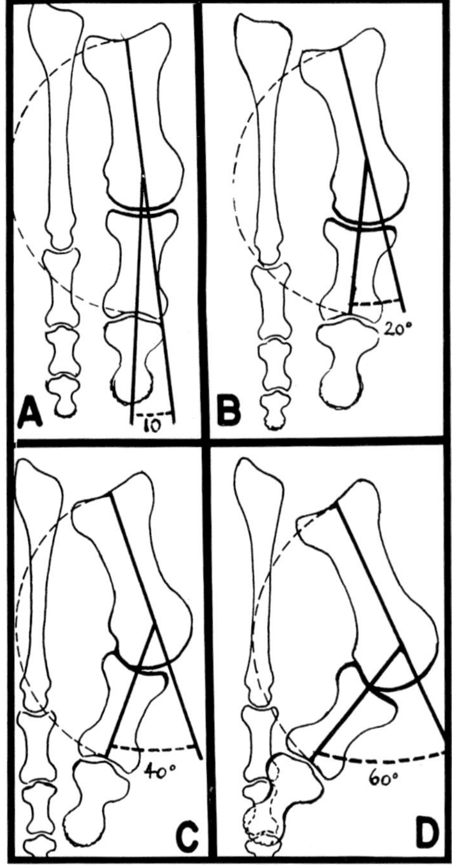

Figure 6–20. Measurements of the degree of valgus of the proximal phalanx of the great toe.

deformity of the first metatarsal. One must not overlook the varus inclination of the second metatarsal, which is more common than is generally suspected. Obviously, the measurement is smaller if the second metatarsal is also inclined inward (Figs. 6–18 and 6–19).

In ascertaining grades of valgus deformity of the great toe itself, the lines representing the long axis of the first metatarsal and of the proximal phalanx are utilized. When extended, these lines form an angle, which opens anteriorly. Owing to a slight medial inclination of the first metatarsal and the deviation of the proximal phalanx in opposite direction, this angle normally measures about 8 to 10 degrees. Any measurement exceeding this amount is considered indicative of hallux valgus; 20 degrees is taken for mild, 30 for moderate, and 40 or more for marked hallux valgus. Increment of lateral deviation of the terminal phalanx at the interphalangeal joint is not taken into consideration in this measurement (Figs. 6–20 and 6–21).

Piggott (1960) distinguished three patterns in the relationship of the articular facets of the proximal phalanx and the metatarsal bone at the first metatarsophalangeal joint. In the first, the two articular surfaces are completely congruous—their central points are opposite each other. In the second, the two surfaces are parallel to one another. In the third, the base of the proximal phalanx has subluxated laterally. These types are respectively referred to as congruous, deviated, and subluxated. The last two usually coexist (Fig. 6–22).

Classification of hallux valgus. This deformity is usually spoken of as being mild, moderate, marked, and severe. From a surgical point of view the following is perhaps a more practical classification:

1. Simple hallux valgus
   A. Without sagittal groove
   B. With sagittal groove
2. Hallux with axial rotation
   A. Reducible
   B. Irreducible
3. Hallux valgus with metatarsus primus varus
   A. Mobile or hypermobile first metatarsal
   B. Fixed varus
4. Hallux valgus with degenerative arthritis of the joint
5. Hallux valgus with mixed deformities

In simple hallux valgus, the outward deviation is not accompanied by axial rotation of the great toe; metatarsus primus varus is negligible. Initially there is no roentgenographic evidence of a sagittal groove dividing the articular surface of the metatarsal head into lateral or "functioning" and medial "nonfunctioning" parts—the portion of the head still in contact with the base of the proximal phalanx from the part that has slipped medially. Axial rotation of the hallux—eversion, pronation—denotes displacement of the abductor hallucis from the medial aspect of the first metatarsal head to down under it, and lateral migration of the sesamoid pad. If the

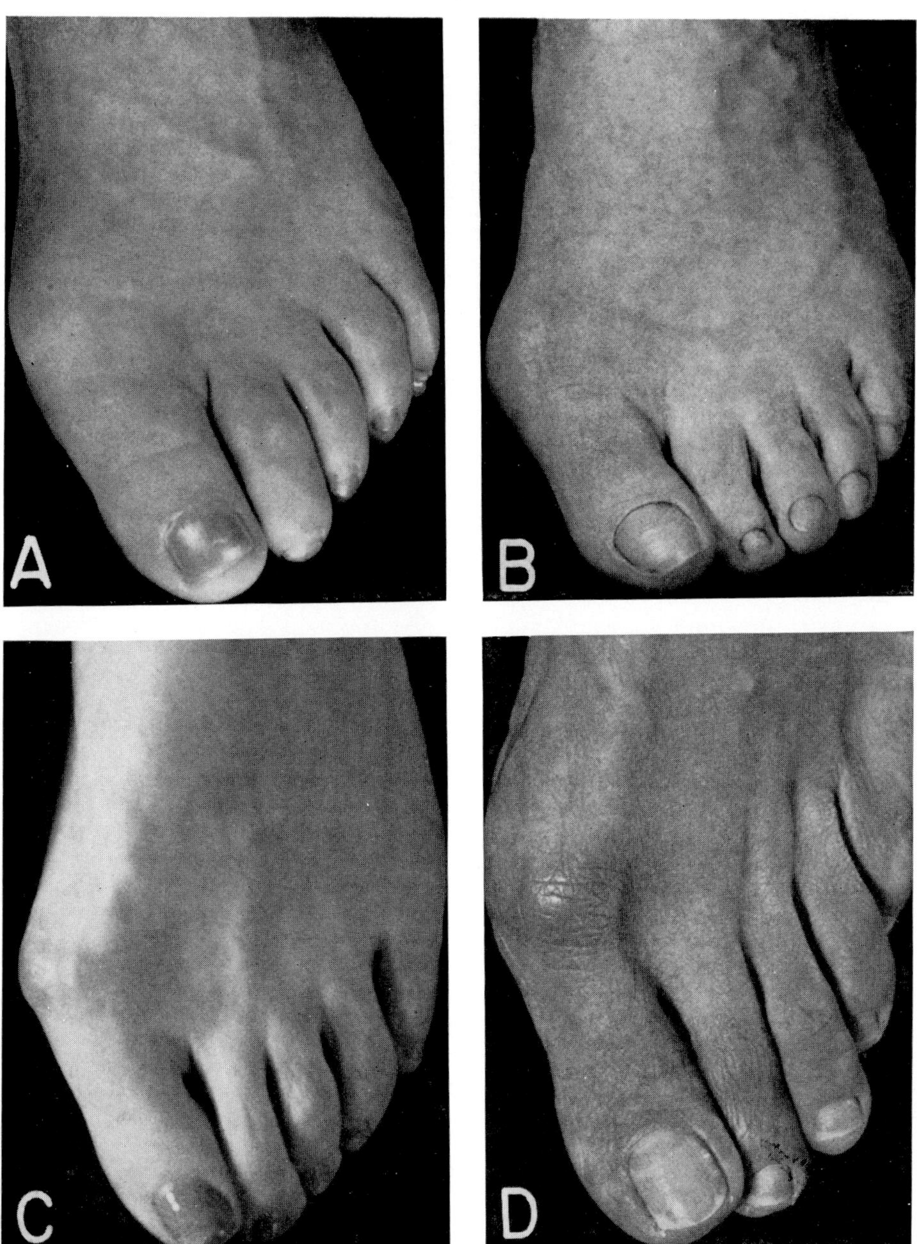

Figure 6–21. Grades of hallux valgus.

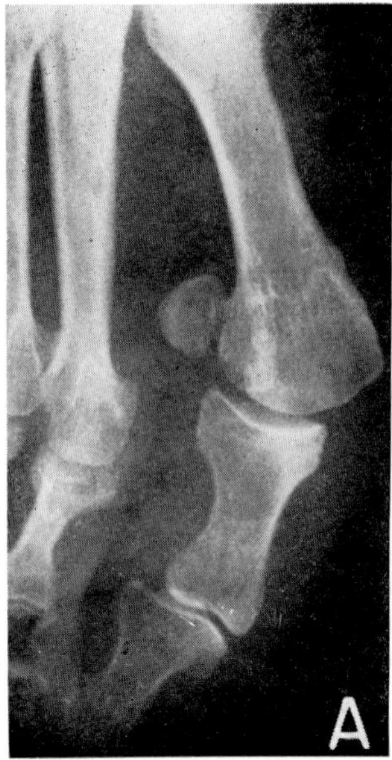

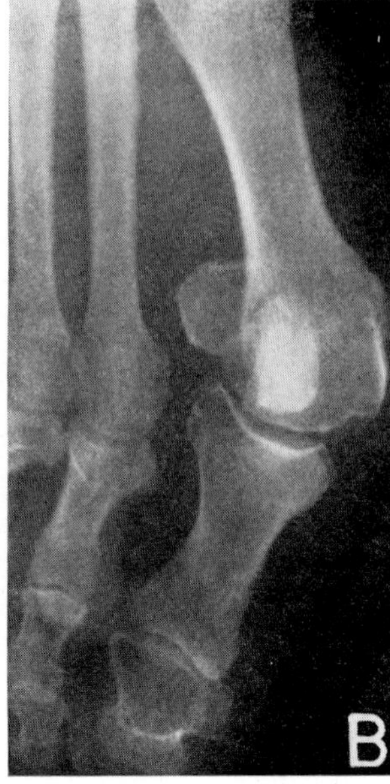

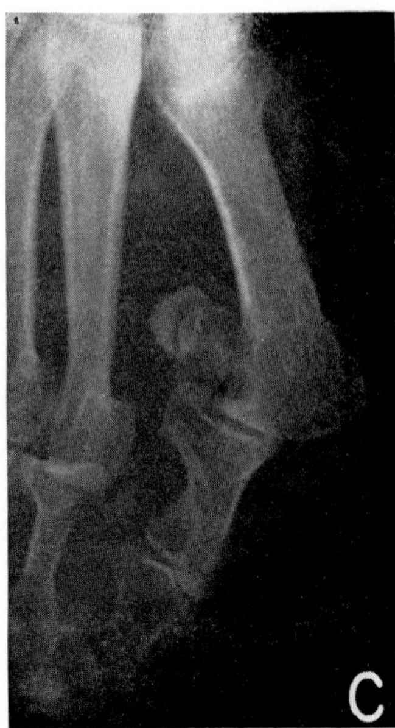

Figure 6–22. Congruous (*A*), deviated (*B*), and subluxated (*C*) joint in hallux valgus.

toe can passively be derotated, the shift of position of the sesamoid pad is reversible. Metatarsus primus varus may likewise be dynamic or fixed. There are various degrees of arthritis. The important point to determine is whether the hallux can be pushed into extension painlessly when the patient rises on his toes as in the take-off phase of walking. In more advanced cases of hallux valgus, outward deviation and axial rotation of the great toe, metatarsus primus varus, osteoarthritis of the joint, deformities of lesser toes, corns, and keratosis coexist.

Varieties of forefoot splaying. The following may serve as a useful classification:

1. Dynamic splaying
   A. Side-to-side spread of the forefoot—metatarsus latus
   B. Reducible plantar bulge of the central metatarsal heads
2. Fixed incarceration of the central metatarsal heads.

Side-to-side splaying is seen mainly in adolescents and young adults with hypermobile marginal metatarsals. These two bones spread out sideways under the body weight—the first metatarsal goes into an exaggerated varus position and the fifth into a valgus position. The hallux may deviate in a lateral direction and the small toe assumes a varus position. The central toes are not hammered or clawed; the heads of the middle metatarsals show no plantar bulge. The patient complains mainly of chafing of the area over the medially displaced first or laterally bulging fifth metatarsal head. In dynamic plantar bulge, the central metatarsal heads may be palpated on the sole of the forefoot, but yield to upward thrust, an indication of intact flexibility at the metatarsophalangeal joints. Fixed incarceration of the central metatarsal heads is characterized by rigidity of the forefoot as a whole, clawing of toes, plantar keratosis, and even ulcers.

REFERENCES

Baker, L. D.: Diseases of the foot. Am. Acad. Orthop. Surgeons *10*:327–343, 1953.

Piggott, H.: The natural history of hallux valgus in adolescence and early adult life. J. Bone Joint Surg. *42*:749–760, 1960.

Chapter Seven

PALLIATIVE MEASURES

Early authors did not make a distinction between corns, calluses, and bunions. Theodorice (1267), the Bishop of Cervia, considered a corn "calloused flesh" that "should be excavated all around, and then extirpated down to its roots with forceps, or scissors or some other instrument. Afterwards the spot should be cauterized and cared for until it heals." Wiseman (1676) advised paring the corn and applying red, soft wax. An unnamed author who chose to call himself *An Experienced Chiropodist* (1818) advised "application of cataplasm of oatmeal and ground linseed, renewed twice a day, until inflammation subsides." He thought this would prepare the "bunnion (sic) for a more convenient extraction. . . . To cut the corn to the quick," he said, "is not to cure it."

Dorsey (1818) wrote: "When the corn is covered with a mass of thickened cuticle, the foot should be soaked in warm water, and this cuticle pared off. A very excellent mode of defending the corn from the pressure of the shoe, when the patient walks, is to spread several small pieces of leather with adhesive plaster; in the center of these leather strips, a hole is to be cut rather larger than the corn. They are to be applied successively over the toe or foot in such a manner that the corn shall be surrounded by the leather, and the shoe will then press upon the leather, the corn remaining untouched. When situated on the sole of the foot, a felt or cork sole should be worn with a hole cut in it opposite to the corn."

For the painful bunion, Aston Key (1836) prescribed the following treatment: "The offending toe is placed in a separate compartment of the stocking, like the finger of a glove: this again is enclosed in a separate part of the shoe, which is contrived by fixing a piece of firm cow-leather in the sole of the shoe so as to form a separate apartment for the toe."

In a book called *Domestic Medicine, or Poor Man's Friend,* Gunn (1837) had this to say about corns: "To get rid of them in the shortest possible time, bathe the foot or feet well in warm water, about half an hour before going to bed. When the corns have become soft from bathing, shave down the horny parts smooth, but not so close to produce blood; then moisten the tops of them with spittle, and rub over them a little lunar caustic, which you can easily procure. This caustic must be gently rubbed on, until a sufficiency of it sticks on the corns to change them first to a dark gray color and next to a deep black. Put a little cotton over them, to prevent the stocking from rubbing them, and in a few days they will come out by the root. . . ."

For what we now call *bunionette,* Durlacher (1845) prescribed the following treatment: "If the bunion has been some years in existence, is covered with thickened cuticle, and studded with corns, the cuticle should be removed, the corn extracted, and soap plasters worn constantly over the joint. Much benefit will be derived from wearing latterly, between the little toe and the projecting point, a piece of buckskin leather spread with adhesive plaster and cut to form a semicircle, of sufficient thickness to keep off the pressure of the shoe from the part."

"The cure of callosities and corns requires, above all things," Chelins (1847) wrote, "the removal of pressure from tight shoes and even from tight stockings. . . . If the corn be upon the sole of the foot, a felt sole must be worn, with a hole in it to receive the corn."

Corns, calluses, and bunions were thus "excavated," "extracted," "cauterized," rubbed with "lunar caustic," "cut to the quick," and protected by pressure pads and plasters.

In his *Practice of Surgery,* Miller (1852) designated five groups of *bunion:* chafing of the skin by the shoe, adventitious bursa, suppurative bursitis, bony enlargement, and joint displacement. The key word in the treatment prescribed was "palliated." Skin irritation was treated by "abstraction of the cause," meaning elimination of badly fitting footwear; by rest and fomentation; and by "subsequent light use of the nitrate of the silver, or solution of the iodine." Acute bursitis was allayed by "antiphlogistics"; "discutient" drugs were prescribed for chronic cases; to equalize the pressure by the shoe, "a thin caoutchouc envelope" was applied. Suppurative bursitis was allowed to become fistulous; "piece of potass" was inserted into the sinus to destroy the "cyst." Afterwards, the granulating sore was "brought to heal under the ordinary means"—rest and simple applications. Bunions of the "aggravated class," characterized by "enlargement of osseous texture," were occasionally blistered, but in general "palliated by able adjustment of the shoe." In the final group belonged cases with partial displacement at the joint, as seen in "the rheumatic and gouty adult, with the toe riding over its fellows and pointing to the outer side of the foot. This, too, is palliated," Miller wrote. He suggested no surgical treatment.

The thinking of the next two decades was tinged by the naturalistic philosophy of the anatomist, Hermann Meyer (1858), who was, as has been noted, an arch crusader against shoes dictated by fashion. It was his contention that deformities of the toes, including those of the hallux, were caused by ill-fitting shoes. "If the great toe is inclined obliquely inward (sic) towards the others," Cleaveland (1862) wrote, "a piece of sponge, or a pledget made with tape . . . of sufficient thickness, should be placed between the great toe and the one next to it so as to bring it in its natural position parallel with the other toes and with the bones of the foot."

Hermann Meyer's American disciple, Peck (1871), drew the inference from the master's writing that toes that were not badly distorted would gradually resume correct position in a shoe with plenty of room. But what about already established deformities? Here again, it was reasoned that if the foot were pliable, removal of external pressure that caused its "wrong shape" would in time allow a return to a "natural shape." To correct the deformity of the great toe, which we now call hallux valgus, a separator was devised. It was fashioned from a strip of "thick tin covered neatly with cloth or with a piece of thin sheepskin or kid leather." It was fastened to the "exact place" on the insole.

The section dealing with this subject in Peck's book was captioned, "How Distorted Great Toe Can Be Straightened." There was a note of overconfidence, both in this title and throughout the discussion that followed. Peck's toeseparator ushered in an era of mechanical contrivances: one ingenious gadget vied with the other. There was Krohn's lever, Bigg's bunionspring, Holden's toepost, Seyre's linen glove stocking, Pitha's sandal, Lothrop's cot, and sundry other contraptions. Each appliance had its ardent advocate and its period of popularity. In due time they were all discarded.

This is not to say that the age of mechanical appliances is over. We have our own bunion shields, pads, and plasters, straps, insoles, and bars. Present-day pressure doughnuts are reminiscent of Miller's "caoutchouc envelope"; gum rubber or synthetic interdigital inserts may be regarded as the direct—somewhat more humane—descendants of Peck's toeseparator or Holden's toepost. Like Miller, in some instances, we too advise suitable adjustment of the shoe—the creation of a stall to comfortably pocket the knuckled joint. We are also in sympathy with Meyer's crusade against the dictates of fashion and would like to see shoes with straighter inner lasts and roomy toe boxes. But we concede—which Meyer would not—that human vanity is far too strong to be subdued with a pamphlet. We do the best we can to repair the ravages of fashion by surgery or prescribe our own brand of corrective shoes, bars, pads, props, and plates. We use these appliances as necessary makeshifts or supplements to surgery and not as substitutes (Figs. 7–1 and 7–2).

In passing we should perhaps say a word about physical therapy. Functional exercises of the toes, especially the hallux, have been recommended by some—in particular by German authors. Thomsen (1944) wrote a book with extensive discussions about exercises to mobilize the toes and correct already established deformities. This book also contains a large section on corrective shoes and supplementary appliances.

"To strengthen the muscles we use exercises of the toe," Hohmann (1951) wrote. He recommended flexion of the toe against resistance with the aid of a strap and pulley arrangement. It was hoped that strengthened flexors would eventually overcome the taut extensors. "The closer to right angle the foot is

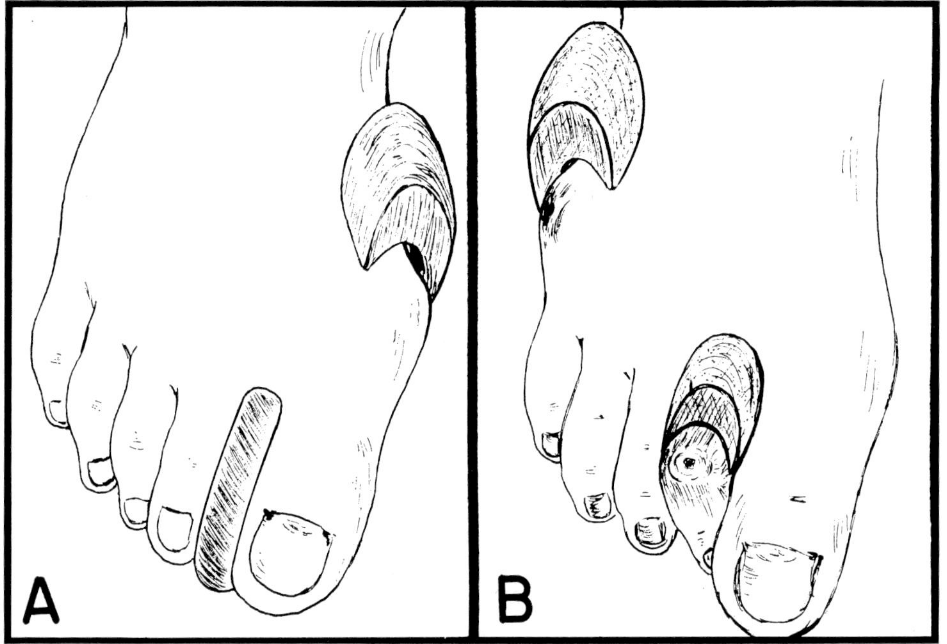

Figure 7–1. Protective pad and interdigital insert for hallux valgus (*A*). Protective pads for hammered toe and bunionette (*B*).

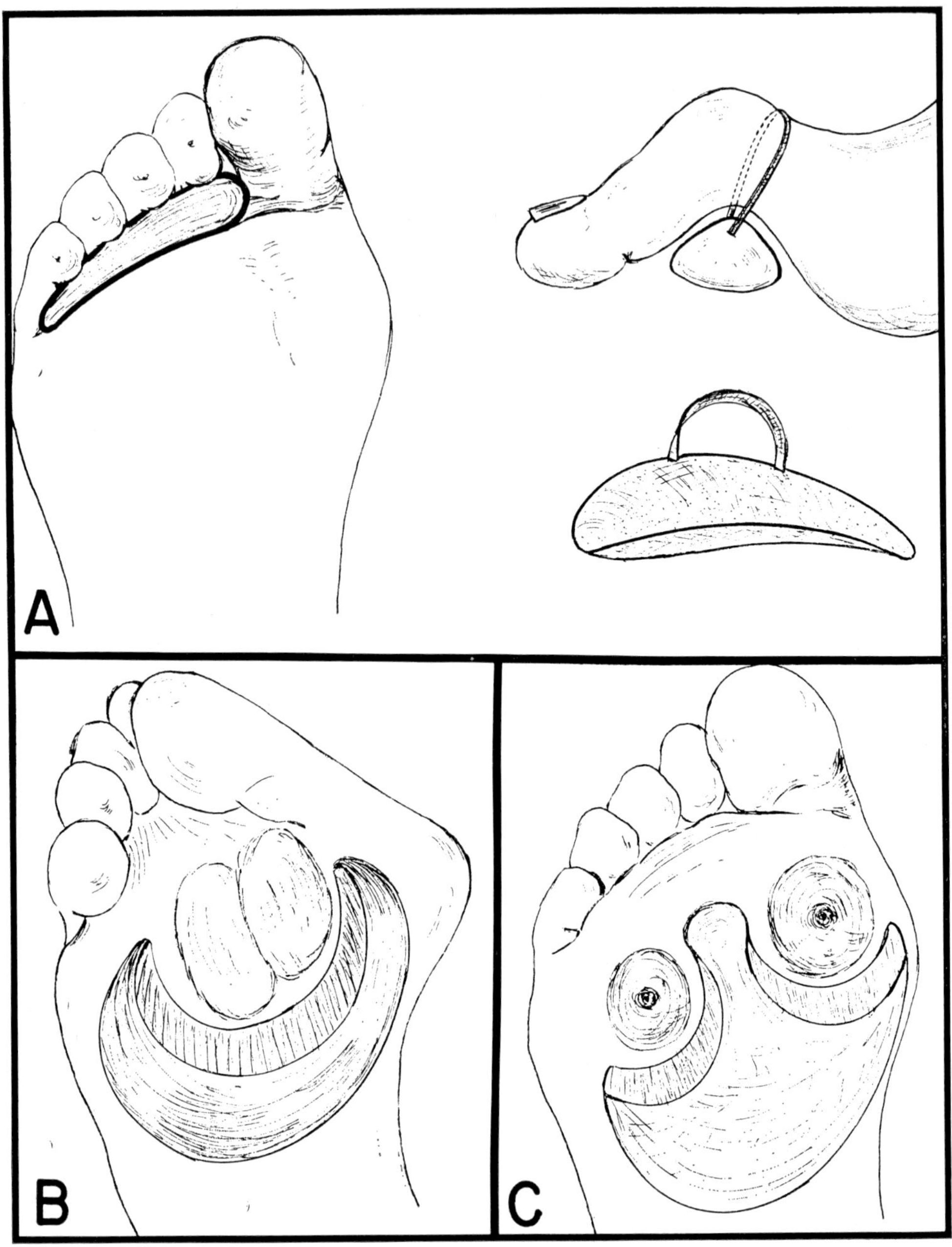

Figure 7–2. Plantar pad to help the toes establish a fixed point from which the flexor tendons can act and lift the metatarsal heads (*A*). Protective pads for plantar keratoses (*B*).

held at the ankle during this exercise," Hohmann continued, "the more efficient will be the flexion (of the toe). Gripping with the toes has also its place. We try to strengthen the muscles of the sole with vigorous massage." Postoperatively Joplin (1964) recommends "toe-curling" exercises.

It is difficult to evaluate the actual benefit derived from physiotherapy. Flexion exercises of the toes are important; if judiciously followed they will often ameliorate metatarsalgia due to reducible plantar protrusion of the central metatarsal heads. All one can say about massage is that, except in infected cases, it can do no harm and may perhaps help.

REFERENCES

Chelins, J. M.: *A System of Surgery* (Tr. from German by J. F. South). Edinburgh, Malachlin, Stewart & Co., Dublin, Fannin & Co., 1847, Vol. 2, p. 668.

Cleaveland, C. H.: *Causes and Cure of Diseases of the Feet.* Cincinnati, Bradley and Webb, 1862, pp. 42–48.

Dorsey, J. S.: *Elements of Surgery for the Use of Students.* Philadelphia, Benjamin Warner, 1818, pp. 346–347.

Durlacher, L.: *A Treatise on Corns, Bunions, the Diseases of Nails and the General Management of the Feet.* London, Simkin, Marshall & Co., 1845, pp. xxii–xxiii and 89–119.

Experienced Chiropodist: *The Art of Preserving the Feet;* or, practical instructions for the prevention and cure of Corns, Bunnions, Callosities, Chilblains, etc. 2nd Ed. London, H. Colburn, 1818, preface and pp. 120–131.

Gunn's *Domestic Medicine or Poor Man's Friend.* 9th Ed., Xenia, Ohio, J. H. Perry, 1837, p. 385.

Hohmann, G.: *Fuss und Bein.* Munich, J. F. Bergmann, 1951, pp. 145–192.

Joplin, R. J.: Sling procedure for correction of splay foot, metatarsus primus varus, and hallux valgus. J. Bone Joint Surg. *46:*690–693, 1964

Key, A.: Some observations on the nature and treatment of ganglion, bunion, etc. Guy's Hosp. Rep. *1:*415–428, 1836.

Meyer, G. H.: *Why the Shoe Pinches* (Tr. by J. S. Graig). New York, R. T. Trall & Co., 1863, pp. 5–35. The German pamphlet was called *Die rightige Gestalt der Schuhe,* Zurich, Myer & Zeller, 1858.

Miller, J.: *The Practice of Surgery.* 2nd Ed., Edinburgh, Adam and Charles Black; London, Longman & Co., 1852, pp. 647–648.

Peck, J. L.: *Dress and Care of the Feet.* New York, S. R. Wells, 1871, pp. 137–149.

Theodorice, B. (Bishop of Cervia): *The Surgery of Theodrice* (Tr. from Latin by E. Campbell and J. Colton). New York, Appleton-Century-Crofts Inc., 1955–1960, Vol. II, p. 110. The original appeared in 1267.

Thomsen, W.: *Kampf der Fusschwaeche.* Munich, J. F. Lehmanns, 1944, pp. 1–277.

Wiseman, R.: *Several Chirurgical Treatises.* London, E. Flesher & J. Macock, 1676, pp. 95–98.

Chapter Eight

AUXILIARY SURGICAL STEPS AND SUPPLEMENTARY CARE

One often hears it said that postoperative care is as important, if not more so, than the actual surgery. This may be true in some instances. As a rule an operation judiciously selected and carried out with commensurate skill need not be followed with elaborate aftercare. Conversely, inadequate preoperative preparation, poorly chosen and poorly executed procedure, will necessitate prolonged postoperative treatment, and it is questionable if the most arduous effort along this line can affect the ultimate result. This is not saying that postoperative care is unimportant. It is. Care should start the moment the patient is examined and be carried through surgery and for some time after.

Cleansing care. In the literature, we find no specific statement as to how the limb should be prepared prior to surgery on the toes—in particular for hallux valgus. Hawkins, Mitchell, and Hedrick (1945) disposed of the subject with the following curt remark: "Two routine orthopedic preparations are required during the twelve hours preceding operation. The feet are again prepared with a suitable antiseptic in the operating room." No one has explained what is meant by "routine orthopedic preparation." At one time it was customary to bathe the limb the night before surgery, treat it with iodine and alcohol, and swathe it in sterile wrappings. Just before the operation the extremity was again painted with iodine and alcohol. The more recent trend is to clip the toenails and shave the leg the preceding night. Just before surgery the extremity is scrubbed for 10 minutes with soap (such as G-11 or hexachlorophene), and water. The leg is painted with one of the newer antiseptics: tinctures of Merthiolate, Zephiran, or Phemerol. We prefer painting the foot, including the interdigital spaces, with a 3.5 per cent tincture of iodine; after this has dried, it is washed with sodium thiosulfate and alcohol solution (40 per cent). Finally we swab the region with ether to obtain a dry field.

Anesthesia. In a report from Guy's Hospital, published in *The Medical Times and Gazette,* July 30, 1853, we read that "the patient being under the influence of chloroform," Hilton resected the first metatarsophalangeal joint. The exact date of this operation was not given. It must have been soon after August 10, 1852, when, we are told, Hilton decided to perform this procedure "in preference to amputation." At the time anesthesia was in its very infancy; ether had been in use only 10 years and chloroform 5 years. No less an exalted person than Queen Victoria was administered chloroform by John Snow–the first professional anesthetist–on the 7th day of April, 1853, 9 months after Hilton had used the newer agent on William Templeman, a common "farm-laborer."

With the advent of local anesthesia–especially suited for surgery of the extremities–it was inevitable that controversy should arise as to which would be more appropriate for hallux valgus surgery. We learn from Bade (1940) that local anesthesia was favored by Cramer, Payr, Redwitz, Wymer, Fragenheim, and Wulfing. Brandes is said to have admitted that an occasional skin slough followed local infiltration, but he persisted with the practice. Sekely is quoted as saying that a hallux valgus operation should never be done with the aid of local anesthesia but with either general or spinal anesthesia.

Bade himself was partial to general anesthesia. In 38 years of hallux valgus surgery he had met with no delayed healing of the surgical wound; he ascribed his good fortune to abstinence from constricting sutures and to careful tissue apposition, but mainly to the use of general–by implication to avoidance of local–anesthesia. Wulfing, from Fragenheim's clinic–where local anesthesia was used–had complained that, after hallux valgus operations, wounds did not heal by primary intention. Pick, from Redwitz' clinic–another haven of infiltration anesthesia–had reported necrosis of skin in almost one out of every two operated cases. "As Wulfing and others have found out," Bade wrote, "the skin overlying the bunion is thin, delicate. The circulation is not very good. If this poorly nourished skin is damaged by local anaesthesia, it obviously will be more susceptible to inflammation than when general anaesthesia had been used. I, therefore, think the question of anaesthesia is important."

A definite advantage of general anesthesia is that it permits temporary use of a tourniquet to secure a bloodless field while reconstructive surgery is being carried out.

Tourniquet. Relatively few authors writing on hallux valgus and allied forefoot deformities mention use of the tourniquet during surgery. Blodgett (1880) reported a case of gangrene of the foot following decapitation of the first metatarsal for hallux valgus. The patient was 75 years old. An Esmarch constrictor had been used during surgery. Gangrene of the foot and the leg followed and the patient died 11 days after the operation. The surgeon who had operated ascribed the disaster to the use of a tourniquet.

Experiences such as this must have induced some earlier surgeons to avoid using a constrictor during operations on the foot. One of the seven pontifical canons Parker Syms (1897) set down for hallux valgus surgery read: "Never use an Esmarch's bandage." He did not mention any other tourniquet. The implication was that none was needed or was dangerous. Roth (1931) also advised against the use of a tourniquet. Porter (1909), Vance (1934), and Stein (1938) thought surgery for hallux valgus could be carried out more expediently with the aid of a constrictor. The second of the ten steps Hawkins, Mitchell, and Hedrick (1945) gave in describing their technique of distal osteotomy of the first metatarsal read: "An Esmarch tourniquet is applied to the lower leg, extending to approximately four inches below the head of the fibula. . . ." We consider this statement as arbitrary as the one enunciated by Syms 48 years earlier. It is not that the pneumatic cuff has now replaced Esmarch's elastic bandage. We are unable to see the rationale of placing the tourniquet on the lower leg where two flanking bones would make it difficult to compress three arterial trunks: the tibialis posterior, the peroneal, and the tibialis anterior.

Except in arteriosclerosis, a tourniquet is now used almost routinely in

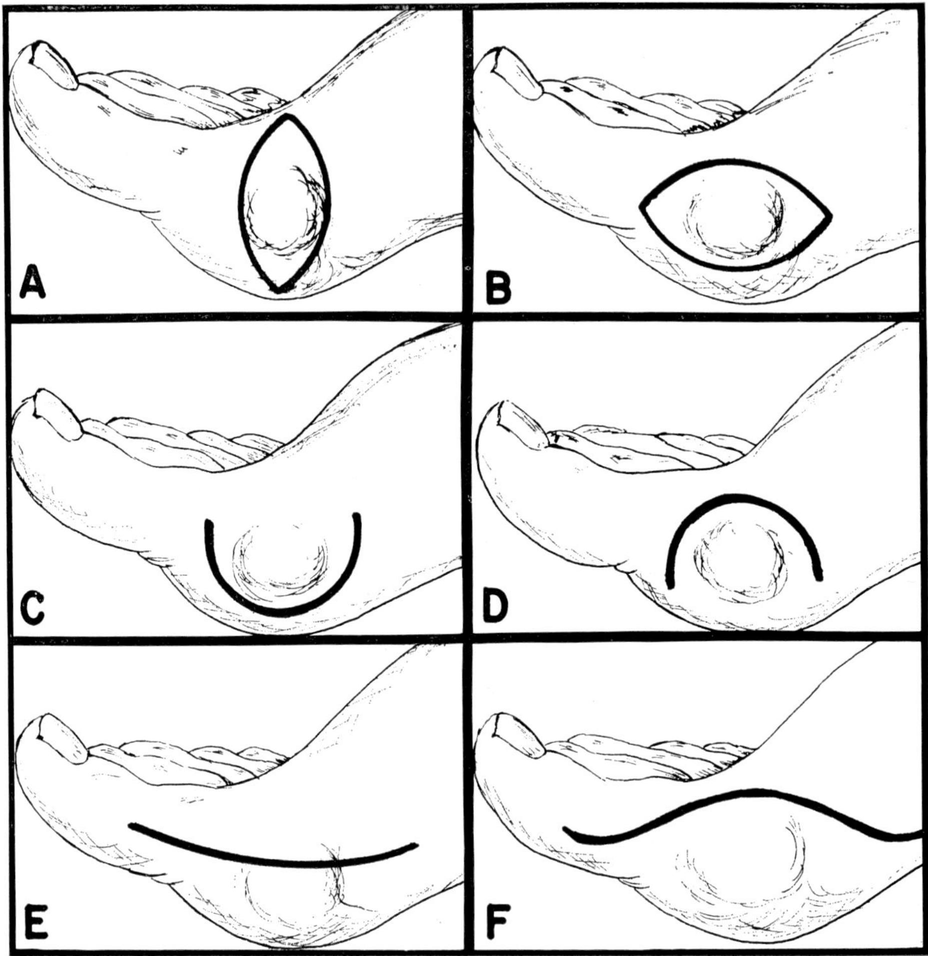

Figure 8–1. Medial incisions.

hallux valgus and allied forefoot surgery. After the usual cleansing preparation the leg is elevated or "milked" with an elastic bandage beginning from behind the toes and going proximally well past the knee. The tourniquet–pneumatic or Esmarch–is then applied around the midthigh. When a pneumatic cuff is used, the pressure should be at least twice the systolic measurement of the arm. The bulk of the thigh is also to be taken into consideration. The pneumatic cuff has an advantage in that it can be deflated and inflated at will. It is good practice to reduce the pressure at the completion of the main reconstructive work, ligate or cauterize the bleeders, and then close the incision. Too much reliance is being placed on pressure bandages to control postoperative bleeding.

Incisions. Earlier operations–such as lancing the bursa or tenotomy–must have been performed through stab wounds. According to Heubach (1897), as early as 1835, Fricke of Hamburg resected the metatarsophalangeal joint of the great toe through "two elliptical incisions." We learn from Moeller (1894) that Max Schede utilized a pair of elliptical skin cuts to resect the medial eminence of the metatarsal head. Roberts (1923) resected the basal joint of the great toe through similar skin cuts. Over a hundred years after Fricke, Treves (1937) approached the first metatarsophalangeal articulation through a pair of elliptical incisions. He placed the skin cuts in a dorsoplantar direction. This incision was described again by Prignacchi and Zanasi (1957).

Hueter (1871) decapitated the first

metatarsal through "a small lengthwise incision . . . on the inside of the foot over the affected part of the capitalum." A medial longitudinal incision was utilized in an extended form by Ludloff (1918), Juvara (1919), Royle (1931), and many others. Weir (1897) made use of a curved incision around the medial eminence; he placed the base of the curve on the dorsal plane, parallel with the long extensor tendon of the great toe. A skin flap was developed that was hinged on its pedicle and turned over the back of the foot. Mayo (1908) reversed the curve of the Weir incision. He placed the base of the skin flap "downwards" along the plantar border of the foot. These "horse-shoe" cuts carried some hazard. The medial cutaneous nerves were in danger of being damaged in undermining the skin, and at the highest point of the curve the margin of the flap sometimes sloughed. A compromise paramedian incision was proposed by Kreuscher and Kelikian (1935). It started over the medial aspect of the first metatarsal and ran longitudinally for about an inch or two. It then traced a mild curve dorsalward toward the extensor hallucis longus tendon, descended gradually plantarward and coursed in axial direction along the inner border of the first phalanx. This incision makes it possible to develop a plantar flap with a broader base and blunter curve. It provides ample room for resection of the medial eminence of the first metatarsal head, excision of the base of the proximal phalanx, enucleation of the sesamoids, release of the tension on the lateral side of the joint, and repair of the medial capsule (Figs. 8–1 and 8–2).

The most ingenious incision for exposing the metatarsophalangeal joint of the great toe was devised by Petersen (1888). He placed the skin cut in the groove between the first and second metatarsal bones. The incision bisected the interdigital web. Petersen originally used this approach to resect the first metatarsophalangeal joint ravaged by tuberculosis. It was subsequently adopted for hallux valgus by Fowler (1889, 1907), Singley (1913), Campbell (1916), Davis (1917), Hagenauer (1927), Stanley and Breck (1935), Arredondo (1946), Fernandez (1947), and Massart (1950). In this exposure, structures attached to the lateral base of the proximal phalanx are severed and the toe is dislocated medially until its direction is completely reversed, which brings the articular surfaces of the metatarsal head and of the phalangeal base into full view, lying next to each other.

Petersen's incision has dual advantages: it places the skin cut in a vascular area where healing is favorable and the scar formed is not subjected to chaf-

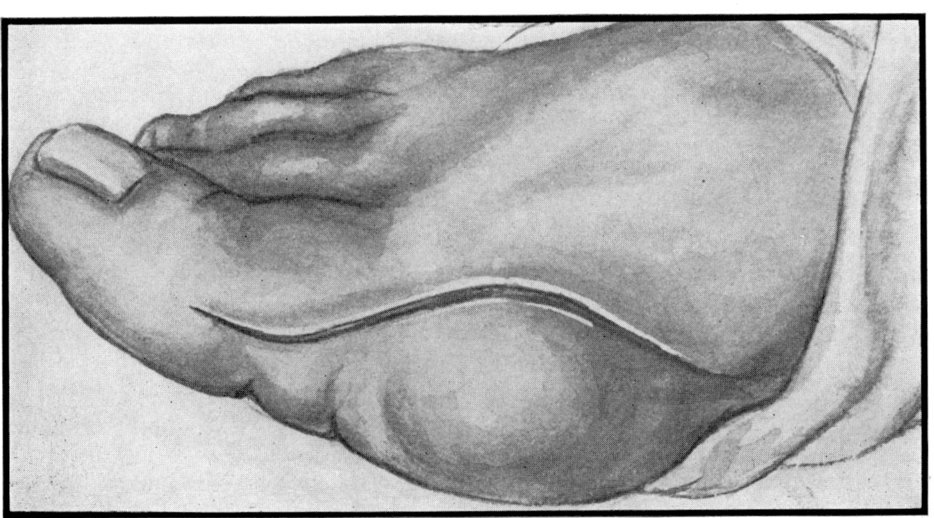

Figure 8–2. Medial curvilinear incision.

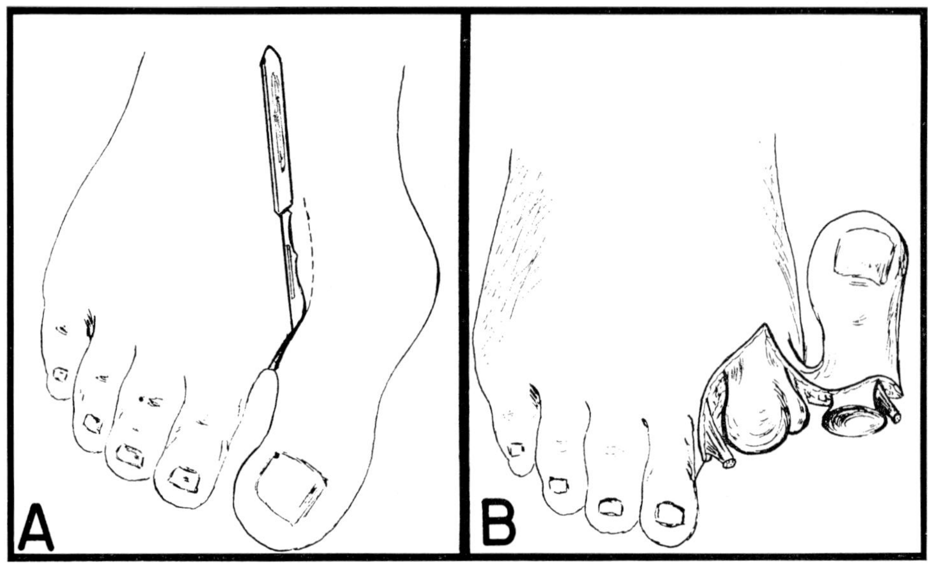

Figure 8–3. Petersen's interdigital approach.

ing by the shoe. The incision is preferable to that along the medial border of the forefoot, when the skin in that area is parchment-thin, precarious. It also offers an alternative approach when there has been previous infection from bursitis or scars due to antecedent surgery. This incision enables one to release the adductor tension on the lateral side of the first metatarsophalangeal joint, resect the medial eminence of the first metatarsal head, and excise the proximal portion of the basal phalanx of the great toe. Through this incision it is also feasible to resect the proximal portion of the first phalanx of the second toe or the distal segment of its metatarsal (Figs. 8–3 and 8–4).

Dorsal incision was first advocated by Syms (1897), who approached the first metatarsophalangeal joint through a small skin cut along the medial margin of the long extensor tendon. Franz Schede (1927) described an **S** shaped cut that started on the medial side of the first metatarsal base and curved laterally toward the innermost intermetatarsal groove. From this point it turned back to terminate over the lateral side of the great toe. McBride (1928) shifted the original dorsal incision of Syms to the lateral side of the extensor tendon and gave it a slight curve. Mauclaire (1933) extended both ends of the dorsal incision transversely, simulating a French window pane. Vance (1934) gave his incision the configuration of **J**. Recently Clayton (1960) described a transverse dorsal incision he utilized to resect the metatarsal heads and the proximal portions of the adjoining phalanges in order to correct clawed toes due to rheumatoid arthritis (Fig. 8–5).

For what was called "severe grades of contracted or clawed toes," Hoffmann (1911) resected the distal extremities of the metatarsal bones through a transverse plantar incision. This approach was described again by Kreuz (1923) for resection of the proximal portions of the basal phalanges of the central toes to correct hammered toes. Balog (1928) and Erlacher (1928) combined transverse and longitudinal plantar skin cuts—"hockey stick" incisions—to correct hallux valgus (Fig. 8–6).

Stein (1938) made use of two more or less parallel skin cuts: a longitudinal intermetarsal and a slight curved paramedian incision. Parra and McKeever (1959) and Simmonds and Menelaus (1960) also utilized two longitudinal incisions—one dorsal, one paramedian. Parallel incisions carry some risk in that the skin between them may be deprived of nutrient supply and slough. The dis-

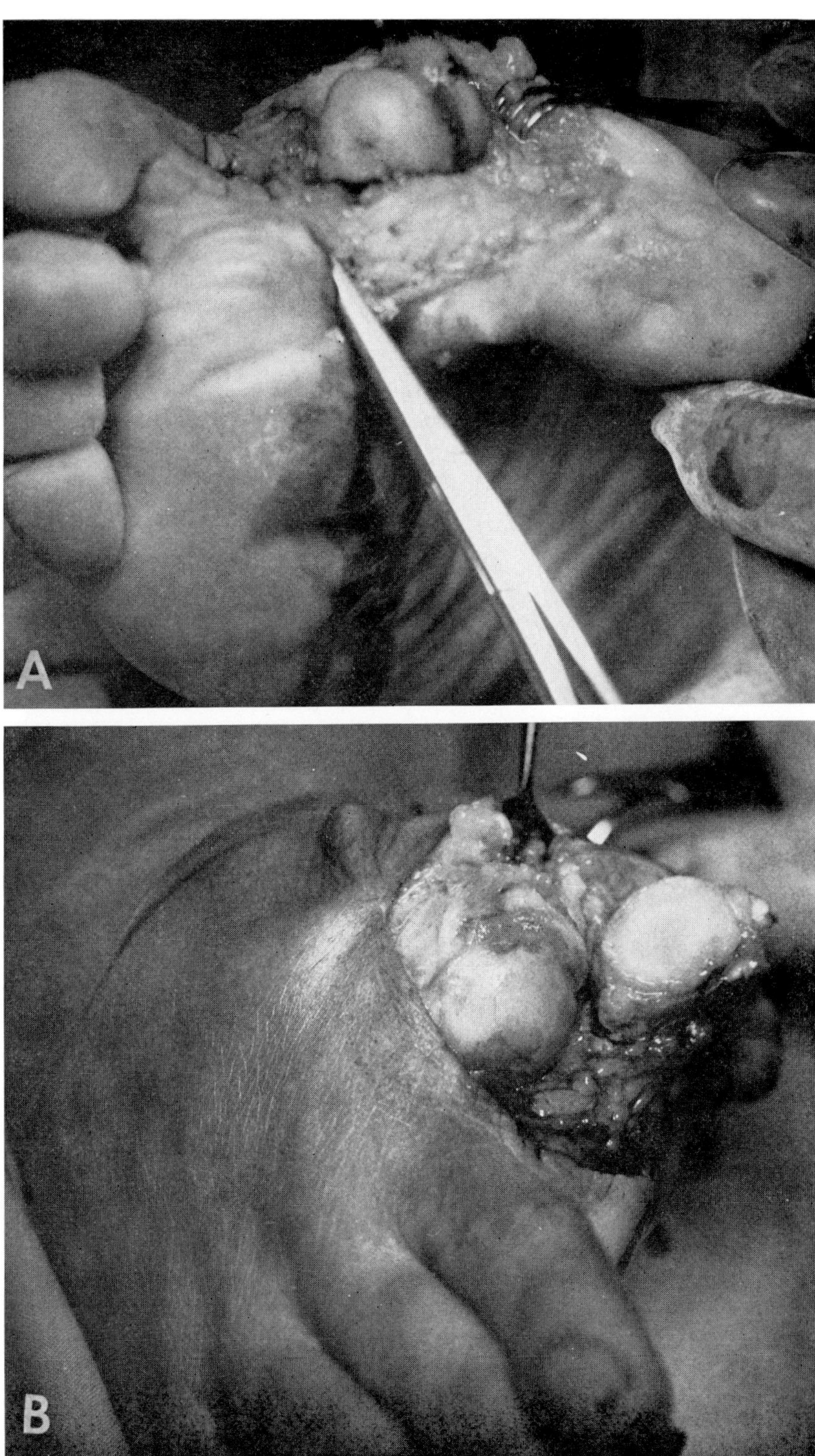

Figure 8–4. Exposure of the first metatarsophalangeal joint by interdigital approach.

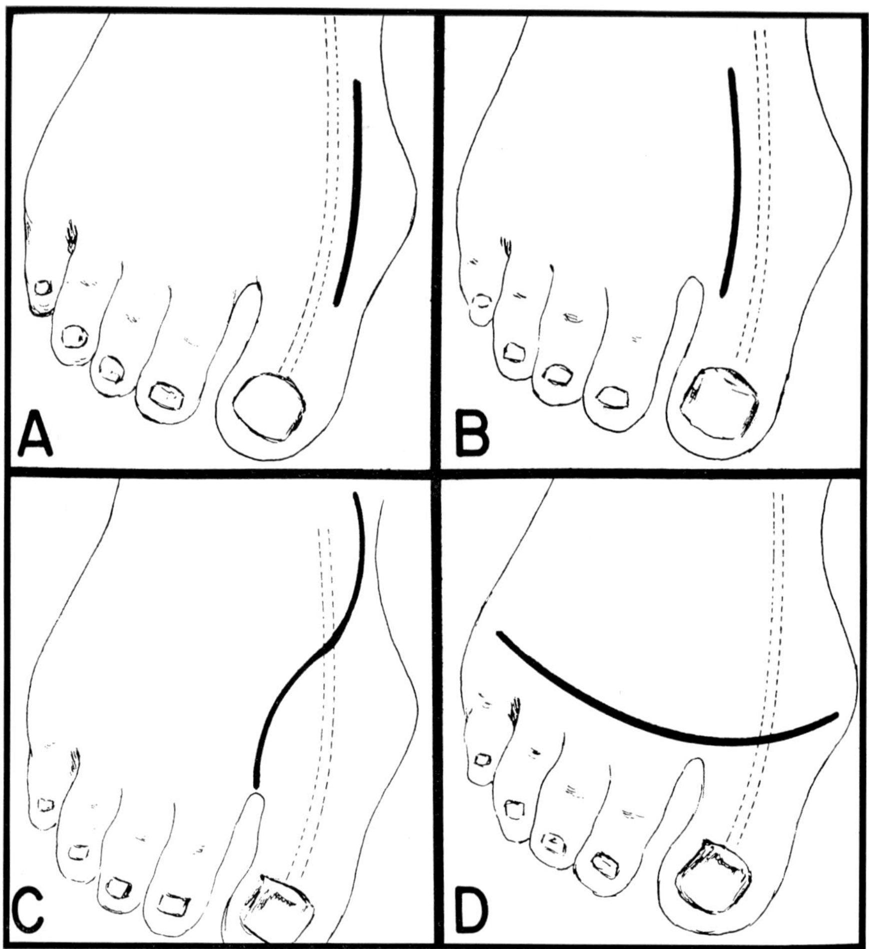

Figure 8–5. Dorsal incisions.

tance between the two cuts should not be less than two-thirds their respective lengths.

Krida (1939) utilized two small curved incisions to carry out his sling operation —one on the medial side of the first metatarsophalangeal joint and another on the lateral aspect of the fifth metatarsophalangeal joint. The "encircling fascial band" used for this operation necessitated two other skin cuts on the side of the thigh over the fascia lata. Joplin's (1950, 1958) sling procedure required five separate incisions.

In summary we may state that surgical procedures for hallux valgus have been carried out through a variety of incisions: (1) elliptical skin cuts—either axial in direction or dorsoplantar; (2) medial longitudinal incisions that may be placed close to the dorsal or plantar surface of the forefoot or midway between them; (3) medial curved incisions with a dorsal or plantar base; (4) medial curvilinear, utility incisions; (5) dorsal incisions—longitudinal, transverse, straight, curved, and so on (6) interdigital incisions; and (7) plantar incisions.

Fascial flaps. John B. Murphy (1904) developed an arthroplastic procedure for major joints in which a locally fashioned fascial flap was turned to cover the denuded articular end of the remodeled bone. Taking his cue from Murphy, C. Mayo (1908) combined this method of coverage with decapitation of the first metatarsal. The flap Mayo described consisted of the medial capsule of the metatarsophalangeal joint of the great toe and the overlying bursa. The flap was cut proximally where it obtained most of its nutrient supply. It was dissected distalward and left attached to the base of the proximal phalanx from where it received only very minute nutrient twigs. The flap then was turned into the space created by resection of the head. In Steindler's (1925) illustration of the Mayo operation, after turning it into the space created by resection and remodeling of the metatarsal head, the base of the distally pedicled fascial flap was shown stitched to the periosteal cuff of the metatarsal stump with multiple mattress sutures that would surely insulate the interposed portion and cut it off from any possible source of nourishment. Bentzon (1935) modified the Mayo operation using two fascial flaps —one pedicled proximally, the other distally—both too thin to survive.

However attenuated, detached, and insulated with sutures, even without pedicle, completely free fascial flaps may survive in a more central and deeply placed joint like the hip. These flaps are not likely to have the same favorable fate in a joint far away from central circulation and located just underneath the skin as is the metatarsophalangeal articulation of the great toe. Metcalf (1912) suggested a fascial flap with proximal attachment. Keller (1912) spoke of the sloughing of the bursa following Mayo's procedure and considered it the main objection to this operation. In the discussion that followed Henderson's (1915) paper on the Mayo procedure, Rugh raised the following objection: "It does not appear to me the best surgery

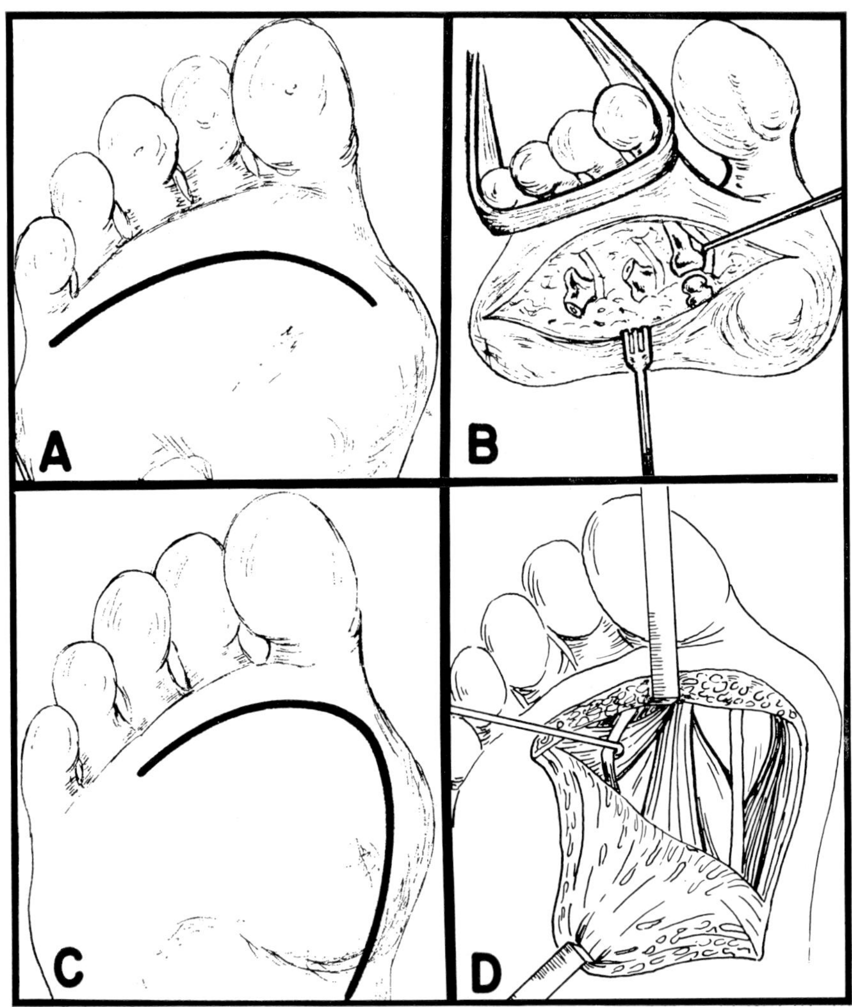

Figure 8–6. Plantar incisions.

to make the base of the flap anteriorly. I always make my flap with the base posteriorly along the side of the metatarsal to guard against sloughing." Rugh suggested that a fascial flap with a proximal pedicle would have a better chance to survive. Sir Robert Jones (1917) wrote: "At one time I used to interpose the whole bursal sac, but nearly twenty years ago several patients developed bursitis in the transposed bursa. The procedure I now adopt, therefore, is to open the bursa and interpose only one wall as a covering for the bone . . . or to obliterate the bursal cavity." In the accompanying illustrations the bursal flap was shown with a proximal pedicle.

Aitken (1921), Royle (1931), Levinthal and Kraft (1953), and Prignacchi and Zanasi (1957) were among many who adopted the proximally pedicled flap of Metcalf and Robert Jones. Silver (1923) prepared a medial capsular flap dissected proximally, leaving its base attached distally to the first phalanx. Hawkins, Mitchell, and Hedrick (1945), Mitchell and his associates (1958), Mikhail (1960), and Simmonds and Menelaus (1960) utilized similar flaps.

Levine (1938) fashioned an H capsular flap. It yielded two leaves: one was used to close the joint defect and the other was utilized as a retention sling for the long extensor tendon. Stein (1938) recommended what he called a "corrective flap." It had a broad base that was continuous with the abductor. Stein's flap is more likely to survive than Silver's, from which it is derived (Fig. 8–7).

Sloughs and infections are not uncommon in hallux valgus operations. The necrosis of the devitalized flap as a source of drainage has not been sufficiently stressed in the literature.

Drains. The question as to whether surgical wounds of the forefoot should be drained or not has often been taken up in the literature. Some surgeons insist on the routine use of drains and others argue against this practice. Fricke (1837) packed the wound with gauze. Hamilton (1874) left it wide open and immersed the foot in warm and hot water. Syms (1897) closed the "wound by suture, without draining." Wilson (1906) considered drainage for 48 hours after surgery a necessity. "The question of drainage," Metcalf (1912) wrote, "should be decided for the individual case. It is ordinarily not needed." Notwithstanding the recent surge of enthusiasm about suction methods, it is generally felt that clean, surgical wounds of the forefoot need not be drained if hemostasis is observed during the operation.

Antibiotics. "Since the introduction of antibiotics," Lapidus (1960) wrote, "we have applied an antibiotic ointment routinely to the suture line and also given the patient an antibiotic starting from one day before the operation and continuing for about one week postoperatively. It was noted that better wound healing was gained with prophylactic use of the antibiotics in surgery." Considering the susceptibility of surgical wounds of the forefoot to infection, it is perhaps wiser to eschew theoretical arguments against the routine use of antibiotics and give the patient the benefit of a broad spectrum antibiotic for the first 5 days after surgery.

Splints and appliances. Mechanical methods have featured prominently in discussions about immediate postoperative care of patients who have undergone hallux valgus surgery. Lothrop (1873) recommended a "cot made of muslin or some soft fabric." Sayre's (1879) stall consisted of buckskin. Porter (1909) used a "cigar box splint" and supplemented this with a plaster cast. Painter (1910) devised an L shaped malleable copper splint. Jarecki (1933) applied a doughnut shaped pad over the medial eminence and a domed cushion under the metatarsal heads. Miltner (1937) advocated use of Japanese type of stocking and sandal. Batts (1941) held the great toe in overcorrected position, in varus position, with the aid of a rubber glove. Mitchell and his associates (1958) initially used a padded tongue depressor and then a cast after transcervical osteotomy of the first metatarsal.

Following modified Silver and Keller procedures, we utilize a convergent, figure-eight, mildly compressive pressure bandage. This bandage consists of inch-wide twilled tape, previously rolled into a bandage and sterilized. The bandage begins to circle the base of the forefoot and is carried from the tibial to the fibular side. It follows a figure-eight pattern, going around the foot and passing along the fibular border of each toe. The bandage is reinforced by strips of adhesive tape to hold the toes in slight flexion. After fusion of the first metatarsophalangeal joint or osteotomy of one of the bones, we apply a short walking cast with the great toe included. If a Kirschner wire has been used for internal fixation, it is removed as soon as the cast hardens. After 5 weeks the cast is removed. If roentgenograms show adequate consolidation of bones, Unna's boot is applied and is replaced in 2 weeks with a tensor bandage. Women appear to be more prone to postoperative edema; they are advised to wear elastic stockings until the swelling subsides (Figs. 8–8 and 8–9).

Internal fixation. Stabilization of osteotomized fragments and articular ends of bones apposed for fusion allays pain, obviates an undesirable shift of position, and promotes early osteosynthesis.

Juvara (1919) secured the osteotomized fragments of the first metatarsal shaft with a nail. In splay foot Bettmann (1924) snugged the tibial four metatarsals together and transfixed them with a screw. Lenggenhager (1935) approximated the medial two metatarsals with a loop of flexible wire. Taylor (1940) used Kirschner wire inserted intramedularly to fuse the first interphalangeal joint of one of the smaller toes. Chapchal (1941–1943) spoke of stabilizing the great toe and osteotomized the first metatarsal with a "needle." After resection of the proximal half of the first phalanx of the great toe, Fitzgerald (1950) recommended stabilization of the hallux with an intramedulary pin. In adolescents with imminent metatarsus primus varus, Ellis (1951) stapled the lateral base of the first metatarsal with the hope of arresting the growth from that side of epiphysial cartilage. In connection with fusion of the first metatarsophalangeal joint, Hulbert (1955) utilized compression clamps, while Wilson (1958) used a miniature Rush nail (Figs. 8–10 to 8–12).

Most of these methods were subsequently adopted by others and quite frequently transposed from one type of

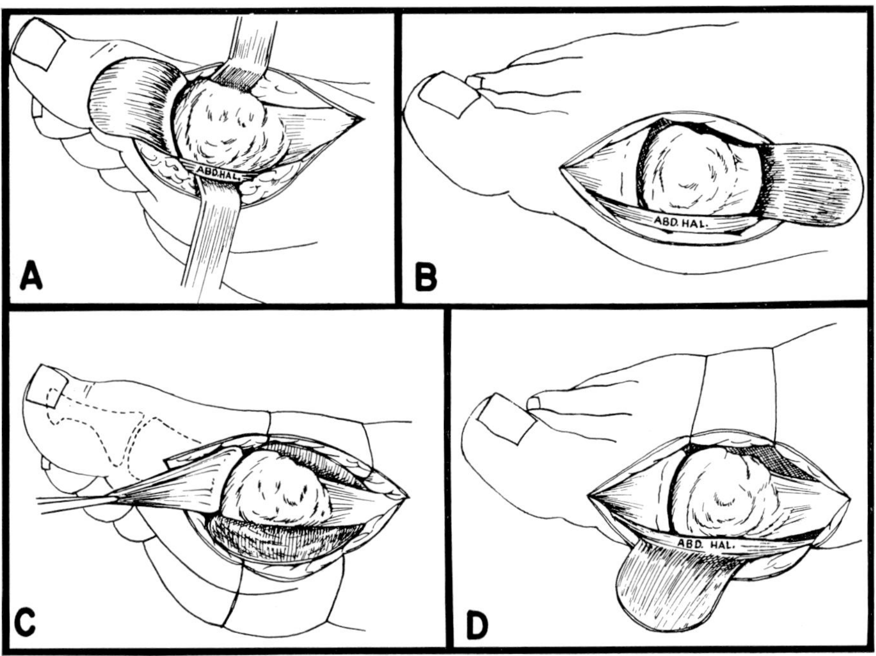

Figure 8–7. Fascial flaps.

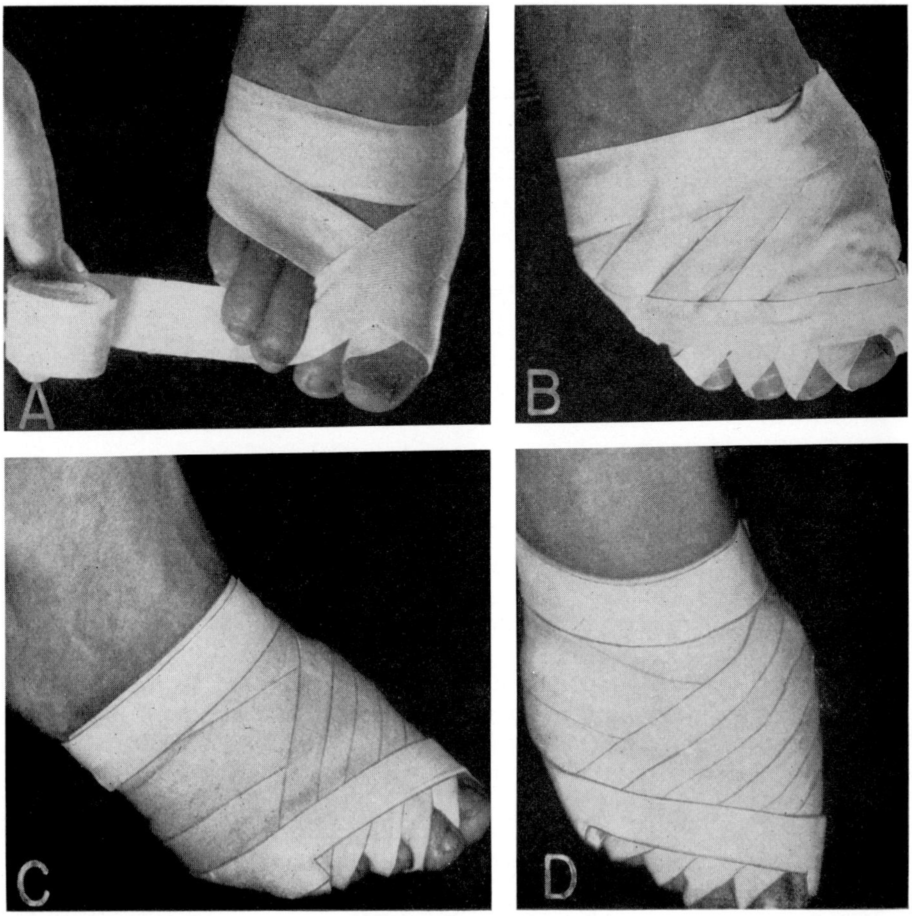

Figure 8–8. Bandage.

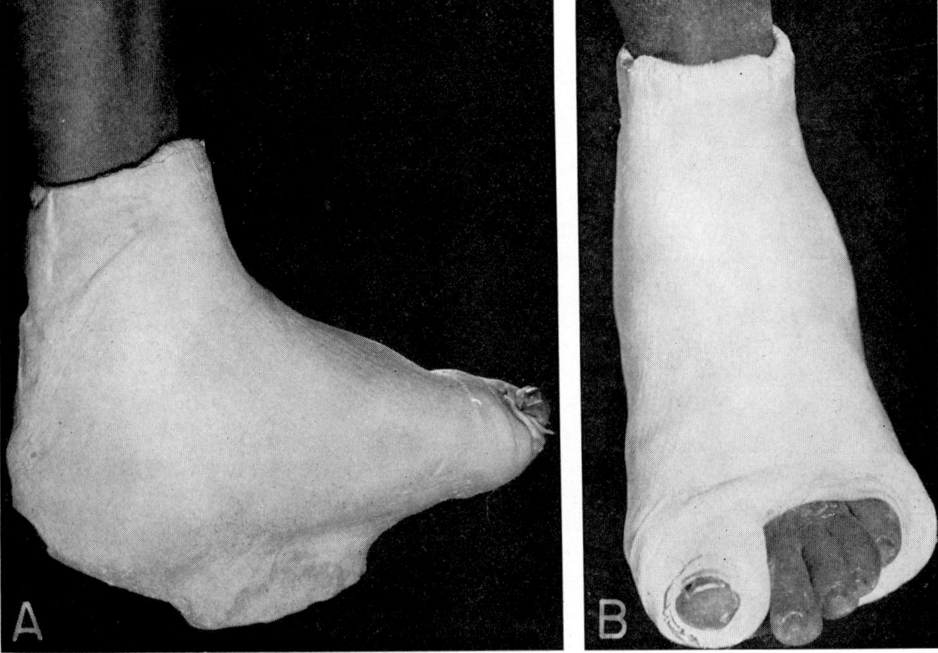

Figure 8–9. Plaster boot.

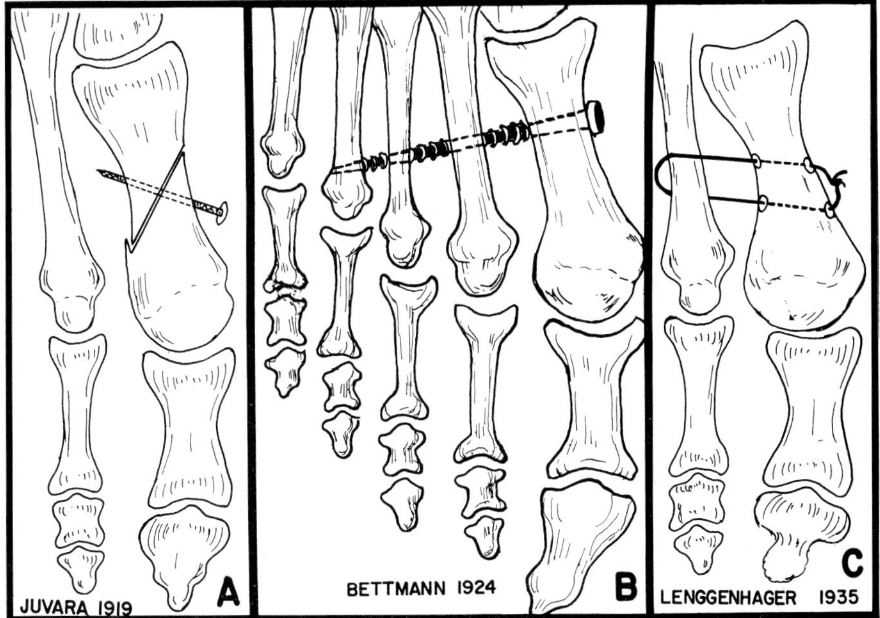

Figure 8–10. Earlier methods of internal fixation.

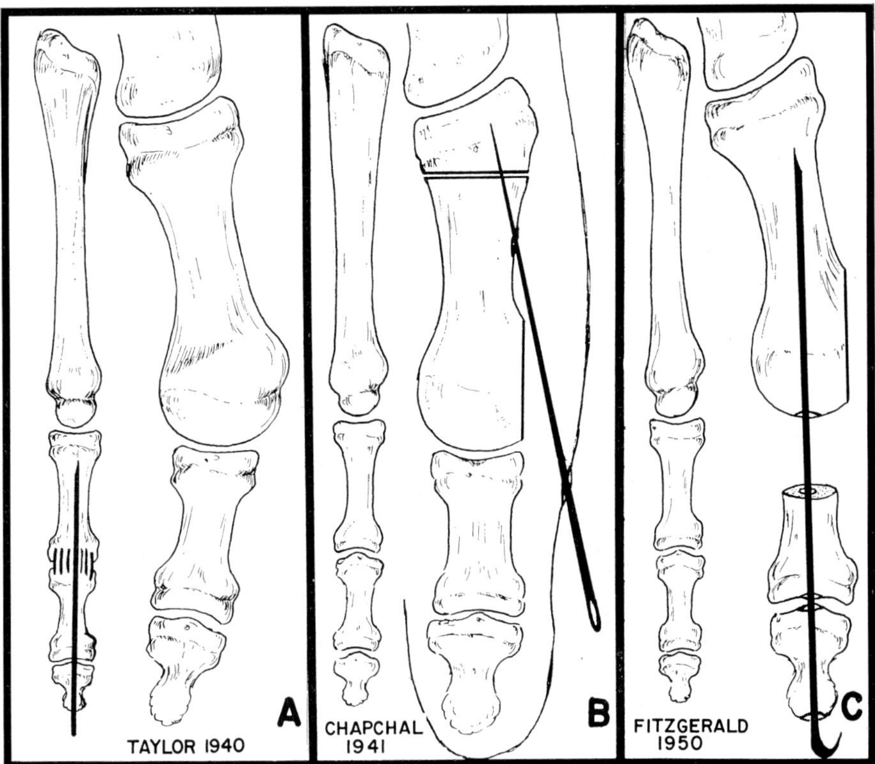

Figure 8–11. Later methods of internal fixation.

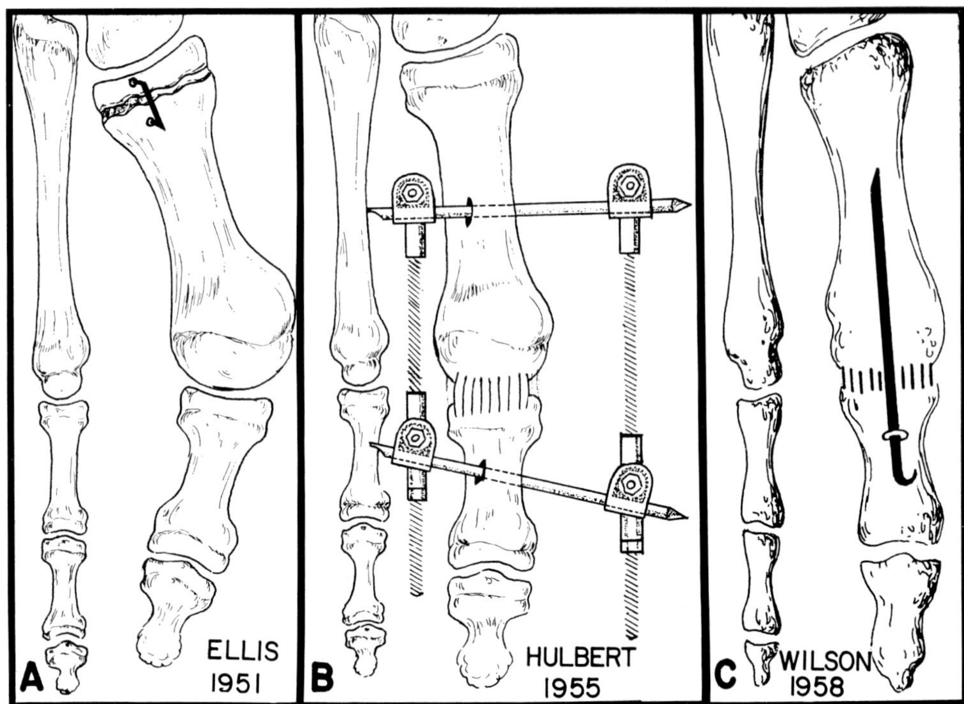

Figure 8–12. Staple (*A*), compression clamp (*B*), and Rush nail (*C*).

procedure to another. McKeever (1952) fused the first metatarsophalangeal joint with the aid of a screw. McBride (1952) attempted to approximate the first and second metatarsal bones with a circumferential suture of No. 2 chromic catgut. After proximal osteotomy of the first metatarsal, Bonney and Macnab (1952) transfixed this bone with its fellow on the lateral side utilizing the same technique that Bettmann had. Gilmore and Bush (1957) described again Fitzgerald's method of Kirschner wire stabilization of the hallux that had been subjected to Keller resection. Intramedulary Kirschner wire fixation was also utilized to stabilize the osteotomized fragments of the first metatarsal by Mizuno and his associates (1956) and others. Harrison and Harvey (1963) utilized the "compression technique" of fusion described earlier by Hulbert. Mikhail (1960) used the same kind of small Rush nail in connection with osteotomy of the first metatarsal that was utilized by Wilson for fusion of the basal joint of the big toe.

Traction. Extension of the great toe had already been advised by Sir Robert Jones (1924) after decapitation of the first metatarsal when Royle (1931) described his "new procedure." It was a modified resection of the head converting the stump of the metatarsal into a cone. "A most important detail in this procedure," Royle wrote, "is to apply toe-nail extension to the great toe." Cotte (1931) used traction after osteotomy of the first metatarsal but did not say what kind. Finochietto (1938) recommended toenail traction. Kranepuhl (1958) described Gocht's arthroplastic resection of the first metatarsal head and postoperatively resorted to pulp traction. Sperling (1958) advocated skeletal traction through the terminal phalanx.

Shoes. The type of footwear to be worn after surgery has also become the subject of controversy. "The patient," Porter (1909) warned, "must never again be allowed to wear taper-toed shoes, but a straight-lasted shoe, with a broad ball, must be insisted upon even with women in the height of fashion. If you cannot dictate the shoes, don't do the operation." Porter's operation consisted of generous resection of the medial eminence and tightening of the inner capsule. Recurrence of hallux valgus was frequent after this type of operation, especially when fashionable footwear was worn postoperatively. Porter had reasons to warn against "taper-toed shoes." Recurrence is less common following resection of articular ends and osteotomy of the first metatarsal. Three to four months after surgery these patients may wear shoes that are esthetically acceptable. To disperse the excessive stress on the metatarsal heads one may have to add a transverse bar to the sole of the shoe or place a metatarsal pad inside it. Men may tolerate the former; women prefer the latter.

Physical therapy. Postoperative massage and manipulation have had ardent advocates, especially in Germany. In his survey of the results of 200 hallux valgus operations, Cleveland (1927) wrote: "The majority of the patients were treated by massage and exercise for two or three months. In twelve cases, postoperative treatment was not instituted, and in many of these the most brilliant results were obtained. In contrast to this, several patients who came to the dispensary over a period varying from a year to eighteen months after operation achieved a poor final result, which shows conclusively that a poor result cannot be improved by massage. Too active massage and manipulation in some cases may be a definite cause of poor end-result." Nelson and Kaplan (1942) wrote: "Postoperative application of various methods of physiotherapy, shoes and mechanical devices indicated that no standard method is in existence. One gathers the impression that there is no scientific conclusive proof based on controls that the addition of various devices in the postoperative period is really necessary and that, in an occasional instance, the advice to wear a pad and special shoes is based mostly on intuition."

There is much that is arbitrary in the aftercare of patients subjected to forefoot surgery. Unless there has been infection or phlebitis, massage cannot do any harm and it may help to subdue the swelling. Manipulation of the toes too soon after surgery is avoided. Active flexion and pressing-down exercises are encouraged. The patient is advised to periodically rise on the tip of his toes, to promote extension, which is perhaps more important than flexion in civilized shoe-wearing people. The initiation of weight-bearing and walking depends on the type of procedure. Following modified Silver and Keller procedures, ambulation may be initiated within the first week. After joint fusion and osteotomy, a plaster shoe is applied and the patient is allowed to walk when postoperative pain has diminished.

REFERENCES

Aitken, D. M.: Hallux valgus, hallux rigidus, hallux flexus. *In Orthopedic Surgery of Injuries* (Sir Robert Jones, ed.). London, Oxford Univ. Press, 1921, Vol. I, pp. 386–389.

Arredondo, F. O.: Hallux valgus. Tratamiento quirúrgico, Operación de Sacco. Rev. Asoc. Méd. Argent. *60:*1009–1010, 1946.

Bade, P.: Der Hallux valgus. Stuttgart, F. Enke, 1940, pp. 1–84.

Balog, A.: Entstehung und Operation des Hallux valgus. Zbl. Chir. *55:*464–468, 1928.

Batts, M.: A simple corrective device for hallux valgus. J. Bone Joint Surg. *23:*183, 1941.

Bentzon, P. G. K.: After-examination of hallux valgus patients treated with arthroplastic resection of the head of the first metatarsal bone. Acta. Orthop. Scand. *6:*195–206, 1935.

Bettmann, E.: Beitrag zur operativen Behandlung des Schmerzhaften Spreizfusses. Verhand. Dtsch. Orthop. Ges. *45:*115–117, 1924.

Blodgett, A. N.: Hallux valgus, with a report of two successful cases. Med. Rec. New York *18:*34–37, 1880.

Bonney, G., and Macnab, L.: Hallux valgus and hallux rigidus; a critical survey of operative results. J. Bone Joint Surg. *34:*366–385, 1952.

Campbell, W. F.: Hallux valgus. Med. Tms. N.Y. *44:*188–200, 1916.

Chapchal, G.: Zur operativen Behandlung des Hallux valgus. Ztschr. Orthop. Grenzgb. *73–74:*47–60, 1941–1943.

Clayton, M. L.: Surgery of the foot in rheumatoid arthritis. Clin. Orthop. *16:*136–140, 1960.

Cleveland, M.: Hallux valgus, final results in 200 operations. Arch. Surg. *14:*1125–1135, 1927.

Cotte, G.: Ostéotomie du premier metatarsien pour hallux valgus. Lyon Chir. *28:*757-758, 1931.

Davis, G. F.: Cure for hallux valgus: the interdigital incision. Surg. Clin. N. Amer. *1:*651–658, 1917.

Ellis, V. H.: A method of correcting metatarsus primus varus. J. Bone Joint Surg. *33:*415–417, 1951.

Erlacher, P. J.: Die Technik des orthopaedischen Eingriffs, Entstehung und Operation des Hallux valgus. Chirurg. *55:*977-978, 1928.

Fernandez, J. C.: Hallux valgus operación de Peterson. Rev. Asoc. Méd. Argent. *613–614:* 677–679, 1947.

Finochietto, R.: Hallux valgus. Extension continua post-operatoria. Prensa Méd. Argent. *25:*1908–1909, 1938.

Fitzgerald, W.: Hallux valgus. J. Bone Joint Surg. *32:*139, 1950.

Fowler, G. R.: Partial resection of the head of the first metatarsal bone for hallux valgus. Med. Rec. *36:*253–255, 1889.

Fowler, G. R.: *A Treatise on Surgery*. Philadelphia, W. B. Saunders Co., 1907, Vol. 2, pp. 621–622.

Fricke, J. L. G.: Exostosis of the ball of the foot. J. Med. Sci. *11:*497–504, 1837.

Gilmore, G. H., and Bush, L. F.: Hallux valgus. Surg. Gyn. Obst. *104:*524–528, 1957.

Hagenauer, G. A.: Operation for bunion. Med. J. Aust. *1:*787, 1927.

Hamilton, F.: The use of warm and hot water in surgery. Med. Rec. *9:*249–252, 1874.

Harrison, M. H. M., and Harvey, F. J.: Arthrodesis of the first metatarsophalangeal joint for hallux valgus and rigidus. J. Bone Joint Surg. *45:*471–480, 1963.

Hawkins F. B., Mitchell, C. L., and Hedrick, D. W.: Correction of hallux valgus by metatarsal osteotomy. J. Bone Joint Surg. *27:*387–394, 1945.

Henderson, M. S.: Operative treatment of bunions by the Mayo method. J.A.M.A. *65:*1356–1359, 1915.

Heubach, F.: Ueber Hallux valgus und seine operative Behandlung nach Edm. Rose. Dtsch. Ztschr. Chir. *46:*210–275, 1897.

Hilton, J.: Resection of the metatarsophalangeal joint of the great toe. Med. Tms. Gaz. *7:*141, 1853.

Hoffmann, P.: An operation for severe grades of contracted or clawed toes. Am. J. Orthop. Surg. *9:*441–449, 1911.

Hueter, C.: *Klinik der Gelenkkrankheiten*. Leipzig, F. C. W. Vogel, 1871, pp. 339–351.

Hulbert, K. F.: Compression clamp for arthrodesis of the first metatarsophalangeal joint. Lancet *1:*597, 1955.

Jarecki, G.: Beitrag zur konservativen Hallux-valgus-Behandlung. Münch. Med. Wchnschr. *80:*56–567, 1933.

Jones, R.: *Notes on Military Orthopaedics*. New York, P. B. Hoeber, 1917, pp. 38–57.

Jones, R.: Discussion on the treatment of hallux valgus and rigidus. Brit. Med. J. *2:*651–656, 1924.

Joplin, R. J.: Sling procedure for correction of splay-foot, metatarsus primus varus, and hallux valgus. J. Bone Joint Surg. *32:*779–785, 1950.

Joplin, R. J.: Some common foot disorders amenable to surgery. Am. Acad. Orthop. Surgeons Lectures *15:*144–158, 1958.

Juvara, E.: Nouveau procédé pour la cure radicale du "hallux valgus." Presse Méd. *40:*395–397, 1919.

Keller, W. L.: Further observations on the surgical treatment of hallux valgus and bunions. New York Med. J. *95:*696–698, 1912.

Kranepuhl, F.: Hallux-valgus-Operationen nach Gocht. Zbl. Chir. *83:*1505–1510, 1958.

Kreuscher, P. H., and Kelikian, H.: Hallux valgus (bunion). Illionis M. J. *67:*453:456, 1935.

Kreuz, L.: Die Hammerzehen und ihre Operation nach Gocht. Arch. Orthop. Unfall-Chir. *21:* 459–472, 1923.

Krida, A.: A new operation for metatarsalgia and splay-foot. Surg. Gyn. Obst. *69:*106–107, 1939.

Lapidus, P. W.: The author's bunion operation from 1931 to 1959. Clin. Orthop. *16:*119–135, 1960.

Lenggenhager, K.: Eine neue Operationsmethode zur Behandlung des Hallux valgus. Chirurg. *7:*689–692, 1935.

Levine, M. A.: An operative technique for hallux valgus. J. Bone Joint Surg. *20:*923–925, 1938.

Levinthal, D. H., and Kraft, G. L.: Disabilities and surgery of the great toe. Surg. Clin. N. Amer. *33:*1511–1521, 1953.

Lothrop, C. H.: Bunion. Boston Med. Surg. J. *88:*641–643, 1873.

Ludloff, K.: Die Beseitigung des Hallux valgus durch die schraege plantodorsale Osteotomie des Metatarsus 1 (Erfahrungen und Erfolge). Arch. Klin. Chir. *110:*364–387, 1918.

McBride, E. D.: A conservative operation for bunion. J. Bone Joint Surg. *10:*735–739, 1928.

McBride, E. D.: Hallux valgus bunion deformity. Am. Acad. Orthop. Surgeons *9:*334–346, 1952.

McKeever, D. C.: Arthrodesis of the first metatarsophalangeal joint for hallux valgus, hallux rigidus, and metatarsus primus varus. J. Bone Joint Surg. *34:*129–134, 1952.

Massart, R.: Le débridement commissural dans la chirurgie du pied. Bull. Mem. Soc. Chir. *40:*248–252, 1950.

Mauclaire, P.: Traitement de l'hallux valgus grave par l'arthroplastie reconstitutive. Rev. Chir. *52:*661–674, 1933.

Mayo, C.: The surgical treatment of bunions. Ann. Surg. *48:*300–302, 1908.

Metcalf, C. R.: Acquired hallux valgus, late results from operative and non-operative treatment. Boston Med. Surg. J. *167:*271–277, 1912.

Mikhail, I. K.: Bunion, hallux valgus and metatarsus primus varus. Surg. Gyn. Obst. *111:*637–646, 1960.

Miltner, L. J.: Care of the feet after bunionectomy. J. Bone Joint Surg. *19:*235, 1937.

Mitchell, L. S., Fleming, J. L., Allen, R., Glenney, C., and Sanford, G. A.: Osteotomy-bunionectomy for hallux valgus. J. Bone Joint Surg. *40:*41–60, 1958.

Mizuno, S., Sima, Y., and Yamazaki, K.: Detorsion osteotomy of the first metatarsal bone in hallux valgus. J. Jap. Orthop. Soc. *30:*105–110, 1956.

Moeller, F.: Beitrag zur operativen Behandlung des Hallux valgus. Jahrb. Hamb. Staatskrankenanst. *3:*306–338, 1894.

Murphy, J. B.: Ankylosis; Arthroplasty, clinical and experimental. Trans. Am. Surg. Assoc. *22:*315–376, 1904.

Nelson, L. S., and Kaplan, E. B.: Hallux valgus: Survey of end results of various operative procedures for correction of hallux valgus performed at the hospital during the past ten years (1931–1940). Bull. Hosp. Joint Dis. *3*:17–25, 1942.

Painter, C. F.: A splint for postoperative hallux valgus. Am. J. Orthop. Soc. *8*:407–408, 1910.

Parra, G., and McKeever, D. C.: An operation for correction of metatarsus primus varus. Clin. Orthop. *14*:162–165, 1959.

Petersen, F.: Ueber Arthrectomie des ersten Mittelfusszehengelenkes. Arch. Klin. Chir. *37*:677–678, 1888.

Porter, J. L.: Why operations for bunion fail, with description of one which does not. Surg. Gyn. Obst. *8*:89–90, 1909.

Prignacchi, V., and Zanasi, R.: La tecnica di Hueter-Mayo nella cura chirurgica dell'alluce valgo. Chir. Org. Mov. *44*:234–242, 1957.

Roberts, P. W.: An operation for hallux valgus. J.A.M.A. *80*:540–542, 1923.

Roth, P. B.: Hallux valgus: a note on operative technique. Brit. Med. J. *1*:443-444, 1931.

Royle, N. D.: Treatment of hallux valgus and hallux rigidus. Aust. N. Z. J. Surg. *1*:88–91, 1931.

Sayre, L. A.: *Lectures on Orthopedic Surgery*. New York, D. Appleton & Co., 1879, pp. 140–141.

Schede, F.: Hallux valgus, Hallux flexus und Fussenkung. Ztschr. Orthop. Chir. *48*:564–571, 1927.

Silver, D.: The operative treatment of hallux valgus. J. Bone Joint Surg. *5*:225–232, 1923.

Simmonds, F. A., and Menelaus, M. B.: Hallux valgus in adolescents. J. Bone Joint Surg. *42*:761–768, 1960.

Singley, J. D.: The operative treatment of hallux valgus and bunion. J.A.M.A. *16*:1871–1872, 1913.

Sperling, E.: Extensionsarthroplastik beim Hallux valgus. Zbl. Chir. *83*:335–343, 1958.

Stanley, L. L., and Breck, L. W.: Bunions. J. Bone Joint Surg. *17*:961–964, 1935.

Stein, H. C.: Hallux valgus. Surg. Gyn. Obst. *66*:889–898, 1938.

Steindler, A.: *A Text-Book of Operative Orthopedics*. New York, D. Appleton & Co., 1925, pp. 148–154.

Syms, P.: Bunion: its aetiology, anatomy and operative treatment. New York Med. J. *66*: 448–451, 1897.

Taylor, R. G.: An operative procedure for the treatment of hammer-toe and claw-toe. J. Bone Joint Surg. *22*:608–609, 1940.

Treves, A.: Difformités du gros orteil. In *Traité de Chirurgie Orthopédique*. (L. Ombrédanne and P. Mathieu, eds.). Paris, Masson et Cie., 1937, Vol. 5, pp. 4045–4061.

Vance, E. B. M.: The treatment of bunions. Med. J. Austr. *1*:202–204, 1934.

Weir, R. F.: The operative treatment of hallux valgus. Ann. Surg. *25*:444–452, 1897.

Wilson, C. L.: A method of fusion of the metatarsophalangeal joint of the great toe. J. Bone Joint Surg. *40*:384–385, 1958.

Wilson, H. A.: An analysis of 152 cases of hallux valgus in 77 patients with a report upon an operation for its relief. Am. J. Orthop. Surg. *3*:214–230, 1906.

Chapter Nine

SO-CALLED CONSERVATIVE OPERATIONS

The term *bunionectomy* should rightly be reserved for the surgical effacement of the swelling at the base of the great toe. The tumefaction is caused mainly by the medially displaced head of the first metatarsal and the overlying inflamed bursa. Historically, attempts at evacuation or extirpation of the bursa preceded the sagittal resection of the medial eminence of the first metatarsal head. Capsuloplasties came later.

Bursectomy. One of the earliest hints of a definitive surgical interference for hallux valgus—then still called *oignon* in France—was given by Boyer (1826). He recommended ablation of the "cyst." Because of the hazard of opening the joint, Boyer preferred to cauterize the lining of the bursal sac, instead of dissecting it out. Brodie (1846) incised the bursa and applied concentrated nitric acid to its inner surface. Ashton (1852) advised drainage of the bursal abscess. Annandale (1866) opened the bursa only if it was filled with pus. Lane (1887) also recommended evacuation of the infected bursa. Goldthwait (1893) thought bursectomy should be performed in conjunction with bone operations. Syms (1897) on the other hand did not think bone surgery should be complicated with bursectomy. He regarded bursectomy unnecessary, even dangerous, because it would stir up infection. Aitken (1921) considered extirpation of the bursa of little use unless an attempt also was made to strengthen the toe.

As a separate operation, bursectomy is now undertaken for gouty and calcareous deposits and when there has been a spontaneous rupture, persistent sinus, and drainage. In infected cases, bursectomy alone is justifiable if the sinogram does not indicate pocketing of pus deeper in the joint or bone. Nonsuppurative bursitis occurring in connection with hallux valgus will subside if the skeletal deformity is rectified. The bursa is removed only when its walls are inordinately thick or studded with villi.

Schede's simple exostectomy. Ever since Reverdin (1881) spoke about it, sagittal resection of the medial eminence of the first metatarsal—or exostectomy—has been carried out in conjunction with numerous procedures: osteotomy of the first metatarsal, resection of the proximal phalanx, capsulorrhaphy, and others. When performed by itself or in connection with bursectomy, the operation has come to be called Schede No. 1 technique. The reference is to Max Schede. Schede No. 2 and No. 3 techniques were devised by Franz Schede. No one seems tc have adopted these last two.

Max Schede himself does not appear to have written about hallux valgus. Moeller (1894) published an extensive monograph reviewing the cases operated in Schede's clinic between 1884 and 1892. Heubach (1897) gave an adequate description of Schede's technique. Both these accounts appeared in the 1890's. Timmer (1930) placed 1904 to Schede's name on the schematic drawing representing various procedures for hallux valgus. Following Timmer, Verbrugge (1933), Khoury (1947), McBride (1952), and Lapidus (1960) gave 1904 as the date of initial announcement of Schede's exostectomy. This is an example of how an error, perhaps a slip of the pen, can be transmitted from one article to another.

Five years prior to Moeller's (1894) report about Schede's operation, Fowler (1889) acknowledged that it was Reverdin who had proposed "to perform partial resection or to simply remove the overgrowth, or exostosis, of the internal portion of the articular head of the metatarsal bone." Reverdin (1881) reported two cases in which he had used this method. Fowler modified Reverdin's "exostectomy" by approaching the first metatarsophalangeal joint through the interdigital incision that Petersen (1888) had described in the preceding year.

According to Heubach, Max Schede approached the first metatarsophalangeal joint through a pair of elliptical skin cuts that met over the medial base of the proximal phalanx. A segment of the bursa and of the capsule was excised to expose the medial eminence. The part of the first metatarsal head no longer in contact with the base of the proximal phalanx was resected. The elliptical incisions were sutured in such a way—apparently perpendicular to their axes—as to "shorten the skin" and bring the toe into "normal position." In his description of Schede's technique, Bromeis (1931) gave a few more details. The curved skin cuts surrounded the medial eminence. If the integument was calloused, it was "elliptically circumcised." The bursa was extirpated. The incision was carried through the periosteum and the joint capsule. The hallux was pushed laterally and the medial portion of the metatarsal head was chiseled off. The resected surface of the bone was smoothed with a rasp; its sharp margins were filed down. The toe was "forcefully" manipulated into correct position. The wound was closed.

Schede's exostectomy came into vogue at the turn of the century. It was variously modified. Syms (1897) advised removing as much bone as was necessary to flatten the prominence of the inner base of the great toe. Wilson (1906) resected the part of the metatarsal head that protruded beyond the base of the proximal phalanx. Porter (1909, 1918) removed two-thirds to three-fourths of the metatarsal head, including "the enlarged inner tuberosity." Stanley and Breck (1935) revived Fowler's (1889) method of resecting the medial eminence through Petersen's (1888) interdigital incision. Fernandez (1947) described the same technique and called it Petersen's operation. It should be noted that this approach necessitates lateral capsulotomy—exostectomy is supplemented with release of the adductor tension (Fig. 9–1).

Resection of the medial eminence has had ardent advocates. Wilson (1906) recommended it for all cases of hallux valgus that necessitated "bone operation." Porter (1909) characterized his method of resection of the medial eminence as an operation "which does not" fail. Kocher (1911) said he "invariably gained satisfactory results from chiseling off the inner half of the first metatarsal." In assessing the results of Schede's "exostectomy," Bromeis (1931) considered painless gait as the sole criterion: he recorded 87 per cent lasting relief and 8 per cent amelioration. "The anatomical position of the toe has nothing to do with the final result," Bromeis wrote. He reported no infection, which

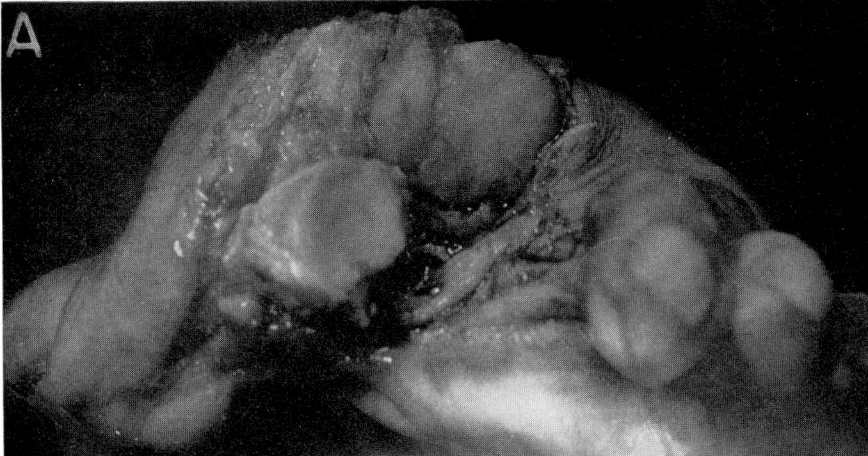

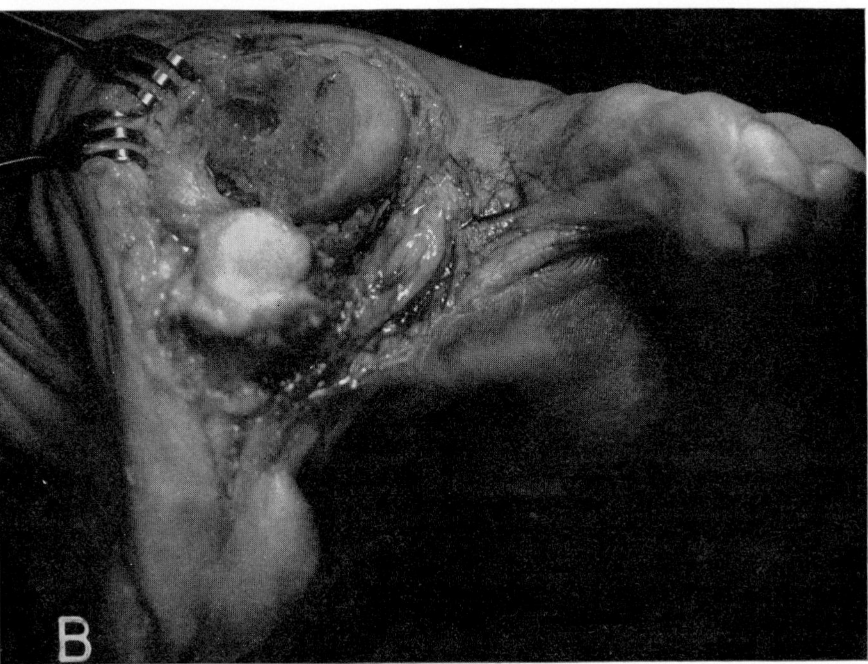

Figure 9–1. Sagittal resection of the medial eminence through Petersen's interdigital incision Conjoined tendon and capsule attached to the lateral base of the proximal phalanx of the great toe have been severed and the hallux jack-knifed medially and plantarward to bring the first metatarsal head into full view (*A*). The medial eminence is chiseled off flush with the inner cortex of the first metatarsal shaft (*B*).

he ascribed to the simplicity of the procedure and to diligent postoperative care —mainly elevation. McElvenny and Thompson (1940) considered "simple exostectomy" a satisfactory procedure for relief of "bunion pain."

Sagittal resection of the medial eminence—Schede's exostectomy—also had its critics. But even those who have denounced the concept of exostosis in hallux valgus as a "myth"—Stein (1938), for one—apparently could not resist the temptation of tampering with the medial eminence. Hohmann (1951) said Schede's exostectomy was no more than a palliative treatment. It merely removed the medially protruding portion of the first metatarsal head; it did not correct the outward deviation of the great toe, nor did it remedy the splaying of the forefoot. All the same, Hohmann conceded that he occasionally performed this operation in the aged and decrepit to dispose of the pain caused by the pressure by the shoe. Storen (1961) reported that more than 50 per cent of patients subjected to simple exostectomy were dissatisfied with the ultimate outcome. Both the pain and bony prominence recurred in time. The method, he concluded, should be reserved for elderly patients, deemed unfit for more elaborate surgery.

Schede's exostectomy should be consigned to the category of temporizing measures. It has one objective: to relieve chafing due to friction by the shoe. It is suitable for older individuals who are not concerned with the correction of the valgus deformity of the great toe. In the aged with already fixed arthritis of the innermost cuneometatarsal joint, one does not anticipate continued increase of varus inclination of the first metatarsal and, hence, recurrence of the medial eminence. In the presence of hypermobile first metatarsal, recurrence is inevitable. The operation should not be attempted in the young with pliable feet. Surgeons who advocate resection of the medial eminence as a satisfactory procedure for hallux valgus claim that it is less traumatic than other operations. This is true. It would not add much to the surgical trauma to release the adductor tension on the lateral side of the joint and shorten the medial capsule, as advised by Silver.

Silver's capsulorrhaphy. If we had to select a relatively recent article on hallux valgus to be placed by the side of the classics of the past, we would seriously consider David Silver's (1923). We may criticize a point or two of his operative technique and cavil about his postoperative management. But for sheer appreciation of the complicated problems of hallux valgus and compact and clear exposition of the available knowledge up to his time, we can think of no other writer who came close to Silver in the earlier decades of the present century. Many surgeons benefited from his teachings. Some— like McBride (1928), Hiss (1931), Lapidus (1934), Stein (1938), Hawkins and *et al.,* (1945), and Mitchell and associates (1958)—utilized Silver's method to supplement theirs.

Silver removed a "thin layer of cortex, together with the periosteum and any exostosis that may be present" as a step in his operation to correct the valgus deformity of the great toe. He released the tension on the fibular aspect of the first metatarsophalangeal joint and reenforced the medial capsule. The last step was designed to reconstruct the medial collateral ligament and at the same time transpose the tendon of the abductor hallucis to a more dorsal position on the inner aspect of the joint. It was hoped that the abductor tendon, which remained continuous with the sesamoid pad, would pull the pad back under the first metatarsal head.

We have already touched on the history of the sagittal resection of the medial eminence—the exostectomy step of the Silver operation. Lothrop (1873)—of Fort Riley, Kansas, later of Lyons, Iowa —was first to mention adductor tenotomy and lateral capsulotomy. Erichsen (1873) suggested sectioning the outer head of the short flexor also. Weir (1897) considered "the complete liberation of the phalanx on its outer side by free section of the binding capsule and other tissues" as most important. Clarke (1900) advised shortening the stretched out medial collateral ligament—a procedure that has been variously described as reefing, plicating, or imbricating. Fuld (1916–1919) detached the abductor hallucis from its insertion and dissected it free, up to its fleshy belly, proximally. He opened the joint capsule, exposed the medial eminence, and chiseled it off. He laid the capsular flap against decorticated bone, closed the joint, slung the abductor tendon obliquely up, and sutured it to a more dorsal point on the inner side of the proximal phalanx.

We learn from the available information that Fuld was primarily an ophthalmic surgeon. It is possible that the idea of abductor transfer was suggested to him by similar operations to restore muscle balance in eye surgery. "I have devised and found . . . feasible," Fuld wrote, "a transplantation of the abduc-

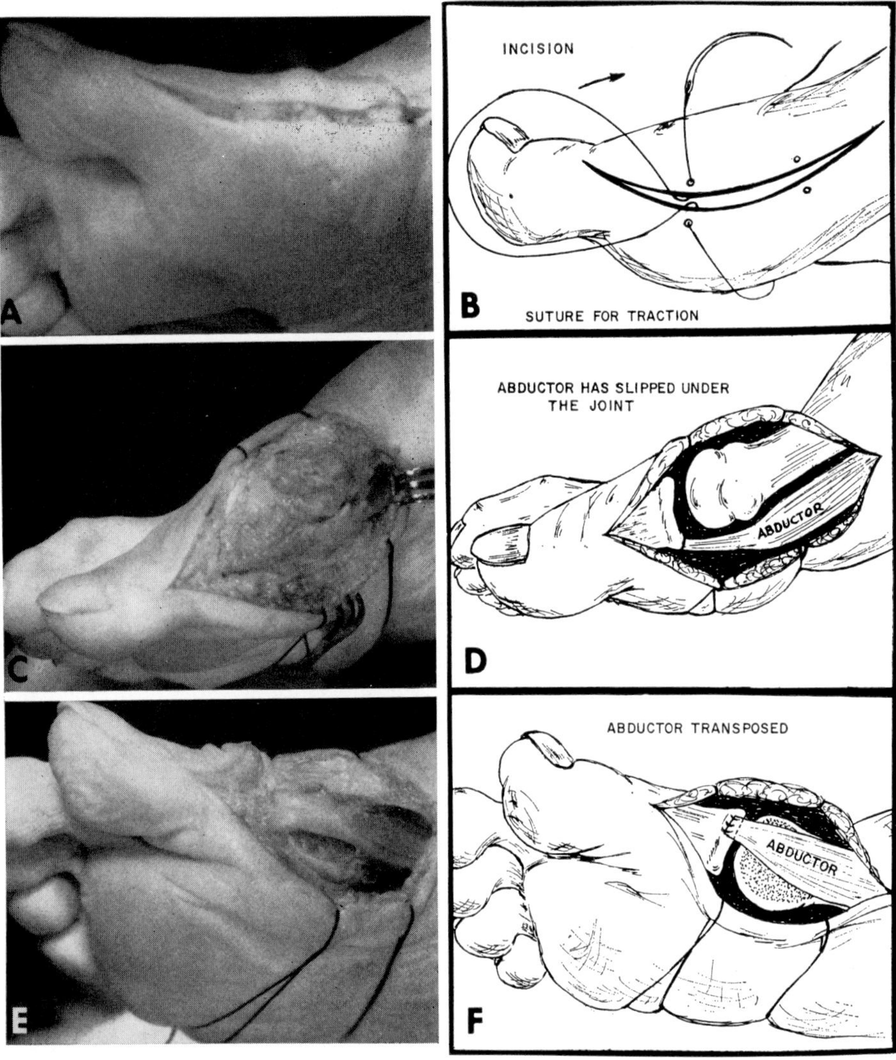

Figure 9–2. Photographs and interpretative diagrams showing combined operation of sagittal resection of the medial eminence and transfer of abductor hallucis from under the first metatarsophalangeal joint to its medial aspect. Incision (*A*). Suture to retract skin edges—the loop passes over the toes and the ends of the suture are tied on the fibular side of the forefoot (*B*). Exposure showing the displaced abductor (*C* and *D*). Resection of the medial eminence and reinsertion of abductor to a more dorsal point on the medial base of the proximal phalanx (*E* and *F*).

tor hallucis from its usual insertion in the plantar surface of the base of the first phalanx to the periosteum covering the middle of the inner surface of the same bone." Fuld had hallux valgus in mind when he assigned the plantar, rather than the inferomedial, surface of the phalangeal base as the point of "usual insertion" of the abductor hallucis. In years to come the concept of restoring *muscle balance* in hallux valgus surgery ran like a red streak through the writings of numerous authors, none of whom mentioned Fuld (Fig. 9–2).

With its fleshy muscle and stout tendon, the abductor hallucis serves more than one purpose. Using the head of the metatarsal as a fulcral point, it prevents the adductors on the other side of the joint from pulling the great toe too far laterally, into a greater valgus position; the abductor also provides the head of the first metatarsal with a medial brace and counteracts its tendency to go into a greater varus position. In more pronounced cases of hallux valgus, when the abductor has slipped from its usual position on the inferomedial aspect of the metatarsal head to down under it, it can no longer counterbalance the action of the adductors, or provide the first metatarsal head with a medial buttress. Bringing the displaced abductor back to the medial side of the metatarsal head is regarded an important step in operations designed to correct hallux valgus—as important as the release of the adductors on the lateral side of the joint.

Silver benefited from Fuld's—as well as Lothrop's and Reverdin's—teachings. Although Silver did not mention these three pioneers, he appropriated their ideas and developed the procedure with which we have come to connect his name. He approached the basal joint of the great toe through a curved medial incision with the convexity of the curve directed toward the sole. The bursa, if inflamed, was removed. A triangular flap was fashioned out of the medial capsule with its pedicle connected distally to the inner base of the proximal phalanx. This flap was freed proximally and reflected distally. From the apex of the triangular cut, the capsular incision was extended proximally. Two other flaps—dorsal and plantar—were developed. The plantar flap was continuous inferiorly with the tendon of the abductor hallucis. The medial eminence was exposed; it was economically resected. To release the adductor tension on the fibular aspect of the joint, the toe was extended, a tenotome was inserted along the dorsal surface of the metatarsal head, and the lateral capsule was slit lengthwise. The toe was flexed—the tenotome was inserted under the metatarsal head and the lateral capsule was cut again in a longitudinal direction. The toe was put under traction to open the joint space and the dorsal and the plantar capsular incisions were connected with a vertical cut (Fig. 9–3).

The toe was held in a 45 degree varus position. The distal triangular flap was laid back on the decorticated surface left by exostectomy and sutured under tension. The first suture was passed through the dorsal flap well back toward its posterior margin and through the upper corner of the distal flap. A second suture was similarly placed between the posterior end of the plantar and the lower corner of the triangular flap. When the two sutures were tied, the distal flap was drawn under the dorsal and plantar flaps thus holding the toes in the overcorrected position; the dorsal and plantar flaps were sutured together, overlapping the distal flap. "In passing these sutures through the plantar flap," Silver stressed, "the abductor tendon should be included. This brings the flexor and extensor tendons, together with the sesamoids, towards the inner side of the joint and pulls the abductor hallucis up into its normal position, thus completing restoration of muscle balance." The skin was closed and compression dressing applied (Fig. 9–4).

Silver's contribution cannot be assessed solely on the basis of the surgical technique he described. Silver understood the complicated problem of hallux valgus as well as any of his contemporaries. He was one of the first to point out that hallux valgus is not a simple deformity, but only a factor in a general distortion of the forefoot. With that went his second aphorism: no method of treatment can be considered sufficient that does not have for its final object the correction of this general distortion and the restoration of foot function. "This means, therefore," Silver wrote, "not only that the operative procedure chosen should be, if possible, one which restores the normal anatomical relations, but also, as is so frequently the case in the treatment of deformities, that the operation itself is only one step in the treatment."

Silver placed great importance on postoperative care. He was not immune to the wishful thinking of his time that periodic strappings, bias bandage, and leather lacing would redress "the spreading of the anterior arch" or walking along the outer border of the foot would "strengthen the arches." The modern trend is to do as much correction as possible at the time of surgery and leave

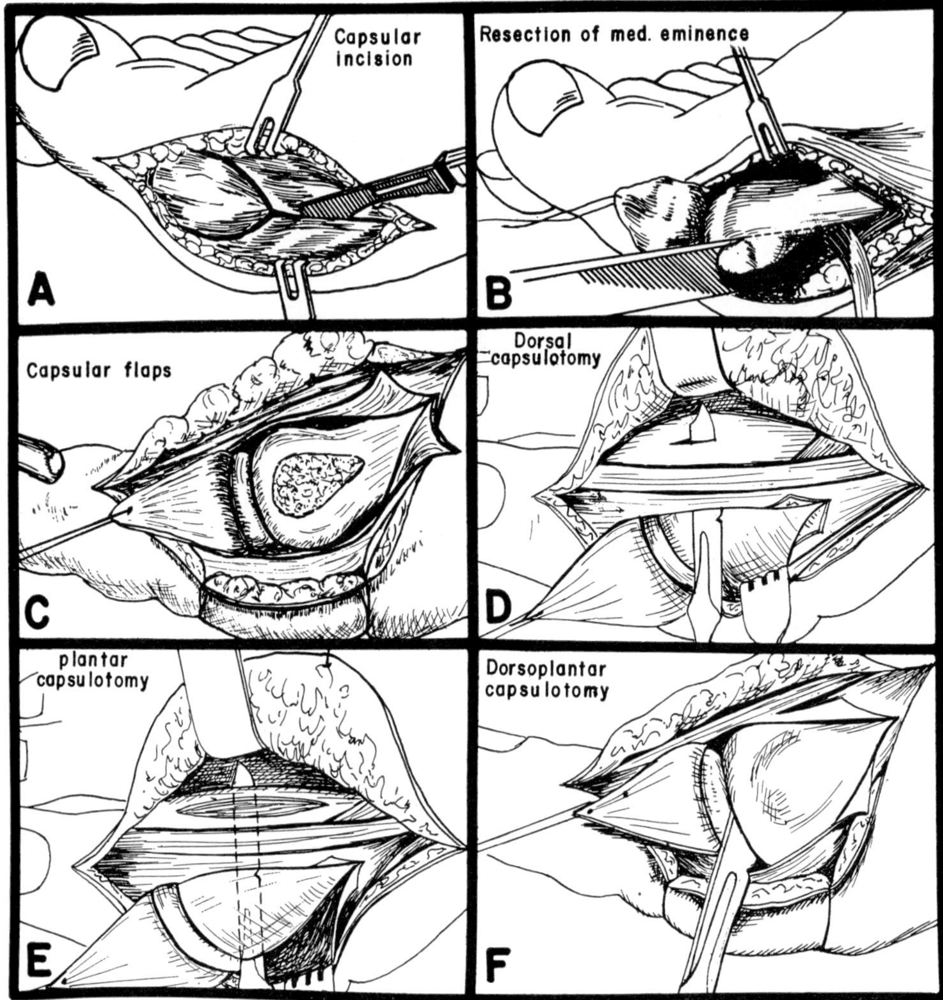

Figure 9–3. Silver operation—preliminary steps. Medial capsular incision (*A*); resection of the medial eminence (*B*); preparation of three fascial flaps (*C*); longitudinal slit of the dorsal capsule (*D*); longitudinal slit of the plantar capsule (*E*); and dorsoplantar cut of the lateral capsule (*F*).

very little for aftertreatment. These days, orthopedic surgeons do not have Silver's patience and younger subjects—for whom Silver considered his operation specially suited—will not submit patiently to the prolonged aftercare as they might have done in his time. Silver said his operation was applicable to any case, whatever the age or degree of severity, in which the articular surfaces did not present gross changes. We have since learned that recurrence is inevitable if the Silver operation is applied to cases of hallux valgus with metatarsus primus varus or hypermobile of the first metatarsal.

McBride's method. Five years after the publication of Silver's paper, Earl McBride (1928) came out with an article entitled *A Conservative Operation for Bunions.* Although Silver's name was not mentioned in this communication, his influence was evident. The method McBride described had much in common with Silver's; there was also definite resemblance of the arguments each author offered in defense of his respective procedure. In his next paper McBride (1935) conceded the similarity of his method to Silver's. McBride's operation differed from Silver's in one basic respect: he transferred the adductor hallucis tendon into the first metatarsal bone.

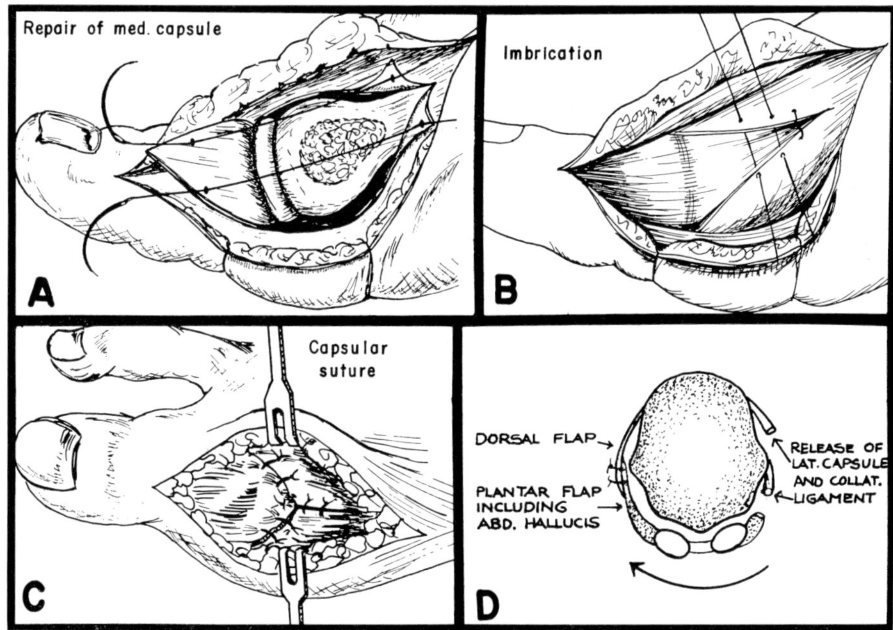

Figure 9–4. Silver operation—reparative steps. Suture to bring the distal triangular fascial flap under the dorsal and plantar flaps (*A*); (*B*) and (*C*) imbrication of fascial flaps; (*D*) diagram showing normal relation between the first metatarsal head and underlying sesamoid bones following the release of tension on the lateral aspect of the joint and capsulorrhaphy on the medial side.

With the popularity of tendon transplantation in the twenties it was inevitable that someone would suggest transference of the adductor hallucis. The suggestion came from Mauclaire (1924). Like most French surgeons of his time Mauclaire utilized the midsagittal line for reference and used *abductor, adductor,* and *internal* conversely to their usage by English-speaking authors. He resected the medial eminence and sectioned the proximal phalanx of the great toe just distal to the articular cortex. He then removed a segment of bone from the distal fragment and tenotomized the long extensor. The long extensor and the lateral conjoined tendon were then inserted obliquely into the first metatarsal head (Fig. 9–5).

We learn from Bade (1940) that as early as 1926 Erlacher had inserted the common adductor tendon into the medial aspect of the first metatarsal head. Erlacher's (1928) paper describing this operation appeared 2 years later. Balog (1928) and McBride (1928) recommended similar procedures. Balog connected the severed adductor to the medial border, while McBride connected it to the lateral border of the metatarsal neck (Fig. 9–6).

McBride approached the first metatarsophalangeal joint through a longi-

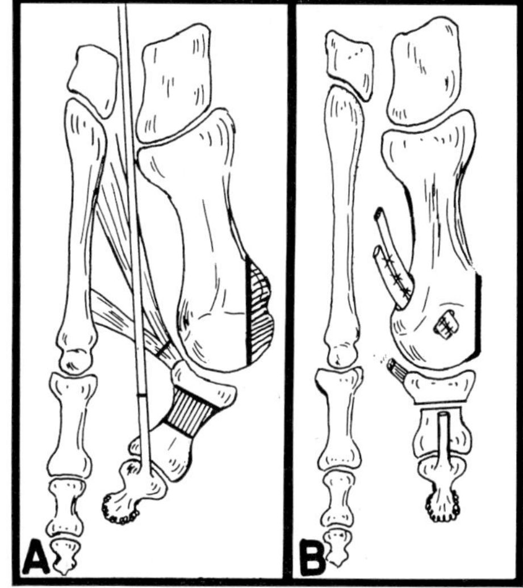

Figure 9–5. Mauclaire's transfer of long extensor and adductor obliquely into the first metatarsal head. The proximal phalanx of the great toe is shortened by removing a segment: tenotomy (*A*); tunneling the tendons obliquely into the metatarsal head (*B*).

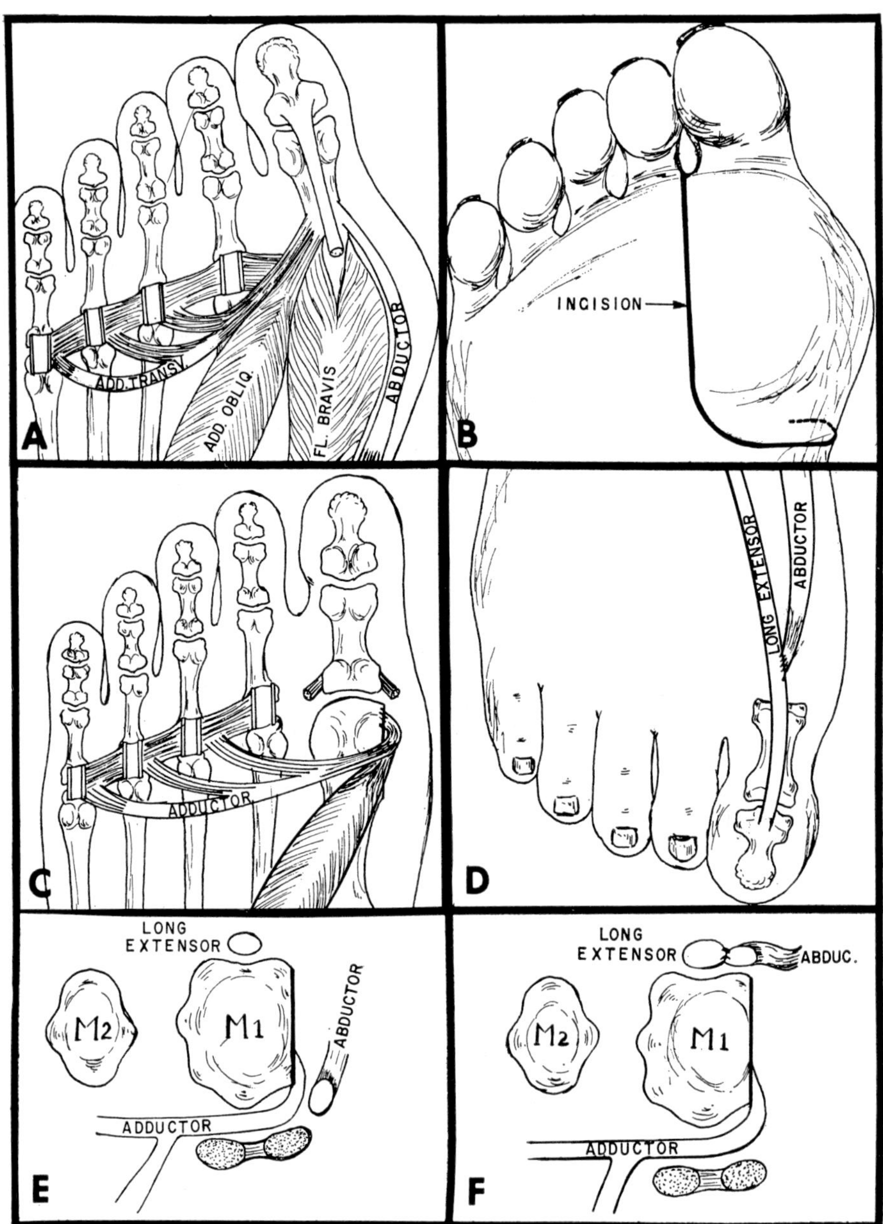

Figure 9–6. Balog operation. Anatomical relations of plantar intrinsic muscles inserting into the proximal phalanx of the great toe (*A*). Plantar "hockey-stick" incision (*B*). The medial eminence has been resected and the detached lateral conjoined tendon is reinserted into the medial aspect of the first metatarsal head (*C*). Dorsal view—the abductor hallucis is connected to the tendon of the long extensor (*D*). Coronal views showing the new points of attachment of adductor and abductor (*E* and *F*).

tudinal incision, about 2 inches long, beginning at the web between the first and second toes and running proximally along the lateral border of the extensor hallucis longus tendon. The incision was deepened plantarward along the fibular aspect of the first metatarsophalangeal joint. The conjoined tendon of the adductor hallucis and the lateral head of the flexor brevis was identified; it was traced to the outer base of the proximal phalanx and severed. The lateral sesamoid was enucleated. The detached conjoined tendon was delivered dorsally, the first metatarsal was pushed close to the second, and the conjoined tendon was sutured subperiosteally to the back of the first metatarsal neck. The incision was retracted medially; the dissection was deepened along the medial side of the joint; the thickened tissue, including the bursa, was extirpated; and the medial eminence was shaved off. From the medial capsule and the abductor tendon a large enough segment was resected so that when the cut edges were approximated the hallux would assume a slight varus position. The incision was closed. A plaster slipper was applied. The cast and stitches were removed in about 10 days. The toe was held in corrected position by adhesive plaster.

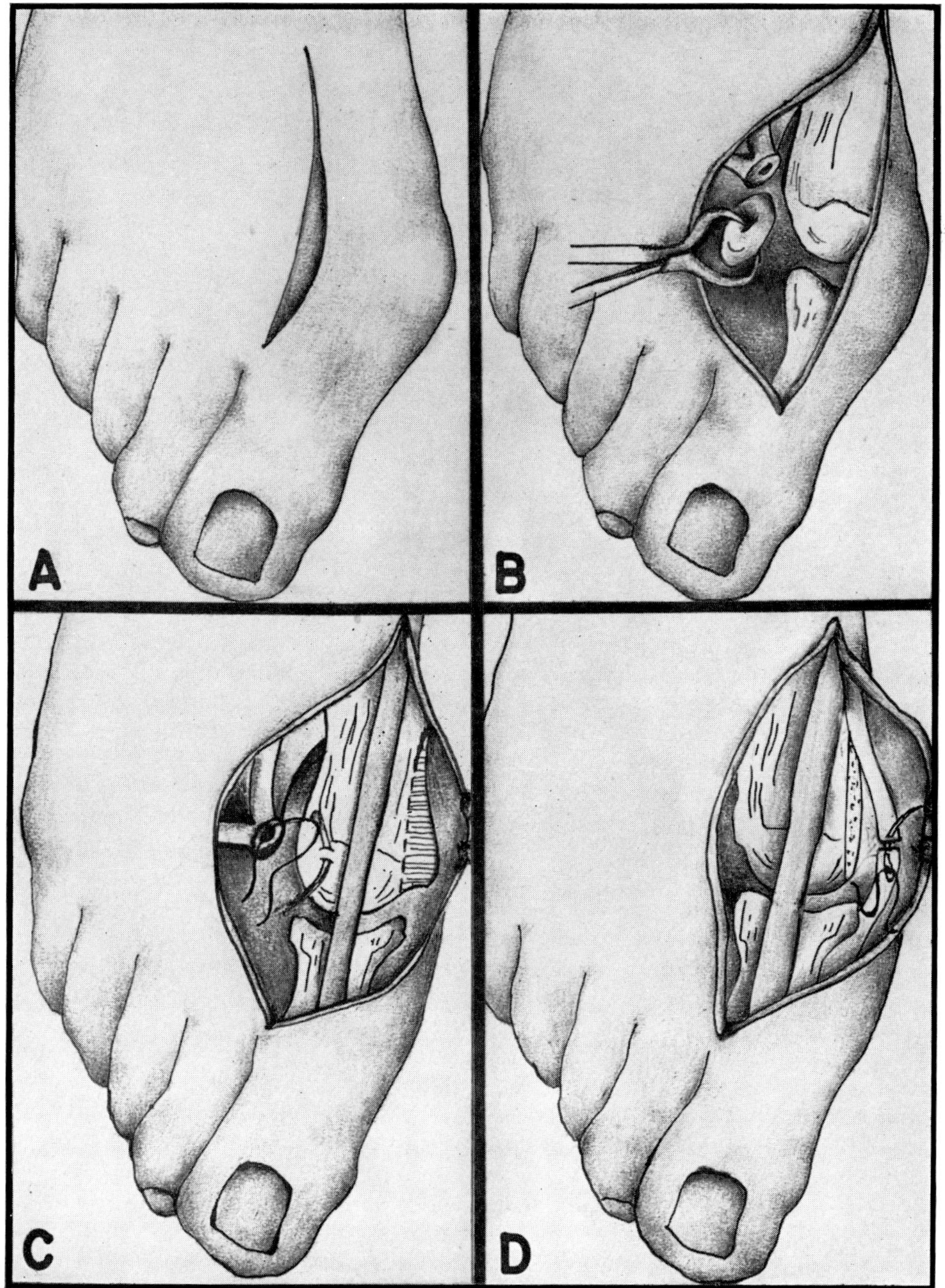

Figure 9–7. McBride operation. Incision (*A*). Detachment of lateral conjoined tendon and enucleation of the outer sesamoid (*B*). Reinsertion of the conjoined tendon into the head of the first metatarsal (*C*). Resection of the medial eminence and shortening of the capsule and the abductor tendon on this side (*D*).

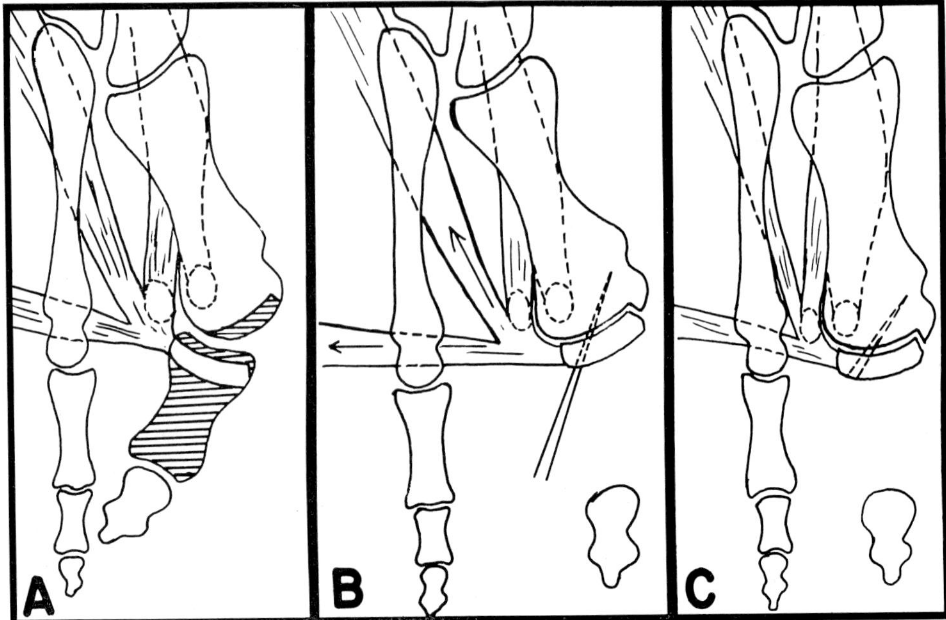

Figure 9–8. Girdlestone-Spooner operation. Resection of all but the base of the proximal phalanx and removal of articular coating of the metatarsal head and the base of the proximal phalanx (*A*). Tacking of the base of the phalanx to the head of the first metatarsal—note the phalangeal base retains its soft tissue attachments (*B* and *C*).

Weight-bearing was allowed at the end of 2 weeks (Fig. 9–7).

McBride's adductor transfer has been adopted by many and variously modified. Girdlestone and Spooner (1937) resected the distal two-thirds of the proximal phalanx of the great toe, removed the medial eminence, and denuded the opposed articular surfaces of the first metatarsophalangeal joint. They approximated the two medial metatarsals, fitted the phalangeal cap on the head of the first bone, and fixed it with a bradawl. The aim of this operation was not to fuse the joint but to transfer the adductor pull to the first metatarsal with the hope of restraining its inward inclination (Fig. 9–8).

Joplin (1950) considered his *sling procedure* a modification of the McBride operation. Joplin said his operation differed from McBride's in that he attached the adductor to the medial rather than to the lateral aspect of the first metatarsal. Joplin inserted the adductor tendon into the metatarsal from the lateral aperture of the drill hole, brought it out on the other side and sutured it to the medial capsule. The part of the tendon passing through bone in time would become incorporated. Ultimately, one ended with a typical McBride attachment of the adductor to the lateral side of the metatarsal neck. All one can say of the Joplin transplant is that it is more likely to take, for the tendon is inserted into the cancellous bone, rather than sutured subperiosteally as it was in the McBride operation (Fig. 9–9).

Stamm (1957) excised the base of the phalanx, resected the medial eminence, performed proximal osteotomy of the first metatarsal, and threaded the common adductor tendon through a tunnel in the metatarsal head. In what he called "my own operation," Lake (1956) utilized a similar technique. Parra and McKeever (1959) attempted to attach the adductor to the medial neck of the first metatarsal—as had Erlacher and Balog years before, but he made no mention of their names. Simmonds and Menelaus (1960) osteotomized the first metatarsal near its base, resected the medial eminence, and threaded the common adductor tendon through a tunnel in the metatarsal head.

Behind all these attempts lurked the

hope that the transplanted adductor would correct, or at least check, the tendency of the first metatarsal to go into a greater varus position. That this would be a difficult feat to accomplish—without capsulotomy of the innermost cuneometatarsal joint or osteotomy of the first metatarsal—does not seem to have occurred to the earlier advocates of adductor transfer. There was another contention implicit in the attempt: the transfer of the adductor into the head of the first metatarsal would restore muscle balance.

At that time there had been considerable discussion concerning the varus deflection of the first metatarsal. It was inferred that by transplanting the adductor into the first metatarsal McBride and his followers tried to approximate this bone closer to its fellow on the fibular side. McBride himself was noncommittal about the reason behind this step. Perhaps, he did not originally intend to convey the impression that in transferring the adductor to the first metatarsal he was aiming to correct metatarsus primus varus. But that impression was widespread. In the course of his discussion of McBride's (1935) paper, Lapidus came out point-blank and said that the transference of the adductor insertion into the first metatarsal was really an attempt to approximate that bone to its immediate neighbor on the fibular side. Hallock (1949) gave a similar interpretation of McBride's operation.

In his second communication McBride again advised early ambulation after surgery. He wrote: "Several of the best results have been obtained when the patient began wearing ordinary shoes with roomy toes, at the end of three weeks. When weight bearing activity is prohibited more than three weeks, persistent symptoms due to the effect of weakness and atrophy are likely to occur."

Those who still nurtured the impression that by transferring the adductor tendon to the first metatarsal McBride aimed to provide an active mechanism to draw this bone closer to its mate on the fibular side should have asked: how long would the precarious suturing (we assume it was with catgut) of the adductor tendon to the periosteum of

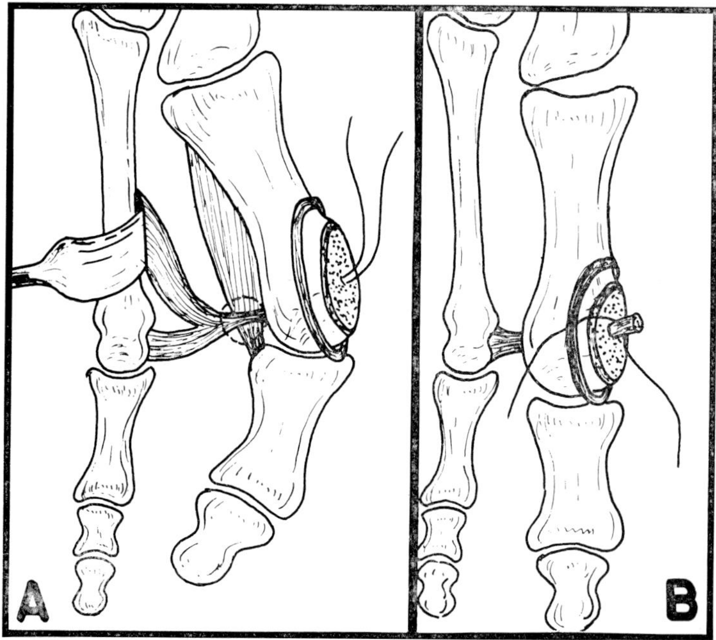

Figure 9–9. Joplin modification of adductor transfer into the head of the first metatarsal. The common adductor tendon is threaded through a tunnel into the first metatarsal head (*A*). The adductor tendon is sutured to the medial capsule of the first metatarsophalangeal joint (*B*).

the first metatarsal hold under the body weight? Even if the first metatarsal were temporarily brought closer to its immediate neighbor, would it not eventually spring back into a varus position?

In the course of his discussion of Joplin's (1950) sling operation, McBride conceded that the transverse portion of the adductor "arises from the plantar metatarsophalangeal ligaments of the third and fourth and fifth toes." The transverse component of the adductor hallucis originates from a yielding substratum and not from a fixed bone. When one arises on the toes, as in the take-off stage of walking, the adductor transversus comes to lie under the entire body weight. Pinned between the metatarsal heads and the ground, the puny little fasciculi of the adductor transversus cannot be expected to contract and adduct the proximal phalanx, much less the first metatarsal. In hallux valgus, Silver (1923) said, it was this muscle that underwent adaptive shortening most—that is, fibrosis. In his discussion of McBride's (1935) paper, Lapidus wondered whether "this little muscle" was capable of holding the two medial metatarsal bones together. Hawkins, Mitchell, and Hedrick (1945) considered "it difficult to conceive that transplantation of the relatively weak adductor hallucis muscle is capable of maintaining the first metatarsal in this more lateral position."

During the same discussion following Joplin's paper, McBride said: "In 1928 and again in 1935, I directed attention to the importance of the adductor hallucis muscle in the correction of hallux valgus. I also stressed that the removal of the lateral sesamoid permitted closure of the side gap between the first and second metatarsal heads. Subperiosteal fixation of the adductor to the first metatarsal head and firm circumferential sutures to bind the first and second metatarsal heads together takes care of the varus of the first metatarsal."

This was the first time McBride explicitly announced his aim in transferring the adductor to the first metatarsal, thus giving the nod of approval to those who had been thinking all along that the purpose of this step was to correct the varus deformity of the first metatarsal.

In a later communication, McBride (1952) let us know that, for circumferential suture he used No. 2 chromic catgut. How long does such a suture last under the body weight? Lenggenhager (1935) had already described this type of circlage. Lenggenhager used wire for this purpose. He is given no mention in McBride's paper. After osteotomy of the first metatarsal, we have utilized Lenggenhager's technique, using 15-gage stainless steel wire for circlage. Months after the osteotomy healed and the patient began to walk the wire broke, owing to the spreading of the first metatarsal under body weight (Fig. 9–10).

In the same article McBride wrote: "Release of adductor tension is gained through transplanting the adductor from the proximal phalanx to the first metatarsal head. This procedure is for the purpose of permitting reduction of the laterally rotated phalanx and not essentially to correct the primus varus of the first metatarsal." McBride was not as certain as he was 2 years previously when he discussed Joplin's paper. In answer to the objection that transplanting the adductor does not relieve the primus varus or splayfoot deformity, McBride commented: "Too much has been expected of the transplanting of the adductor. The prime object is to release its deforming effect on the proximal phalanx."

We excerpt the following from McBride's (1954) later communication: "The motor power of the great toe is focused on its proximal phalanx. The first metatarsal remains a rigid pronglike base where the forces originating from the tarsals and the outer four metatarsals gradually pull the sesamoids and the phalanges into valgus . . . In the presence of severe hallux valgus, rotation is added to the lateral stress, so that degenerative joint changes cause the deformity. The development of hallux valgus and bunion is said to be a struggle between the abductor and adductor forces in which the adductor forces win. . . ."

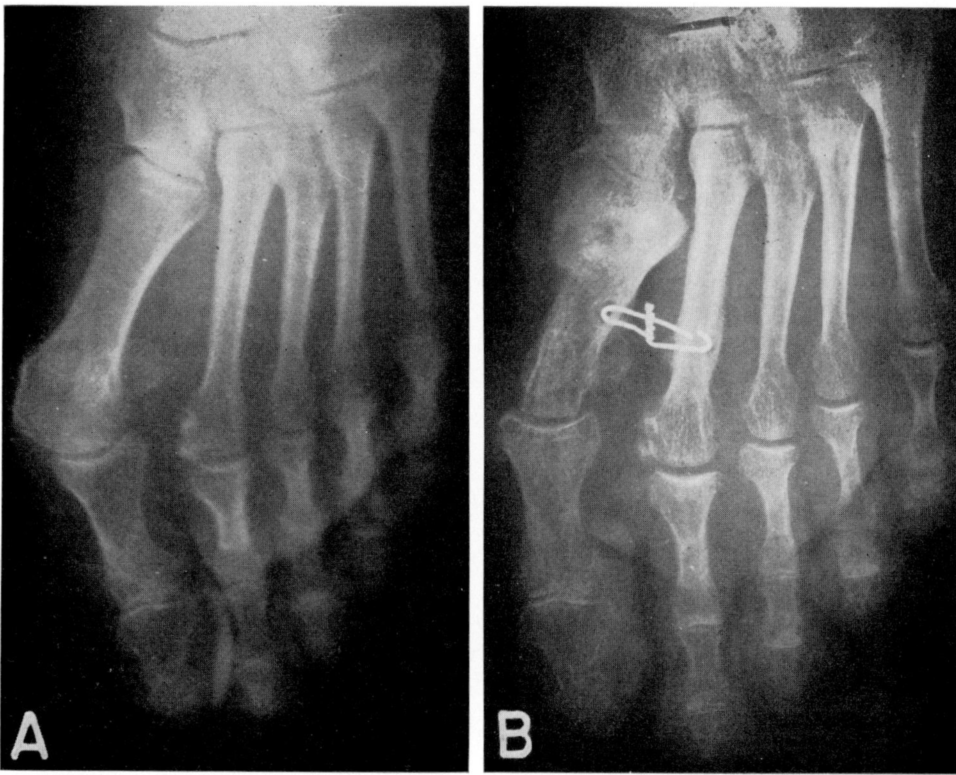

Figure 9–10. Broken circlage wire. Hallux valgus with metatarsus primus varus treated by resection of medial eminence, proximal osteotomy of the first metatarsal and circlage by 15-gage wire—the latter was threaded through two drill holes in the first metatarsal shaft and encircled second metatarsal (*A*). Six months after the operation the wire broke where it went around the second metatarsal bone (*B*).

McBride now recommended his procedure for "severe hallux valgus with moderate articular changes." Earlier he had considered his operation unsuitable for cases of "marked changes in the articular surface or extreme deformity. . . ." Are we justified in inferring that the removal of the outer sesamoid and the transplantation of the adductor benefit moderate arthritics? And how does an operation that years ago was regarded unsuitable for cases of marked changes in the articular surface and extreme deformity become suitable for severe hallux valgus with moderate articular changes? Where is one to draw the line between *marked* and *moderate* arthritis of the first metatarsophalangeal joint and severe hallux valgus and extreme deformity?

McBride also wrote: "The essential feature of the operation is release of adductor tension in order to permit realignment of the phalanges on the first metatarsal. The adductor is detached from the lateral margin of the proximal phalanx and is transplanted to the neck of the first metatarsal. Reattachment of the first metatarsal serves no essential purpose except to assure release from the adductor forces of the phalanges."

We again ask: if reattachment of the adductor to the first metatarsal serves no essential purpose, why go to the trouble of doing it? Release of the proximal phalanx is accomplished by lateral capsulotomy and tenotomy of the conjoined tendon. How does the reattachment of the tendon to the metatarsal assure this release any more than tenotomy has already done? Is it implied that if left unattached the adductor will migrate forward and reattach itself to the base of the proximal phalanx? Do not tendons retract when sectioned?

McBride was aware of the fact that adductor transversus does not originate from bone but from ligamentous structures. Yet, he spoke of "forces originating . . . from the outer four metatarsals." In the same sentence he described the first metatarsal as a rigid pronglike base. But he indicated that this rigid bone could permanently be held closer to the second metatarsal by a circlage suture consisting of No. 2 chromic catgut. For what he called "immutable Hallux Valgus," in which "the joint as well as the bursa shows marked degenerative changes," McBride recommended removal of both sesamoids.

Several years later, in the course of his discussion of a paper by Mitchell and his associates (1958), McBride finally came around and bestowed a reserved nod of approval to osteotomy of the first metatarsal. He also appeared to agree with his critics as to the inadequacy of his procedure in correcting "the primus varus or splayfoot deformity." But he was not willing to concede that release of lateral tension is gained through sectioning of the adductor tendon, which was initiated by Lothrop (1873) and Erichsen (1873) and practiced by many, and not "through transplanting the adductor from the proximal phalanx to the first metatarsal"—the only feature that distinguishes McBride's procedure from numerous other "plastic" operations.

On the credit side we must mention the fact that, after Blodgett (1880), McBride (1935) was one of the few authors who spoke of circulatory complications in connection with hallux valgus surgery, and with undeniable integrity recorded such postoperative mishaps as skin slough, slow healing, persistent sinus, intractable pain, hallux varus, flexion deformity of the distal phalanx, and metatarsalgia. McBride warned against surgery in the presence of "endarteritis."

McBride insisted on excision of the fibular sesamoid. If wedged between the first and second metatarsal and if it hinders their approximation, the lateral sesamoid should be extirpated before an attempt is made to bring the two flanking bones together—after osteotomy of the first metatarsal. It must also be acknowledged that the transfer of adductors to the head of the first metatarsal may temporarily hold this bone closer to its fellow on the fibular side, provided it has been osteotomized at some point proximal.

The indications for McBride's operation do not differ from those of Silver's: hallux valgus uncomplicated with metatarsus primus varus and interlocking arthritis of the first metatarsophalangeal joint. While in the Silver procedure an attempt is made to bring the abductor hallucis to a more dorsal position on the medial aspect of the first metatarsal head and thereby correct the rotation of the hallux, in McBride's operation the medial capsule and the abductor tendon are merely shortened to correct the outward deviation of the great toe.

Some other derivatives of Silver's operation. The three basic tenets of Silver's procedure—sagittal resection of the medial eminence, adductor release, and transposition of abductor hallucis —have been adopted by many and variously modified. As is usually the case, what is most recent or fashionable attracts greater attention and lends itself to experimentation. Lothrop's (1873) release of adductor tension and Reverdin's (1881) resection of the medial eminence had undergone all imaginable renovation by the time Silver introduced his procedure. Fuld's (1916–1919) transfer of abductor hallucis was relatively recent and could stand some modification.

Hiss (1931–1949) described a procedure he called "base correction method," or "the author's tendon balance operation." It differed from Silver's procedure only in the way the abductor hallucis was transposed. The displaced tendon was delivered from under the joint, severed, and reattached to the medial base of the proximal phalanx. It was implied that in case one wanted to augment the action of the flexors, one would reanchor the abductor to a more plantar point on the medial base of the phalanx. If it was desired that the extensors should be reinforced, the abductor was transplanted to a more dorsal point. The illustrations included in the latest edition of his book show the abductor tendon lying against the decorticated surface left after the resection of the medial eminence. After this procedure, the transposed tendon was likely to adhere to the decorticated portion of the metatarsal head and the contractions of the abductor would fail to move the proximal phalanx. The outcome would be tenodesis of the first metatarsophalangeal joint, with the transposed tendon reinforcing the medial capsule, which in itself is desirable. However, one cannot speak of restoring muscle balance as is claimed. Fuld (1916–1919), the originator of abductor transfer, interposed a capsular flap between the transposed tendon and decorticated surface left after the resection of the medial eminence.

Stein (1938) considered hallux valgus a "contractural deformity" with "primary deforming elements" being located on the "contracted side"—meaning the lateral aspect of the first metatarsophalangeal joint. He singled out the following structures: "(1) adductor obliquus attachments to the lateral sesamoid, (2) the external lateral ligament, (3) the capsule between the two structures, (4) frequently, the lateral head of the flexor brevis muscle." The division of these structures would, Stein said, permit unresisted correction of the valgus deformity and allow the sesamoids to slip into place. Although he denounced "exostosis" removed at operation as a "myth," Stein advised removing "secondary hypertrophic changes of the medial margin of the metatarsal head" as well as "osteophitic processes." He fashioned what he called a corrective flap from the medial capsule of the joint. This flap was left attached inferiorly to the tendon of the abductor hallucis. By pulling the flap up and backward, the abductor tendon was brought to the side of the joint; it stayed in that position when the capsular flap was sutured to its newer locations (Figs. 9–11 to 9–13).

Brooke (1941) performed a **Z**-plasty of the long extensor tendon. "By retracting backwards the inner margin of the incision," he wrote, "the inner part of the abductor hallucis, which in this region is partly tendinous comes into view. The tendinous portion is traced downwards to its attachment to the inner sesa-

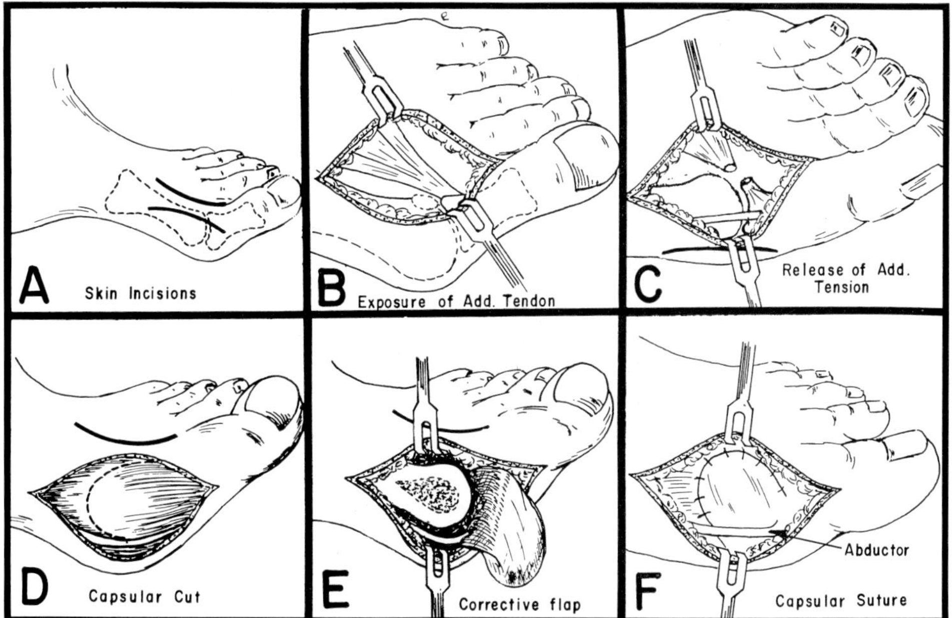

Figure 9–11. Stein operation. Skin incisions (*A*); exposure of lateral conjoined tendon (*B*); release of adductor tension (*C*); medial capsular cut (*D*); corrective flap and resection of the medial eminence (*E*); and capsuloplasty to bring the abductor tendon from under the metatarsal head to the inner side of it (*F*).

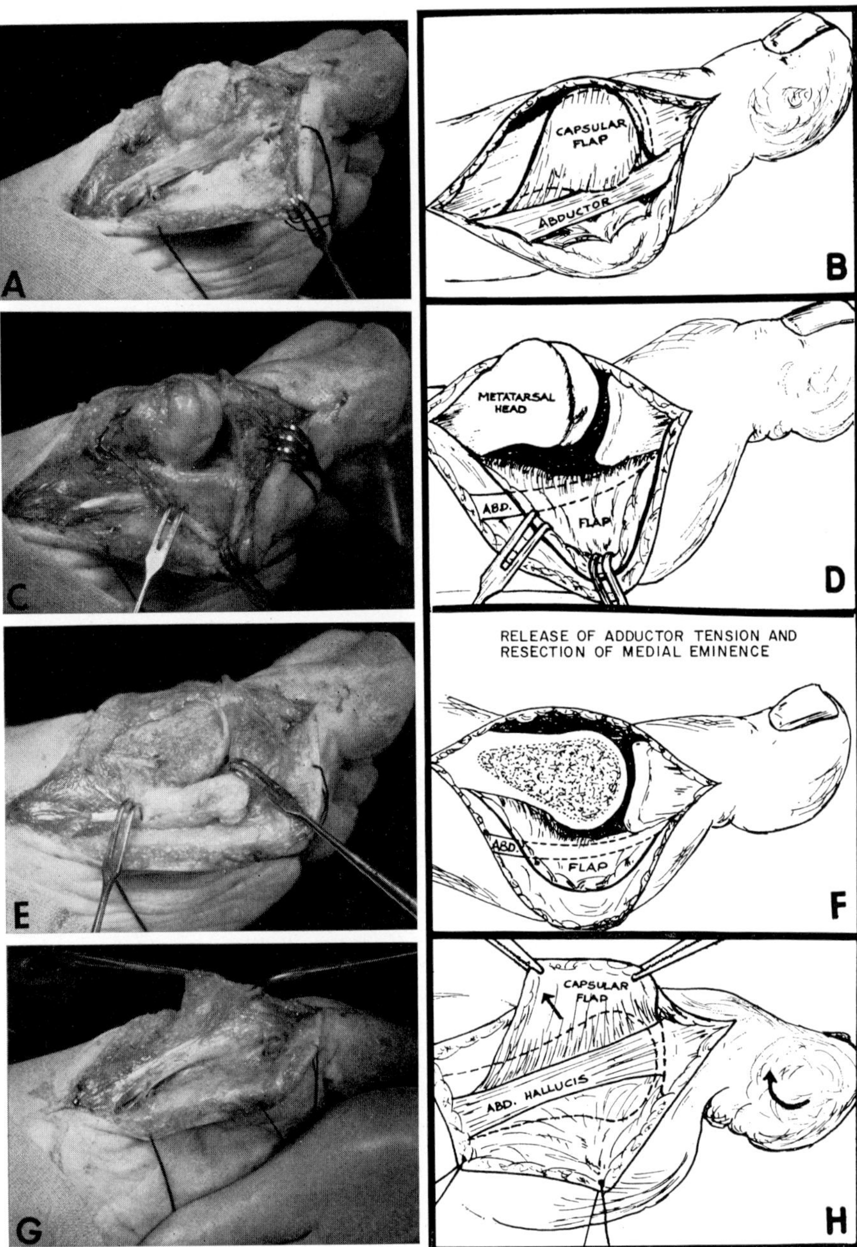

Figure 9–12. Photographs and interpretative diagrams to illustrate some of the steps of modified Stein operation. The position of the displaced abductor hallucis (*A* and *B*). Plantar reflection of capsular flap (*C* and *D*). Resection of the medial eminence and release of adductor tension (*E* and *F*). When the capsular flap is pulled up, the abductor tendon shifts from under the metatarsal head and comes to lie on its inferomedial aspect (*G* and *H*). The sesamoid pad moves with the abductor.

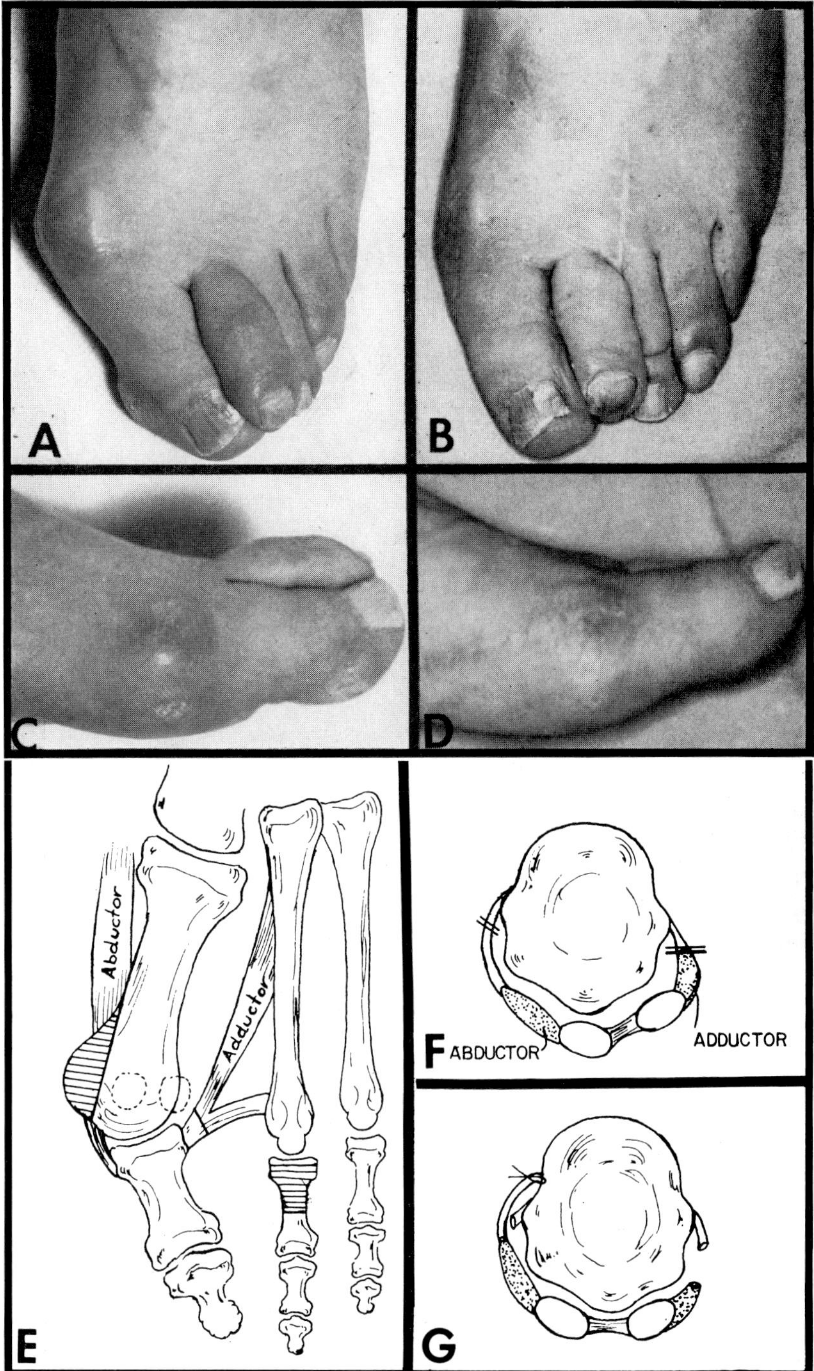

Figure 9–13. Representative case. Woman in her forties. Unilateral hallux valgus with mild axial rotation of the great toe; dorsal subluxation of the second toe at the metatarsophalangeal joint. Surgery: Stein operation; resection of proximal portion of the basal phalanx of the second toe and syndactylia of this digit with its fellow on the lateral side. Dorsal view before surgery (*A*); after surgery (*B*); preoperative side view (*C*); postoperative side view (*D*); interpretative diagrams (*E, F* and *G*). The patient was satisfied with the result.

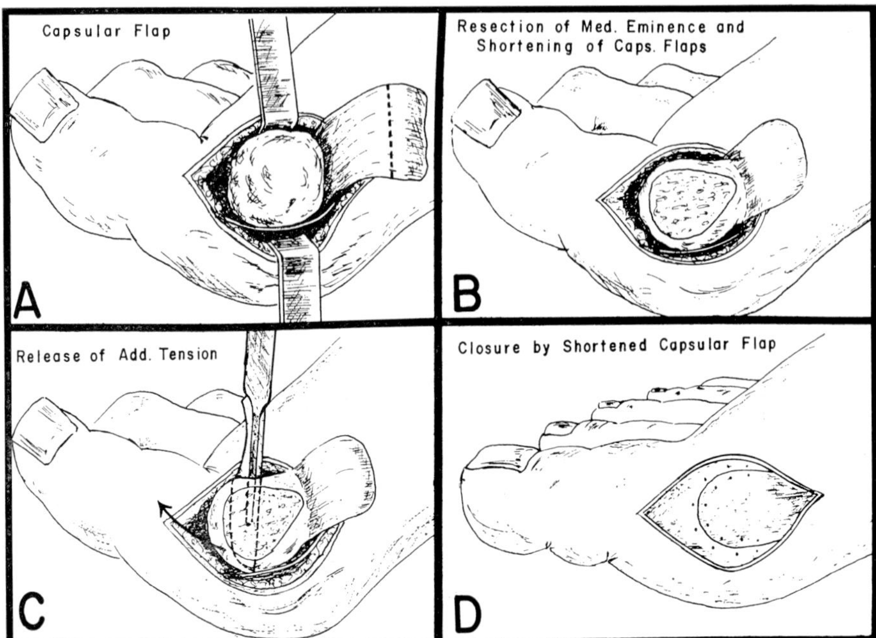

Figure 9–14. Operation for hallux valgus without axial rotation of the great toe. Proximally based fascial flap (*A*); sagittal resection of the medial eminence and shortening the fascial flap (*B*); release of adductor tension (*C*); suturing the shortened capsular flap (*D*).

moid bone, and is then incised horizontally over a distance of one and a half inches, rather nearer the anterior than the posterior margin of the tendon. The smaller anterior portion of the muscle and tendon can be pulled forward, and will form a loop through which the divided extensor hallucis longus is threaded from deep to the superficial aspect, put on the stretch in the overcorrected varus position, and sewn again to the proximal end with three or four interrupted stitches of fine silk-worm gut. The innermost tendon of the extensor digitorum brevis is divided and the wound closed."

In what he called his "technique," Hauser (1939, 1950) disconnected the abductor insertion as had Fuld and reattached it to the inner base of the proximal phalanx "subperiosteally." In his latest modification of *"sling procedure"* Joplin (1958) passed the terminal segment of the long extensor of the fifth toe over the neck of the first metatarsal and then "beneath the superficial fibers of the abductor hallucis" to lift the latter "to a more nearly normal position on the medial side of the joint."

A suggested modification of Silver's procedure. Silver's method of severing the contracted structures on the lateral aspect of the first metatarsophalangeal joint was awkward and the viability of his distal triangular flap precarious. This flap was severed proximally from where it received most of its nutrient supply and left attached with a distal pedicle to the inner base of the first phalanx. Occasionally one has to resect the overhanging medial lip of the base of the first phalanx, which means cutting off the source of nourishment of the fascial flap completely. We prefer a flap with proximal pedicle or one attached inferiorly to the abductor tendon. We also like to resect more bone from the medial eminence than Silver did. In performing medial capsuloplasty, Silver utilized the same technique for both hallux valgus in which the great toe deviated only in an outward direction and for the deformity in which the toe was also rotated around its long axis.

In hallux valgus without axial rotation, one only has to tighten the inner capsule of the first metatarsophalangeal joint and need not transpose the abductor hallucis. The joint is approached through a medial curvilinear incision. A U-shaped capsuloperiosteal flap with a broad proximal base is developed. It is severed distally and left attached to the shaft of the first metatarsal. The hallux is pushed toward the second toe. The osteotome is placed lateral to the strip of erosion—the sagittal groove—separating the surface of the metatarsal head still in contact with the base of the proximal phalanx from the portion that has slipped medially. The blade of the osteotome is tilted so as to remove more bone from the dorsal than from the plantar aspect of the metatarsal head. The medial eminence is shaved flush with the inner cortex of the shaft. All structures attached to the fibular side of the proximal phalanx are severed. The U-shaped flap is shortened

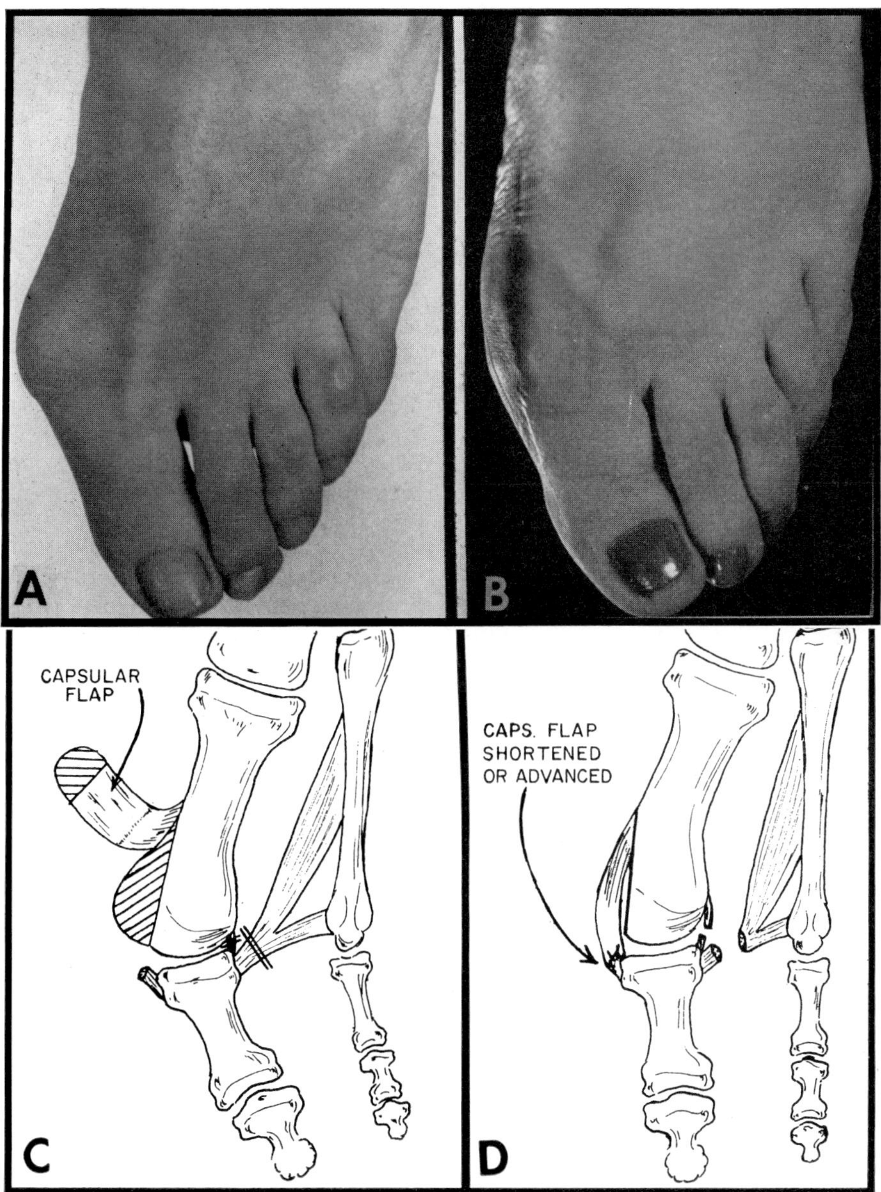

Figure 9–15. Woman, 53 years of age; hallux valgus with no axial rotation of the great toe. Surgery: sagittal resection of the medial eminence, release of adductor tension, and shortening of the medial capsule. Preoperative photograph (*A*); after recovery (*B*); interpretative diagrams (*C* and *D*). The patient was satisfied.

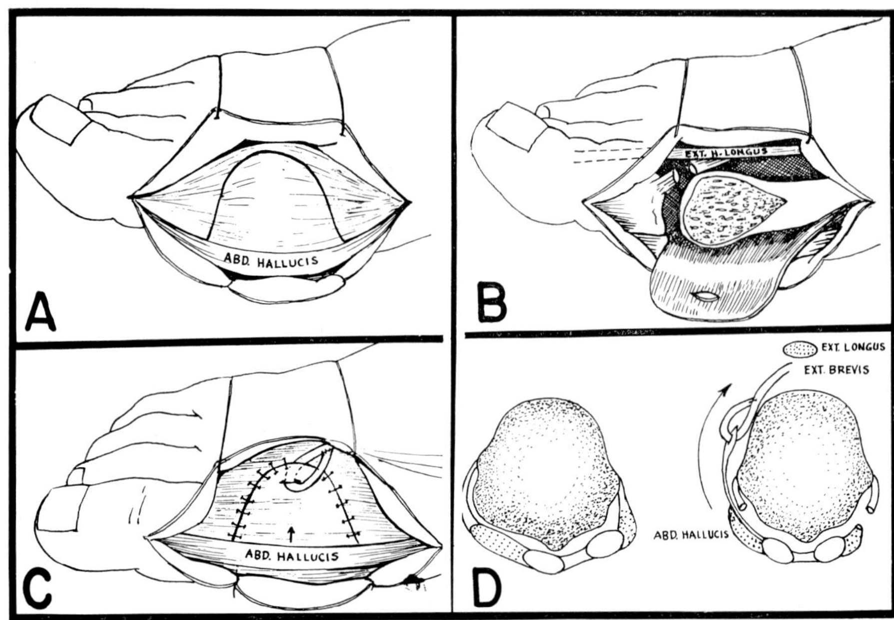

Figure 9–16. Operation for hallux valgus with resilient axial rotation eversion of the great toe. Outline of the plantarly based capsulofascial flap (*A*). The flap has been reflected plantarward and fenestrated, the extensor brevis is detached from the dorsal base of the proximal phalanx, adductor tension on the lateral side of the joint has been released, and the medial eminence chiseled off (*B*). The tendon of the short extensor is threaded through the fascial flap to pull it and the abductor hallucis up (*C*). Restoration of the sesamoid pad to its normal position under the metatarsal head (*D*).

and reattached to the medial base of the phalanx. Overcorrection is avoided (Figs. 9–14 and 9–15).

More often the outward deviation is also accompanied with axial rotation—eversion—of the great toe, in which instance one must suspect plantar migration of the abductor hallucis and a variable degree of lateral shift of the sesamoids. In such a case an attempt should be made to bring the abductor hallucis from under the metatarsal head to its inner side. If the sesamoids are not eroded, mushroomed, or incarcerated, they should also be restored to their usual position under the metatarsal head. The first metatarsophalangeal joint is again approached by way of a medial curvilinear incision. A capsular flap—similar to one suggested by Stein (1938)—is developed. This flap is semicircular, with convexity up; it is continuous below with the abductor tendon, which is left attached to the proximal phalanx. Sagittal resection of the medial eminence and release of the adductor tension are carried out as in hallux valgus without axial rotation. In addition, the fibular collateral ligament holding the lateral sesamoid to the metatarsal head is severed. The extensor hallucis brevis is disconnected at its insertion into the dorsal aspect of the base of the proximal phalanx and is dissected free proximally. A slit is made into the base of the previously prepared abductor flap and the cut end of the extensor brevis tendon is threaded through it; the eversion of the hallux is corrected and the end of the extensor brevis is sutured to its stem. If taut, the tendon of the long extensor is lengthened by Z-plasty (Figs. 9–16 to 9–20).

The foregoing procedure is only effective when the axial rotation of the great toe is resilient—when one can manually correct the rotation of the hallux. In fixed eversion of the great toe, one must suspect adhesions surrounding the sesamoids or incarceration of these ossicles in their displaced position. In such an instance, the sesamoids are usually worn out and arthritic. It is unwise to pull them back under the bearing surface of the metatarsal head. One is then left with two alternatives. When they are

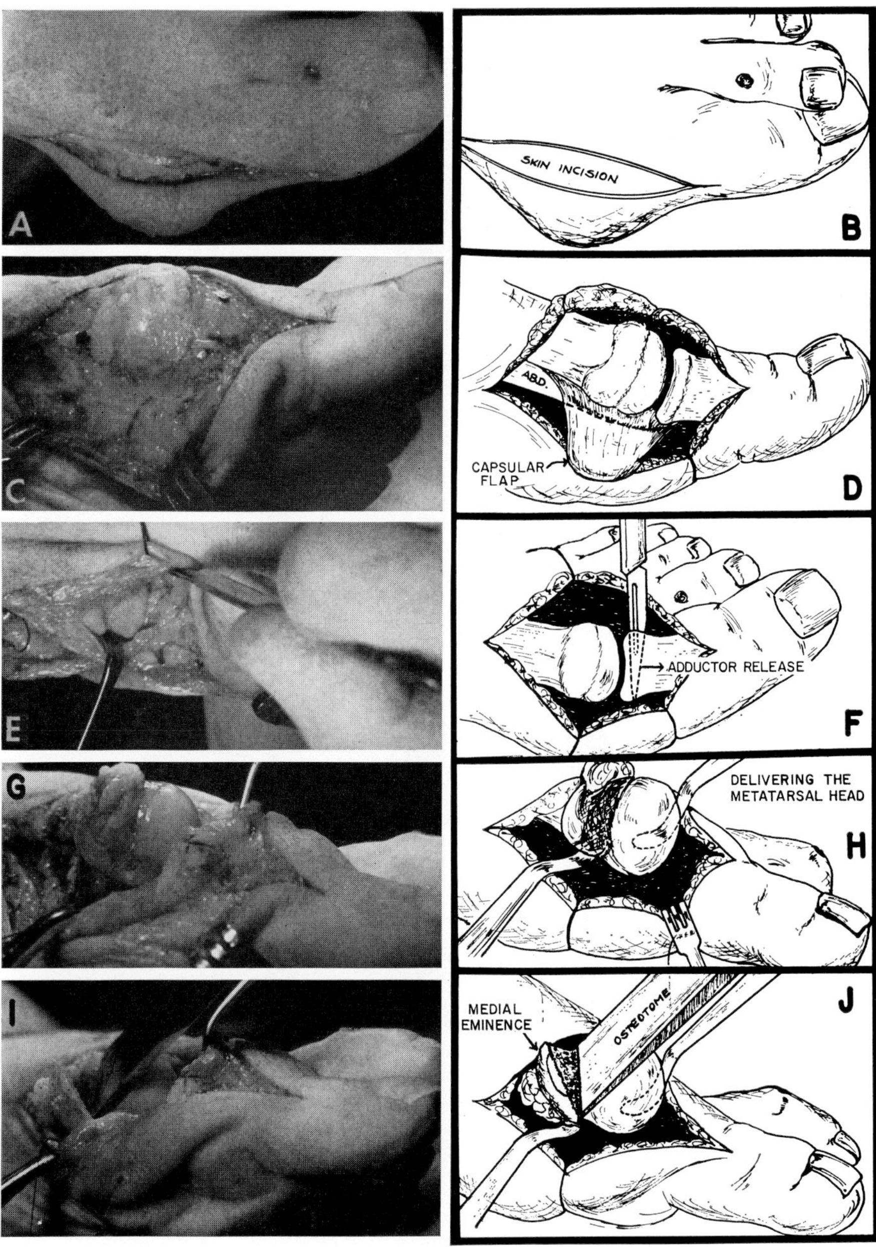

Figure 9–17. Photographs during surgery and interpretative diagrams demonstrating the steps of operation for cases of hallux valgus with resilient axial rotation of the great toe. Incision (*A* and *B*); exposure of the medial eminence with overlying capsular tissue (*C*); plantarly based capsular flap (*D*); release of adductor tension on the lateral side of the first metatarsophalangeal joint (*E* and *F*); levering the head out of the wound—note the deep sagittal groove (*G* and *H*); sagittal resection of the medial eminence (*I* and *J*).

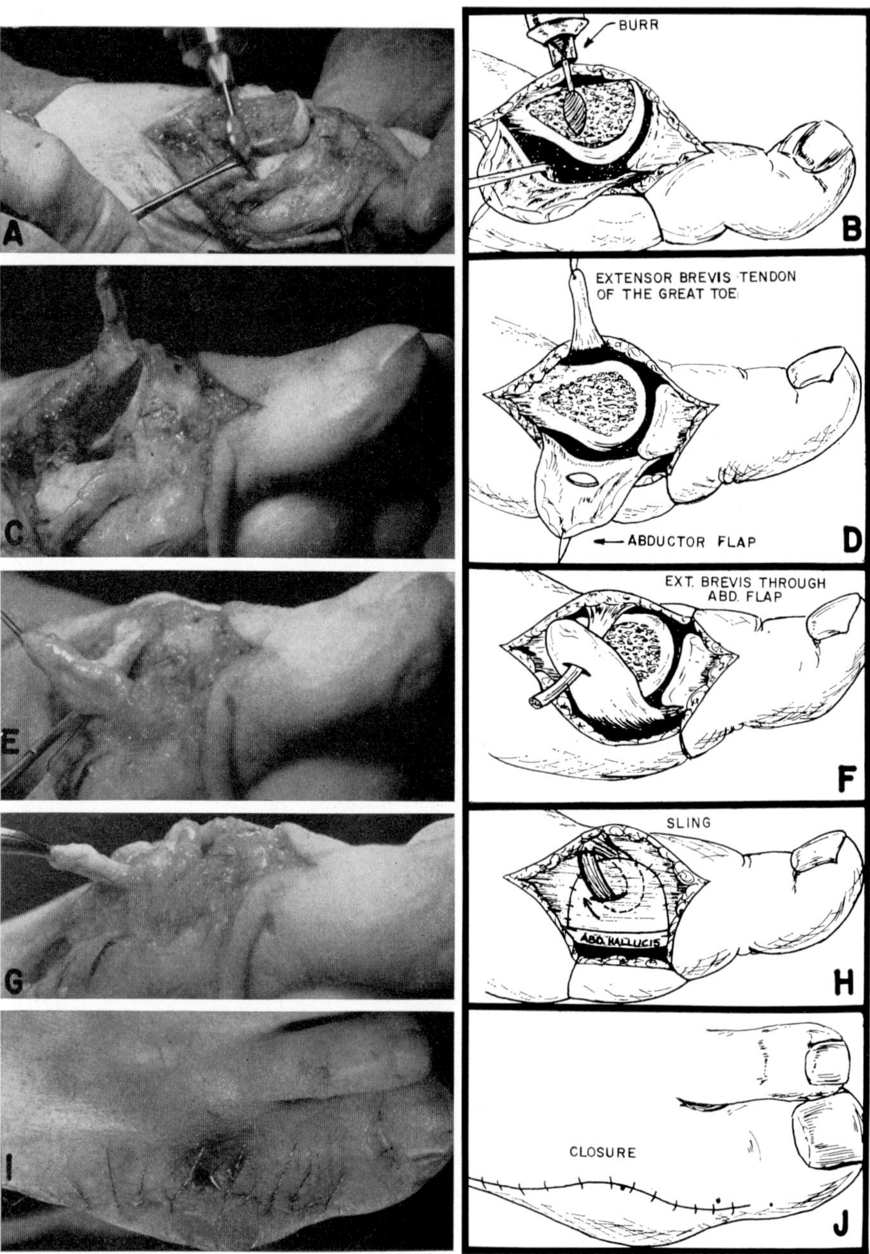

Figure 9–18. The same as Figure 9–17. Decorticated surface left after the sagittal resection of the medial eminence is smoothed (*A* and *B*); detachment and dissection of extensor brevis tendon, which is threaded through a slit in the abductor flap (*C* and *D*); extensor brevis threaded through abductor flap (*E* and *F*); abductor pulled up and extensor brevis sutured to itself (*G* and *H*); closure (*I* and *J*).

suspected of causing metatarsalgia, the sesamoids are shelled out. In the absence of subsesamoid pain, these small ossicles are left in their displaced position; the abductor tendon is delivered from under the joint, it is severed, dissected free from the medial head of the flexor brevis, and reinserted into a more dorsal point on the medial base of the proximal phalanx.

Silver's operation and numerous modifications of it, including our own, should not be tried: (1) in the presence of degenerative arthritis of the first metatarsophalangeal joint with limited—less than 30 degrees—extension of the great toe, (2) when the axial rotation of the great toe is fixed, (3) when the hallux rides over or has slipped under the second toe, (4) when there is more than 15 degrees of metatarsus primus varus, and (5) when the first metatarsal is hypermobile or fans medially on weight-bearing.

A modification of Silver's procedure may be attempted in comparatively young adults who do not have sufficient time for prolonged postoperative convalescence that other procedures—for example, osteotomy of the first metatarsal—necessitate. Roentgenographic evidence of a sagittal groove separating the smooth lateral metatarsal head still in contact with the base of the proximal phalanx from the portion that has slipped medially justifies the "exostectomy" part of the original Silver operation, or of one of its many modifications. Release of adductor tension on the lateral side of the joint and medial capsuloplasty corrects the outward deviation of the great toe; transposition of abductor hallucis to a more dorsal position on the

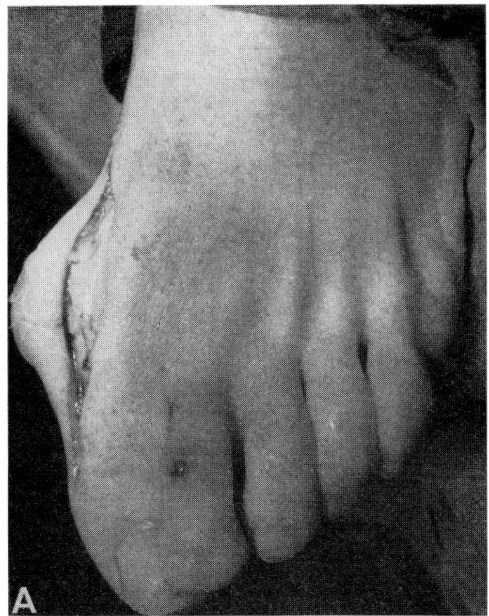

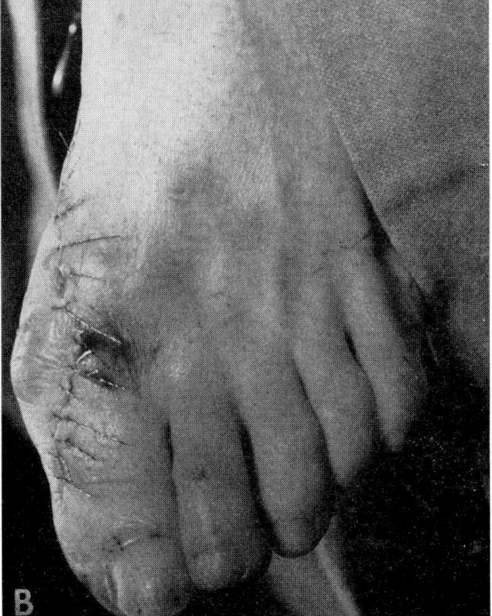

Figure 9–19. The same as Figures 9–17 and 9–18, showing the position of the hallux at the beginning of surgery (*A*) and after closure (*B*).

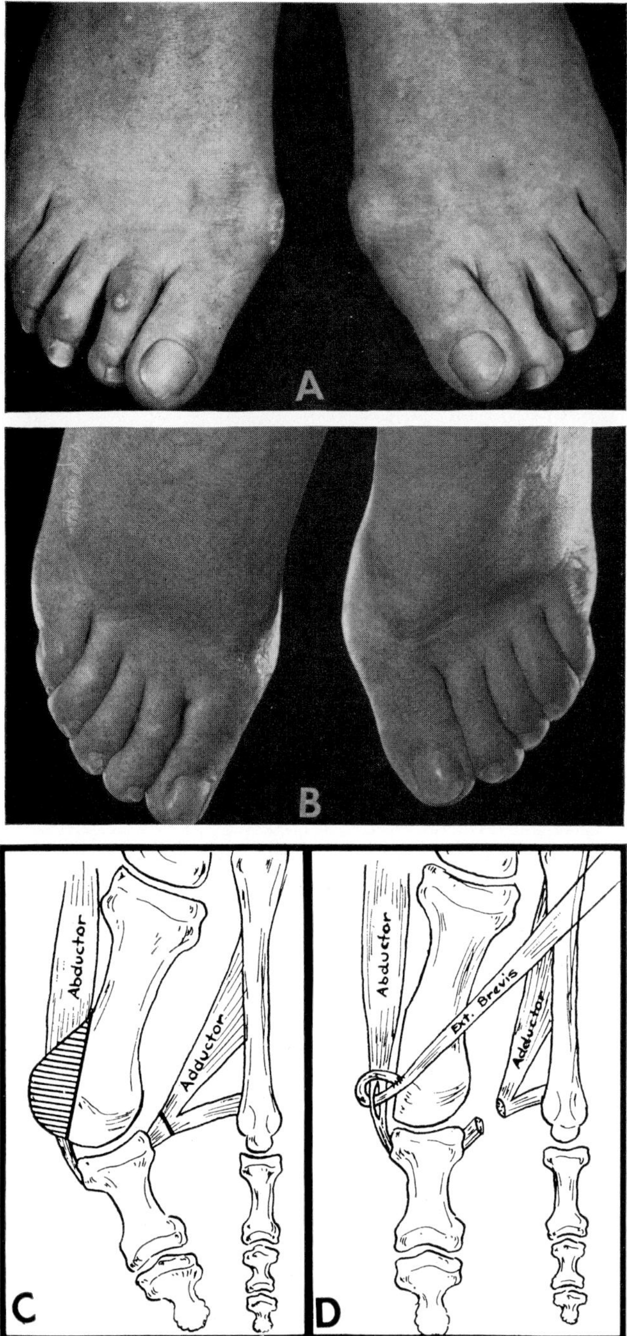

Figure 9–20. Woman, 54, bilateral hallux valgus with resilient axial rotation of great toes. Preoperative photograph (*A*); photograph after recovery (*B*)—the axial rotation of the right foot does not appear to have been corrected sufficiently but this appearance is partly due to the position of the foot at the time of photography; interpretative diagrams (*C* and *D*). The patient has not registered any complaint and is content with the outcome. Better cosmetic result could have been obtained by osteotomy of the first metatarsal.

inner aspect of the metatarsal head may rectify axial rotation—eversion—of the great toe, provided this deformity is not fixed. In the absence of a sagittal groove—especially when there is also definite metatarsus primus varus—osteotomy of the first metatarsal offers a better prospect.

REFERENCES

Aitken, D. M.: Hallux valgus, hallux rigidus, hallux flexus. In *Orthopedic Surgery of Injuries* (Sir Robert Jones, ed.). London, Oxford University Press, 1921, Vol. 1, pp. 386–389.

Annandale, T.: *The Malformations, Diseases and Injuries of the Fingers and Toes.* Philadelphia, J. B. Lippincott Co., 1866, pp. 110–127.

Ashton, T. J.: On corns and bunions. Med. Tms. Gaz. *5*:232–234 and 260–261, 1852.

Bade, P.: Der Hallux valgus. Stuttgart, F. Enke, 1940.

Balog, A.: Entstehung und Operation des Hallux valgus. Zbl. Chir. *55*:464–468, 1928.

Blodgett, A. N.: Hallux valgus, with a report of two successful cases. Med. Rec. *18*:34–37, 1880.

Boyer, A.: *Traité des Maladies Chirurgicales.* 3rd Ed., Paris, 1826, Vol. 2, pp. 73–76.

Brodie, B. C.: *Clinical Lectures on Surgery.* Philadelphia, Lea & Blanchard, 1846, pp. 126–134.

Bromeis, H.: Unsere Erfahrungen mit der Hallux valgus-Operation nach M. Schede. Chirurg. *3*:465–471, 1931.

Brooke, R.: Treatment of hallux valgus deformity in soldiers. Brit. Med. J. *2*:605–606, 1941.

Clarke, J. J.: Hallux valgus and hallux varus. Lancet *1*:609–611, 1900.

Erichsen, J. E.: *The Science and Art of Surgery.* Philadelphia, H. C. Lea, 1873, Vol. 2, pp. 311–312.

Erlacher, P. J.: Die Technik des Orthopaedischen Eingriffs, Entstehung und Operation des Hallux valgus. Chirurg. *55*:977–978, 1928.

Fernandez, J. C.: Hallux valgus operación de Petersen. Rev. Asoc. Méd. Argent. *61*:677–679, 1947.

Fowler, G. R.: Partial resection of the head of the first metatarsal bone for hallux valgus. Med. Rec. *36*:253–255, 1889.

Fuld, J. E.: Transplantation of the abductor hallucis tendon in the surgical treatment of hallux valgus. Surg. Gyn. Obst. *23*:626–628, 1916.

Fuld, J. E.: Hallux valgus. New York Med. J. *106*:265–267, 1917.

Fuld, J. E.: Surgical treatment of hallux valgus and its complications. Am. Med. *14*:536–539, 1919.

Girdlestone, G. R., and Spooner, H. J.: A new operation for hallux valgus and hallux rigidus. J. Bone Joint Surg. *19*:30–35, 1937.

Goldthwait, J. E.: The treatment of hallux valgus. Boston Med. Surg. J. *129*:533–535, 1893.

Hallock, H.: The surgical treatment of common mechanical and functional disabilities of the feet. Am. Acad. Orthop. Surgeons *6*:160–173, 1949.

Hauser, E. D. W.: *Diseases of the Foot.* Philadelphia, W. B. Saunders Co., 1939, pp. 119–151.

Hauser, E. D. W.: *Diseases of the Foot.* 2nd Ed., Philadelphia, W. B. Saunders Co., 1950, pp. 87–125.

Hawkins, F. B., Mitchell, C. L., and Hedrick, D. W.: Correction of hallux valgus by metatarsal osteotomy. J. Bone Joint Surg. *27*:387–394, 1945.

Heubach, F.: Ueber Hallux valgus und seine operative Behandlung nach Edm. Rose. Dtsch. Ztschr. Chir. *46*:210–275, 1897.

Hiss, J. M.: Hallux valgus; its causes and simplified treatment. Am. J. Surg. *11*:50–57, 1931.

Hiss, J. M.: *Functional Foot Disorders.* Los Angeles University Press, 1937, pp. 263–294.

Hiss, J. M.: *Functional Foot Disorders.* 3rd Ed., Los Angeles, Oxford Press, 1949, pp. 531–599.

Hohmann, G.: *Fuss und Bein.* Munich, J. Bergmann, 1951, pp. 145–192.

Joplin, R. J.: Sling procedure for correction of splay-foot, metatarsus primus varus, and hallux valgus. J. Bone Joint Surg., *32*:779–785, 1950.

Joplin, R. J.: Some common foot disorders amenable to surgery. Am. Acad. Orthop. Surgeons *15*:144–158, 1958.

Khoury, C.: *Hallux Valgus.* Buenos Aires, Lopex and Etchegoyen, 1947.

Kocher, T.: *Text-Book of Operative Surgery* (tr. by H. J. Stiles and C. B. Paul). 3rd English Ed., New York, MacMillan Co.; London, A. and C. Black, 1911, Vol. 1, p. 281.

Lake, N. C.: Hallux valgus. Ann. Roy. Coll. Surgeons *19*:23–35, 1956.

Lane, W. A.: The causation, pathology and physiology of the deformities which develop during young life. Guy's Hosp. Rep. *44*:307–317, 1887.

Lapidus, P. W.: The operative correction of the metatarsus varus primus in hallux valgus. Surg. Gyn. Obst. *58*:183–191, 1934.

Lapidus, P. W.: The author's bunion operation from 1931 to 1959. Clin. Orthop. *16*:119–135, 1960.

Lenggenhager, K.: Eine neue Operationsmethode zur Behandlung des Hallux valgus. Chirurg. *7*:689–692, 1935.

Lothrop, C. H.: Bunion. Boston Med. Surg. J. *88*:641–643, 1873.

McBride, E. D.: A conservative operation for bunions. J. Bone Joint Surg. *10*:735–739, 1928.

McBride, E. D.: The conservative operation for "bunions". J.A.M.A. *105*:1164–1168, 1935.

McBride, E. D.: Hallux valgus bunion deformity. Am. Acad. Orthop. Surgeons *9*:334–346, 1952.

McBride, E. D.: Hallux valgus, bunion deformity: its treatment in mild, moderate or severe stages. J. Internat. Coll. Surgeons *21*:99–105, 1954.

McElvenny, R. T., and Thompson, F. R.: A clinical study of one hundred patients subjected to simple exostectomy for relief of bunion pain. J. Bone Joint Surg. *22*:942–951, 1940.

Mauclaire, P.: Ostéoplasties, arthroplasties et transplantations tendineuses combinées pour traiter l'hallux valgus. Rev. d'Orthop. *11*:305–313, 1924.

Mitchell, L. S., Fleming, J. L., Allen, R., Glenney, C., and Sanford, G. A.: Osteotomy-bunionectomy for hallux valgus. J. Bone Joint Surg. *40*:41–60, 1958.

Moeller, F.: Beitrag zur operativen Behandlung des Hallux valgus. Jahrb. Hamb. Staatskrankenanst. *3*:306–338, 1894.

Parra, G., and McKeever, D. C.: An operation for correction of metatarsus primus varus. Clin. Orthop. *14*:162–165, 1959.

Petersen, F.: Ueber Arthrectomie des ersten Mittelfuss-Zehen-Gelenkes. Arch. Klin. Chir. *37*:677–678, and Fig. 6 at end of volume, 1888.

Porter, J. L.: Why operations for bunion fail, with description of one which does not. Surg. Gyn. Obst. *8*:89–90, 1909.

Porter, J. L.: Some further notes on the treatment of bunions. Surg. Gyn. Obst. *26*:460–463, 1918.

Reverdin, J.: De la déviation en dehors du gros orteil (hallux valgus, vulg. "oignon," "bunions," "Ballen.") et de son traitement chirurgical. Tr. Internat. Med. Congr. *2*:408–412, 1881

Silver, D.: The operative treatment of hallux valgus. J. Bone Joint Surg. *5*:225–232, 1923.

Simmonds, F. A., and Menelaus, M. B.: Hallux valgus in adolescents. J. Bone Joint Surg. *42*:761–768, 1960.

Stamm, T. T.: The surgical treatment of hallux valgus. Guy's Hosp. Rep. *106*:273–279, 1957.

Stanley, L. L., and Breck, L. W.: Bunions. J. Bone Joint Surg. *17*:961–964, 1935.

Stein, H. C.: Hallux valgus. Surg. Gyn. Obst. *66*:889–898, 1938.

Storen, G.: Removal of exostosis in hallux valgus (in Norwegian). Nord. Med. *65*:365–368, 1961.

Syms, P.: Bunion: its aetiology, anatomy and operative treatment. New York Med. J. *66*:448–451, 1897.

Timmer, H.: *Die Behandlung des Hallux valgus.* Leipzig, J. A. Barth, 1930, p. 9.

Verbrugge, J.: *Pathogénie et Traitement de l'Hallux Valgus.* Mem. Bull. Soc. Belge d'Orthop. pp. 3–40, 1933.

Weir, R. F.: The operative treatment of hallux valgus. Ann. Surg. *25*:444–453; See also discussion on pp. 480–485, 1897.

Wilson, H. A.: An analysis of 152 cases of hallux valgus in 77 patients with a report upon an operation for its relief. Am. J. Orthop. Surg. *3*:214–230, 1906.

Chapter Ten

OSTEOTOMY

The contention that hallux valgus can be rectified by surgical fracture of one of the bones of the innermost ray germinated during the last quarter of the past century. Initially the first metatarsal was osteotomized, then the adjoining cuneiform and finally the proximal phalanx of the great toe.

Reverdin's angulation osteotomy. In Bick's (1948) *Source Book of Orthopaedics,* in connection with hallux valgus, we read: "Barker advocated osteotomy of the first metatarsal. After him came Schede, Reverdin, Kleinberg and Hohmann who developed modification of the varus position by osteotomy." A glance at the bibliography Bick has appended to the end of the chapter dealing with hallux valgus would reveal that Reverdin preceded Barker by three years. Of the others mentioned, only Hohmann carried out osteotomy of the first metatarsal.

"On May 4, 1881," Bade (1940) wrote, "J. L. Reverdin gave a report to the Medical Society of Genfer concerning the anatomy and the surgery of hallux valgus. He made a curved incision on the medial side of the extensor hallucis, over the so-called exostosis. He incised the periosteum, chiseled off the exostosis and removed a wedge of bone from behind the capitalum of the metatarsus. He then straightened the toe, sutured the bone with catgut and applied Listers's dressing . . . this operation is the predecessor of all operations which aim to correct hallux valgus by a wedge resection behind the capitalum. . . ."

Reverdin repeated his speech at the seventh session of the International Medical Congress, which was held in London between August 2 and 9, 1881. In two cases of hallux valgus, he had resected the medial eminence but was not satisfied with the results. Reverdin thought he could do much better. He proposed a procedure that not only would dispose of the bony prominence but would also correct the outward deviation of the great toe. He excised the medial eminence and leveled the remaining surface. He then carried out a cuneiform resection through the distal portion of the first metatarsal. The base of the wedge of bone removed was directed medially and its apex touched the lateral cortex; the toe was straightened and the capital piece was sutured to the shaft. Reverdin used catgut for this purpose but indicated that a metallic suture might assure a more exact coaption of the osteotomized fragments (Fig. 10–1).

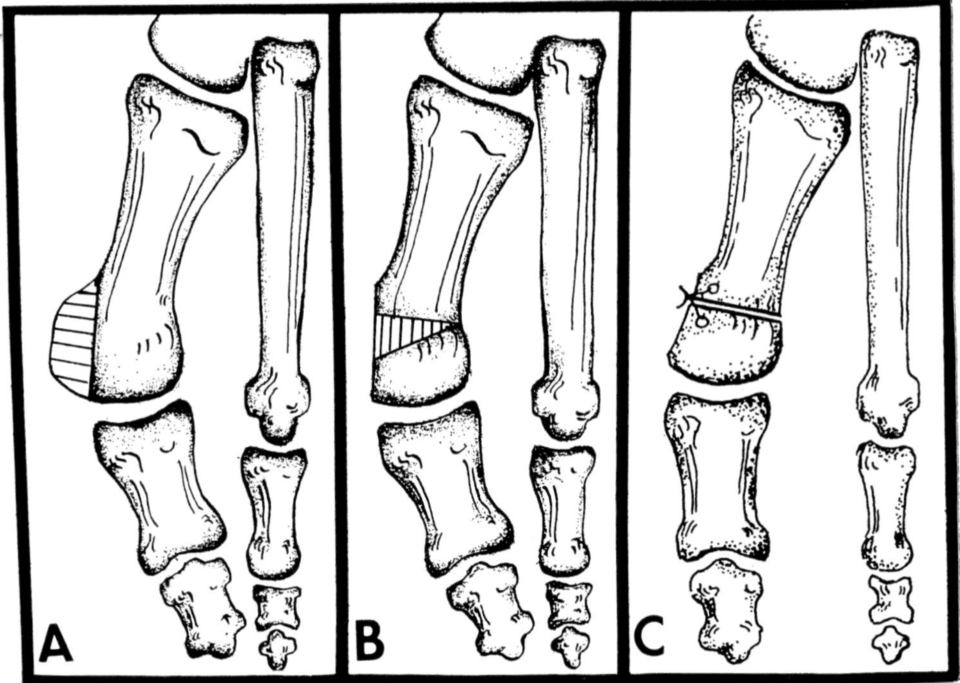

Figure 10–1. Reverdin's operation: resection of the medial eminence (*A*), excision of a wedge (*B*), and coaptation and suture (*C*).

The transactions of the International Medical Congress were published in London in 1881. The volume that contained Reverdin's speech on hallux valgus included other classics: Little's essay on congenital clubfoot, Kocher's description of the famed method of reducing dislocated shoulder, and Ollier's article on joint resection. It is conceivable that A. E. Barker, an active surgeon in London, did not attend the meeting of the Medical Congress or failed to read the published transactions.

Barker (1884) "cut with a chisel a small wedge-shaped piece of bone from the shaft just above the head, the base of the wedge being on the inner surface of the bone." The apex reached the lateral cortex, but did not section it. "Then by forcibly adducting the great toe," Barker wrote, "I snapped the uncut remainder of the metatarsal bone and brought the whole member into a straight line. . . . This little operation," Barker continued, "may have been done before but I cannot find any record of such a procedure. If it be original in this case the merit of the suggestion lies with one of my students at the University College Hospital." Unwittingly perhaps, Barker pointed a way to disclaim precedence and assure for himself the credit of an operation he was not the first to perform. In years to come Barker's coy remark—"this little operation, etc."—was repeated by many with slight change of wording (Fig. 10–2).

Barker's report was published in London. Across the ocean, in New York, *The Medical Record* (1884) reviewed this operation as follows: "Dr. Barker relates in *The Lancet,* No. 15, 1884, the case of a young man suffering from aggravated hallux valgus, in whom every remedial measure had failed to give relief. He was unwilling to resort to amputation, and at the suggestion of a student, Mr. Hoar, determined to try osteotomy. A wedge-shaped piece was removed from the inner side of the metatarsal bone just above the head. The great toe was then forcibly adducted (with reference to the median line), the remaining uncut portion of the bone being fractured by the manipulation. The toe was maintained in position by splints attached to the inner border of the foot, and the wound dressed antiseptically. The result was very satisfactory, and the patient now has a straight toe, and is relieved of all the troubles formerly experienced." No mention was made of Reverdin.

Ever since, with perhaps one or two exceptions, most English-speaking authors have ignored Reverdin and regarded Barker as the originator of metatarsal osteotomy. Continental writers resented the oversight and attempted to straighten the record. Mauclaire (1901) stated that the cuneiform osteotomy of distal end of the first metatarsal, with a medial base, was practiced and described by Reverdin before Barker. Mouchet (1922) resented the fact that, in some books, Barker's name was coupled with Reverdin. Barker, Mouchet pointed out, reported this osteotomy 3 years after Reverdin. Mouchet added that a volume would not suffice to contain the names of those who have adopted Reverdin's procedure.

Reverdin's osteotomy was utilized by numerous surgeons. Bradford (1914) conceived the idea of opening a wedge from the fibular aspect of the first metatarsal head to correct the valgus deformity of the great toe. This was not an intelligent move; it lengthened the bone and put the soft tissues under greater tension. The gap created between the osteotomized fragments would take a longer time to be spanned than if the bones were apposed together. No one else appears to have adopted this method.

Reverdin's own countryman, Roux (1920) of Switzerland, reverted to the original procedure and provided the capital fragment with a long lateral spike. Keszly (1923) performed a classic Reverdin osteotomy and appropriated Barker's concept of not sectioning the bone "through entirely, but only to the cortical layer of the external surface, thus leaving it and its periosteal covering untouched." Keszly extirpated the bursa, resected the medial eminence, and smoothed its matrix. He insisted that the wedge be removed as near the metatarsal head as possible. He also split the long extensor tendon lengthwise and at-

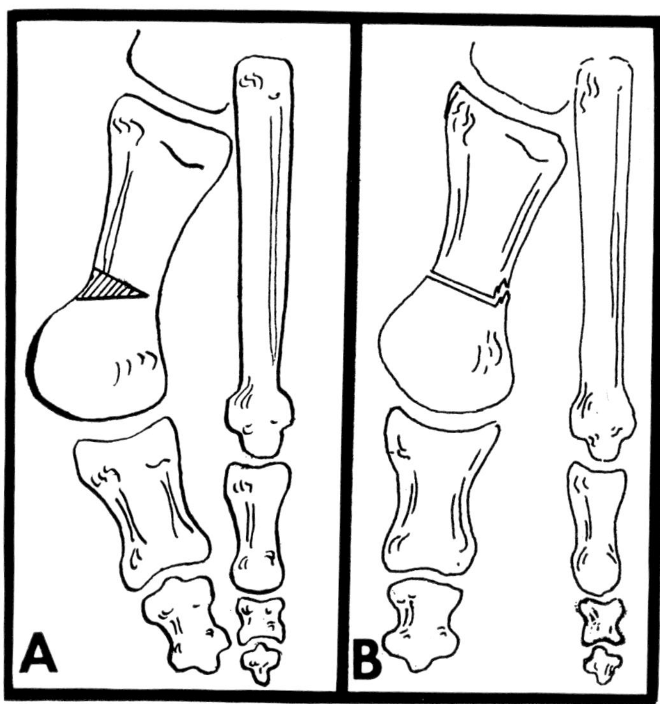

Figure 10–2. Barker's osteotomy: wedge resection short of cutting the lateral cortex (*A*), and coaptation (*B*).

tached the inner slip to the base of the proximal phalanx. Individual modifications were also introduced by Peabody (1931), Gallie (1956), and some others.

In the course of the discussion that followed Bentzon's (1935) paper on hallux valgus, Waldenström reaffirmed his faith in Reverdin's osteotomy. "I think it is important," Waldenström said, "to get plane cut surfaces in as close apposition as possible. To this end I begin by detaching the periosteum, then I carry a Gigli saw round the diaphysis. The proximal portion of the diaphysis is lifted out of the wound and cut off with an Albee saw, so as to get shortening of about 1 cm. The two fragments are drilled, a catgut thread is inserted through these holes and so tied that the cut surfaces are forced close against one another. . . ." We learn from d'Avignon (1942) that at the Orthopedic Institute of Stockholm, the operation has come to be known as the Reverdin-Waldenström method.

Viewed from a historical point of view, Reverdin's operation is a significant stride in the right direction. Reverdin introduced several steps that were new at the time. He was the first to resect the medial eminence and osteotomize the metatarsal. He also sutured the bones with catgut—a procedure that was revived years afterward by Peabody (1931), Wilhelm (1934), Waldenström (1935), Hawkins, *et al.* (1945), Durman (1957), and Mitchell and his associates (1958). This much must be said about Barker's modification of the Reverdin osteotomy: he broke the fibular cortex of the metatarsal manually to assure periosteal continuity on that side of the bone. Inadvertently perhaps, the capital fragment was provided with a lateral beak of bone, which made the osteotomy more secure and stable. In Barker's modification, greater area of surface contact was obtained, which hastened union of the osteotomized pieces.

The aim of angulation osteotomy—Reverdin's or Barker's—was to correct the valgus deformity of the great toe. Varus position of the first metatarsal was overlooked. Instead of diminishing the distance between the heads of the first and second metatarsals, angulation osteotomy actually increased it. No attempt was made to correct the dorsal tilt of the first metatarsal, which we have since learned, usually accompanies metatarsus primus varus and contributes to the pain under the outer metatarsal heads. Angulation osteotomy has limited applications: hallux valgus with no axial rotation of the great toe, no metatarsus primus varus, nor interlocking arthritis of the first metatarsophalangeal joint. This procedure has been greatly improved on by more recent modifications.

Hohmann's dual plane displacement osteotomy. Hohmann (1921–1951) proposed an operation that not only would correct the valgus deformity of the great toe, but would also amend the splaying of the forefoot as a whole. He started with an incision on the medial side of the proximal phalanx and extended it to the base of the first metatarsal. He undermined the plantar edge of the skin until the abductor hallucis came into view. The abductor was dissected free from the medial head of the flexor brevis, detached from its insertion into the base of the proximal phalanx, and reflected proximally. The joint was not opened. The head of the first metatarsal was disconnected from the shaft by a trapezoid or cuneiform osteotomy. The trapezoid piece removed was wider on the medial aspect; the base of the wedge also lay on that side. The capital fragment was pushed closer to the second metatarsal and depressed toward the sole. The hallux was straightened. The redundant medial capsule was pulled proximally, past the osteotomy site, and sutured to the periosteum of the metatarsal shaft. The severed end of the abductor hallucis was reattached to a more dorsal point on the medial side of the base of the phalanx.

When hallux valgus was complicated with splaying of the fifth metatarsal and a bunionette along the lateral border of the foot, Hohmann osteotomized the neck of this bone and pushed the capital fragment closer to the fourth metatarsal. He then brought the abductor of the small toe to the lateral side of the capsule of the fifth metatarsophalangeal joint, fastening the two with catgut. Postoperatively, Hohmann manipulated the deformed smaller toes. He also applied a scantily padded cast from above the malleoli down to the tips of the toes. The cast was molded, creating a depression behind the metatarsal heads, the toes being held in flexion (Figs. 10–3 to 10–5).

Hohmann's operation has been variously interpreted and quite frequently misinterpreted. Peabody (1931) and his spiritual descendants–Hawkins, Mitchell, and Hedrick (1945)–leveled the following objections against Hohmann's procedures: The painful exostosis was not removed; the joint was not visualized; plastic repair of the capsule was not carried out; and stable internal fixation of the metatarsal fragments was not attempted.

Hohmann denied the existence of a "true exostosis" in hallux valgus. By pushing the capital fragment laterally he reduced the prominent medial eminence. Hohmann did not think much was gained by entering the joint. On the contrary, he thought it added to the surgical trauma, invited infection, and paved the way for postoperative stiffness. Hohmann did tighten the medial capsule and reinforced it with the abductor hallucis. Of the four objections to Hohmann's operation, only the last may be considered valid.

Peabody wrote: "Hohmann, in his own report, included the technique of plastic shortening of the tendon of the adductor hallucis." According to Hawkins and his associates, in Hohmann's operation, "the adductor hallucis tendon was shortened in a further effort to prevent recurrence of the deformity." These authors either confused the adductor hallucis for the abductor, or (which is unlikely) adopted the old Continental standard of naming these muscles. In Chapter One we pointed out that Steindler, who had a German education but

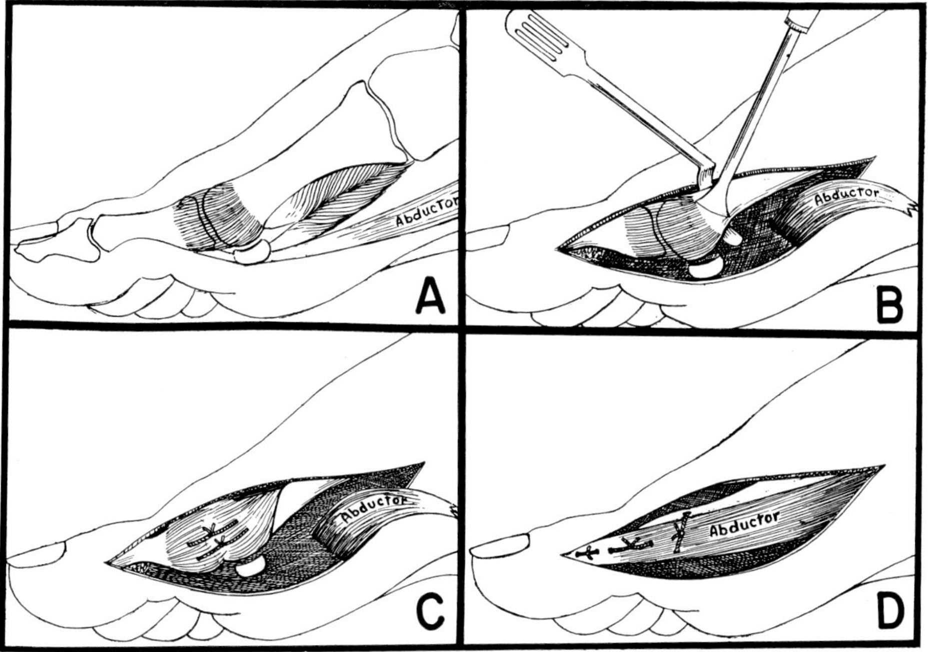

Figure 10–3. Hohmann's transposition of abductor hallucis: Anatomical relations of displaced abductor (*A*). Abductor severed; reflected chisel indicates the site of osteotomy (*B*). Redundant capsule is sutured to the periosteum of the metatarsal shaft past the osteotomy site (*C*). Abductor hallucis is transposed from its displaced position under the first metatarsophalangeal joint to a more dorsal point on its medial aspect (*D*).

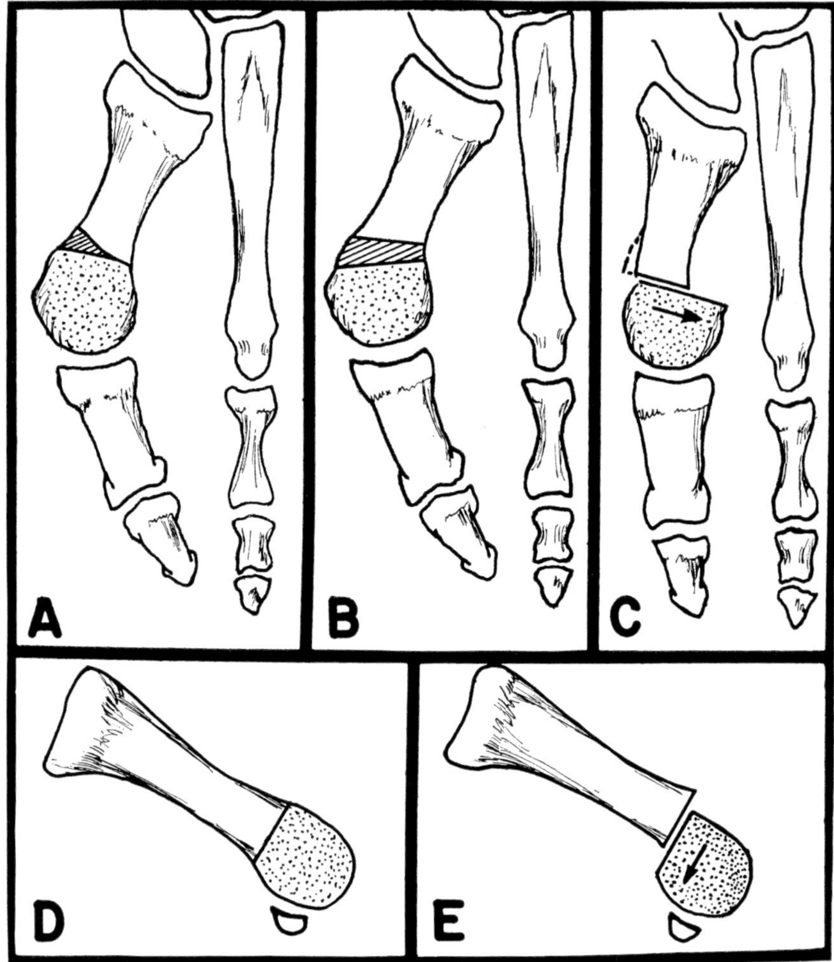

Figure 10–4. Hohmann's method of displacing capital fragment of the osteotomized first metatarsal laterally and plantarward.

wrote mainly in English, was subject to similar confusion. Steindler (1943) interpreted Hohmann's operation correctly except in one respect. He said Hohmann removed the *exostosis.* Hohmann resected the medial eminence only on rare occasions. He did this as a palliative measure in older individuals. More rarely, Hohmann opened the joint and severed adhesions along the plantar aspect of the metatarsal head and sometimes resected a dorsal spur. Exostectomy–by this we understand resection of the medial eminence of the metatarsal head–was not an integral part of Hohmann's procedure.

In hallux valgus, Hohmann argued, the medial part of the metatarsal head slips out of contact with the base of the proximal phalanx. It becomes displaced toward the midsagittal plane, presenting a spherical mass along the tibial border of the foot. Beside the exaggerated inward inclination, the first metatarsal is also rotated around its longitudinal axis, or *supinated.* "The torsion of the first metatarsal," Hohmann wrote, "can easily be seen in a dorsoplantar x-ray film. We see the marginal rim of the capitalum. . . . We see the epicondylus medialis. . . . This is the exostosis of hallux valgus literature. A real exostosis does not exist. It is the epicondylus."

Hauser (1950) also said Hohmann removed "the exostosis on the medial side of the head of the first metatarsal bone." Commenting on the position of the capital fragment after Hohmann's osteotomy, Hauser stated: "The head of the first metatarsal bone is displaced plantarward and medially." Unless the axis of the foot itself and not the midsaggital line was used for reference, this interpretation of Hohmann's operation contains a grave error. Would Hohmann, who wanted to correct the inward inclination of the first metatarsal, push the osteotomized head medially and thereby aggravate the deformity he aimed to correct? "The caput," Hohmann wrote, "should be pushed laterally to obtain a good reduction. A medial angulation is wrong."

Hohmann's basic concept—that the surgical treatment of hallux valgus must aim at the correction of the overall deformity of the splayfoot and redress the *supinatory dorsal tilt* of the first metatarsal as well as its varus inclination—was endorsed by many. Some of Hohmann's followers introduced individual variations of the operative technique. In Hohmann's osteotomy the trapezoid segment of the resected bone was broader on the medial aspect than on the lateral aspect. Sazepin (1926) reversed these dimensions: the piece of bone removed had a broader base on the fibular than on the tibial side. When the gap was closed, the capital fragment came closer to the second metatarsal simply by angulation, without displacement. The surface area of bony contact was greater than in Hohmann's dual displacement method. To correct the valgus deformity of the great toe, Sazepin tenotomized the short extensor and lengthened the long tendon by Z-plasty. Sazepin overlooked the principle of depressing the head in a plantar direction.

Komza (1950) described an osteotomy providing the capital fragment with a long lateral beak of bone. Gielzinski (1958) characterized Komza's operation as an excision of the medial eminence and plastic osteotomy of the first metatarsal neck with lateral and plantar displacement of the head. He contended that the transposition of the abductor and of one-half of the extensor hallucis longus tendon to the base of the proximal phalanx improved the results. Mommsen (1953) provided the capital fragment with a medial spike. The cancellous core of the stump of the shaft was excavated. The capital piece was shifted laterally until its spike contacted the lateral cortex of the proximal fragment. The head was thus displaced closer to the second metatarsal (Figs. 10–6 and 10–7).

Mizuno, Sima, and Yamazaki (1956) described what they called *detorsion os-*

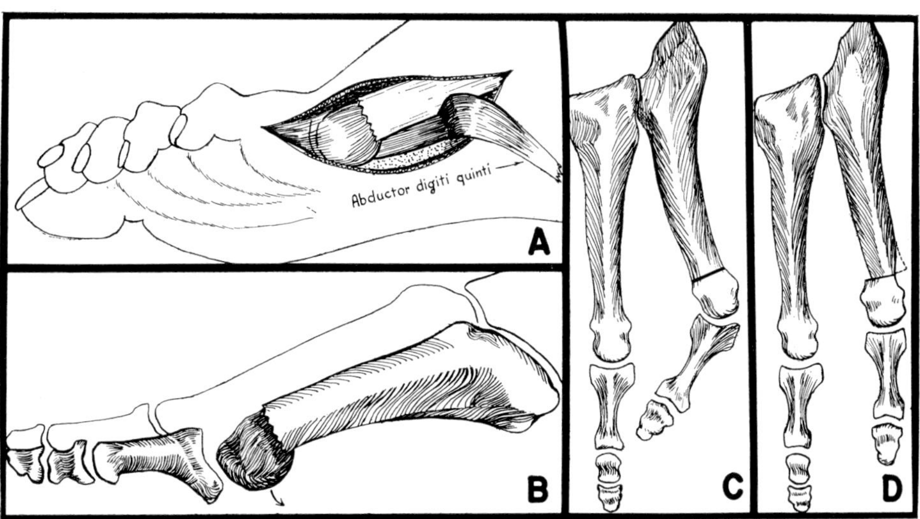

Figure 10–5. Hohmann's operation for metatarsus quintus valgus.

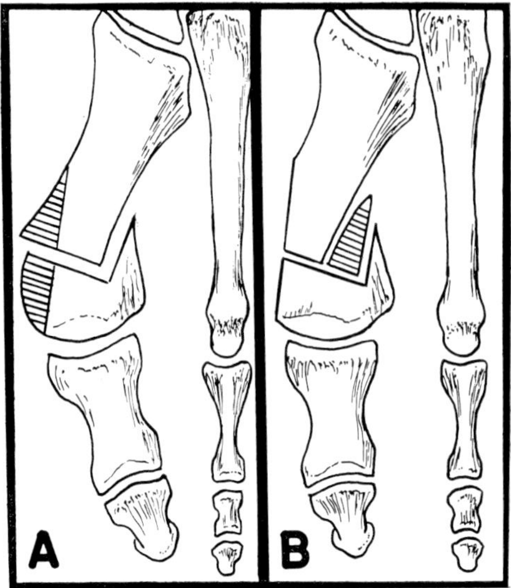

Figure 10–6. Komza's osteotomy.

teotomy of the first metatarsal. They advised fixation of the fragments by a "longitudinally inserted K-wire." Ortiz (1956) insisted that the osteotomized head should be held in the desired position with the aid of a Kirschner wire that penetrated the proximal fragment obliquely and secured the capital piece. Urbanek and Dvorak (1958) transfixed the fragments with a pin passing in reverse direction from that described by Ortiz. In cases of hallux valgus and metatarsus primus varus, Mikhail (1960) advised a trapezoid osteotomy. The configuration of the resected segment of bone was reminiscent of the one described by Sazepin (1926): it was broader on the fibular than on the tibial side. The main fragments were apposed together and transfixed with a small Rush nail. Basically this is a lateral angulation osteotomy. As had Sazepin, Mikhail overlooked Hohmann's principle of plantar depression of the capital fragment (Fig. 10–8).

Hohmann's concept of shifting the head of the first metatarsal closer to the second metatarsal and depressing it toward the sole is sound. This in itself was a major contribution. The same cannot be said about Hohmann's technique. He sectioned the metatarsal through its neck, which possesses less osteogenic potentiality than the cancellous head. The dual plane displacement considerably curtailed the area of surface contact between the fragments and contributed to delayed union. Hohmann depended on external immobilization only. He did admit that the capital fragment sometimes slipped out of position and vitiated the final result. Hohmann's operation might have been supplemented advantageously by internal fixation, as has been suggested by more than one author. Of late the concept of interlocking the osteotomized fragments has come into practice, making for greater security.

Thomasen's peg-and-hole osteotomy. Perhaps the best modification of dual plane—lateral and plantar—displacement osteotomy of the distal end of the first metatarsal is that described by Mygind (1952, 1953) and credited to Thomasen.

This operation made use of the principle of interlocking the osteotomized fragments. It is not without an antecedent. Tierny (1926) described a similar method for correction of hammered toe. In a second paper Tierny (1930) called this operation the procedure of *bilboquet*—which in literal translation means *cup-and-ball*—and suggested its application to hallux valgus. Eick (1931) sectioned the distal end of the first metatarsal across the neck, spiked the stump of the proximal bone, and invaginated it into the capital fragment. In a treatise entitled *A New Operation for the Cure of Hallux Valgus,* David (1934) described a similar method for which he gave the credit to his "master," L. Bazy. The first metatarsal was sectioned across its neck, the capital fragment was gouged out, the cut end of the shaft was tapered, and the two fragments were locked. Lance (1936) inserted the spiked end of the proximal bone into a socket on the medial aspect of the capital piece, as had been suggested by Tierny (1930). Lelièvre (1952) has named this operation *bilboquet of Bazy and Lance.* The aim of each of these procedures was to correct the valgus of the great toe; no attempt was made to redress varus deformity of the first metatarsal and the dorsal tilt of its head (Fig. 10–9).

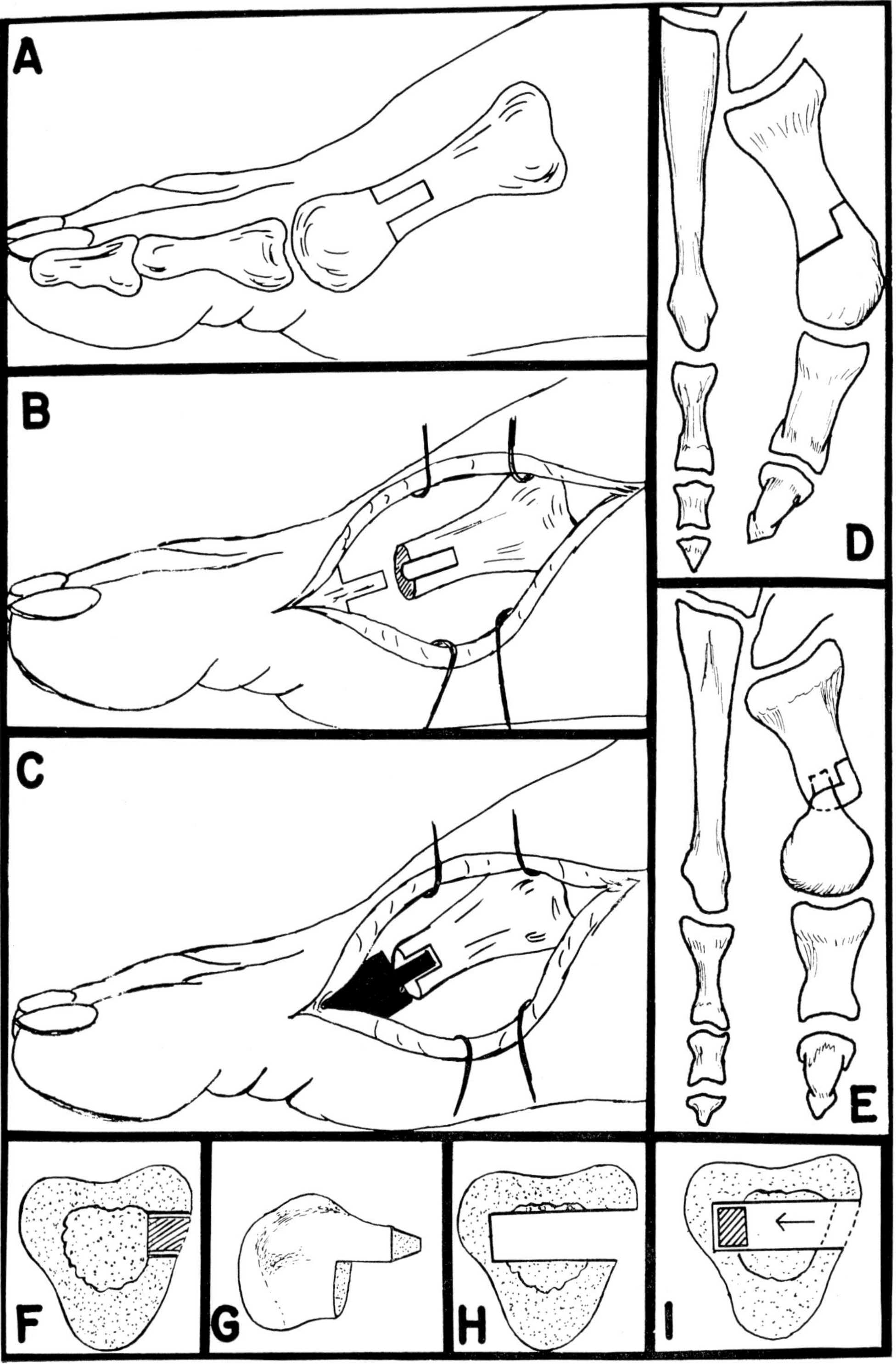

Figure 10–7. Mommsen's lateral displacement method.

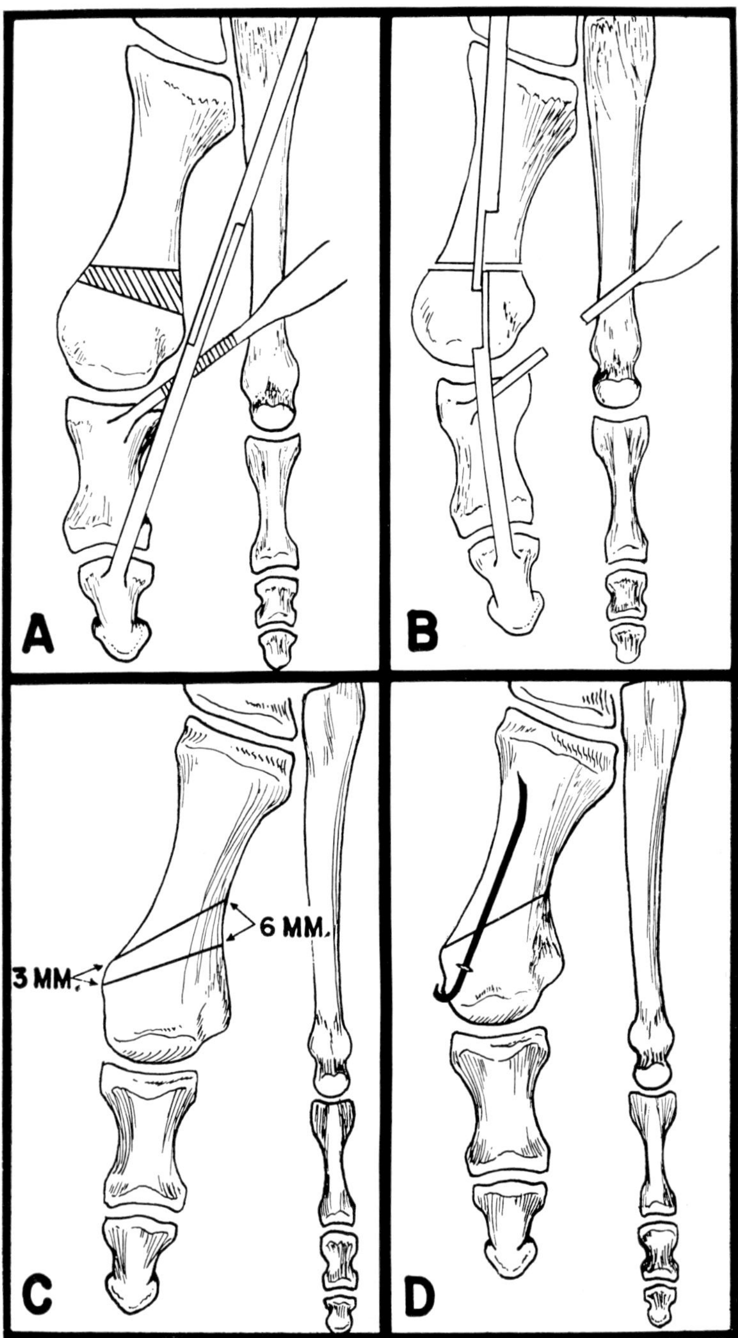

Figure 10–8. Sazepin's method (*A* and *B*). Mikhail's method (*C* and *D*).

In the August, 1952, issue of the British edition of the Journal of Bone and Joint Surgery a brief abstract appeared. It summarized Mygind's report of 535 cases of hallux valgus. The best results were said to have been obtained by the *peg-and-hole* osteotomy of Thomasen. A year later Mygind (1953) described Thomasen's technique in some detail.

After a personal communication with Thomasen himself, we have evolved the following method. The distal end of the first metatarsal is approached through a small medial or dorsal longitudinal incision. The bone is sectioned obliquely providing the shaft fragment with a longer fibular cortex. A peg is fashioned from the plantar portion of this cortex and inserted into a hole in the dorsomedial sector of the capital piece. After the two fragments are locked, the first metatarsal head comes to lie closer to its neighbors on the fibular side and nearer the sole. The capital fragment is thus shifted laterally and plantarward. The fragments are transfixed by intramedullary wire (Figs. 10–10 to 10–17).

In his presidential address to the section of orthopedics of the Royal Society of Medicine, Cholmeley (1958) spoke about Mygind's report and referred to his published paper. "In 1952," Cholmeley said, "Mygind of Copenhagen reported at a meeting of the Danish Orthopedic Association 535 cases of hallux valgus operated on by different methods and stated that the best results had been obtained by an oblique osteotomy of the first metatarsal close to the head, which was displaced laterally and plantarwards on the shaft and kept in place by the hole and the peg devised by Thomasen. . . . Mygind also published in the following year a paper on this subject. . . . In 1953 Mortens of Copenhagen was working at the Royal National Orthopedic Hospital and introduced this operation to the staff of the hospital. . . ."

More recently Gibson and Piggott (1962) described a method they called the *spike technique* of osteotomy. In no essential point does this procedure differ from the *peg-and-hole* osteotomy credited to Thomasen by both Mygind and Cholmeley. "Metatarsal-neck osteotomy has been carried out occasionally at the Royal National Orthopedic Hospital," Gibson and Piggott wrote. "The technique at first resembled that described by Hohmann (1947), but modifications have been introduced by several surgeons, notably J. A. Cholmeley." Had

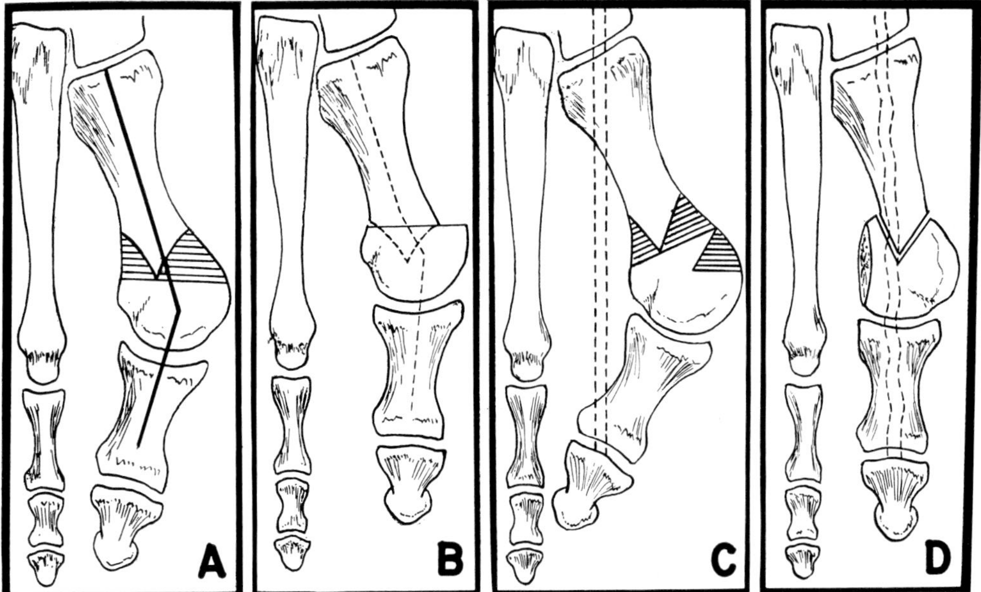

Figure 10–9. Bilboquet operation: Bazy's method (*A* and *B*); Lance's method (*C* and *D*).

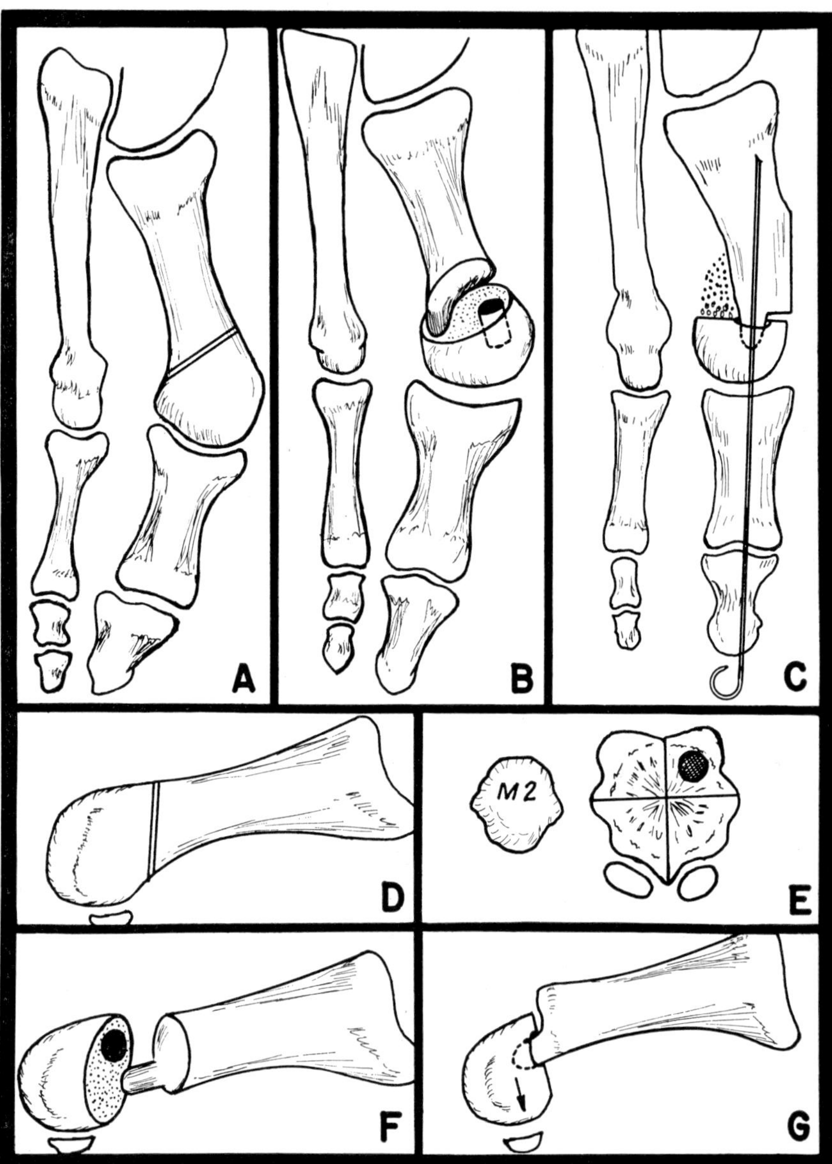

Figure 10–10. Thomasen's peg-and-hole osteotomy, modified: oblique osteotomy of the distal end of the first metatarsal (*A*); spiking the stump of the proximal fragment and excavating a hole into the capital piece (*B*); lateral displacement of the capital fragment, interlocking, piling up bone chips on the lateral aspect of the surgical fracture and transfixation of fragments with an intramedullary K-wire (*C*); osteotomy seen from the side (*D*); location of the hole on the medial and superior sector of the capital fragment (*E*); peg-and-hole seen from the side (*F*); plantar shift of the capital fragment (*G*).

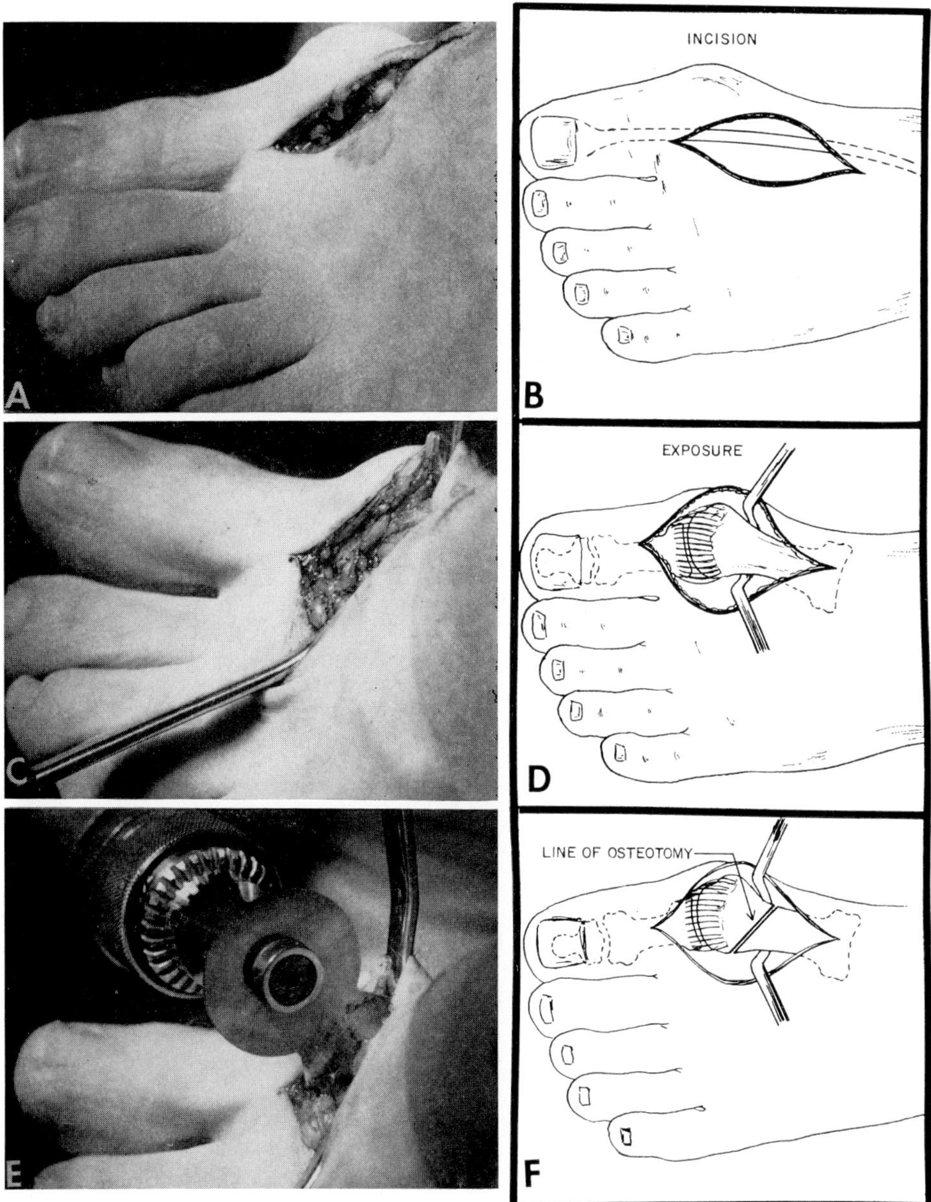

Figure 10–11. Photographs and interpretative diagrams illustrating the main steps of *peg-and-hole* method of correction of hallux valgus.

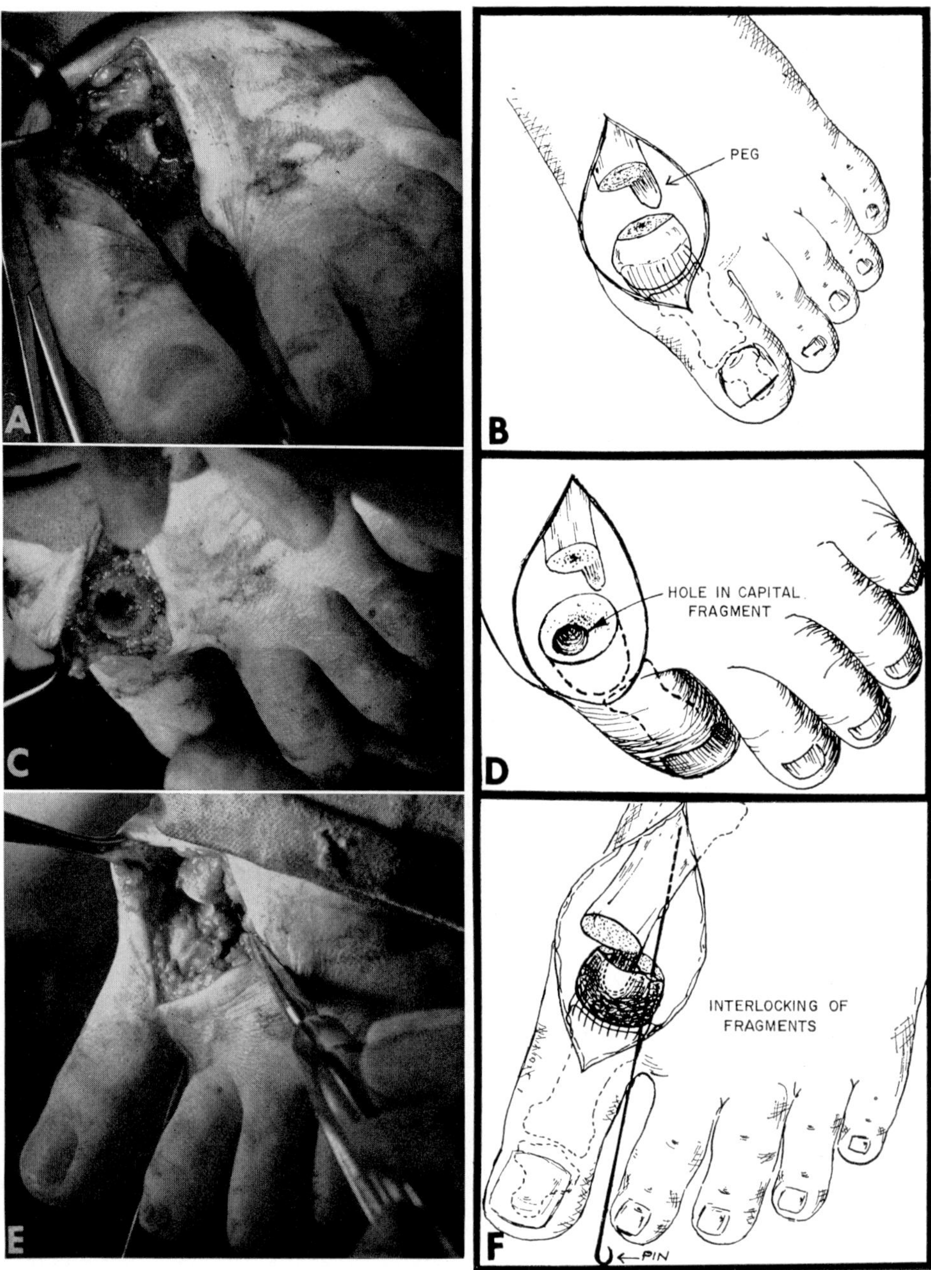

Figure 10–12. A continuation of Figure 10–11.

Gibson and Piggott read Mygind's report they might have avoided the error of attributing the operation to Cholmeley. Had they heard Cholmeley's own speech, they would have known how Cholmeley learned about the modification of Hohmann's technique that he was supposed to have introduced.

Gibson and Piggott stressed the importance of adequate lateral displacement of the capital fragment. "To achieve this," they wrote, "the osteotomy must be as far distal as possible, in the broadest part of the neck. It is most important to avoid dorsal angulation of the metatarsal head: thus the spike on the proximal fragment must be towards the plantar aspect and the great toe must be immobilized in slight plantar flexion."

Unquestionably, Thomasen's peg-and-hole procedure is an improvement on Hohmann's operation: the osteotomy is more secure and the area of surface contact between the surgically severed fragments is greater. Invagination of the spiked end of the shaft into the capital piece does not guarantee against postoperative displacement. Mygind reported one nonunion. Gibson and Piggott reported another. Beside external immobilization with a cast, additional security may be obtained with the aid of an intramedullary pin.

Peg-and-hole osteotomy is primarily indicated in adolescents and young adults with hallux valgus and metatarsus primus varus; it may also be attempted in older individuals with good circulation of the foot, and at least 30 degrees of painless extension of the great toe. Since the medial eminence is not resected and the capsule is not disturbed, one runs no risk of causing avascular necrosis of the capital fragment. Axial rotation of the great toe can be remedied by turning the capital fragment around the spike of the shaft. The varus deformity of the first metatarsal is redressed by shifting the capital fragment fibulaward. The head of the first metatarsal is also depressed plantarward. This last step may relieve mild metatarsalgia under the second and third metatarsal heads.

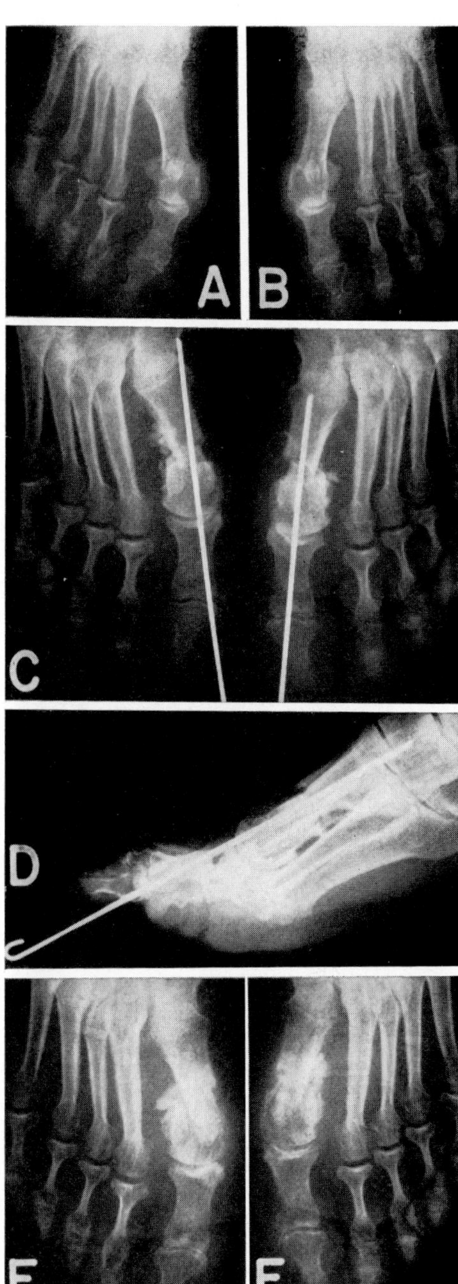

Figure 10–13. Roentgenograms of the forefeet of a woman in her early forties, showing bilateral hallux valgus and mild metatarsalgia. Surgery: modified peg-and-hole procedure. Dorsoplantar view before surgery (*A* and *B*); the same showing lateral displacement of the capital fragments and transfixation by Kirschner wire (*C*); side view of one foot showing plantar shift of the capital fragment (*D*); roentgenograms showing solid osteosynthesis 8 weeks after surgery (*E* and *F*).

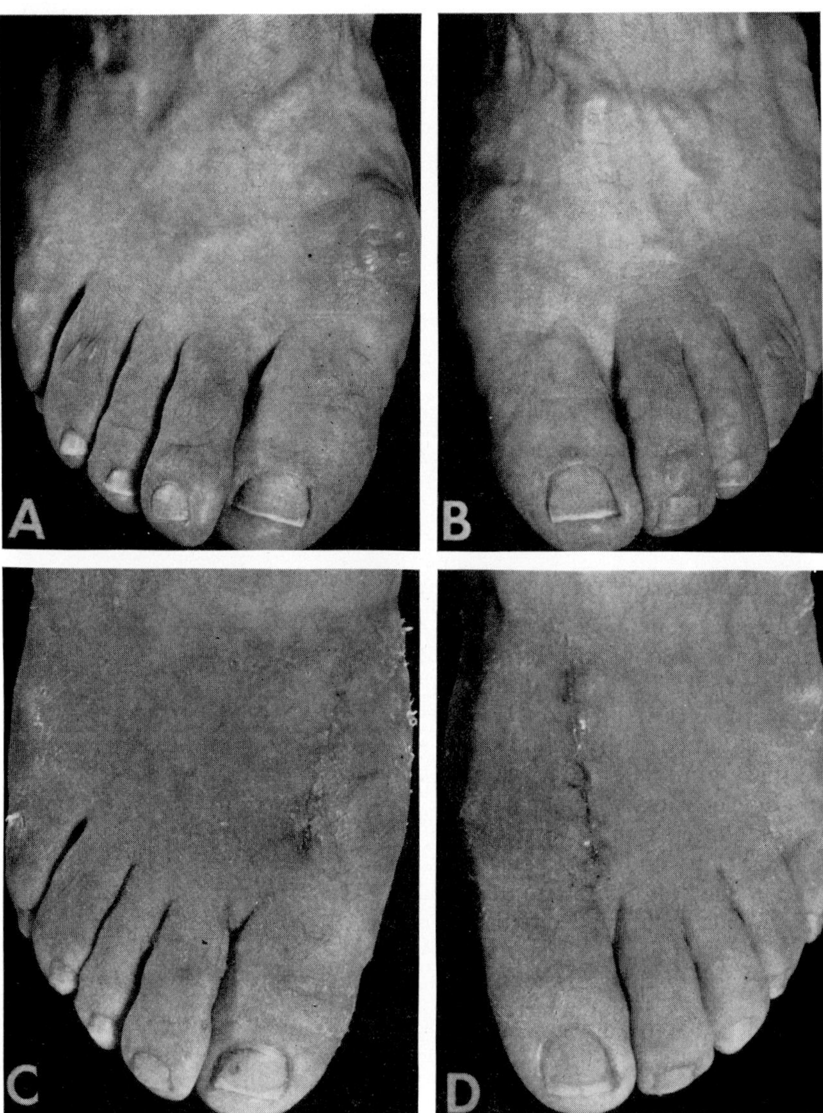

Figure 10–14. The same case as in Figure 10–13: Right and left feet before surgery (*A* and *B*); the same after surgery (*C* and *D*). This patient works as a saleslady, 8 hours a day on her feet.

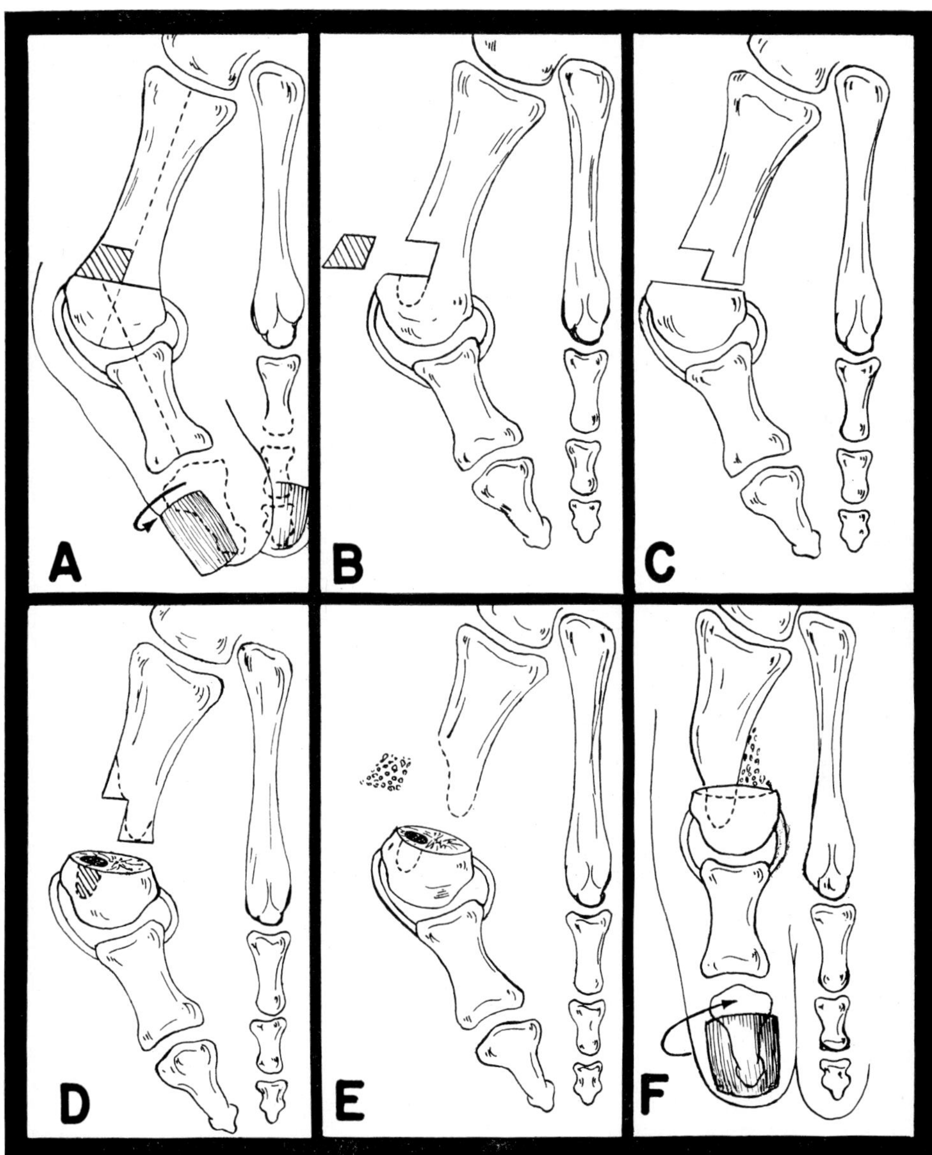

Figure 10–15. Diagrams illustrating peg-and-hole method for correction of hallux valgus metatarsus primus vatrus and axial rotation of the great toe.

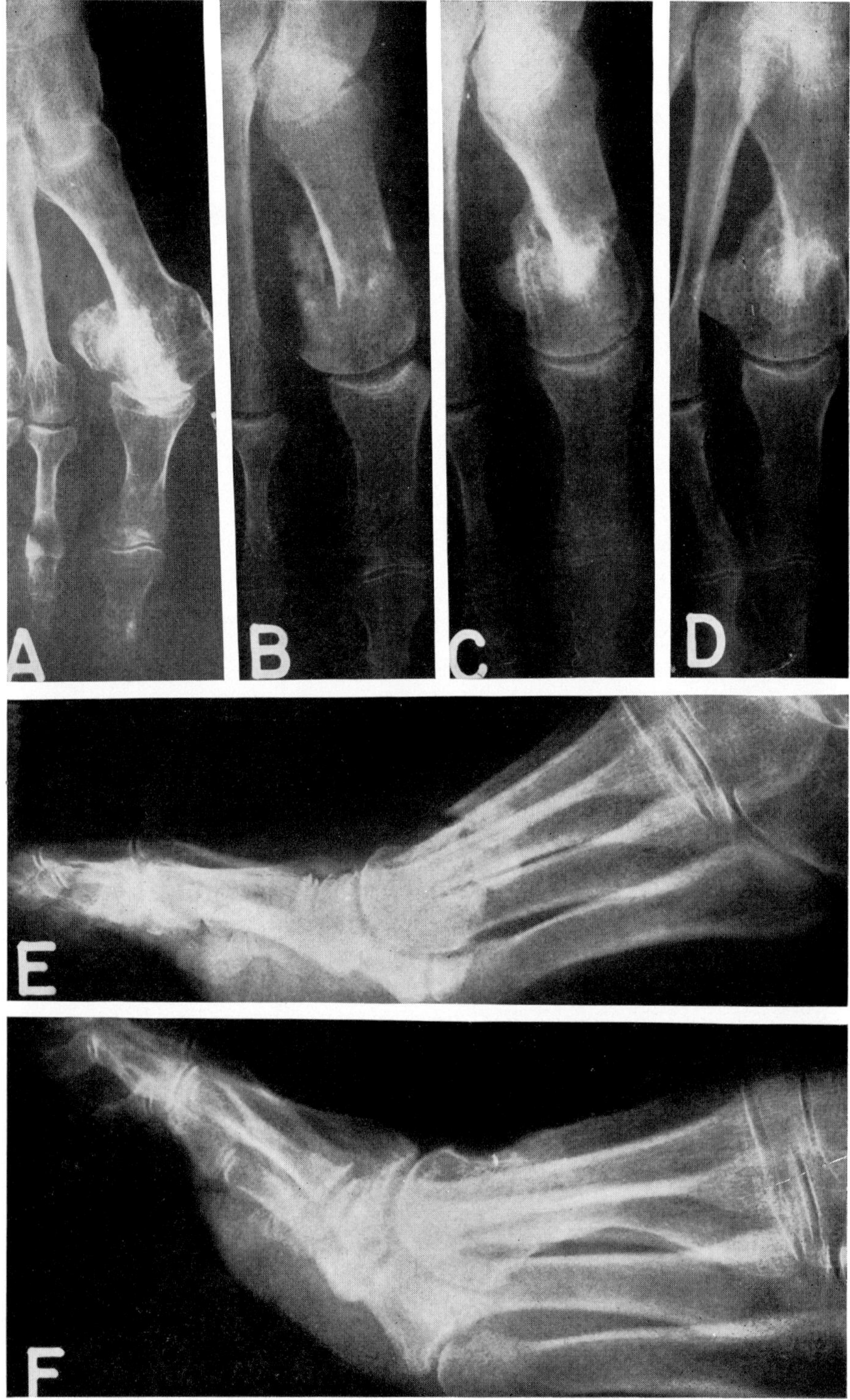

Figure 10–16. Roentgenograms of the forefoot of a woman, 66 years of age but with good circulation, showing hallux valgus and mild metatarsalgia: before surgery (*A*); 4 weeks later (*B*); 8 weeks later (*C* and *D*); side view showing plantar displacement of the capital fragment (*E*); side view after osteosynthesis (*F*).

Peg-and-hole osteotomy is contraindicated in the presence of painful interlocking arthritis of the first metatarsophalangeal joint. It also should not be attempted when the hallux rides over or has slipped under the second toe, or when the outer metatarsal heads are incarcerated causing severe pain and pressure keratoses.

Mitchell's double-transverse osteotomy. In the course of his discussion of a paper by Mitchell (1958), what Hammond—and McBride who followed him—called "The Mitchell Operation," Hawkins, Mitchell, and Hedrick (1945) traced to Peabody, and Peabody (1931) himself conceded priority to Hohmann and Reverdin. By his own admission Peabody learned about the Reverdin and Hohmann procedures secondhand from Taylor and Steindler. Peabody gave the following as the essential points of his operation: "(1) preliminary excision of exostosis; (2) cuneiform or trapezoid resection just proximal to the articular surface; (3) realignment of joint without sacrifice of any part of it; (4) reconstruction of medial collateral ligament."

"The writer's operation," Peabody wrote, "differs from that of either Reverdin or Hohmann in that the wedge resection to correct the valgus is done not in the lower end of the shaft, where the bone is narrow, but in the head where wider surfaces of apposition will prevail and where osteogenesis is more active, so that it is not an extra-articular operation. It differs again in that, whenever the resection is a pure wedge (Reverdin) or more of a trapezoid (Hohmann), it does not quite traverse the entire width of the bone, but leaves the articular or capital fragment prolonged by a thin segment from the lateral (interdigital) side of the neck and the shaft, and at this side there is undisturbed continuity of capsule and periosteum. Furthermore, no mention is made in the technique of these two surgeons of any means of maintaining position and apposition of the bone fragments, such as is obtained in the writer's technique by the fixation suture. Finally, the removal of the painful exostosis secured by our method is not attempted in the Hohmann operation."

Obviously, Peabody was reluctant to part with his claim of originality. In his zeal to establish a precedent, Peabody

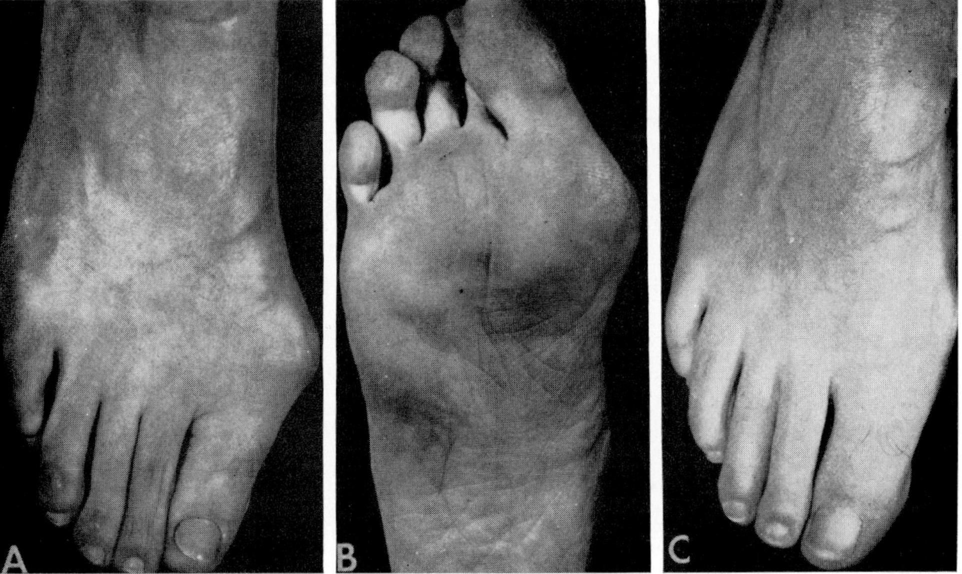

Figure 10–17. The same case as in Figure 10–16: dorsal and plantar view before surgery (*A* and *B*); dorsal view after surgery (*C*). Patient reported: "No pain now, discomfort or complaints. Completely satisfied with the result. Wear regular shoes."

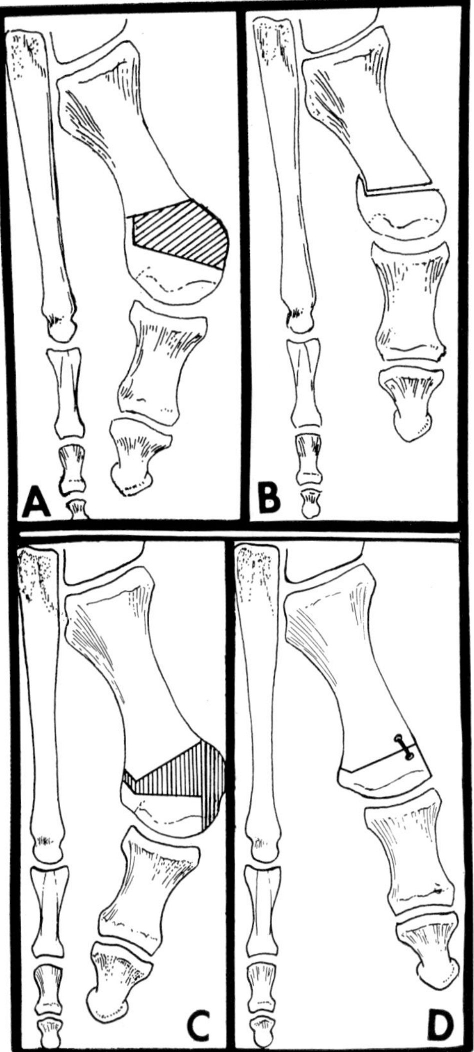

Figure 10–18. Modification of Reverdin's operation: by Roux in 1920 (*A* and *B*); by Peabody 11 years later (*C* and *D*).

committed several mistakes; we have already recorded some of them in connection with Hohmann's operation. Had Peabody read the original Reverdin communication, or numerous articles about it, he would have known that the Swiss surgeon not only secured the bone fragments with catgut—the material Peabody favored—but said he would have preferred a metallic suture that would assure more exact coaptation. Moreover, Reverdin osteotomized the metatarsal head through the cancellous head, as did Peabody himself.

We would have conceded a point of originality to Peabody in not carrying the osteotomy through the lateral cortex. But, as noted, Barker (1884) was the first to stop short of osteotomizing the lateral cortex with a chisel, and Reverdin's own countryman, Roux (1920), interpolated in his article several drawings (Figs. 17 and 18 in Roux's paper) showing the capital fragment provided with a long lateral beak. Peabody made no mention of Barker, Roux, or the many others who had made use of the same principles (Fig. 10–18).

Three years after the appearance of Peabody's paper, Wilhelm (1934) came out with a procedure in which a transverse segment of bone was removed from around the neck of the first metatarsal by two parallel cuts. The remaining fragments were reapposed and sutured together. The purpose of this procedure was to shorten the first metatarsal. Wilhelm also resected a generous portion of the medial eminence (Fig. 10–19).

Hawkins, Mitchell, and Hedrick (1945) bypassed Wilhelm and linked their operation to Peabody's. As had Peabody, they provided the capital piece with a lateral beak and secured the fragments with catgut. They shifted the osteotomy site further proximally, toward the shaft. Even though Mitchell was one of the three authors of the article—not the first one at that—his name became identified with the double transverse osteotomy of the first metatarsal neck (Fig. 10–20).

"A preliminary report of an original operation for hallux valgus was published in 1945," Mitchell and his associates (1958) wrote. "The paper emphasized the role played by metatarsus varus in the etiology of hallux valgus. The operation consisted in a lateral displacement-angulation osteotomy of the first metatarsal neck to correct metatarsus primus varus and medial capsulorrhaphy to correct hallux valgus."

Obviously Mitchell had forgotten that in the preliminary report alluded to, he coauthored the ensuing statements: "Peabody in 1931 reported a bunionectomy which was the forerunner of the operation we shall describe," and that, "in 1923 Hohmann reported for the first time an osteotomy operation devised for the correction of hallux valgus. It was a radical departure from the accepted bunionectomies of the time. . . . It was basically sound," and so on. By a curious coincidence, it was in this same year, 1923, that Silver described the capsulorrhaphy part of Mitchell's "original" operation.

In the more mature Mitchell procedure the first metatarsophalangeal joint was approached through a medial curvilinear

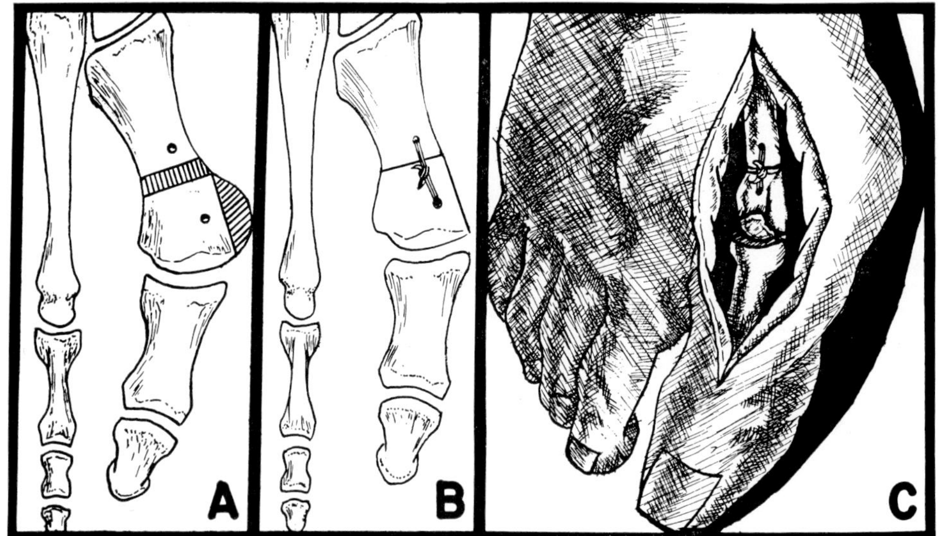

Figure 10–19. Wilhelm's sagittal resection of the medial eminence and double transverse osteotomy of the first metatarsal neck.

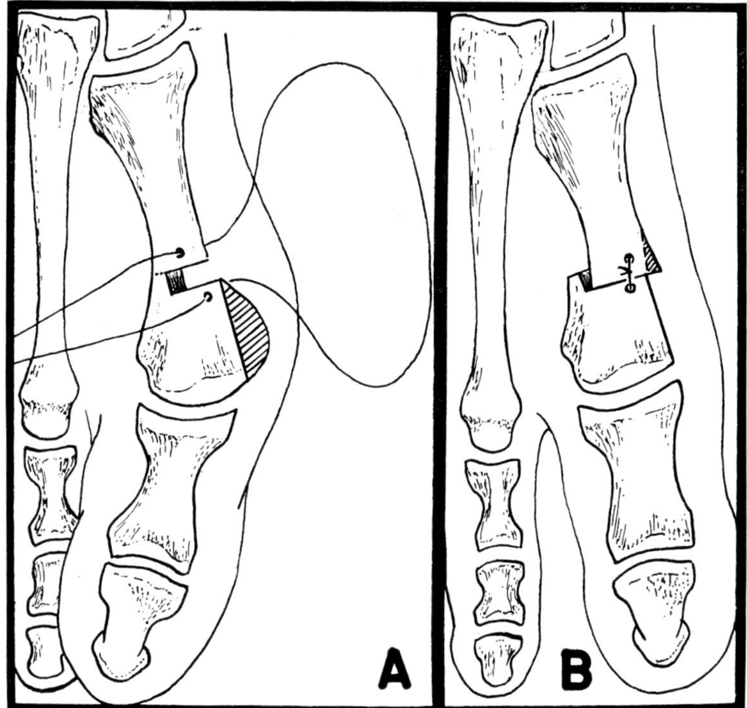

Figure 10–20. Hawkins, Mitchell, and Hedrick double transverse osteotomy of the first metatarsal neck.

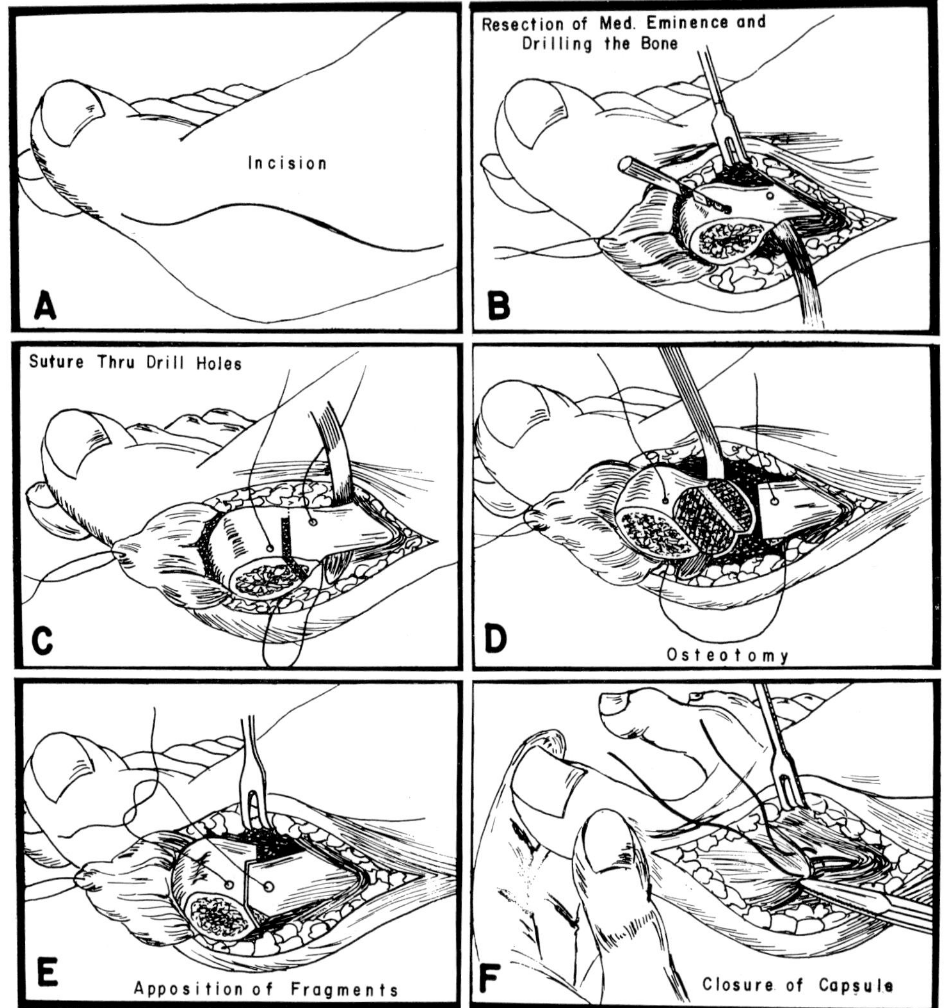

Figure 10–21. Mitchell's operation: incision (*A*); sagittal resection of the medial eminence and drill holes into the distal metatarsal (*B*); catgut threaded through drill holes and double transverse osteotomy carried up to the lateral cortex (*C*); osteotomy completed (*D*); fragments locked (*E*); the capsular flaps sutured (F).

incision. As in the Silver operation, three flaps were fashioned from the medial capsule: distal, superior, and inferior flaps. The medial eminence was resected flush with the inner cortex of the shaft. Two drill holes–the first hole half an inch and the second one inch from the articular surface of the metatarsal head –were drilled. The drill holes traversed the metatarsal bone in a dorsoplantar direction. The distal hole was placed slightly medial to the proximal hole so that the two apertures would be in line when the capital fragment was displaced laterally. A strand of No. 1 chromic catgut was threaded through these holes. A double incomplete osteotomy was carried out. The distal cut lay about three-quarters of an inch from the articular surface of the metatarsal head. The two osteotomy lines were placed between the drill holes described. The thickness of the bone between the osteotomy cuts depended on the amount of shortening of the metatarsal necessary to relax the contracted lateral structures. Usually about 2 to 3 mm. (one-eighth of an inch) of bone was removed. The size of the lateral spur depended on the amount of metatarsus primus varus to be neutralized. In moderate deformity, one-sixth and in severe metatarsus varus one-third of the width of the shaft was left to form the lateral spur. The proximal osteotomy was completed with a thin saw blade. The capital fragment was shifted fibulaward until the lateral spur locked over the shaft; it was tilted toward the sole. The previously inserted catgut suture in the drill holes was tied. The hallux was held in slight overcorrection and the medial capsule and the collateral ligament were constructed as in Silver's procedure (Figs. 10–21 and 10–22).

In what Mitchell called a preliminary report, no mention was made about angulation of the capital fragment in a plantar direction. This idea appears to have come as an afterthought, a discovery. The advantage of a plantar tilt of the head seems to have been suggested to Mitchell's group in the course of their assessment of the end results. In one case the capital fragment had slipped medially and angulated plantarward; the valgus position of the great toe recurred but the patient was completely relieved of the metatarsalgia. It was inferred that if the capital fragment was depressed, the discomfort under the second metatarsal head would likely be alleviated. Conversely, if the head was elevated, metatarsalgia would be aggravated. "The presumptive explanation for this," Mitchell and his associates wrote, "is that if the first metatarsal takes its normal share of the weight, the second metatarsal will not be overloaded. . . . For many years the senior author has insisted that the toe be splinted in slight flexion and this study lends justification to this view."

For many years—if we may borrow this phrase—to be exact, since the early twenties, Hohmann had been promulgating the principle of lateral and plantar shift of the capital fragment, and postoperatively he kept the great toe as well as lesser digits in flexion with a cast. One discerns a naïve note in the statement by Mitchell and company that "as far as can be determined by an extensive search of world literature, it was first described by the senior author and associates in 1945. . . ."

The "extensive search of the world literature" appears to have bypassed numerous publications by Hohmann (1921–1951); articles by Matheis (1927)

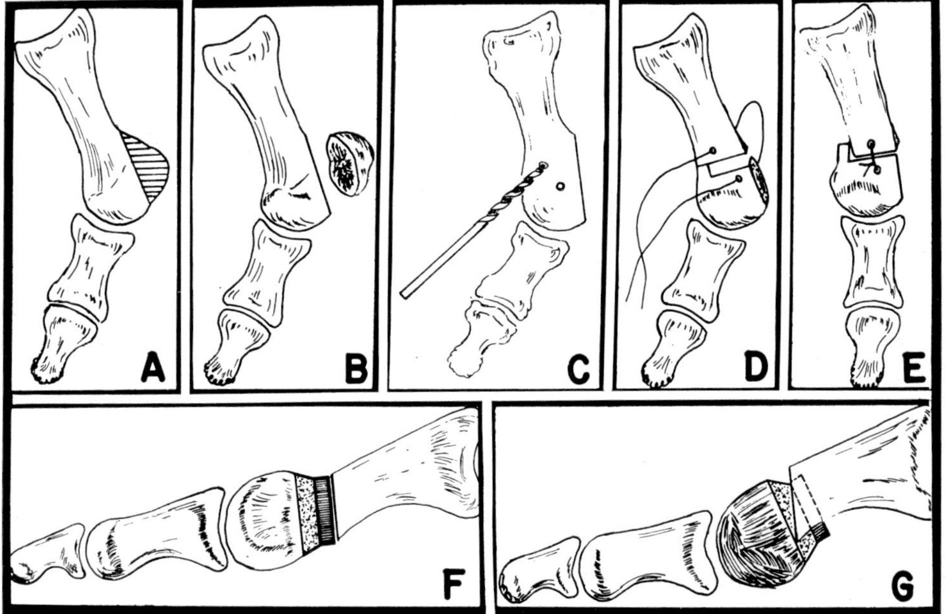

Figure 10–22. Mitchell's operation showing lateral (*E*) and plantar (G) displacement of the capital fragment.

and Cotton (1935), who also insisted that the first metatarsal should be depressed toward the sole; Mayr's (1940) article; Chapchal's (1943) description of van Ness' procedure; Komza's (1950) communication; Mygind's (1953) formal articles—one in Danish and the other in English; the *detorsion osteotomy* of Mizuno, Sima, and Yamazaki (1956); and the modification of Hohmann's operation by Ortiz (1956).

The latest communication by Mitchell and his associates contains a comprehensive postoperative follow-up. These authors gathered data from 59 patients. They considered the result excellent when both the patient and the surgeon were satisfied. Moderate recurrence, exostosis formation, and metatarsalgia that developed or was worse after the operation relegated the case to the category of *fair* results. Eight of the nine *poor* results were due to degenerative joint changes. These patients were all over 40 years of age at the time of surgery. Two patients developed aseptic necrosis of the head and four came back with severe recurrence due to medial angulation at the osteotomy site. The results were rated good or excellent in 82 per cent, and 80 per cent of the patients were totally satisfied. Better results were accompanied by definite diminution of the varus position of the first metatarsal.

Mitchell's operation provides greater area of surface contact for the osteotomized fragments than Hohmann's: nonunion is less likely to occur. On the other hand, the hazard of avascular necrosis of the capital fragment is greater. Capsular flaps have to be lifted and the medial eminence is resected, all of which contributes to the isolation of the head from its nutrient supply. Mitchell's operation necessitates opening the joint, which in part contributed to the stiffness following surgery. In Mitchell's operation the provision of a lateral ledge of bone minimizes the hazard of medial displacement of the capital fragment but not its dorsal tilt. Notwithstanding the claim that "the surprising stability" is procured by the catgut suture, we consider it safer if a firm strand of wire is used instead. One could obtain even better internal fixation with an intramedullary pin.

Mitchell's osteotomy is not as secure as Thomasen's. The axial rotation—eversion, *pronation*—of the great toe can better be corrected by the *peg-and-hole* method. Mitchell's operation has one advantage over Hohmann's or Thomasen's: it disposes of the medial eminence. It is, therefore, applicable to cases of hallux valgus with roentgenographic evidence of a deep sagittal groove separating the articular surface of the metatarsal head still in contact with the base of the proximal phalanx from the portion that has slipped medially. Neither Thomasen's nor Mitchell's method should be attempted in the presence of interlocking arthritis of the joint.

Osteotomy of the first metatarsal shaft. Ludloff (1918) obliquely osteotomized the shaft of the first metatarsal. The line of section ran from the dorsum of the base down and forward and terminated under the neck. Frejka (1924) described what he called the mediolateral oblique osteotomy of Chlumsky. Mau (1926) reversed the direction of Ludloff's osteotomy: he sectioned the bone from above the head obliquely down and backward. Petri (1940) reverted to the original Ludloff osteotomy and held the distal fragment closer to the second metatarsal by an encircling band of fascia (Fig. 10–23).

Many authors—including Mouchet (1922) and McBride (1952)—have lumped Juvara's operation with the cuneiform osteotomy of the proximal end of the first metatarsal. Juvara (1919–1932) himself classified his method under osteotomy of the diaphysis. He cut the metatarsal shaft at about the junction of the middle and proximal thirds. It was, as he said "double oblique section of the metatarsal." He described two versions. In one the osteotomy lines started at the medial cortex of the first metatarsal shaft and progressed laterally and distally; in the other this direction was reversed. In both, osteotomy lines divirged as they approached the fibular

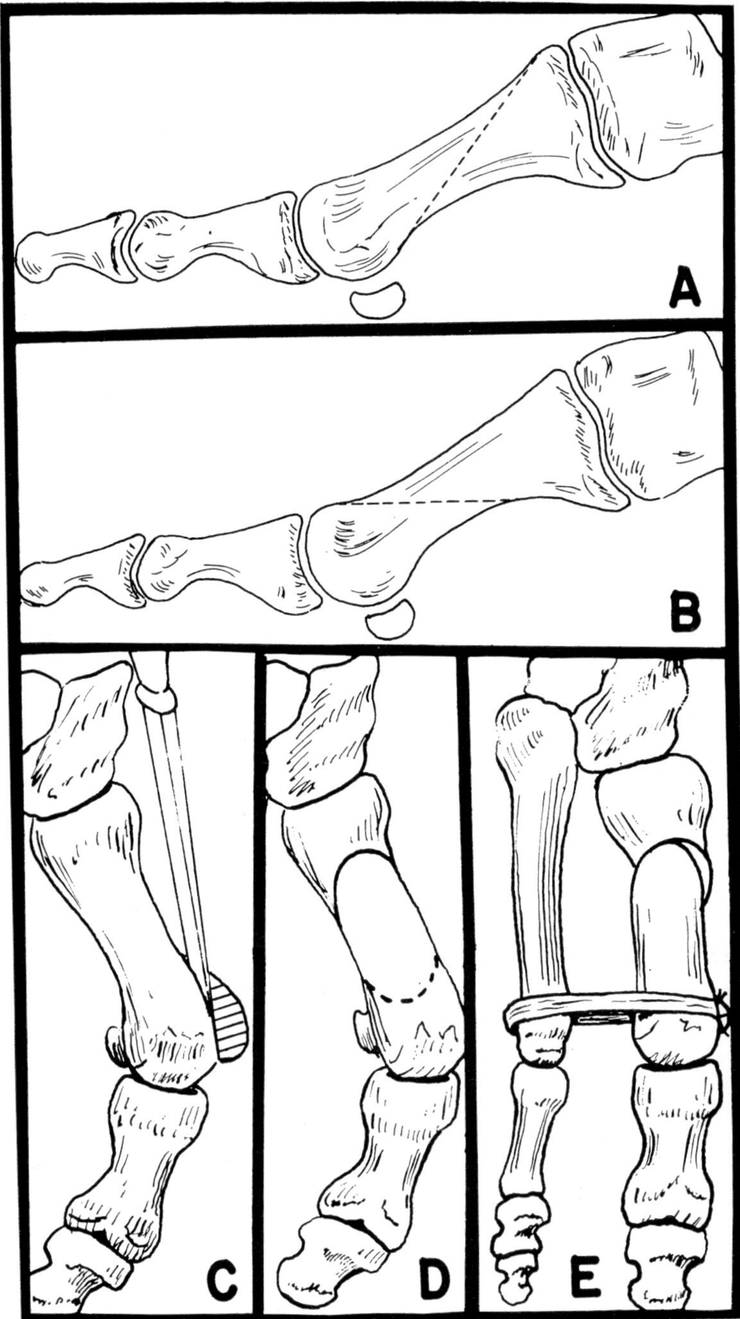

Figure 10–23. Oblique osteotomy of the metatarsal shaft: Ludloff's method (*A*); Mau's method (*B*); Petri's modification (*C, D* and *E*).

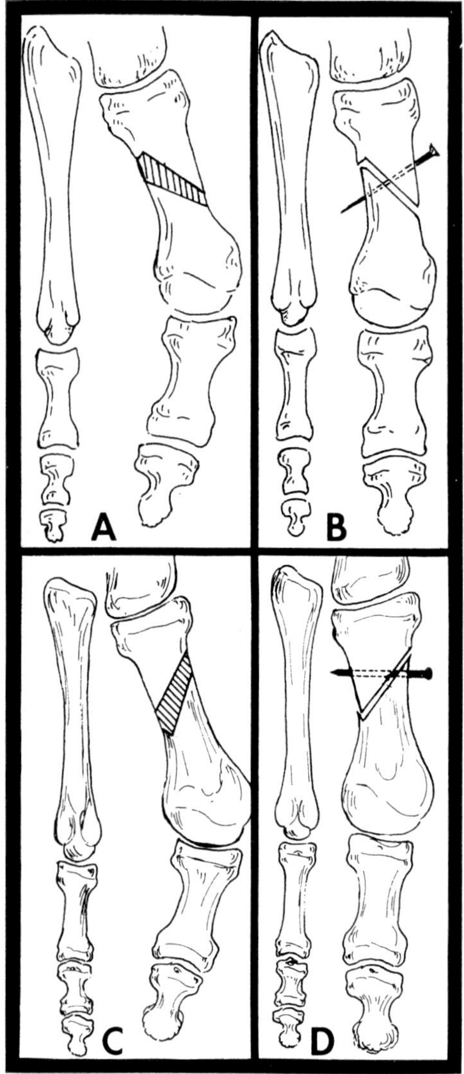

Figure 10–24. Juvara's double osteotomy: first version (*A* and *B*); second version (*C* and *D*).

cortex. The shape of the resected bone was trapezoid: it had a broader lateral base than medial. The fragments were snugged with an encircling wire and transfixed with a nail (Fig. 10–24).

Meyer (1926) carried out a **Z**-osteotomy of the metatarsal shaft. Schotte (1929) from Kotzenberg's clinic described a **V**-osteotomy of the first metatarsal, the apex of the **V** being directed toward the base of the first metatarsal. Cotte (1931) conceived the idea that the cuneiform piece of bone, with the base of the wedge looking laterally, could be turned around and reinserted as a graft from the medial side to correct the inward inclination of the first ray.

Of the shaft osteotomies, Kotzenberg's is the only one that has survived. In the original **V**-osteotomy the bone was sectioned from the medial to the lateral side; it could also have been osteotomized from above down, in a dorsoplantar direction. This latter method is more suitable for correction of metatarsus varus; metatarsus elevatus is better corrected by the former method. Correction of either deformity is easier if the **V** is reversed with the apex pointing distally toward the great toe. Medially and dorsally protruding margins of the proximal end of the distal fragment are nipped off, and the small pieces of bone are packed on the lateral side of the surgical fracture. Kirschner wire is used for internal fixation. The end of the pin comes out of the skin and is incorporated in a cast. The pin is removed after the cast has been applied. When only correction of metatarsus varus is attempted, the necks of the two adjacent bones may also be approximated by stainless steel wire circlage. To avoid slipping we pass the wire through two drill holes across the neck of the first metatarsal and tie the ends over the intervening bridge of bone. **V**-section is perhaps the best osteotomy of the metatarsal shaft. It is stable and provides extensive area surface contact and assures earlier consolidation (Figs. 10–25 to 10–27).

Osteotomy of the proximal end of the first metatarsal. Numerous methods have been devised to correct the varus inclination of the first metatarsal by surgical fracture at or near its base. We may perhaps group them as follows: (1) resection of a cuneiform piece with the base of the wedge looking toward the fibular border of the forefoot, (2) prying open a wedge from the tibial side of the bone, (3) providing one of the osteotomized fragments with a peg, and (4) **V**-osteotomy.

1. For correction of hallux valgus with marked inward inclination of the first metatarsal, Loison (1901) suggested linear or cuneiform osteotomy of the proximal end of the first metatarsal at

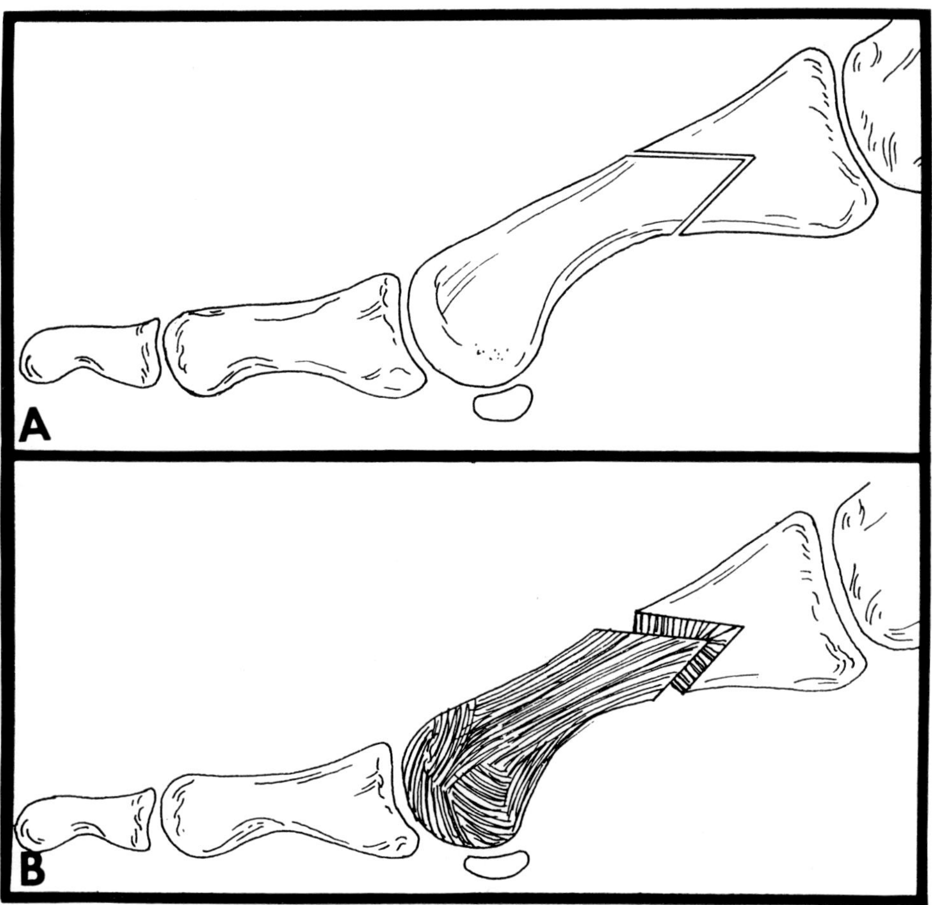

Figure 10–25. Kotzenberg osteotomy of the first metatarsal shaft.

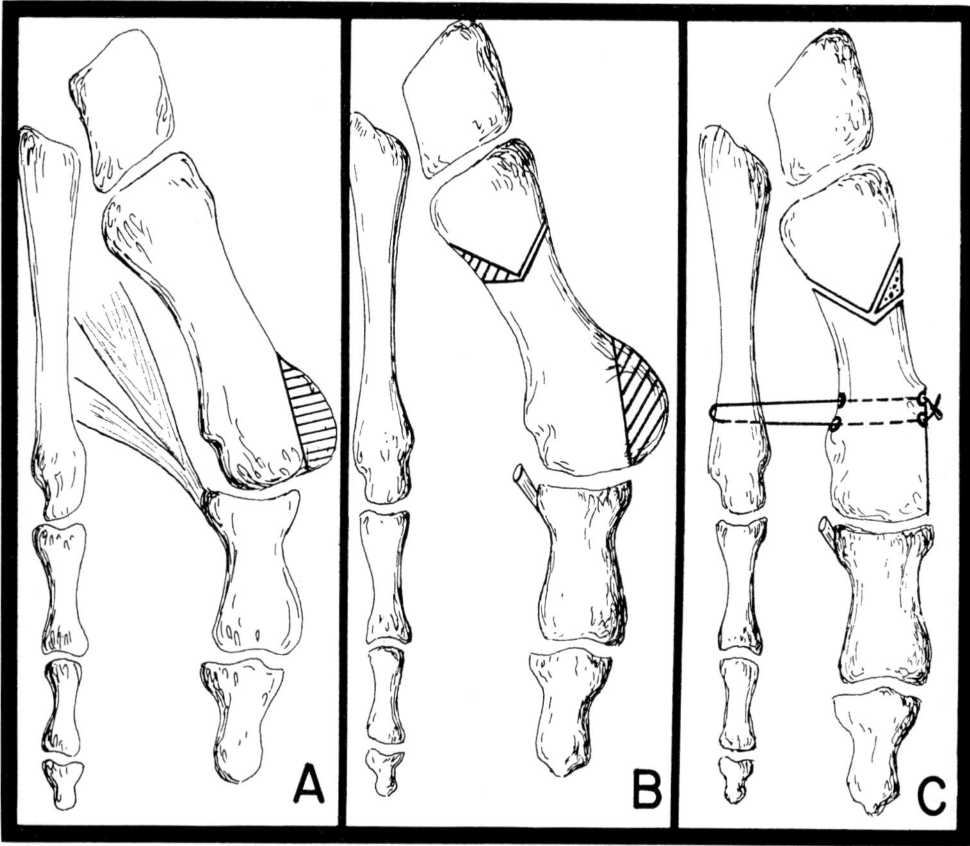

Figure 10–26. Sagittal resection of the medial eminence supplemented with V osteotomy of the first metatarsal shaft and wire circlage.

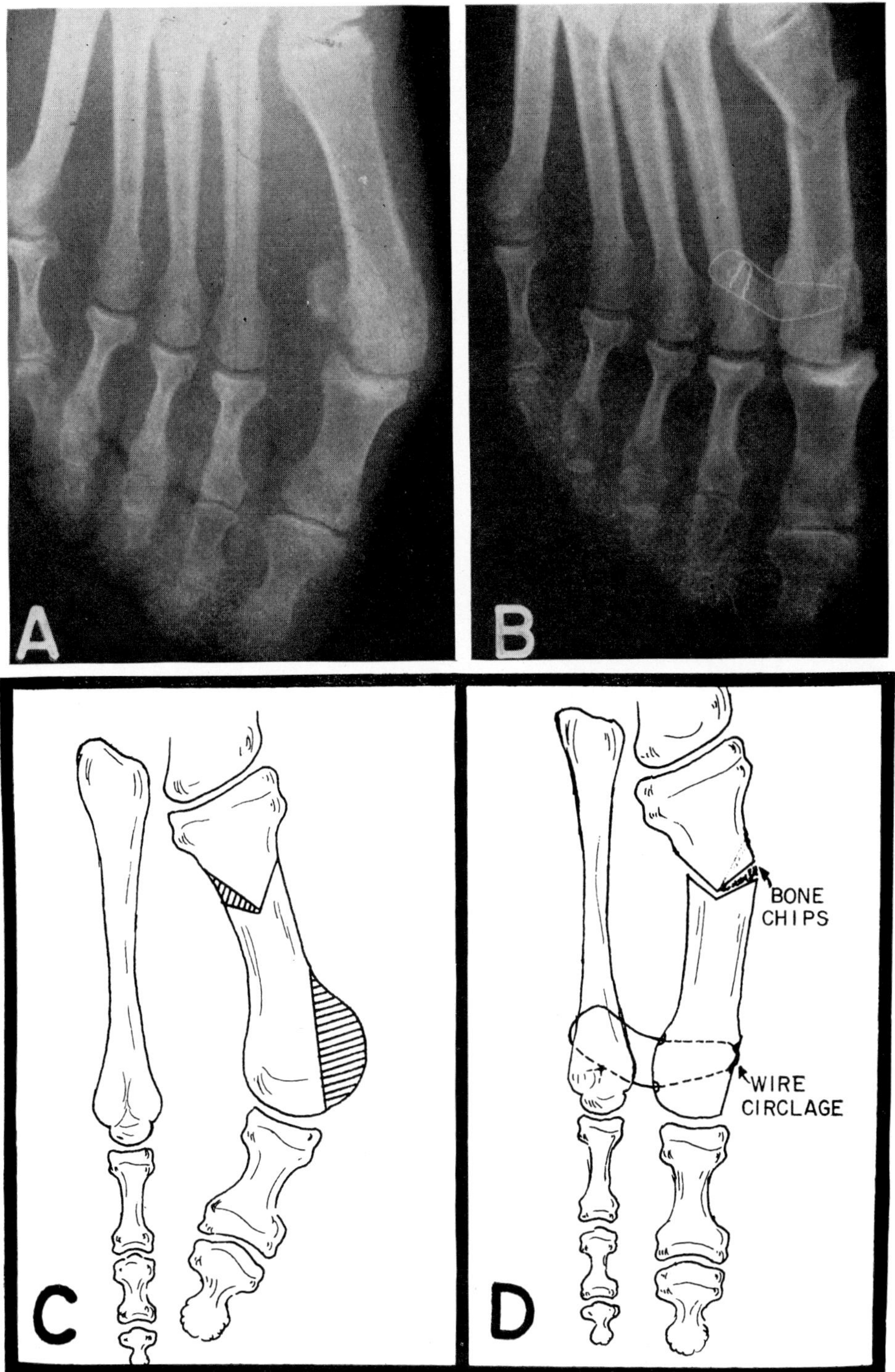

Figure 10–27. Roentgenograms and interpretative diagrams of a case operated by V osteotomy, sagittal resection of the medial eminence, and wire circlage of first and second metatarsals.

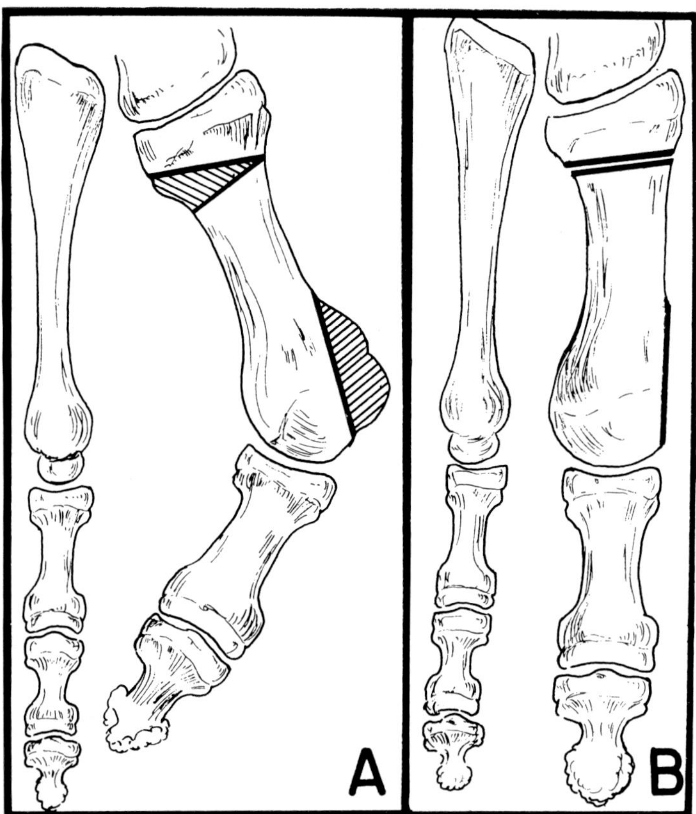

Figure 10–28. Loison-Balacescu operation.

a point just distal to the insertion of the long peroneal tendon. Loison did not perform this procedure; he merely advised it. Balacescu (1903) was the first to carry out this operation. He placed the base of the resected wedge of bone laterally, facing the fibular border of the foot. Chapchal (1943) described the *van Nes method* as follows. A wedge of bone was resected from the lateral and inferior aspect of the base of the first metatarsal. An attempt was then made to correct the three displacements: the varus position of the first metatarsal, its dorsal tilt, and its *supination.* The distal fragment was pushed closer to the second metatarsal; it was displaced plantarward and derotated, or *pronated.* The fragments were temporarily immobilized by a "precutaneous needle." The deformity at the metatarsophalangeal joint was redressed by resection of the medial eminence, adductor release, and transposition of the abductor (Figs. 10–28 and 10–29).

2. Trethowan (1923) recommended prying open a wedge on the tibial side of the first metatarsal base. He plugged the gap by a "shaped-up" cuneiform piece of bone obtained from the resected medial eminence. Almost 30 years later, Trethowan, Bonney, and Macnab (1952) repeated this operation, supplementing it with screw fixation of the two medial metatarsals. Stamm (1957) appropriated the Trethowan technique, but instead of utilizing the piece of bone obtained from the medial eminence, he carved a wedge out of the excised base of the proximal phalanx of the great toe and plugged it into the gap of the osteotomy. Exactly 30 years later Trethowan, Varney and associates (1953) reverted to the original technique but called it "our procedure" (Figs. 10–30 to 10–32).

3. For hallux valgus and marked metatarsus primus varus in adolescence, Rocyn Jones (1948) advised a peg-and-hole type of osteotomy. Cuneiform osteotomy was initiated in the proximal

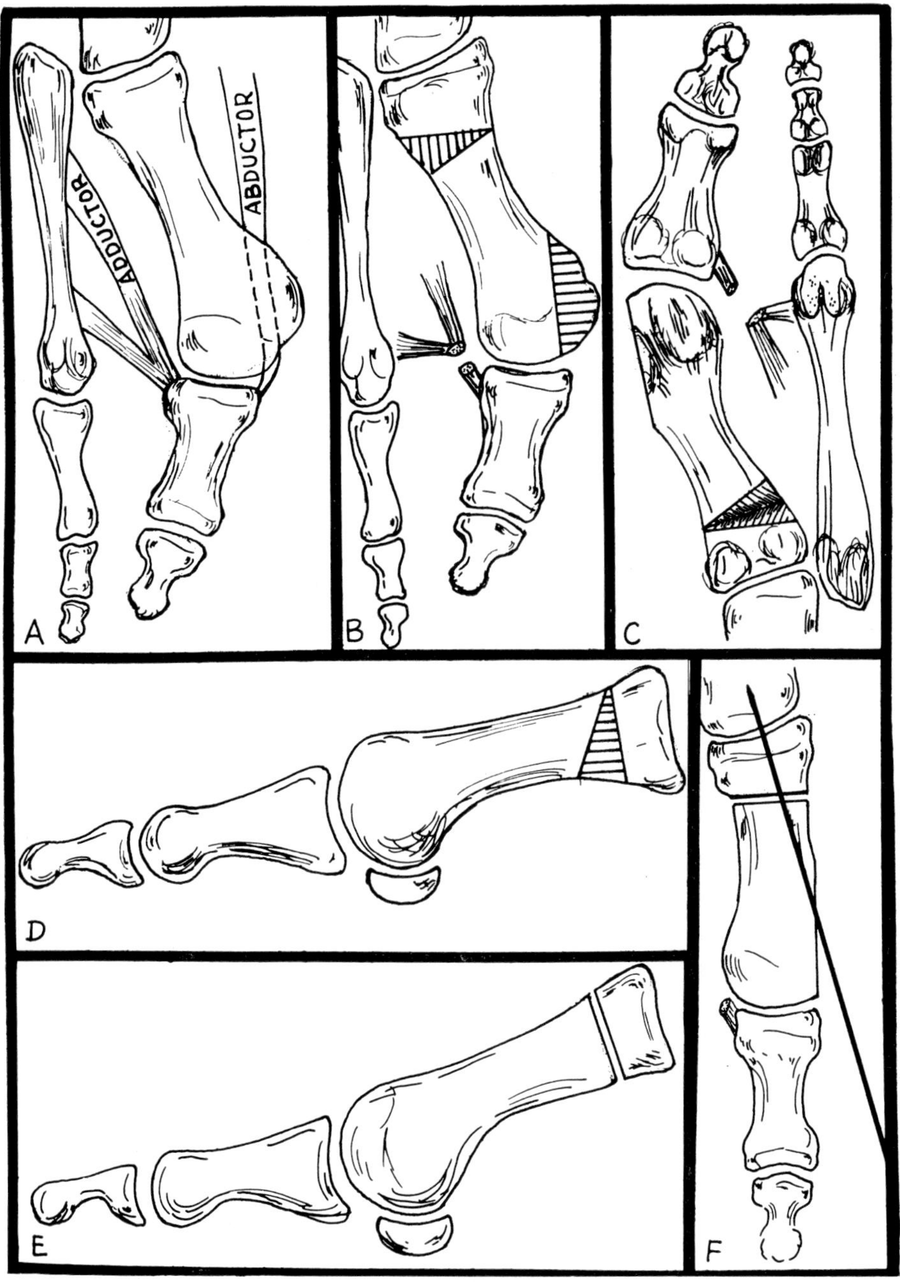

Figure 10–29. Van Nes method.

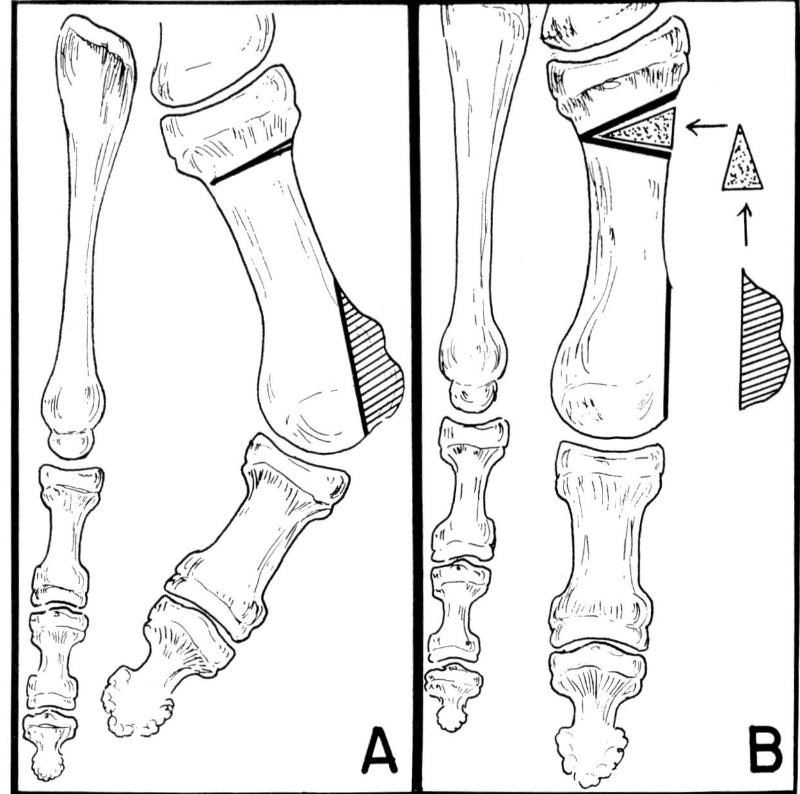

Figure 10–30. Trethowan's operation.

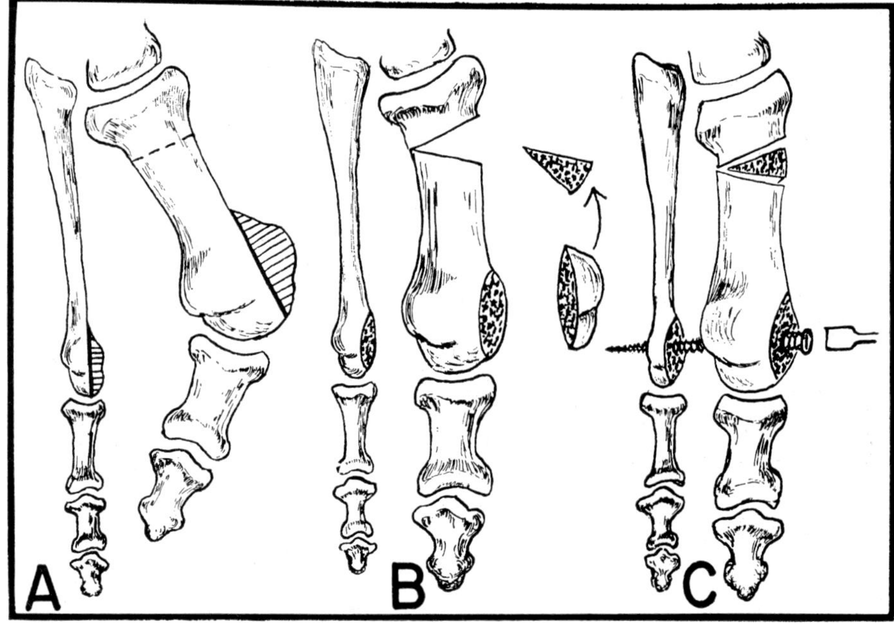

Figure 10–31. The Bonney and Macnab modification.

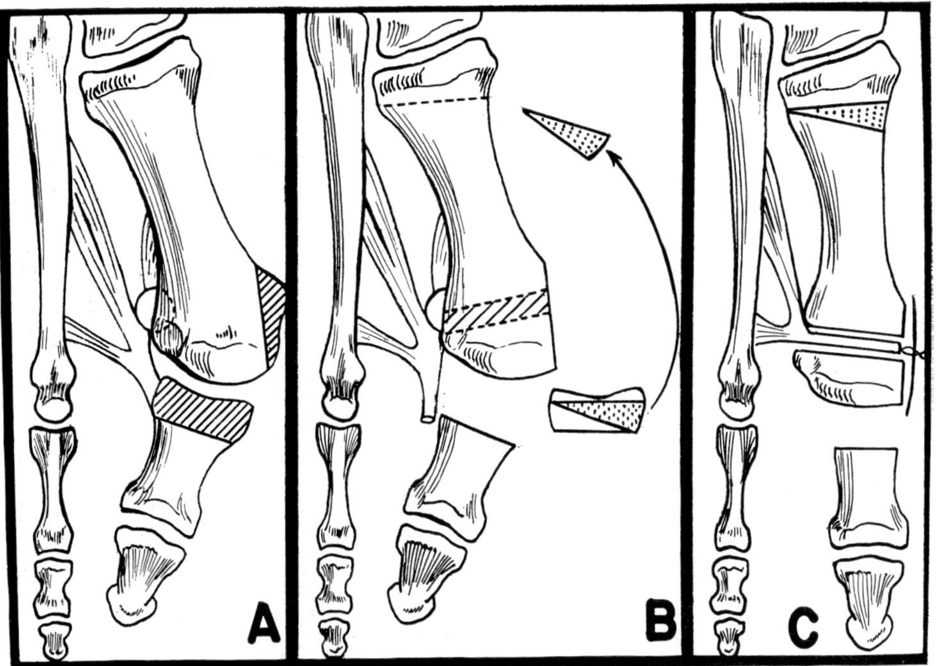

Figure 10–32. Stamm's operation.

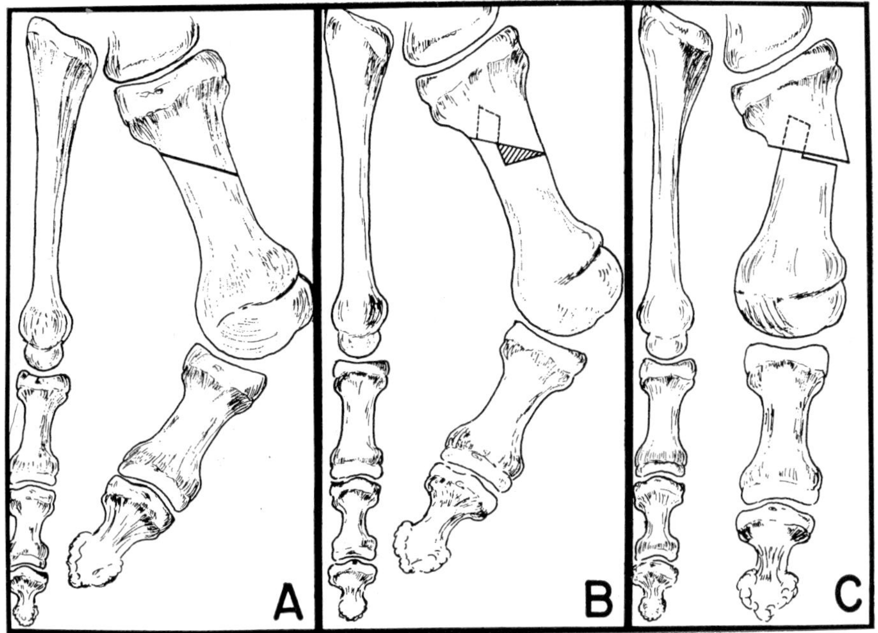

Figure 10–33. Rocyn Jones' operation.

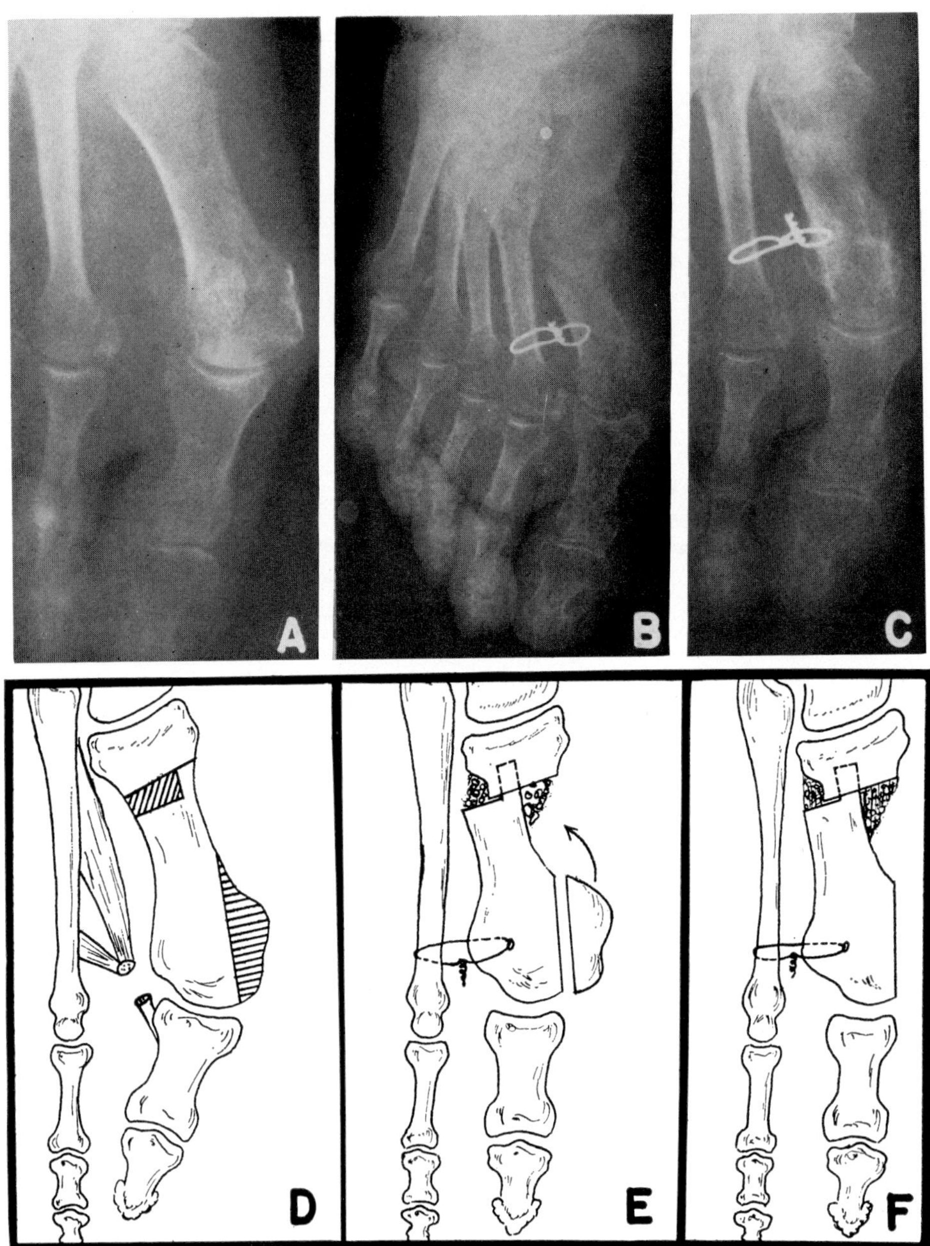

Figure 10–34. Woman, 54, subjected to the Silver procedure. Within a month, while still in the hospital, she complained of inadequate correction of hallux valgus that was due to failure to correct metatarsus primus varus. Roentgenogram before surgery (*A*); soon after proximal osteotomy (*B*); after osteosynthesis (*C*); interpretative diagrams (*D*, *E* and *F*). This patient is completely satisfied with the final result.

extremity of the first metatarsal. Only a part of the wedge was removed and the rest was left as a spike to be impacted into the proximal fragment. "This device," Jones wrote, "secures complete stability of the broken fragments whilst at the same time enabling angulation to take place as a means of correction of the adduction." By adduction he meant the varus position of the first metatarsal. Golden (1961) used a proximal osteotomy that resembled Roux's (1920), Peabody's (1931), or Mitchell's (1958) in that the smaller fragment was provided with a lateral lip of bone. Golden confessed he owed this "device" to one of his assistants. One recalls Barker (1884) and his student. Golden supplemented this osteotomy with sagittal resection of the medial eminence and release of adductor tension on the lateral aspect of the metatarsophalangeal joint (Figs. 10–33 to 10–35).

4. Lenox D. Baker (1953) described his *fishtail osteotomy,* which is reminiscent of Kotzenberg's V-cut described by Schotte (1929) almost a quarter of a century earlier (Fig. 10–36).

The original Loison-Balacescu osteotomy provided greater area of surface contact between the fragments than the later modification by Trethowan and his followers. When a wedge is pried open and the gap is plugged with a piece of bone, the surface contact of the main fragments is reduced radically and union is delayed. The osteotomies of Rocyn Jones, Lenox Baker, and Golden provide a large area of surface contact; they are, in addition, more stable. The only objection one could level against them—as against all osteotomies in close proximity to a joint—is that one might crack the adjoining articular plate and pave the way for traumatic arthritis.

The question arises: when should one resort to proximal in preference to distal osteotomy of the first metatarsal? At the same sitting, one should not detach the medial capsule and resect the eminence on that side, strip the lateral capsule, release the adductor tension, and then

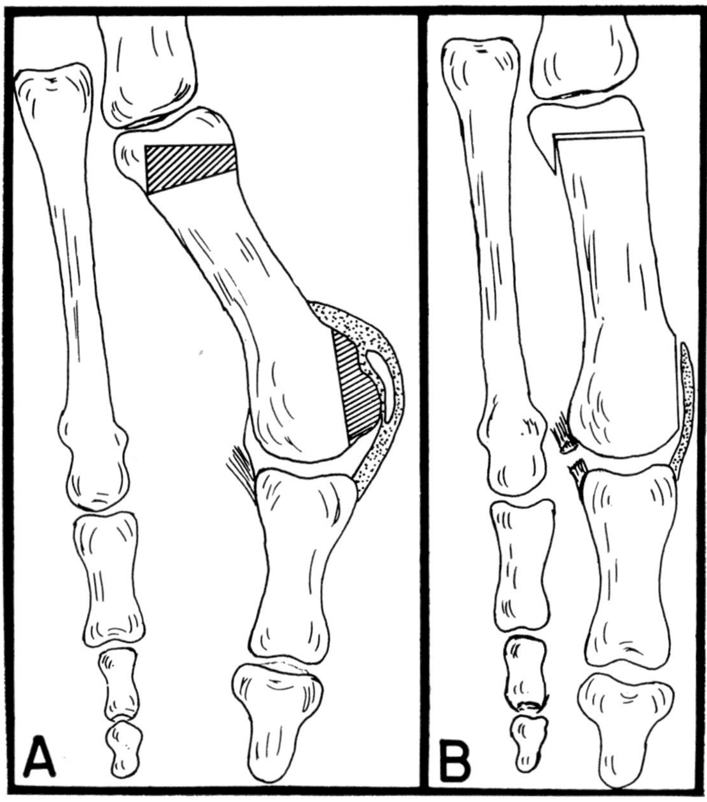

Figure 10–35. Golden's operation.

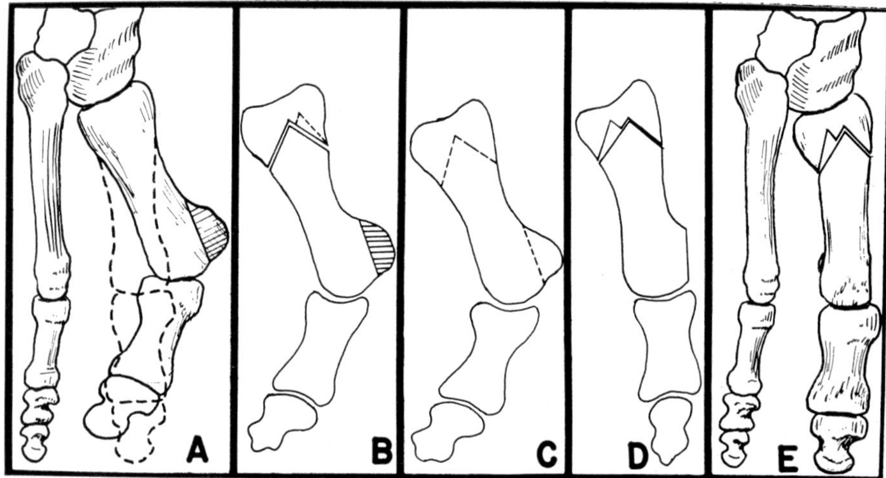

Figure 10–36. Lenox Baker's fishtail osteotomy.

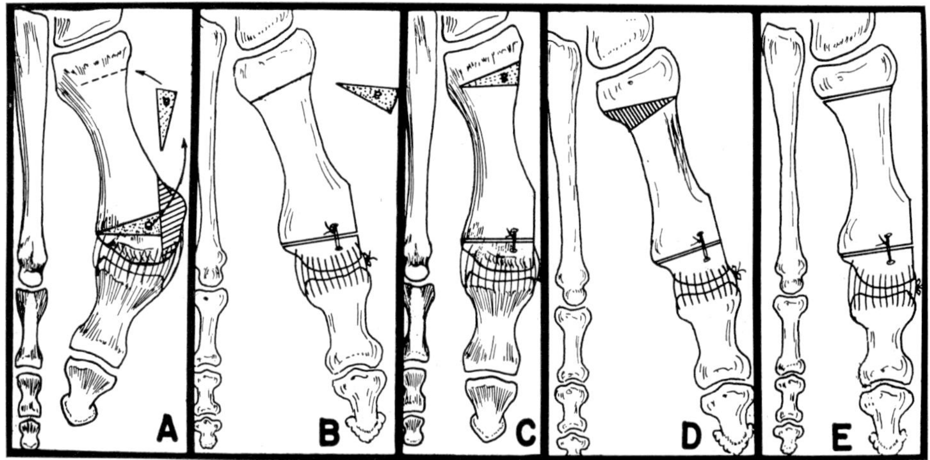

Figure 10–37. Logroscinó's double osteotomy.

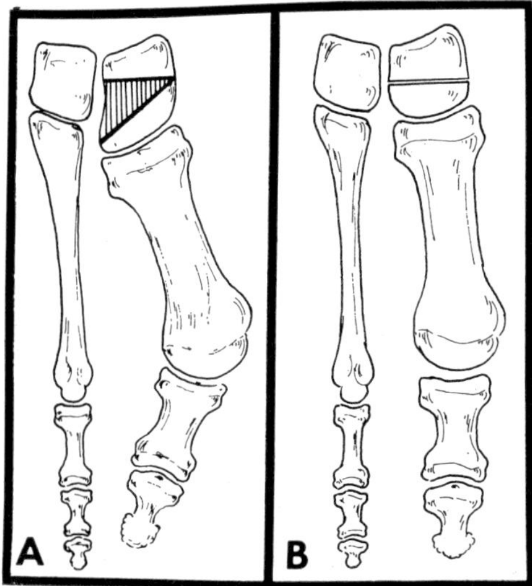

Figure 10–38. Riedl's osteotomy of the innermost cuneiform.

disconnect the head of the first metatarsal from its shaft. These multiple procedures may completely cut off the nutrient supply of the capital fragment and jeopardize its viability. In the presence of fixed hallux valgus, with unyielding adductor tension, a deep sagittal groove, and metatarsus primus varus, plastic procedures at the distal joint should be coupled with proximal osteotomy of the first metatarsal.

Double osteotomies. Logroscinó (1948) advised double osteotomy of the first metatarsal: one at the proximal end, the other at the distal. The operation on the proximal end of the bone at times simulated Balacescu's and at other times Trethowan's; the procedure at the distal extremity of the bone was like Reverdin's. We fail to see the advantage

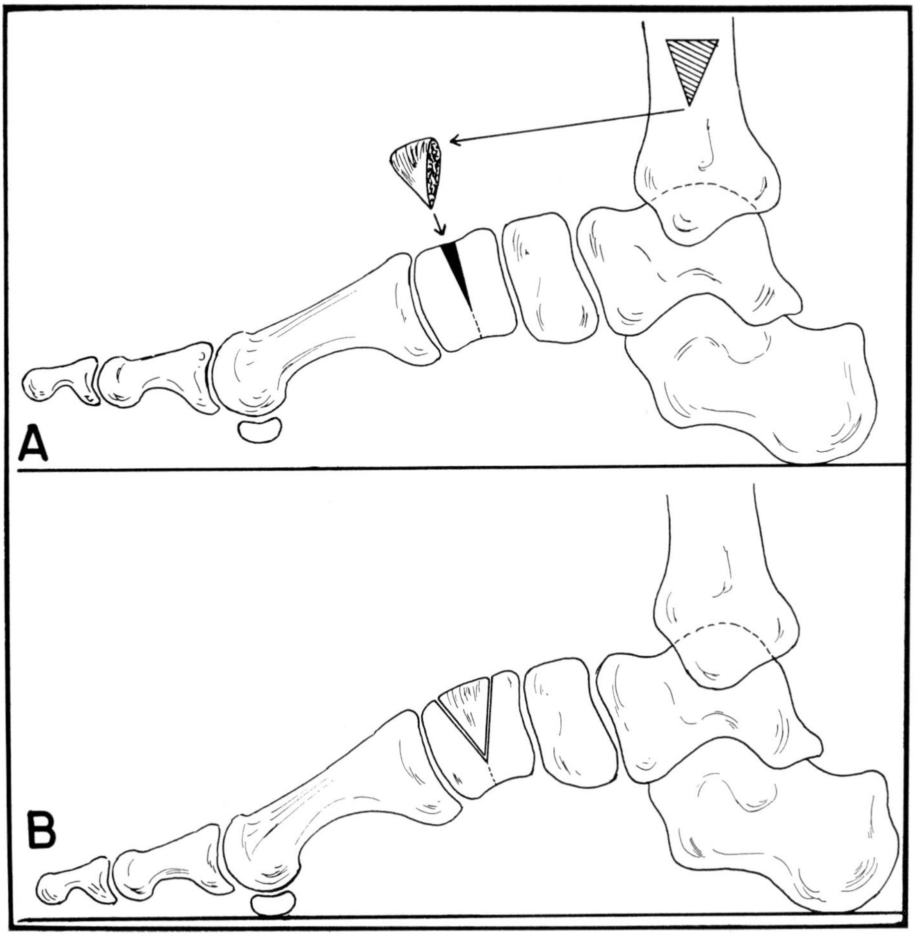

Figure 10–39. Cotton's osteotomy of the innermost cuneiform.

of these double osteotomies. They create unnecessary problems of maintenance of position and prolong the convalescence, to say nothing of the added surgical trauma (Fig. 10–37).

Osteotomy of the first cuneiform. Riedl (1909), from Brenner's clinic in Linz, recommended wedge osteotomy of the innermost cuneiform for correction of the exaggerated varus deformity of the first ray. He placed the base of the wedge laterally. Cotton (1935) split the first cuneiform from its dorsal aspect, opened a wedge, and plugged it with a block of bone. In the latest modification of his sling operation, Joplin (1958) pried a wedge from the medial aspect of the innermost cuneiform and spanned the gap with a bone graft (Figs. 10–38 to 10–40).

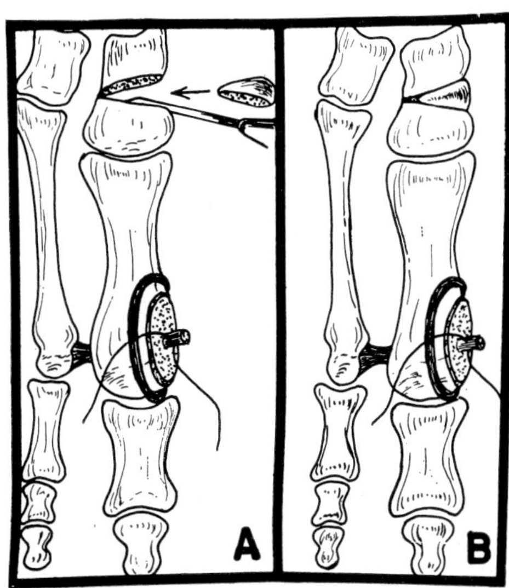

Figure 10–40. Joplin's osteotomy of the innermost cuneiform.

Osteotomies of the innermost cuneiform bone have no advantage over those

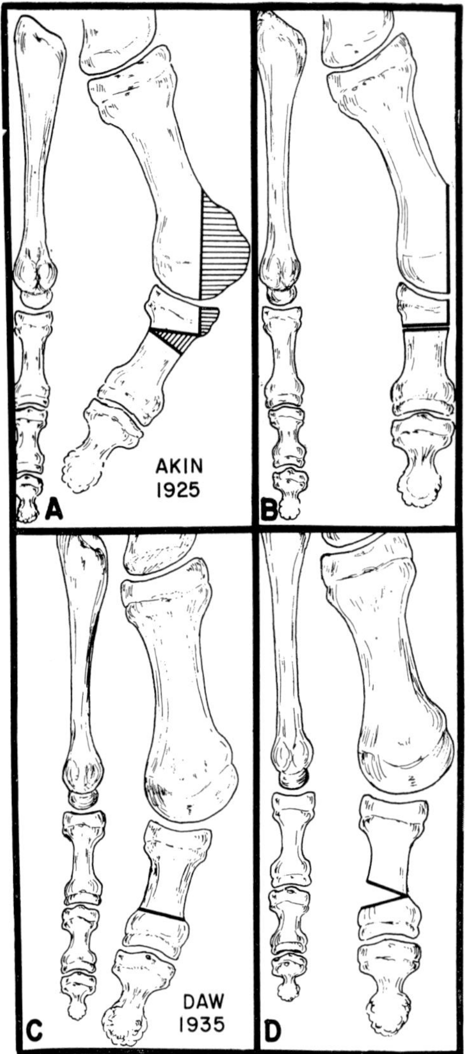

Figure 10–41. Osteotomy of the proximal phalanx of the great toe: Akin's method (*A* and *B*); Daw's method (*C* and *D*).

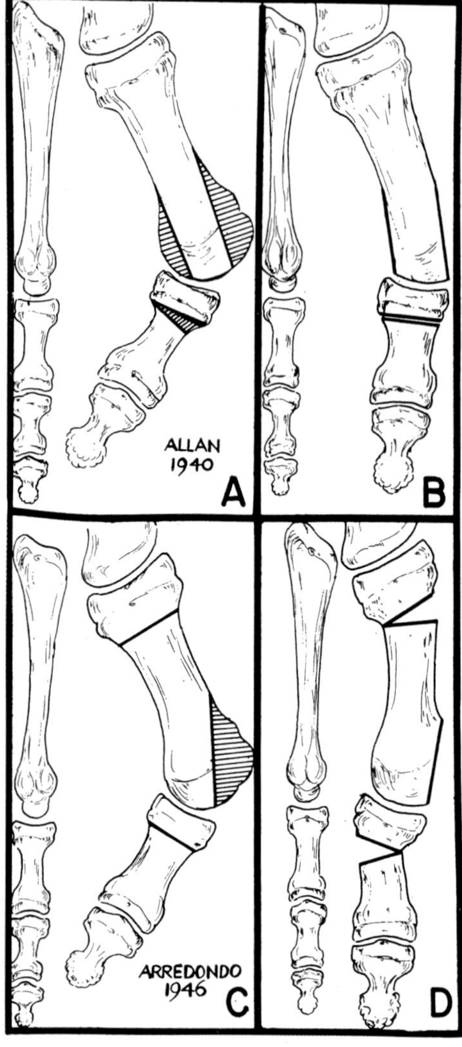

Figure 10–42. Osteotomy of the proximal phalanx of the great toe: Allan's method (*A* and *B*); Arredondo's double osteotomy (*C* and *D*).

of the first metatarsal. One unnecessarily runs the risk of traumatizing the joint between middle and medial cuneiform bones.

Osteotomy of the proximal phalanx. Akin (1925) described what he called "a new operative procedure" for hallux valgus. It consisted of resection of the medial eminence of the first metatarsal and the adjacent lip of the proximal phalanx. The phalanx was subjected to cuneiform osteotomy. Daw (1935) corrected *hallux valgus interphalangeus* by a linear osteotomy toward the distal end of the proximal phalanx. For excessive valgus position of the great toe, in addition to trimming the metatarsal head, Allan (1940) advised removal of a wedge from the medial aspect of the base of the proximal phalanx. In what he called the Sacco operation, Arredondo (1946) described opening a wedge on the medial base of the first metatarsal and lateral side of the proximal phalanx. "When the big toe joint was mobile," Jamieson (1952) thought, "there was a place for osteotomy of the proximal phalanx." Bourdillon (1957) spoke of Butler's operation for hallux valgus, "which consisted of a spokeshave to remove the protruding part of the metatarsal head, and osteotomy of the base

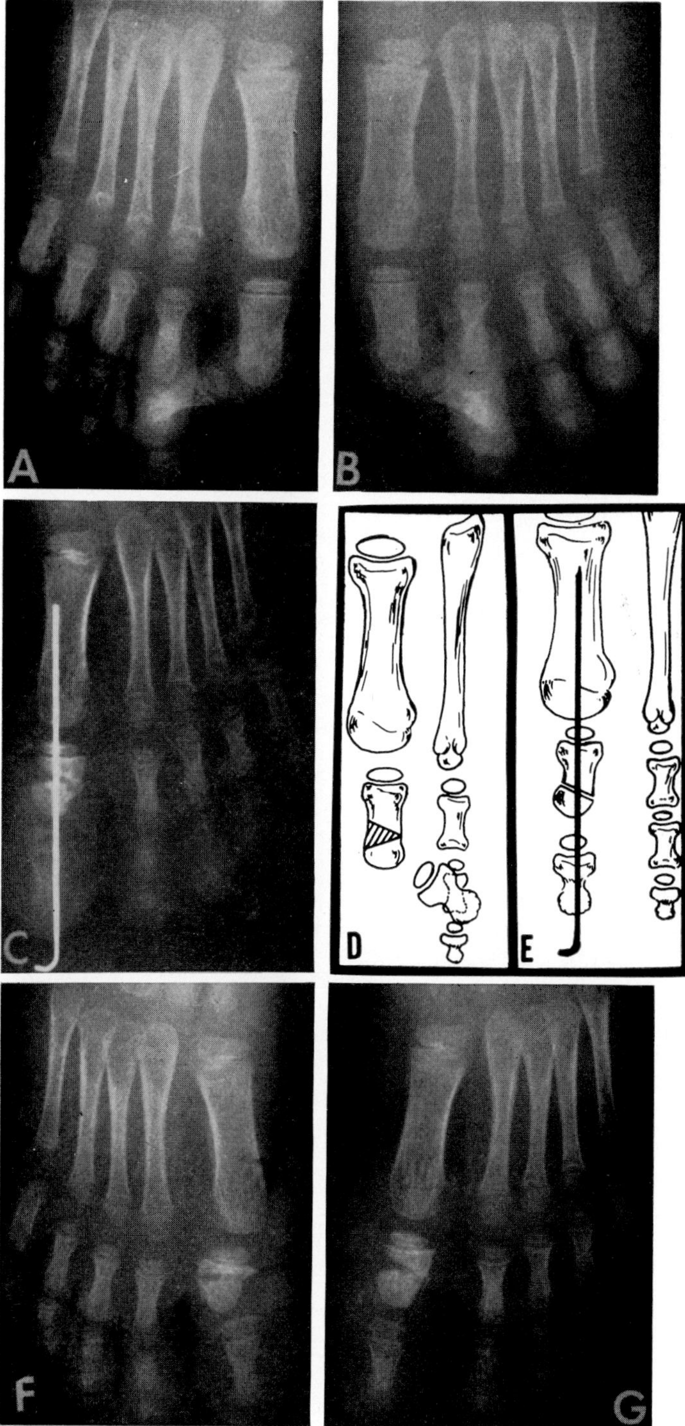

Figure 10–43. Bilateral hallux valgus interphalangeus seen at birth, in boy, 1 year of age: roentgenogram before surgery (*A* and *B*); after osteotomy of the proximal phalanx of the great toe on one side and transfixation with Kirschner wire (*C*); interpretative diagrams (*D* and *E*); osteosynthesis after 4 weeks (*F* and *G*).

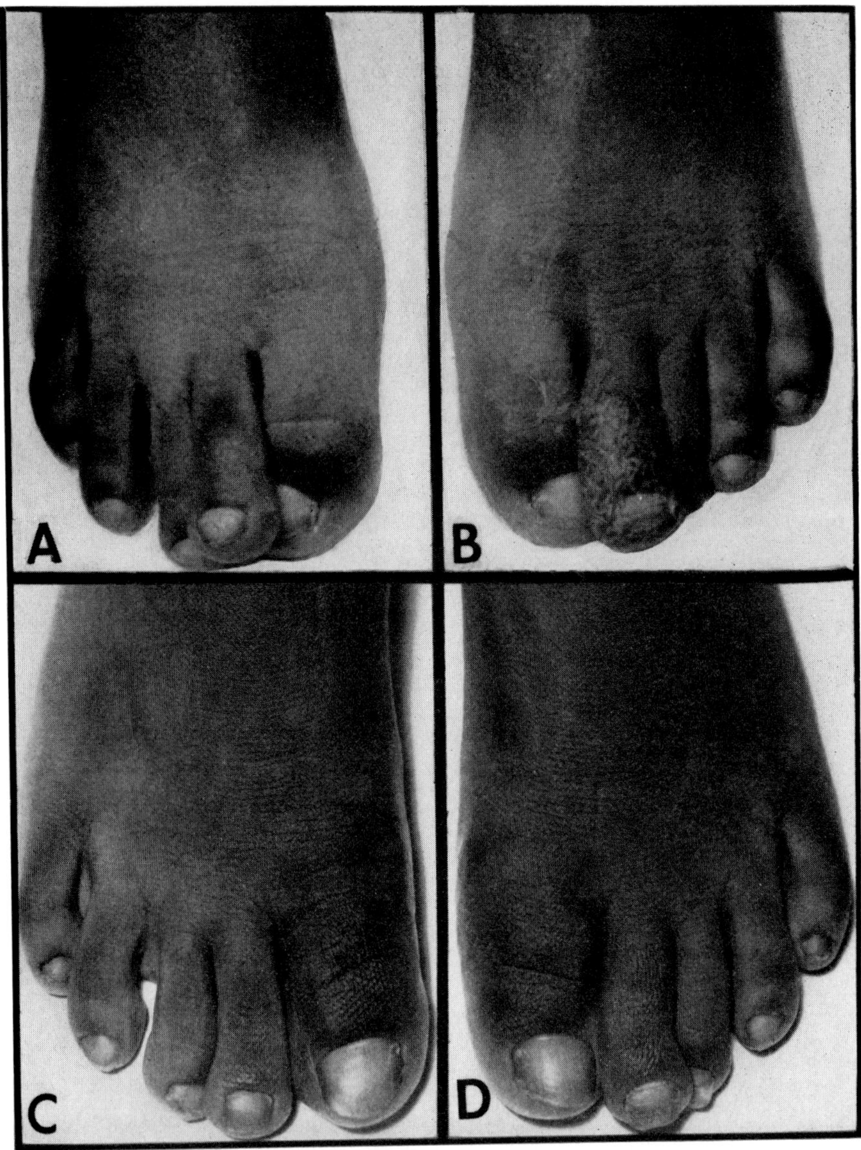

Figure 10–44. Photographs of the case in Figure 10–43 before surgery (*A* and *B*); after surgery (*C* and *D*).

of the proximal phalanx to realign the great toe." More recently, Butterworth and Clary (1963) described a combined resection of the medial eminence of the first metatarsal head and removal of a wedge from the inner aspect of the proximal phalanx. They credited John Vann of Norfolk, Virginia, for this operation; they said that the only information they had about the procedure was a "description at the local medical meetings" in the course of a casual conversation on bunions. The caption under the title of the article characterized this operation as being "previously undocumented." One wonders.

Osteotomy of the proximal phalanx of the great toe has a justifiable indication in hallux valgus interphalangeus (Figs. 10–41 to 10–44).

REFERENCES

Akin, O. F.: The treatment of hallux valgus—a new operative procedure and its results. Med. Sentinel *33*:678–679, 1925.

Allan, F. G.: Hallux valgus and rigidus. Brit. Med. J. *1*:579–581, 1940.

Arredondo, F. O.: Hallux valgus. Tratamiento quirurgico, Operación de Sacco. Rev. Asoc. Méd. Argent. *60*:1009–1010, 1946.

d'Avignon, M.: Examen subséquent des patients opérés du hallux valgus suivant une modification de la méthode opératoire. Reverdin. Acta Chir. Scand. *87* (supplément 76–77): 97–102, 1942.

Bade, P.: *Der Hallux valgus.* Stuttgart, F. Enke, 1940.

Baker, L. D.: Diseases of the foot. Am. Acad. Orthop. Surgeons *10*:327–343, 1953.

Balacescu, J.: Un caz de hallux valgus simetric (in Rumanian). Rev. Chir. *7*:128–135, 1903.

Barker, A. E.: An operation for hallux valgus. Lancet *1*:655, 1884.

Bentzon, P. G. K.: After-examination of hallux valgus patients treated with arthroplastic resection of the head of the first metatarsal bone. Acta Orthop. Scand. *6*:195–206, 1935.

Bick, E. M.: *Source Book of Orthopaedics.* 2nd Ed., Balitmore, Williams & Wilkins Co., 1948, pp. 262–265.

Bonney, G., and Macnab, L.: Hallux valgus and hallux rigidus; a critical survey of operative results. J. Bone Joint Surg. *34*:366–385, 1952.

Bourdillon, J.: Butler's operation for hallux valgus. J. Bone Joint Surg. *40*:346, 1958.

Bradford, E. H.: Linear osteotomy in hallux valgus, etc. Am. J. Orthop. Surg. *12*:169–182, 1914.

Butterworth, R. D., and Clary, B. B.: A bunion operation. Virginia Med. Monthly *90*:11–14, 1963.

Chapchal, G.: Zur operativen Behandlung des Hallux valgus. Ztschr. Orthop. Grenzgb. *73–74*:47–60, 1941–1943.

Cholmeley, J. A.: Hallux valgus in adolescents. Proc. Roy. Soc. Med. *51*:903–906, 1958.

Cotte, M. G.: Ostéotomie du premier métatarsien pour hallux valgus. Lyon Chir. *28*:757–758, 1931.

Cotton, F. J.: Foot statics and surgery. Tr. New Eng. Surg. Soc., *18*:181–208, 1935.

David, P.-É.-M.: *Une Nouvelle Opération pour la Cure de l'Hallux Valgus.* Thesis. Paris, Librairie Louis Arnette, 1934, pp. 1–76.

Daw, S. W.: An unusual type of hallux valgus (two cases). Brit. Med. J. *2*:580, 1935.

Durman, D. C.: Metatarsus primus varus and hallux valgus. A.M.A. Arch. Surg. *74*:128–135, 1957.

Eick, K.: Beitrag zur operativen Behandlung des Hallux valgus. Chirurg. *58*:326–330, 1931.

Frejka, B.: Mediolateral oblique osteotomy of Chlumsky (in Czech). Bratisl. Lek. Listy *3*: 329–335, 1924.

Gallie, W. E.: Avascular necrosis involving articular surfaces. J. Bone Joint Surg. *38*:732–738, 1956.

Gibson, J., and Piggott, H.: Osteotomy of the neck of the first metatarsal in the treatment of hallux valgus. J. Bone Joint Surg. *44*:349–355, 1962.

Gielzinski, A.: Results of the treatment of hallux valgus by Komza's method (in Polish). Oddz. Ortop. Urazowego, Chorzow, Chir. Narzad, ruchu. *23*:427–430, 1958.

Golden, G. N.: Hallux valgus, the osteotomy operation. Brit. Med. J. *1*:1361–1365, 1961.

Hauser, E. D. W.: *Diseases of the Foot.* 2nd Ed., Philadelphia, W. B. Saunders Co., 1950, p. 102.

Hawkins, F. B., Mitchell, C. L., and Hedrick, D. W.: Correction of hallux valgus by metatarsal osteotomy. J. Bone Joint Surg. *27*:387–394, 1945.

Hohmann, G.: Symptomatische oder physiologische Behandlung des Hallux valgus? Münch Med. Wchnschr. *33*:1042–1045, 1921.

Hohmann, G.: Über ein Verfahren zur Behandlung des Spreizfusses. Zbl. Chir. *49*:1933–1935, 1922.

Hohmann, G.: Über Hallux und Spreizfuss, ihre Entstehung und physiologische Behandlung. Arch. Orthop. Unfall-Chir. *21*:525–550, 1923.

Hohmann, G.: Zur Hallux valgus-Operation. Zbl. Chir. *51*:230–231, 1924.

Hohmann, G.: Der Hallux valgus und die uebrigen Zehenverkruemmungen. Ergeb. Chir. Orthop. *18*:308–348, 1925.

Hohmann, G.: *Fuss und Bein.* Munich, J. F. Bergmann, 1951, pp. 145–192.

Jamieson, E. S.: Hallux valgus. J. Bone Joint Surg. *34*:328, 1952.

Jones, A. R.: Hallux valgus in the adolescent. Proc. Roy. Soc. Med. *41*:392–393, 1948.

Joplin, R. J.: Some common foot disorders amenable to surgery. Am. Acad. Orthop. Surgeons *15*:144–158, 1958.

Juvara, E.: Nouveau procédé pour la cure radicale du "hallux valgus." Presse Méd. *40*:395–397, 1919.

Juvara, E. Cure radicale de l'hallux-valgus par la résection cunéiforme de la portion moyenne de la diaphyse du métatarsien, suivie de l'ostéosynthèse des fragments. Lyon Chir. *23*: 429–442, 1926.

Juvara, E.: L'hallux-valgus; son traitement opératoire. Rev. Chir. *5*:321–348, 1932.

Keszly, S.: Eine neue Modifikation der operativen Behandlung des Hallux valgus. Zbl. Chir. *50*:91–94, 1923. Abstract in J. Bone Joint Surg. *5*:617, 1923.

Komza, J.: The operations of the big toe (in Polish). Pol. Przegl. Chir. *22*:153–170, 1950.

Lance, M.: Le traitement chirurgical de l'hallux valgus par le procédé du "bilboquet." Gaz. Hôp. *109*:1628–1630, 1936.

Lelièvre, J.: *Pathologie du Pied.* Paris, Masson et Cie., 1952, pp. 319–331.

Logroscinó, D.: Il trattamento chirurgico dell'-alluce valgo. Chir. Org. Mov. *32*:81–96, 1948.

Loison, M.: Note sur le traitement chirurgicale du hallux valgus d'après l'étude radiographique de la déformation. Bull. Mem. Soc. Chir. *27*:528–531, 1901.

Ludloff, K.: Die Beseitigung des Hallux valgus durch die schraege planto-dorsale Osteotomie des Metatarsus I (Erfahrungen und Erfolge). Arch. Klin. Chir. *110*:364–387, 1918.

McBride, E. D.: Hallux valgus bunion deformity.

Am. Acad. Orthop. Surgeons *9:*334–346, 1952.
Matheis, H.: Die Entstehung und ursaechliche Behandlung des Hallux valgus. Ztschr. Orthop. Chir. *48:*1–21, 1927.
Mau, C., and Lauber, H. T.: Die operative Behalung des Hallux valgus (Nachuntersuchungen). Dtsch. Ztschr. Chir. *197:*361–377, 1926.
Mauclaire, P.: Déviation des orteils. *Traité de Chirurgie de Dentu et Delbet.* Paris, J. B. Baillière et Fils, 1901, Part II, pp. 1185–1200.
Mayr, O.: Über Hallux valgus–Operationen im Kriege. Arch. Orthop. Unfall-Chir. *40:*485–491, 1940.
Med. Rec. *25:*640, June 7, 1884. (Editorial.)
Meyer, M.: Eine neue Modifikation der Hallux valgus Operation. Zbl. Chir. *53:*3215–3268, 1926.
Mikhail, I. K.: Bunion, hallux valgus and metatarsus primus varus. Surg. Gyn. Obst. *111:*637–646, 1960.
Mitchell, C. L., Fleming, J. L., Allen, R., Glenney, C., and Sanford, G. A.: Osteotomy-bunionectomy for hallux valgus. J. Bone Joint Surg. *40:*41–60, 1958.
Mizuno, S., Sima, Y., and Yamazaki, K.: Detorsion osteotomy of the first metatarsal bone in hallux valgus. J. Jap. Orthop. Soc. *30:*105–110, 1956.
Mommsen, F.: Eine neue Operationsmethode zur Behandlung der leichten Formen des Hallux valgus. Dtsch. Gesundh. *8:*121–123, 1953.
Mouchet, A.: Pathogénie et traitement des difformités du gros orteil. Rev. d'Orthop. *9:*582–637, 1922.
Mygind, H. B.: Operations for hallux valgus. J. Bone Joint Surg. *34:*529, 1952.
Mygind, H. B.: Operative treatment of hallux valgus (in Danish). Ugeskr. Laeg. *115:*236–239, 1953.
Mygind, H. B.: Some views on the surgical treatment of hallux valgus. Acta Orthop. Scand. *23:*152–158, 1953.
Ortiz, D.: Hallux valgus. Operación de Hohmann modificada. Bull. Soc. Argent. Ortop. Traum. *21:*65–74, 1956.
Peabody, C. W.: The surgical cure of hallux valgus. J. Bone Joint Surg. *13:*273–282, 1931.
Petri, C.: Zur Behandlung von Vorfussdeformitaeten. Ztschr. Orthop. Grenzgb. *70:*343–349, 1940.
Reverdin, J.: Anatomie et opération de l'hallux valgus. Internat. Med. Congr. *2:*408–412, 1881.
Reverdin, J.: De la déviation en dehors du gros orteil (hallux valgus, vulg. "oignon," "bunions," "Ballen") et de son traitement chirurgical. Tr. Internat. Med. Congr. *2:*408–412, 1881.
Riedl, H.: Osteotomie des Keilbeines bei Hallux valgus. Arch. Klin. Surg. *88:*565–575, 1909.
Roux, C.: Aux pieds sensibles. Rev. Méd. Suisse Rom. *40:*62–83, 1920.
Sazepin, T.: Operative Therapie des Hallux valgus. Zbl. Chir. *53:*134–138, 1926.
Schotte, M.: Zur operativen Korrektur des Hallux valgus im Sinne Ludloffs. Klin. Woch. *50:* 2333–2334, 1929.
Silver, D.: The operative treatment of hallux valgus. J. Bone Joint Surg. *5:*225–232, 1923.
Stamm, T. T.: The surgical treatment of hallux valgus. Guy's Hosp. Rep. *106:*273–279, 1957.
Steindler, A.: *Orthopedic Operations.* Springfield, Ill. Charles C Thomas, 1943, p. 218.
Thomasen: Personal communication.
Tierny, A.: Traitement de l'orteil en marteau. Rev. d'Orthop. *33:*445–452, 1926.
Tierny, A.: La correction de l'orteil en marteau et de l'hallux valgus par le procédé du Bilboquet. Paris, La Clinique, 1930, pp. 211–212.
Trethowan, J.: Hallux valgus. In *A System of Surgery* (C.C. Choyce, ed.). New York, P. B. Hoeber, 1923, pp. 1046–1049.
Urbanek, K., and Dvorak, J.: The late results of operative treatment of hallux valgus (in Czech). Acta Chir. Orthop. Traum. *25:*240–244, 1958.
Varney, J. H., Cocker, J. K., and Cawley, J. J.: Bunion treatment by greenstick osteotomy, metatarsal base. West. J. Surg. Obst. Gyn. *61:*36–38, 1953.
Waldenström: See Bentzon (1935).
Wilhelm, R.: Ein einfaches Operationsverfahren bei Hallux valgus. Zbl. Chir. *61:*2424–2425, 1934.

Chapter Eleven

ARTHROPLASTIC RESECTIONS

When hallux valgus is complicated with painful arthritis of the first metatarsophalangeal joint and with erosion and interlocking of the opposed articular surfaces, one is left with two alternatives: resection of the articular bones or fusion. Resection has for its aim preservation of motion. For this reason it has acquired the epithet *arthroplastic.* In most instances no attempt is made to remodel the ends of remaining bones or provide them with coverage. When the head of the first metatarsal and the base of the proximal phalanx are excised in the same operation, the procedure is spoken of as *joint resection* or *arthrectomy.* Both terms imply more than what is actually done. Resection of the articular extremities of the two main bones entering into the first metatarsophalangeal joint together with the sesamoids has come to be known as the *Edmond Rose method.* When only the head of the first metatarsal is excised, the operation is called *Hueter resection.* Excision of the proximal portion of the first phalanx of the great toe is identified with Keller's name.

Edmond Rose's resection. In the May, 1837, issue of *The Dublin Journal of Medical Sciences,* there is a section entitled *Dr. Fricke's Report on the Hamburg Hospital for the First Quarter of 1836.* Dr. Fricke, we are told, operated on two cases of "exostosis of the ball of the foot, which greatly obstructed walking. . . . Excision of the bones, which form the metatarsodigital joint of the great toe, was performed with perfect success." We may remember that 2 years earlier Froriep (1834) had given the name *exostosis* to what was then known as *Ballen* in Germany, which in the 1870's, was renamed by Hueter *hallux valgus.*

Heubach (1897) described Fricke's operation as follows: "Two eliptical incisions were drawn around the swelling, the soft tissue was retracted and the joint approached by blunt dissection. The articulation was opened; with a saw, the head of the first metatarsal and the base of the proximal phalanx were resected. The wound was packed with gauze, the foot was bandaged on a board, with a pad of gauze under the toes, heavier under the first." Examination of the resected parts revealed "adhesions between the two bones and severe degeneration of the articular cartilage."

Sporadic cases of the first metatarsophalangeal joint resection were reported by Pancoast (1844), Hilton (1853), But-

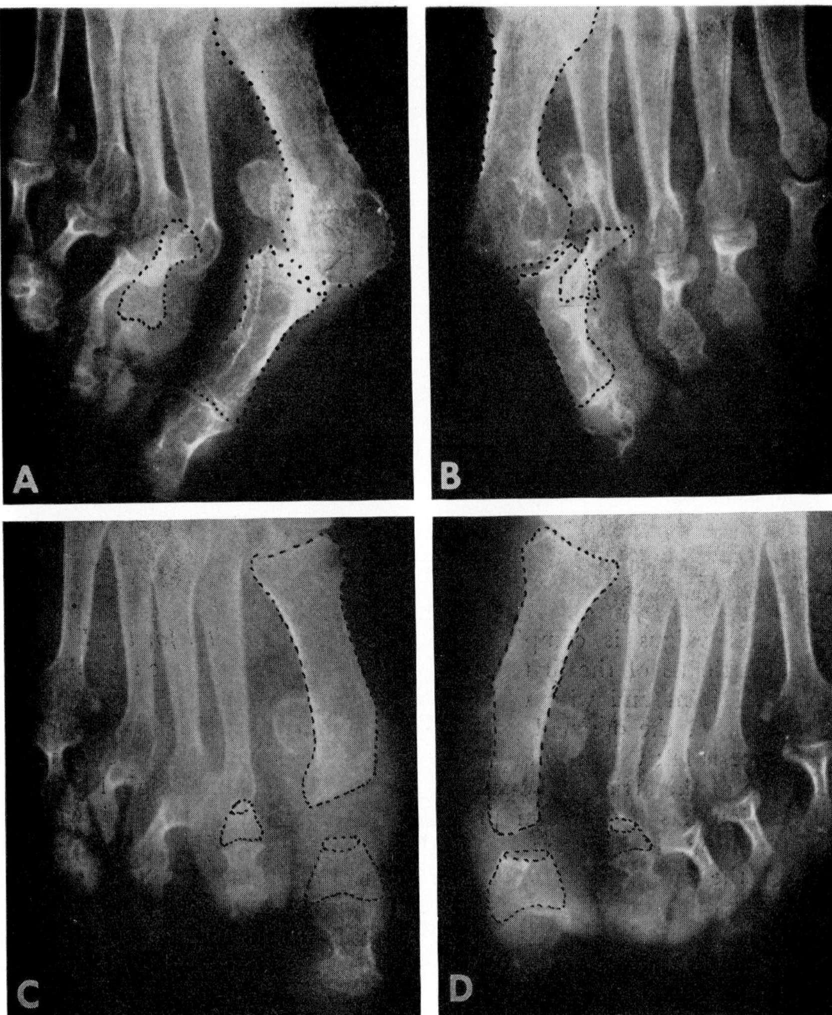

Figure 11–1. Woman, 62, afflicted with generalized rheumatoid arthritis, bilateral hallux valgus, dislocated second toes. Surgery: resection of the first metatarsophalangeal joints and excision of the basal portion of the proximal phalanges of both second toes; surgical syndactylia of first and second toes. The third, fourth, and fifth toes, though deviated, had not been causing any discomfort. They were left alone. Preoperative roentgenograms (*A* and *B*); exposures after surgery (*C* and *D*).

cher (1859), and some others. In most instances the reason given was *caries*—a ubiquitous term meaning decay—which was used indiscriminately in the past to include almost every type of bone and joint disease, including hallux valgus complicated with degenerative arthritis.

Hilton excised "the articular extremities of the metatarsal and the first phalanx . . . together with the two sesamoid bones" for what was described as "inflammatory disorganization of the joint of the great toe." Sayre (1879) specifically recommended joint resection for hallux valgus. Heubach (1897) called this procedure "the operation of Edmond Rose" and went into great detail to point out its advantages over the other methods then in practice. Edmond Rose extirpated the sesamoids in addition to resection of the head of the first metatarsal and the base of the proximal phalanx—exactly what John Hilton had done earlier.

Resection of the first metatarsophalangeal joint was practiced sporadically during the earlier decades of the present century. Singley (1913) exposed the joint through Petersen's (1888) interdigital incision. He excised the metatarsal head, and reamed and rounded the remaining stump. He removed the base of the proximal phalanx and concaved the remaining surface. From around the first intermetatarsal space he obtained a flap of fatty tissue and interposed it between the two bones.

At present, resection of the main articular bones entering into the formation of the metatarsophalangeal joint of the great toe is practiced only in marked

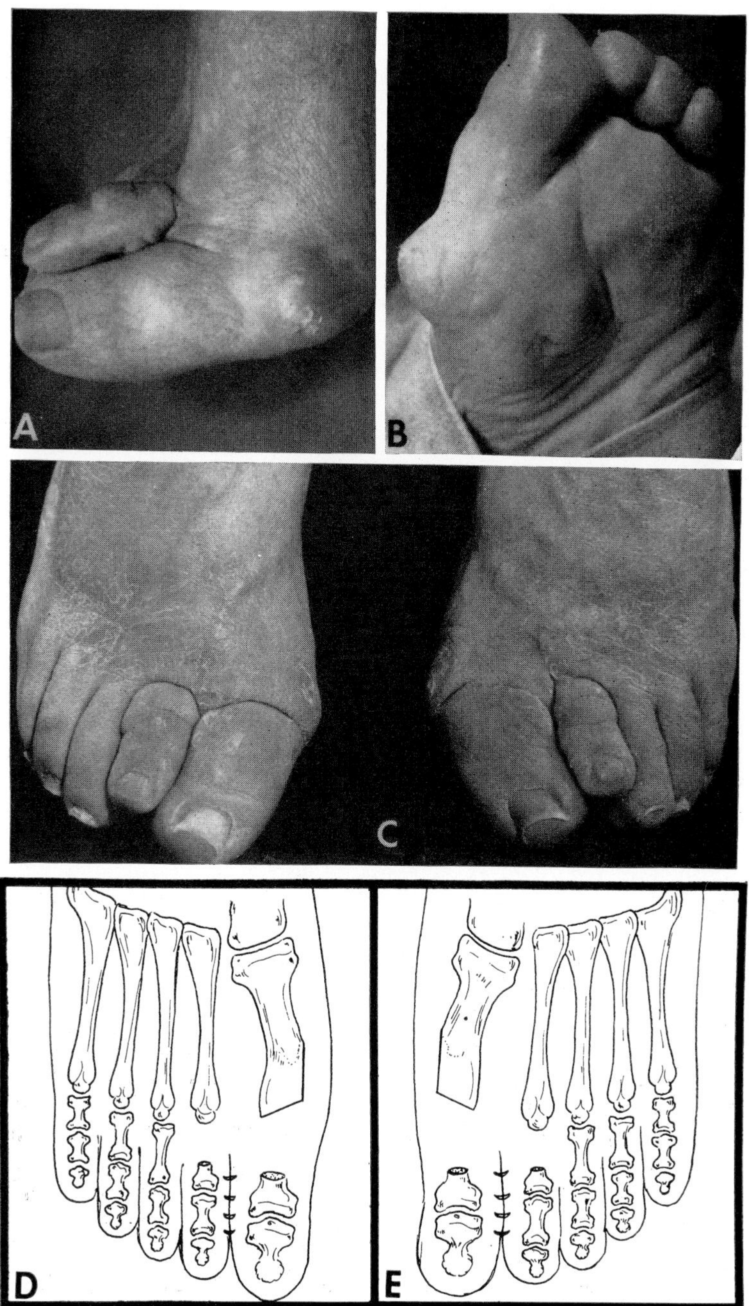

Figure 11–2. The same patient shown in Figure 11–1. Profile view photographs of right forefoot, seen from the medial side just before surgery (*A*). Plantar view of left forefoot (*B*). Both feet seen from the dorsal aspect several months after surgery (*C*). Interpretative diagrams (*D* and *E*). This patient reported no discomfort and no pain; she stated she wears ordinary shoes without any trouble.

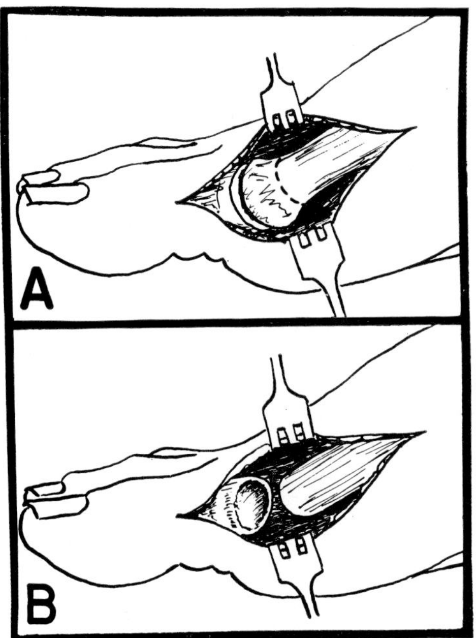

Figure 11–3. Hueter resection: line of resection (*A*); rounding the stump after the head of the first metatarsal had been removed (*B*).

hallux valgus due to rheumatoid arthritis. Ordinarily, either the head of the first metatarsal or the adjoining portion of the proximal phalanx is removed (Figs. 11–1 and 11–2).

Hueter's resection. Oskar Heyfelder (1861) mentioned Kramer and Roux as having decapitated the first metatarsal in 1826 and 1829 respectively. The reason given in both instances was *caries;* the final result was recorded as good. In 1837 Pétrequin went on a trip to Italy. He saw Professor Regnoli of Pisa resect the head of the first metatarsal. On his return, Pétrequin (1838) wrote: "I saw decapitation of the first metatarsal bone. This resection kept intact the big toe and its tendons and the form of the foot." It was in this same year (1838) that Carl Hueter, whose name is linked with the resection of the first metatarsal head, was born.

Hueter (1871) recommended resection of the first metatarsal head for infected hallux valgus. A. Rose (1874) of New York (not to be confused with Edmond Rose) approved of Hueter's operation but pointed out that Hueter resected the head of the first metatarsal when hallux valgus was complicated with joint infection. "So far as I know," Rose wrote, "the first resection in a case of simple hallux valgus uncomplicated with abscess or caries of the joint was made at St. Francis Hospital, in this city, by Frank H. Hamilton, April 17, 1873." Hamilton had planned to resect the articulating ends of both bones when Rose told him about Hueter's operation. Hamilton decapitated the first metatarsal. A year later, Hamilton (1874) reported this case and added a few more; Blodgett (1880) and Post (1882) reported some more.

Hueter's technique was simple and expeditious. The first metatarsophalangeal joint was approached through a small longitudinal incision along the medial aspect. The capsule and the periosteum were incised. The metatarsal head was levered out of the surgical wound and resected with a chain saw (Fig. 11–3).

In the ensuing decades, Hueter's resection was variously modified. Perhaps taking his cue from Murphy (1904), Halstead (1906) suggested interposition of a "slip of the extensor sheath" between the decapitated metatarsal and the base of the proximal phalanx. Mayo (1908, 1920) covered the metatarsal stump with a locally fashioned pedicled flap. This flap consisted of the medial capsule of the joint and the overlying bursa. Mayo thought that removal of all or nearly all of the head of the first metatarsal was too radical. He advised excising "one-quarter of an inch of articulating surface" and supplemented this with sagittal resection of the medial eminence (Fig. 11–4).

Surgical virtuosity was in its heyday. Edenhuizen (1913) covered the end of the metatarsal with free fascial graft. Lexer (1917) turned in a layer of fat. Mauclaire (1920) capped the stump with the cartilage of the resected head. Rafarin (1920) wrote his thesis about a similar operation for which he credited his teacher Gernez and called it "a new procedure for the treatment of hallux valgus." Fessler (1926) shaved off the medial eminence and the lateral corner of the metatarsal head, but left the plantar, weight-bearing surface intact. Bentzon (1930) fashioned two fascial flaps: one from the bursa and the adjoining periosteum that was used to cover the raw surface of the resected stump; the other from the medial capsule to line the base of the proximal phalanx. Kruimel (1931) excised a square block from the portion of the metatarsal head still in contact with the base of the phalanx and hinged the remaining medial segment laterally to cover the raw bone. Soresi (1931) gouged the interior of the metatarsal head, leaving only a thin shell of articular cortex and cartilage to collapse. Royle (1931) said he had "devised a new operative procedure," the distinctive features of which were shaping the metatarsal head into a cone and covering it with a proximally-based fascial flap. Hove (1951) suggested replacing the first metatarsal head with an acrylic prosthesis. Seiffert (1953) used nylon for interposition. Radulesku and Robnesku (1956) reverted to Hove's method and substituted the head with an acrylic prosthesis. Prignacchi and Zanasi (1957) resected the head through a pair of dorsoplantar elliptical skin cuts, on the medial aspect of the joint. They covered the metatarsal stump with a proximally pedicled fascial flap. Recently, Bingham (1960) described a method that he credited to Stone. The plane of resection of the metatarsal head slanted obliquely so as

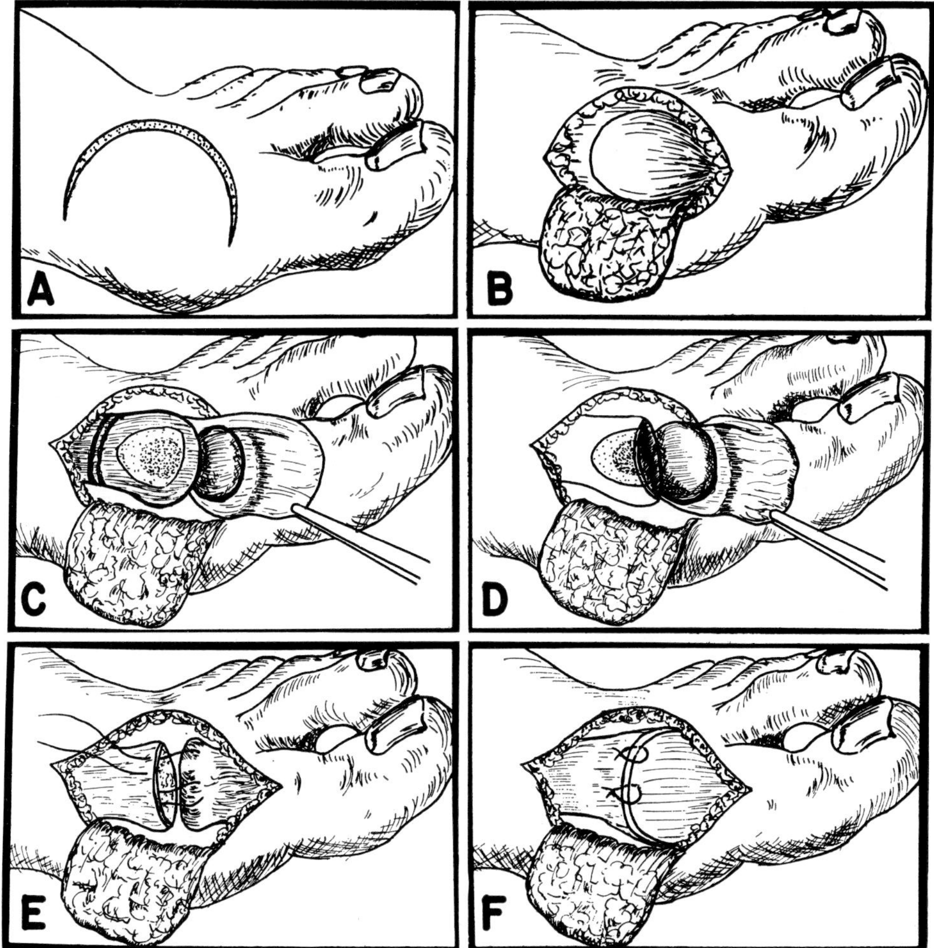

Figure 11–4. Mayo's operation: incision (*A*); distally pedicled capsulobursal flap (*B*); sagittal resection of the medial eminence (*C*); minimal decapitation of the first metatarsal (*D*); interposition of bursal flap (*E*); suturing the base of the flap to the periosteum of metatarsal stump (*F*).

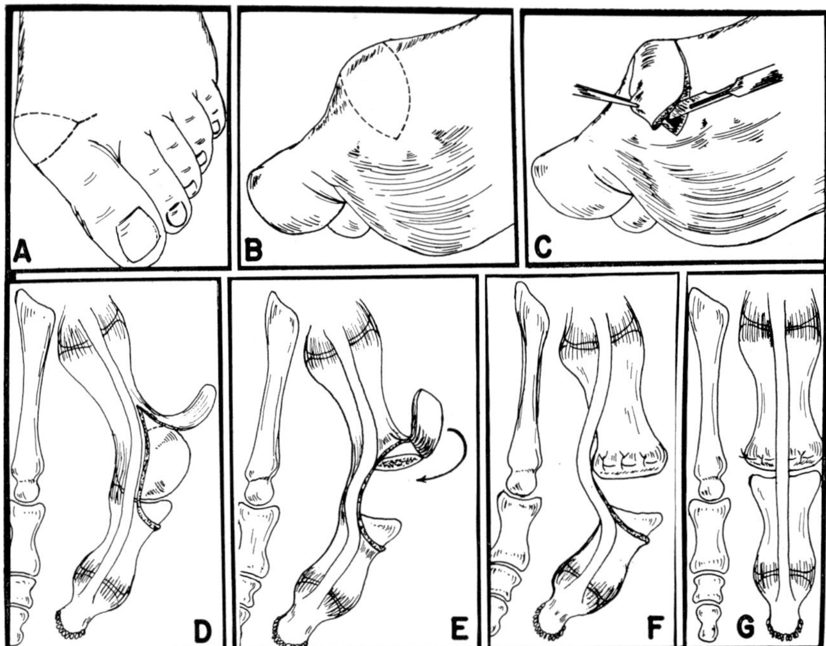

Figure 11–5. Prignacchi and Zanasi modification: elliptical skin cuts (*A, B,* and *C*); proximally pedicled fascial flap (*D*); the stump of the decapitated metatarsal is covered with the fascial flap (*E* and *F*); the toe is straightened (*G*).

to leave more cartilage-coated bone on the plantar aspect; the medial eminence was resected flush with the inner cortex of the shaft. The sharp margins of the remaining bone were rounded. It was advised that approximately three-fourths inch of space be left between the metatarsal and the phalanx. Of these operations, the one described by Prignacchi and Zanasi and that ascribed to Stone can be said to enjoy a measure of popularity (Figs. 11–5 and 11–6).

Hueter's *Grundriss der Chirurgie* was posthumously revised by Lossen (1884), who warned against resection of too great a segment of the distal metatarsal as it would deprive "the arch of the foot of one of its major points of support." Riedel (1886) considered decapitation of the first metatarsal justifiable in persons with flatfoot in which the entire sole rested on the ground and the first metatarsal had long lost its usefulness as a bearing point. He advised against this procedure in patients with high insteps on the basis that it would disturb the normal weight distribution in the forefoot and interfere with locomotion. It would cause pain in *planta pedis,* or what a few years later was labeled by Pollosson (1889) *anterior metatarsalgia.*

Fowler (1889) leveled the following criticism against Hueter's resection: "it shortens the inner margin of the foot unnecessarily, and by removing the inner support of the anterior extremity of the plantar arch, forces the body weight in walking upon the heads of the metatarsal bones of the other toes. These soon develop a painful condition, due to crowding against the sole of the shoe."

Hueter's resection had its share of criticism. The Mayo modification was due for some. We already have recorded the objection to using the proximally detached, distally pedicled fascial flap that Mayo used to cover the stump of the decapitated first metatarsal. In the discussion that followed Harding's (1927) paper, Gallant said: "I have seen a number of cases of Mayo operation and the patients had painful feet afterwards, some of them lasting more than a year. This procedure should be completely eliminated from the list of operations."

Notwithstanding, modified Hueter

procedures continued to attract enthusiastic followers—Perkins (1927), Bankart (1935), and many others. Nilsonne, who discussed Bentzon's (1935) paper, preferred Mayo-Bentzen's arthroplasty to Schede's or Hohmann's operation. According to Nilsonne, the recovery period was shorter, the cosmetic outcome equally good, and the functional result excellent. Lloyd (1936) resected the first metatarsal head in 20 cases and the basal half of the proximal phalanx in an equal number of patients. The results following decapitation of the first metatarsal were as satisfactory as those after partial proximal phalangectomy. Veyrassat and Patry (1946) favored Hueter's resection. But they warned against resecting too large a segment—8 to 10 mm. was considered optimum. Platzgummer and Jud (1952) thought the Mayo plastic resection was easier to perform and yielded better cosmetic results than the Brandes plastic resection, a variant of Keller's resection.

The original Hueter resection, without refinements, is still used in severely deformed great toe, especially when the head of the first metatarsal has been irreparably eroded by arthritis. Interposition of bursal flap, fascia lata, fat, cartilaginous cap, nylon, and acrylic have all been tried needlessly. Adhesions and spurs are more likely to form postoperatively when resection is carried through the cancellous head, as was done by Mayo, than when the line of section passes proximally through cortical bone. In hallux valgus occurring in the wake of burnt-out rheumatoid arthritis in which the other metatarsophalangeal joints also are involved, nothing short of decapitation of five bones yields anything approaching a functionally useful forefoot. In hallux valgus proper, with degenerative joint changes, partial resection of the proximal phalanx of the great toe is considered more appropriate.

Keller's resection. Spiers (1920) spelled Keller's name as Kell*a*r. This error has been perpetuated by Watson-Jones (1927), Harding (1927), Manwaring (1930), Agnew (1936), Creer (1936), Hiss (1937), Nelson and Kaplan (1942), Milch (1942), again by Hiss (1949), and Watson-Jones (1957).

William J. Keller was an army surgeon; when he wrote his first article on hallux valgus he was stationed at Fort Riley, Kansas, the cavalry center. It was another cavalry surgeon from Fort Riley, Charles H. Lothrop (1873), who originally introduced the concept of adductor release for the treatment of hallux valgus. It cannot be said that Keller was the first to advocate the operation with which we have come to connect his name (Fig. 11–7).

There are several versions as to who first put into practice resection of the proximal portion of the first phalanx of the great toe as a method of treatment for hallux valgus. In the course

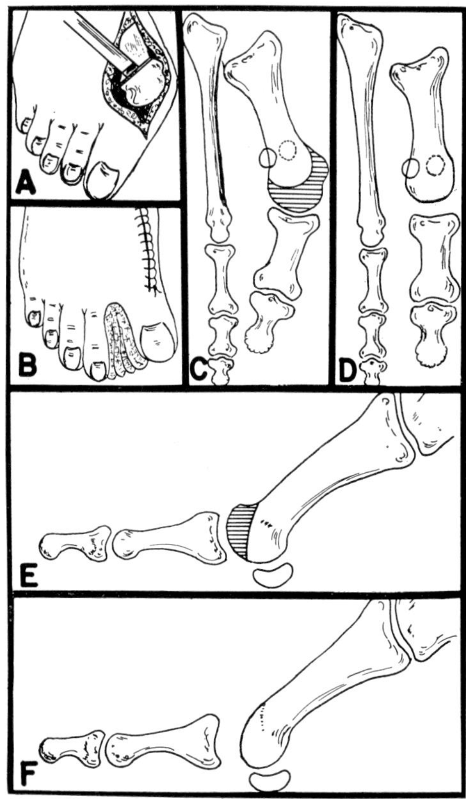

Figure 11–6. Stone's operation: exposure and the line of bone resection (*A*); closure and interdigital pad (*B*); shaded area showing the part of the bone to be resected (*C*); rounding the remaining stump (D); skeletal elements seen from the side, with shaded area showing that more bone is resected from the dorsum of the metatarsal head than from its plantar aspect (*E*); the same after rounding the stump (*F*).

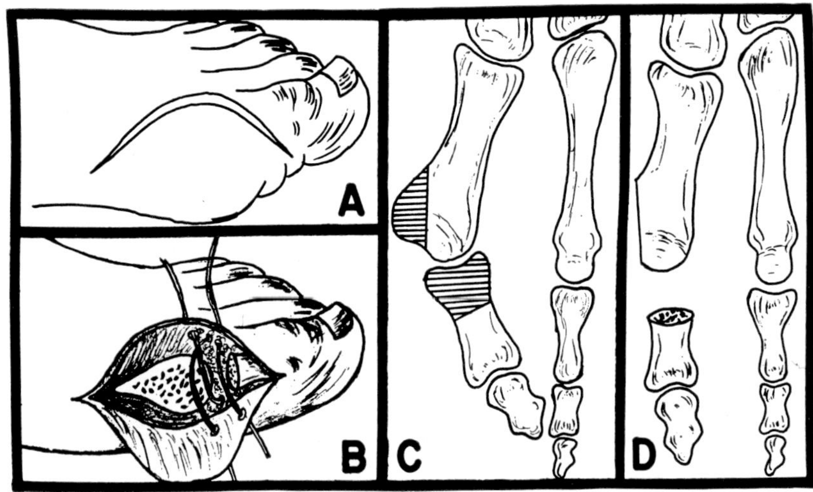

Figure 11–7. Keller resection: incision (*A*); resection of the medial eminence and basal portion of the proximal phalanx—the interval is being closed with the aid of two figure-8 sutures (*B*); shaded areas indicate parts of the bones to be resected (*C*); remaining bones (*D*).

of the discussion of a paper on hallux valgus by Ezra Jones (1940), Ober evoked the name of a nonexistent surgeon, Walsh M. Hughes, which appears to be a phonetic perversion of Walsham and Hughes (1895). These two authors wrote a book on the deformities of the foot and, in passing, mentioned resection of the phalanx. Sir Robert Jones (1924) credited Davies-Colley for this procedure and most English authors subscribe to this view. The editors of Campbell's (1956, 1963) *Operative Orthopedics* summoned the testimony of Osmond-Clarke to the effect that this operation was described by Davies-Colley of Guy's Hospital in 1887. In the year mentioned, a short notice appeared in The British Medical Journal. It was about a lecture Davies-Colley had delivered before the Clinical Society of London. The essayist had discussed a condition that he called *hallux flexus* and that later was renamed *hallux rigidus*. For treatment he advised excision of the proximal half of the basal phalanx of the great toe. He said nothing about resecting the medial eminence of the first metatarsal head, which Keller was to recommend in 1904.

The combined resection of the medial eminence and the base of the proximal phalanx, as a method of treatment for hallux valgus, was first advocated by Riedel (1886), who made his recommendation in a formal article that preceded the sketchy report of Davies-Colley's lecture. Riedel operated on four patients with hallux valgus by this method—two more than Davies-Colley had done for hallux flexus or rigidus. Davies-Colley deserves credit as he was the first to specify resecting the proximal half of the phalanx instead of just its base. He sectioned the bone across the cortical midshaft, where osteogenesis is minimal and postoperative joint stiffness less likely.

Riedel's, or Davies-Colley's, operation was widely discussed during the last decade of the past century. Riedel's student, Cornils (1890), wrote his inaugural dissertation about this procedure. Hoffa (1894) spoke of the combined resection of the medial eminence and excision of the proximal phalangeal base. Walsham and Hughes (1895) said partial proximal phalangectomy was preferred by Davies-Colley to decapitation of the first metatarsal head because it did not interfere with the "tripod strength of the foot." Wackerhagen (1895) mentioned Riedel and described his operation in some detail. Syms (1897) did likewise. In the course of a discussion that followed Weir's (1897) paper on hallux valgus, Willy Meyer discussed Riedel's operation. Steele (1898) pointed out the advantage of resecting the base of the proximal phalanx over decapitation of the first metatarsal, for it avoided removing "one of the points of the tripod" on which the foot rested. Clarke (1899) wrote: "Riedel (quoted by Hoffa) and Davies-Colley recommended removal of the base of the first phalanx: this measure has the disadvantage of leaving the deformed head of the metatarsal bone." Apparently Clarke was not aware that Riedel had disposed of his objection by recommending resection of the medial eminence of the metatarsal head in addition to excision of the base of the proximal phalanx—the combined procedure identified with Keller's name.

Keller (1904, 1912) wrote two articles on hallux valgus; both appeared in the New York Medical Journal—the same periodical in which Syms (1897) had previously described Riedel's operation. The method Keller advocated was basically identical to the one described by Riedel two decades earlier. Keller must have known this procedure had been practiced before and frequently discussed in the literature, but he acknowledged no precedence. Nor did he seem to have any qualms about calling it his operation. But there is ample evidence that Keller was influenced by the teachings of his predecessors; at least he reflected their views. As had Riedel, Keller considered the resection of the first metatarsal head justifiable only in "flat-footed" individuals, but not in those with high insteps. Davies-Colley's and Steele's image of the *tripod of the foot* cropped up in both of Keller's communications about hallus valgus.

Reading Keller's articles after Riedel's affects one the same way as listening to a jazz version of a composition by Chopin when the original is still remembered. Keller referred to the "lateral" enlargement of the metatarsal head when he meant *medial.* He spoke of resecting the "articular head of the first phalanx" when he should have said *the proximal articular end* or merely *the base.* The head of the phalanx is the part that enters into the formation of the interphalangeal, and not the metatarsophalangeal, joint of the toe. Keller advised freeing "flexor longus hallucis" from the base of the proximal phalanx when it is *the short,* and not the long, flexor that is attached to this portion of the bone and needs to be freed.

Keller claimed the operation he described did not disarrange "the normal levels of the foot," nor did it disturb "the tripod upon which the foot rests." He gave the following description: "A longitudinal incision, two inches in length, is made along the inner side of the foot, exposing the first metatarsophalangeal articulation. The skin and tissues over the head of the metatarsal bones are retracted; the joint is then opened and opposing articular ends are separated; the periosteal covering over the lateral (sic) enlargement and adjoining part of bone are pushed back; and the exostosis with one-eighth of an inch of bone is removed by a rongeur forceps, or preferably, with a small saw. The tendon of the flexor longus hallucis (sic) is freed by blunt dissection from under the surface of the base of the first phalanx, sufficiently to pass a Gigli saw around the bone; the periosteum is pushed back, disarticulation accomplished, and the articular head (sic) of the first phalanx is removed. Particular care should be taken throughout the operation to protect the periosteum from needless destruction, and an effort should be made to preserve enough of it to cover the exposed surface of the bone."

In 1904 Keller reported four patients operated on by the aforementioned method. By curious coincidence this was exactly the number of patients Riedel had similarly treated in 1886. In his next article, Keller (1912) again stressed the inviolability of the *tripod of the foot.* He now approached the joint through an incision similar to the one described by Mayo (1908) and advocated excision of half the proximal phalanx as had been advised by Davies-Colley (1887), whom he did not mention.

In the decades that followed his last communications on hallux valgus, Keller appears to have diverted his attention to other surgical problems—to chest surgery, varicose veins, and skin graft.

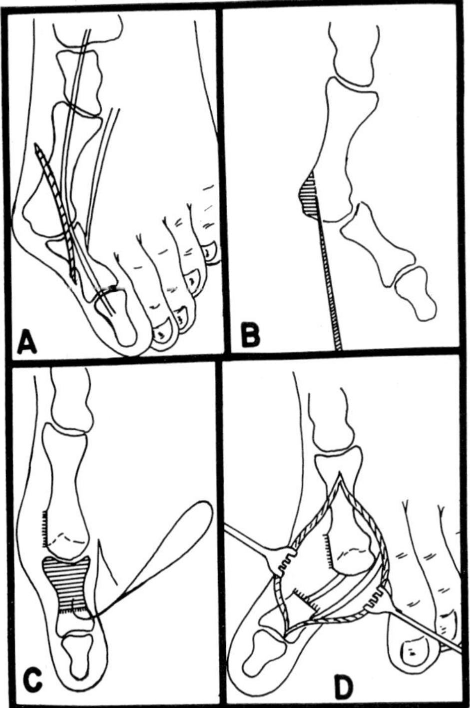

Figure 11–8. Brandes resection: incision (*A*); resection of the medial eminence (*B*); excision of the proximal two-thirds of the basal phalanx of the great toe (*C* and *D*).

Meanwhile, his operation for hallux valgus was practiced by many with numerous reports of favorable results: Spiers (1920), Olivecrona (1924), Anderson (1929), Brandes (1929), Schanz (1929), Gottlieb (1930), Kaspar (1933), McMurray (1936), Galland and Jordan (1938), Haggart and Toomey (1939), Schein (1940), Starr (1942), Nelson and Kaplan (1942), Cleveland and his associates (1944, 1950), Perrot (1946), McElvenny (1947), Hallock (1949), DeRacker (1951), Jordan and Brodsky (1951) all registered their approval. Brandes (1929) resected the proximal two-thirds of the first phalanx of the great toe. Endler (1951) substituted the base of the proximal phalanx with acrylic prosthesis. More recently Joplin (1964) spoke of replacing the articular end of this bone with "a Vitallium-stem prosthesis." Brandes popularized his subtotal proximal phalangectomy on the continent, where he is given credit for having originated what in English-speaking countries has come to be known as Keller's resection (Fig. 11–8).

It can now safely be said that Keller's resection is the most popular procedure for hallux valgus. But it would be erroneous to convey the impression that this operation has met with universal approval. Rogers and Joplin (1947) were dissatisfied with the results of the Keller operation. They wrote: "While the Keller procedure eliminates pain at the great toe joint and makes easier fitting of shoes, it does not restore the power of the great toe lost through the deformity and does not arrest the progress of degenerative joint changes." Joplin (1950) leveled the same criticism a few years later. Keller's resection, he argued, yielded a weaker postoperative push-off mechanism; it increased the tendency to splayfoot and the calluses under the metatarsal heads persisted. "A survey in 1947 of the end results of operation for hallux valgus at the Massachusetts General Hospital revealed that," Joplin wrote, "Keller operation, employed for the most part up to that time, hardly gave satisfactory results. Similar observations have been made recently by Cleveland and Winant. . . ." In the article by Cleveland and Winant (1950), we find the following conclusion: "Arthroplasty of the metatarsophalangeal joint of the great toe by the Keller procedure gave good or excellent results in ninety-three percent," which by any standards would be regarded as more than satisfactory, as results of hallux valgus surgery go.

Bonney and Macnab (1952) were critical of Keller's operation. In one of their cases, despite adequate excision of the proximal phalanx and the wide space between the resected bone and the metatarsal head, there was almost complete lack of movement following surgery; the hallux would not extend. Bonney and Macnab found the results of Keller's operations performed in the presence of a growing epiphysis uniformly bad, which is understandable. No surgeon in his senses should subject a growing child or adolescent to a Keller resection—an operation designed primarily for older adults with more than moderate hallux valgus and variable degrees of arthritic change at the joint.

D. J. Morton (1952) pointed out that following resection of the phalangeal base and detachment of the short flexors, the sesamoid bones shifted backward, toward the heel; they no longer supported the head of the first metatarsal. The resulting metatarsalgia was similar to that produced by a short metatarsal bone. Lapidus (1960) was also critical of the "Keller-Brandes procedure." According to him, after this operation the great toe often became converted into a short, dangling appendage held above the ground, and its important "shove-off" function was permanently lost. If one wished to obtain, as close as possible, restoration of normal anatomic and physiologic relations, Lapidus argued, one could not accept the "Keller-Brandes operation."

Some of the criticism leveled against Keller's resection would be valid if the operation is performed—as it should not be—on a young patient with intact, intrinsic muscle power and a great toe capable of contacting the proffered surface and pressing down on it with power. The patient who is subjected to Keller's resection usually is past 50 years of age. The great toe is in marked outward deviation; it is rotated around its long axis and has slipped under, or rides over, the second toe—the hallux does not touch the supporting surface. The first metatarsophalangeal joint is arthritic and interlocked, and the intrinsic muscles have long lost their power of contraction. When Keller's resection is carried out in comparatively young adults, an attempt should be made to provide the abductor and adductor hallucis and flexor brevis with an anchorage.

Suggested modifications of Keller's resection. Keller did not even surmise that by removing the base of the proximal phalanx, to which the intrinsic muscles of the great toe are attached, he released the adductor tension and at the same time put five muscles out of function. His aim was to shorten the skeletal framework of the toe to allow the extrinsic muscles—the long flexor and the extensor—gain in relative length. Keller did not seem to be aware of the existence of the intrinsic muscles, much less their function. The turn of his mind was mechanical; he thought of the foot primarily as a static structure—a tripod, rigid and unyielding.

We now think that the intrinsic muscles attached to the base of the proximal phalanx serve a purpose. They stabilize the proximal phalanx of the great toe and thus augment the pressing-down action of the hallux. In older individuals with long-standing hallux valgus, especially when this deformity is complicated with arthritis and these muscles have undergone irreversible fibrosis, it matters little if the muscles are left detached after a Keller resection. As noted, in the relatively young and robust an attempt should be made to provide these muscles an anchorage.

We have been practicing the following modification of the standard Keller technique: A broad, **U** shaped flap consisting of the medial joint capsule and the tendon of the abductor hallucis is fashioned. The base of the flap is placed proximally; it is separated from the bone past the flare of the medial eminence. The medial eminence is resected flush with the inner cortex of the shaft. The proximal portion of the phalanx is dissected free past the midshaft; the desired segment of the bone is resected. The sesamoids are inspected; if arthritic or mushroomed, they are shelled out. After proximal phalangectomy, sesamoidectomy offers no difficulty. An attempt is then made to reconstruct a tendinous sling for the metatarsal head. The fasciotendinous flap is split lengthwise into two halves. The plantar slip includes the abductor tendon and is continuous with its muscular belly. The inferior edge of the plantar slip is sutured to the severed end of the flexor brevis. The distal end is connected to the detached common adductor tendon on the lateral side of the joint. When the stitches are tied, the head of the metatarsal is provided with a hammock. The toe now is brought in to neutral position, as far as varus and valgus, everted and inverted positions are concerned. The superior

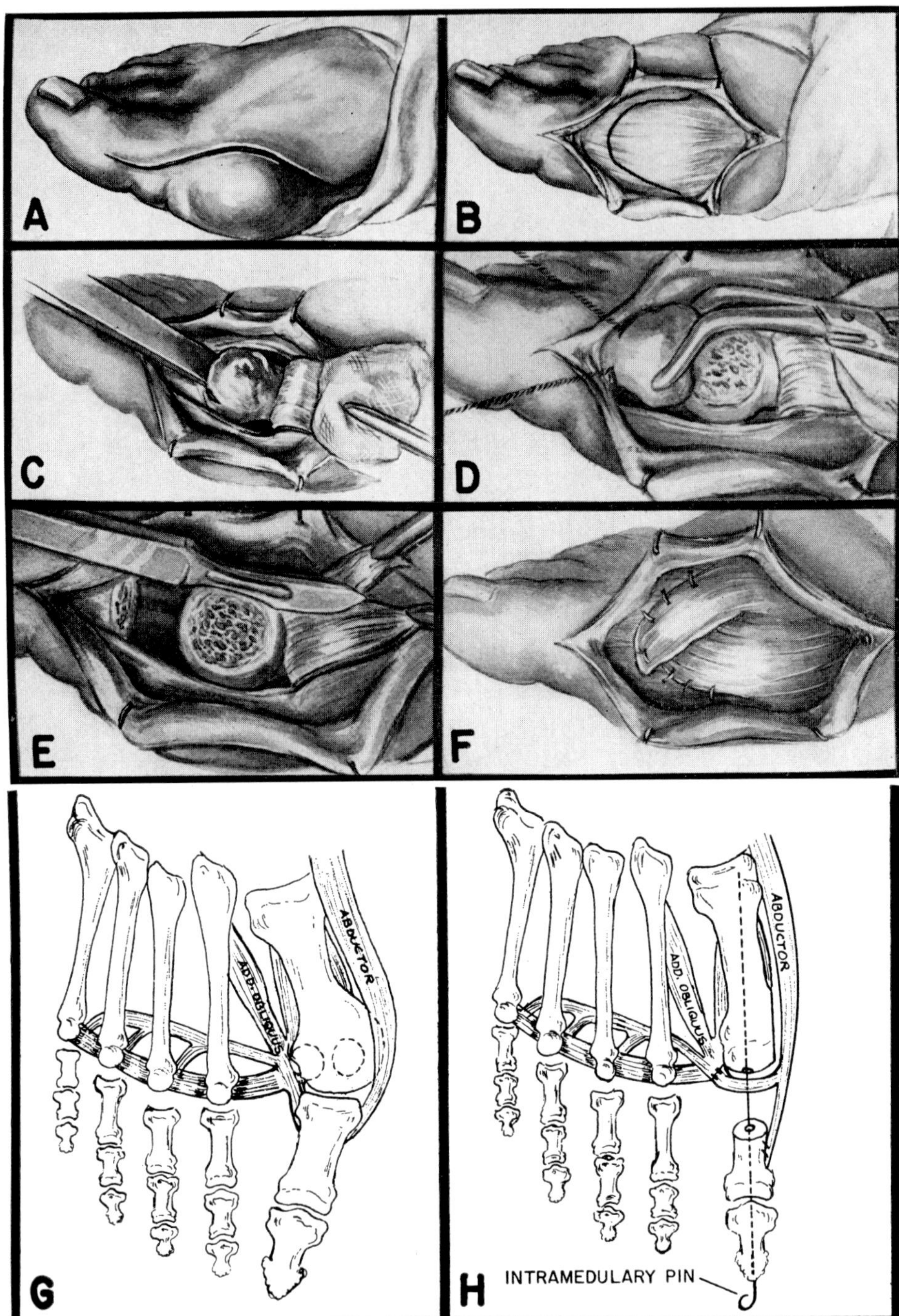

Figure 11–9. Modified Keller resection: incision (*A*); fascial flap (*B*); sagittal resection of the medial eminence (*C*); excision of the basal half of the proximal phalanx (*D*); splitting the fascial flap into two slips (*E*); the plantar muscular slip is sutured to the flexor brevis and to the common tendon of adductor transversus and obliquus (*F*); the dorsal fascial slip is sutured to the periosteum of the stump of the proximal phalanx; the attachment of intrinsic muscles to the base of the proximal phalanx (*G*); providing the intrinsic muscles with an anchorage and temporary stabilization of the toe with Kirchner wire (*H*).

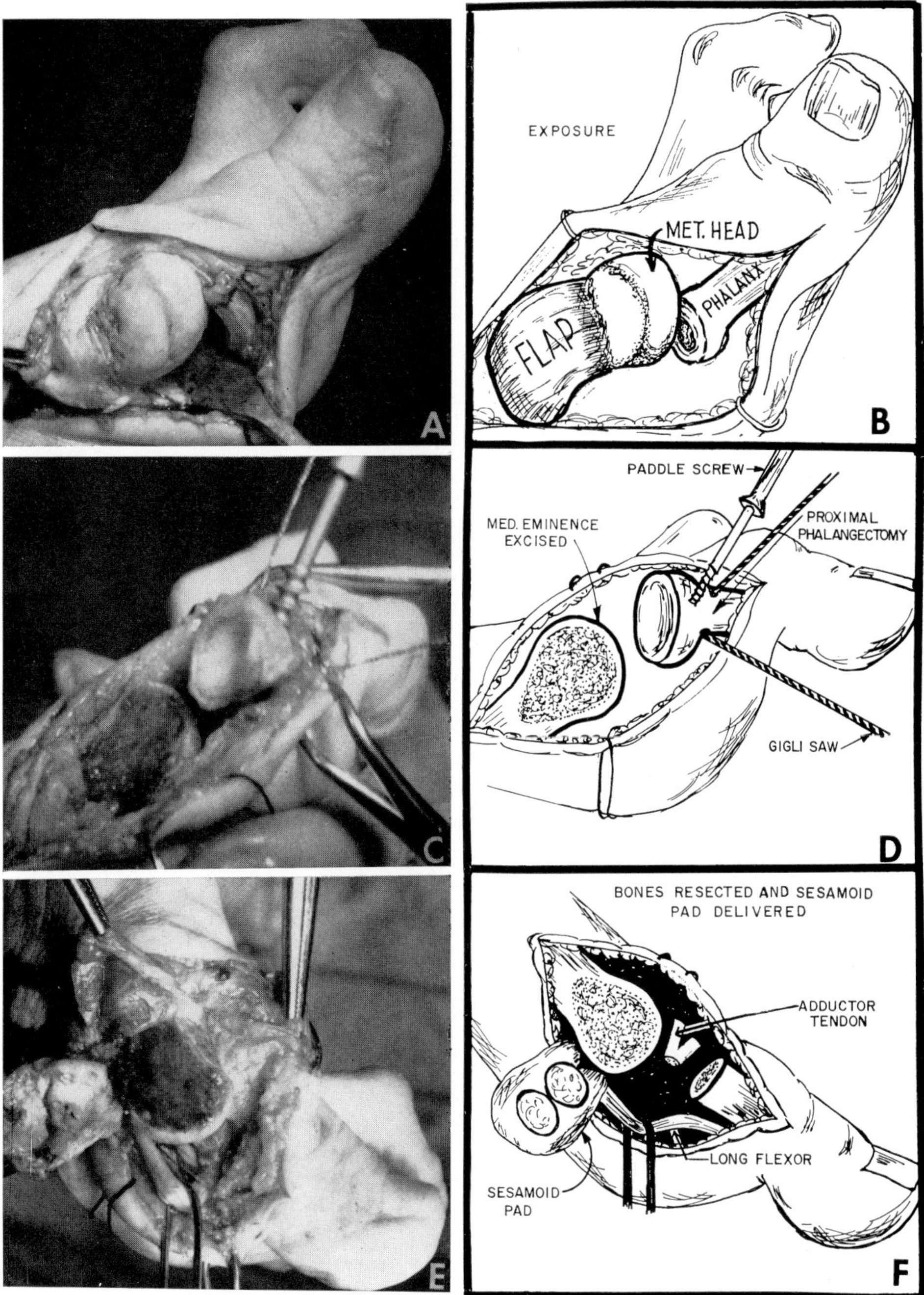

Figure 11–10. Modified Keller resection: photographs during surgery and interpretative diagrams.

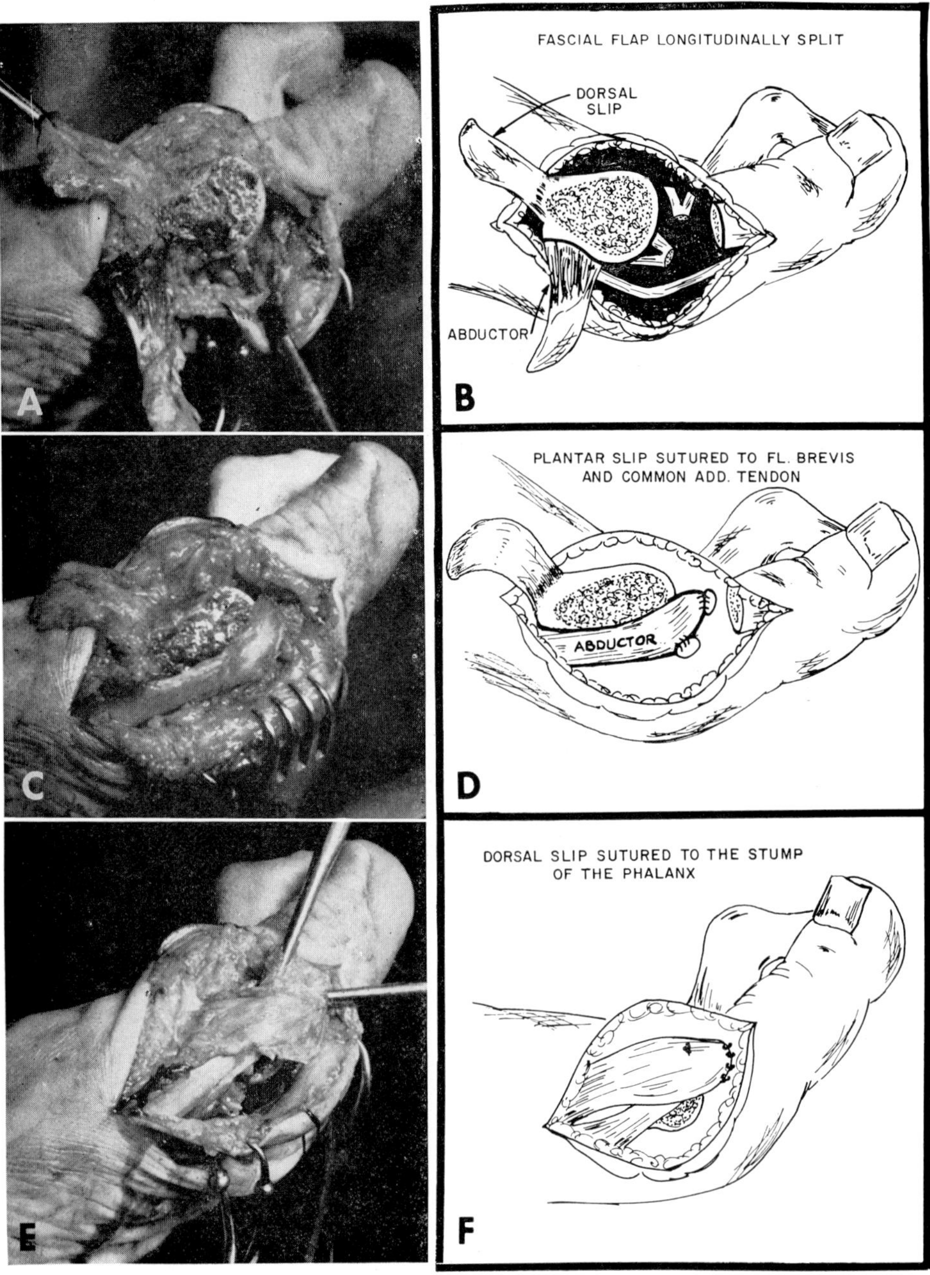

Figure 11–11. Modified Keller resection, continued from Figure 11–10.

slip of the fascial flap is sutured to the medial periosteum of the remainder of the proximal phalanx. Overcorrection is avoided (Figs. 11–9 to 11–18).

In case the skin on the medial aspect of the first metatarsophalangeal joint seems precarious, or the hallux does not appear to possess sufficient pressing-down power, the Keller resection is carried out through a Petersen (1888) interdigital incision and the two toes are surgically syndactylized. This method also is utilized when the hallux has slipped under or rides over the second toe or when the second toe is hammered. Another indication for a Keller resection and surgical syndactylia of the two medial toes is when the distal end of the second metatarsal has to be resected because of localized metatarsalgia or plantar keratosis. The great toe gains power when it is connected with the second digit: its pressing-down action is augmented (Figs. 11–19 to 11–25).

After a Keller operation, postoperative pain can be minimized considerably if the great toe is temporarily transfixed to the first metatarsal by an intramedullary Kirschner wire. This recommendation first came from Fitzgerald (1950). Gilmore and Bush (1957) followed. Thomas (1962) advised the use of one of the two types of "distractor"–intramedullary wire and external staple–to

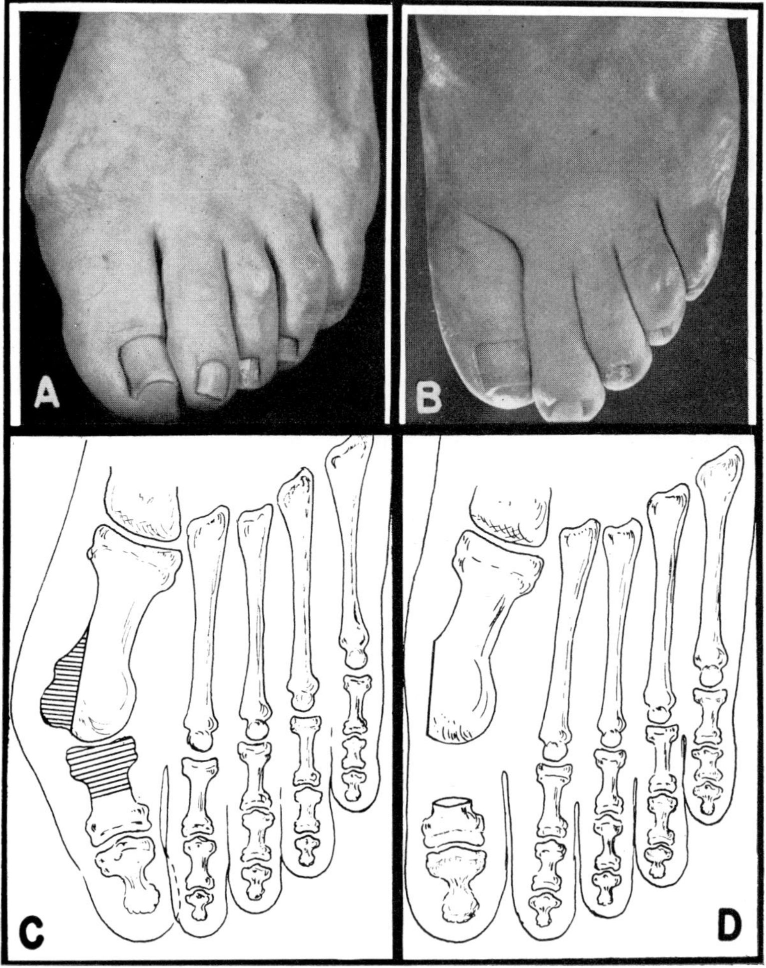

Figure 11–12. Woman, 63, with unilateral hallux valgus and limited extension of the great toe. Before surgery (*A*); after recovery (*B*); interpretative diagrams (*C* and *D*). Patient reported complete satisfaction with the outcome.

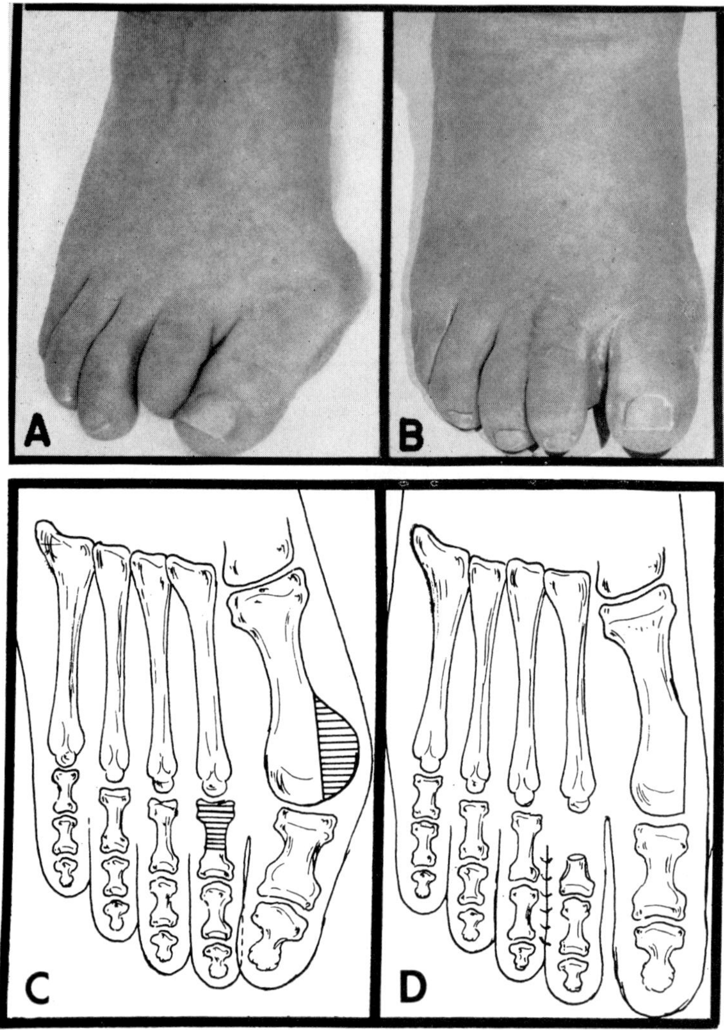

Figure 11–13. Woman, 65, with hallux valgus, arthritis of the first metatarsophalangeal joint, and hammered second toe. Surgery: modified Keller resection and excision of proximal half of the basal phalanx of the second toe and surgical syndactylia of this digit with its neighbor on the lateral side. Before surgery (*A*); after recovery (*B*); interpretative diagrams (*C* and *D*). This patient reported wearing "dress shoes" since recovery without any discomfort.

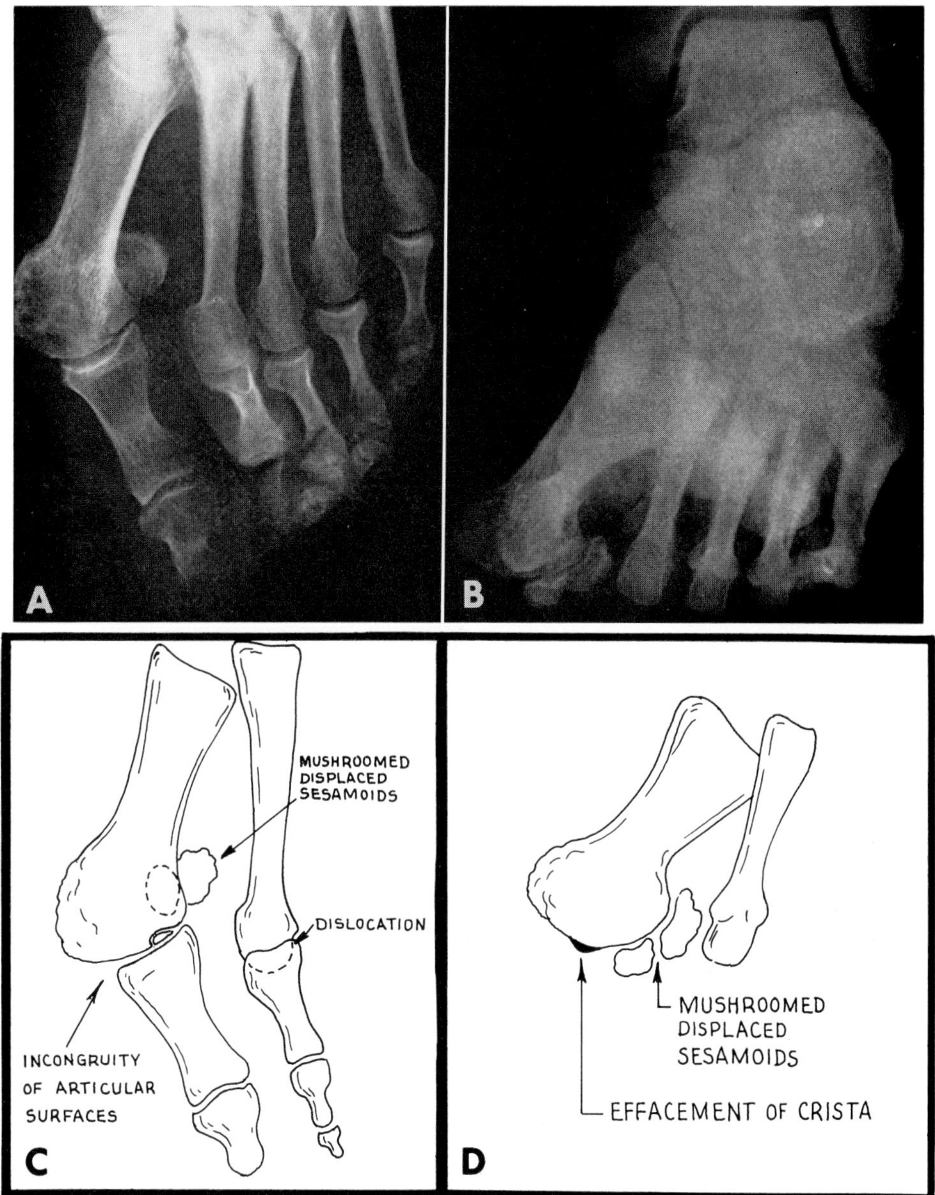

Figure 11–14. Woman, 54, with unilateral hallux valgus, limited extension but good pressing-down action of the great toe, hammered second digit, and subsesamoid pain. Dorsoplantar roentgenogram showing irregularity of the articular cortex of the first metatarsal head and subluxation at the second metatarsophalangeal joint (A). Sesamoid view–note the effacement of crista under the first metatarsal head, the outward shift of sesamoids, and mushrooming of the lateral ossicle (*B*). Interpretative diagrams (*C* and *D*).

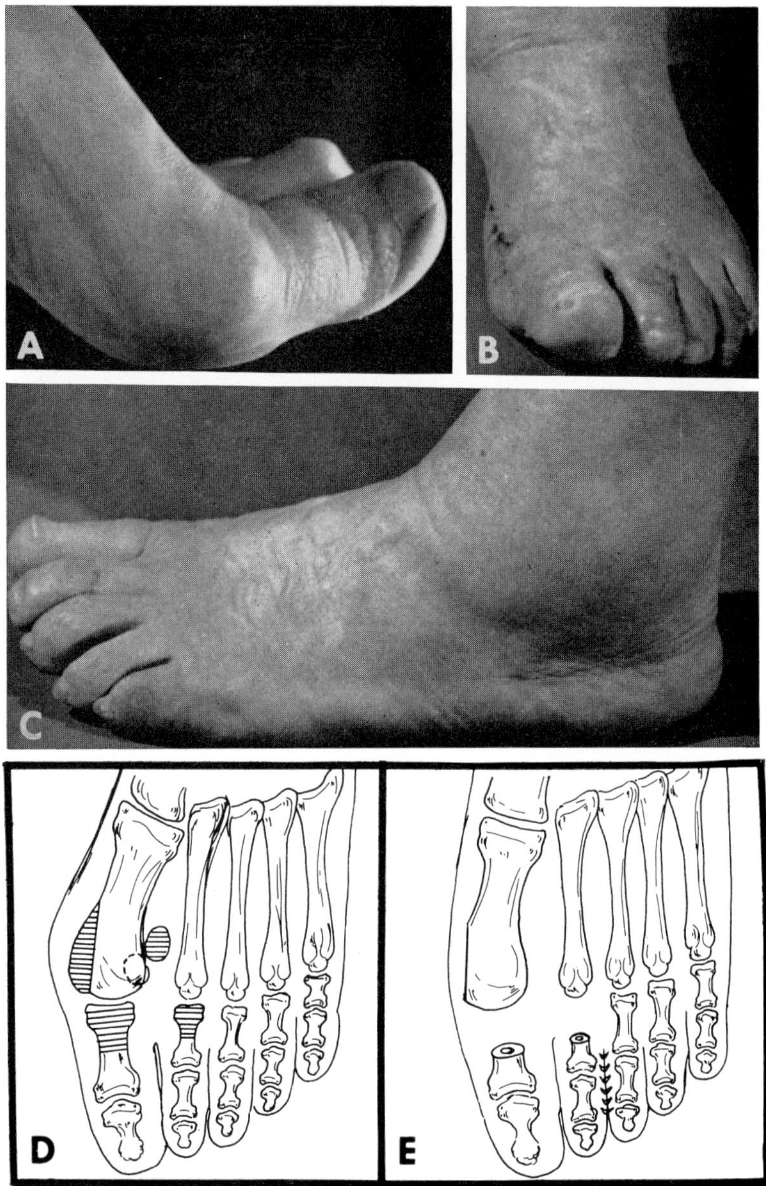

Figure 11–15. The same as in Figure 11–14. Forefoot, from the medial aspect just before surgery (*A*); from the dorsal aspect after recovery (*B*); from the lateral aspect after recovery (*C*). Diagrams for interpretation of the modified Keller resection, sesamoidectomy, resection of basal half of the proximal phalanx of the second toe, and syndactylia of this digit with its neighbor on the lateral side (*D* and *E*). The patient was content with the cosmetic and functional results.

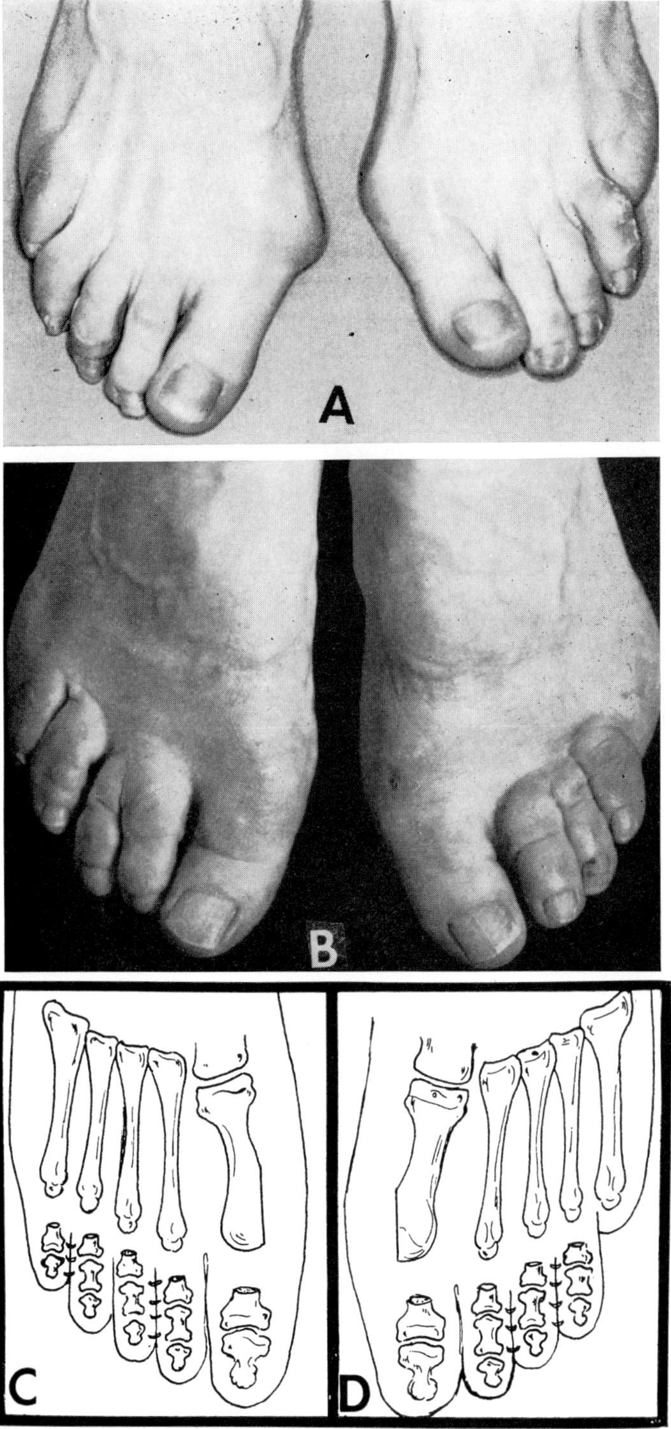

Figure 11–16. Woman, 53, with bilateral hallux valgus, limited extension at the first metatarsophalangeal joints, and hammered lesser toes. The small toe on the left side had been amputated earlier in life for a deformity said to have been caused by injury. Surgery: modified Keller resection, partial proximal phalangectomy of second to fifth toes on the right and second to fourth toes on the left, and surgical syndactylia of the adjacent digits on both sides. Preoperative photograph (*A*); after recovery (*B*); interpretative diagrams (*C* and *D*). The patient is completely content with the outcome.

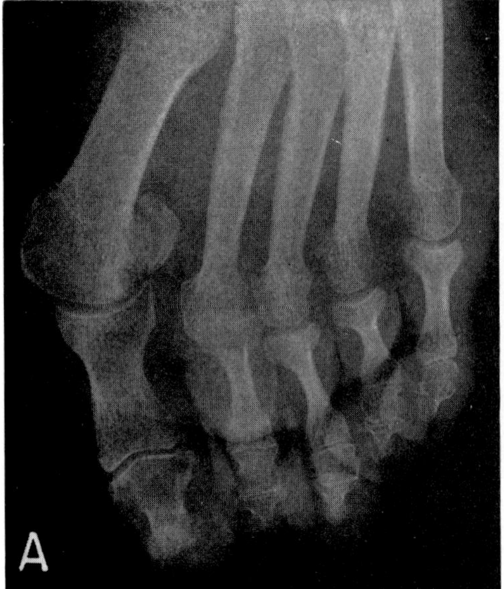

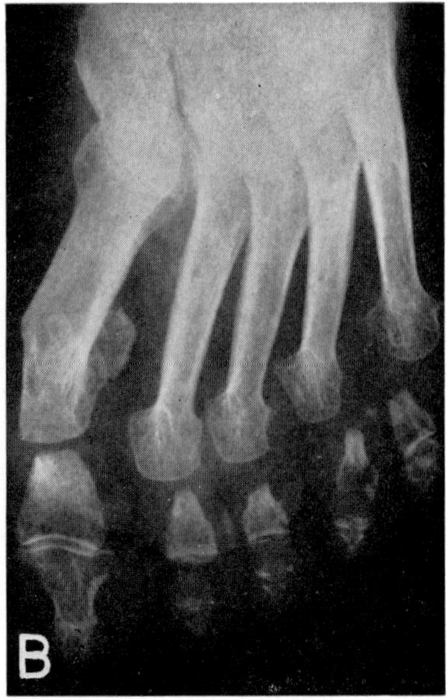

Figure 11–17. Woman, 49, with bilateral hallux valgus, arthritis of the first metatarsophalangeal joints, and hammered lesser toes. Surgery: modified Keller resection, partial proximal phalangectomy of the lesser toes, and surgical syndactylia of adjacent digits. Roentgenogram of the left foot before surgery (*A*). Note the incongruity of the articular surfaces of the first metatarsophalangeal joints and the subluxation at the second metatarsophalangeal joints. Roentgenogram after surgery (*B*).

procure rest and maintain the length of the great toe for 3 weeks after operation.

A definite drawback to the Keller resection is that if less than the proximal half of the first phalanx is removed or if the bone is sectioned through the cancellous base, there is likely to be postoperative proliferation and formation of painful osteophytes. If a greater segment is resected, the second toe gains in relative length, buckles against the tip of the shoe, and goes into a hammer type of deformity. The first phalanx of the great toe should be sectioned through its tubular shaft and the second toe subjected to partial proximal phalangectomy. Occasionally the third toe also is shortened and the two adjacent digits are surgically syndactylized to avoid dangling and retraction.

Arthritis of the first metatarsophalangeal joint with limited—less than 30 degrees—extension of the great toe remains the most legitimate indication for a Keller resection. Age is another factor. Older patients—persons past 60 years—seem to tolerate a Keller resection better than Silver's operation or one of its numerous variants. The angle of outward deviation of the great toe also enters into consideration. When this angle exceeds 40 degrees, correction is easier by Keller's than by Silver's operation. Keller resection is suitable when the hallux rides over or has slipped under the second toe. Fixed axial rotation of the great toe may also be corrected by a Keller resection.

McMurray (1936) contended that when pressure exerted by the base of the proximal phalanx is removed, the varus position of the first metatarsal corrects itself. This is not true. Keller resection does not affect metatarsus primus varus. One gets a false impression from roentgenograms taken soon after surgery —before the patient has walked or been relieved of compressive bandages. Keller resection, including our modification, is contraindicated in marked metatarsus primus varus and in the presence of severe metatarsalgia. Holden (1954) wrote: "When there is severe deformity of the hallux and of the other toes, the Keller procedure gives poor results. In selected cases, arthrodesis of the first metatarsophalangeal joint with correction of toe deformities and excision of the displaced metatarsal heads gives gratifying results."

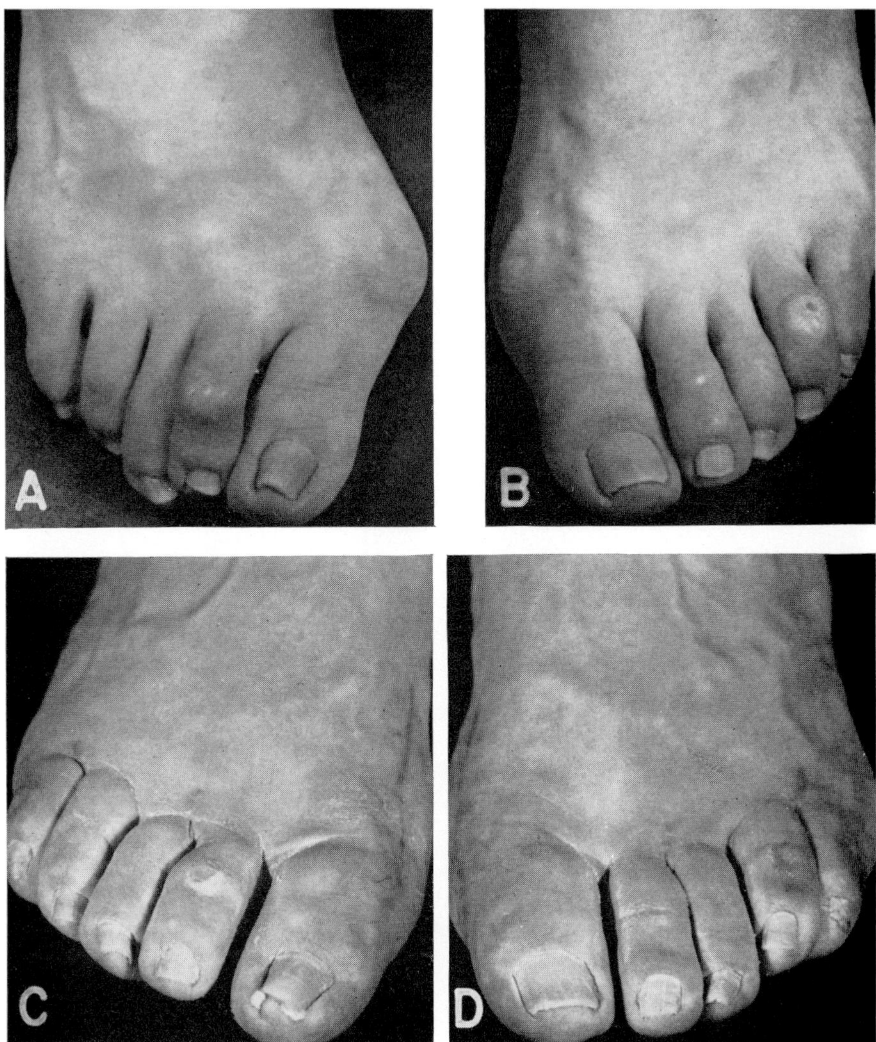

Figure 11–18. The same patient as in Figure 11–17: the forefoot before surgery (*A* and *B*); after recovery (*C* and *D*). The patient is completely satisfied.

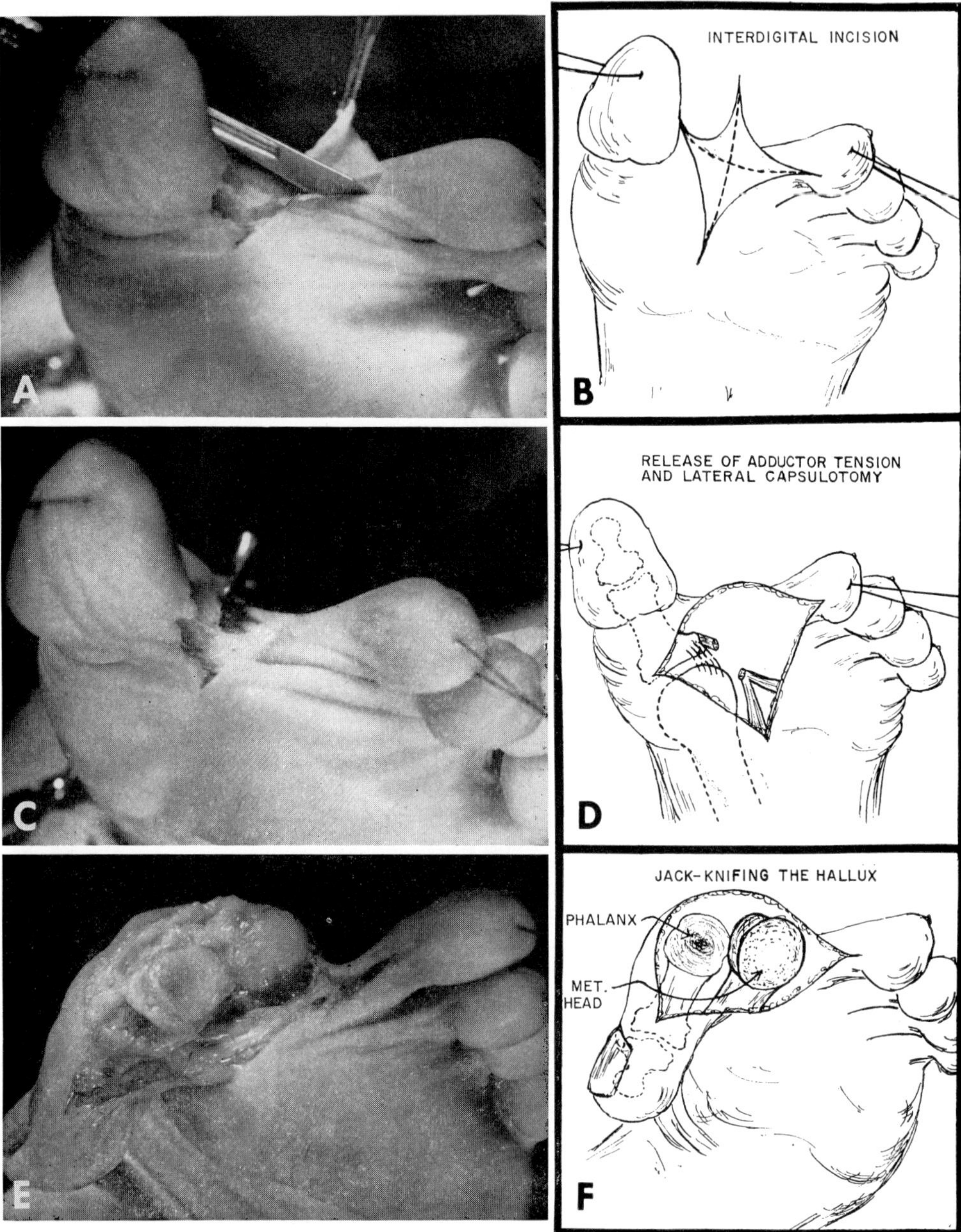

Figure 11–19. Keller resection through an interdigital approach: skin incision in preparation of surgical syndactylia of the first and second toes (*A* and *B*); lateral capsulotomy and release of adductor tension (*C* and *D*); jack-knifing the hallux until the base of the proximal phalanx comes to lie next to the metatarsal head.

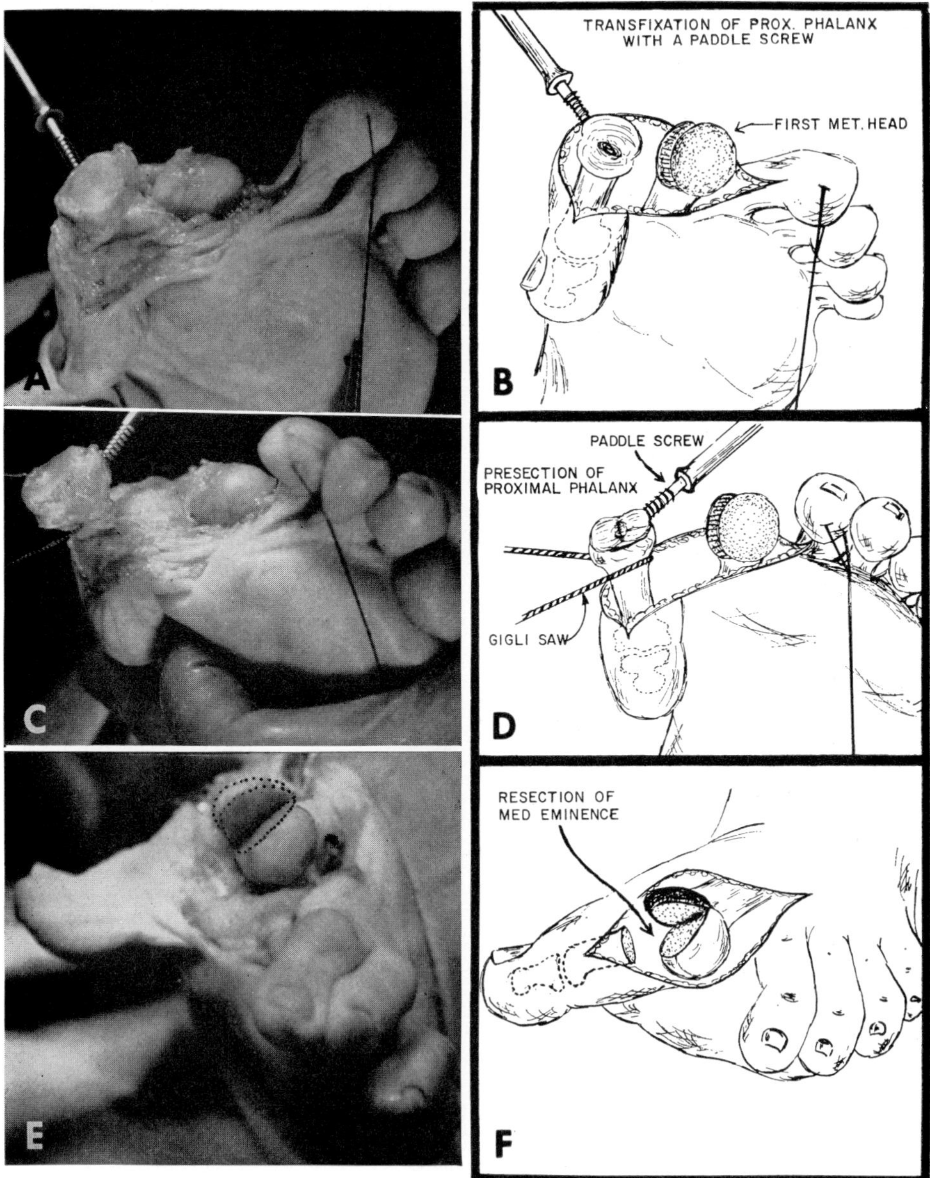

Figure 11–20. Keller resection continued from Figure 11–19: the basal portion of the proximal phalanx is transfixed and dissected free (*A* and *B*); resection of the proximal portion of the phalanx (*C* and *D*); sagittal resection of the medial eminence (*E* and *F*). As in modified Keller resection, the severed abductor is sutured to the flexor brevis and to the common adductor tendon. The first and second toes are syndactylized together.

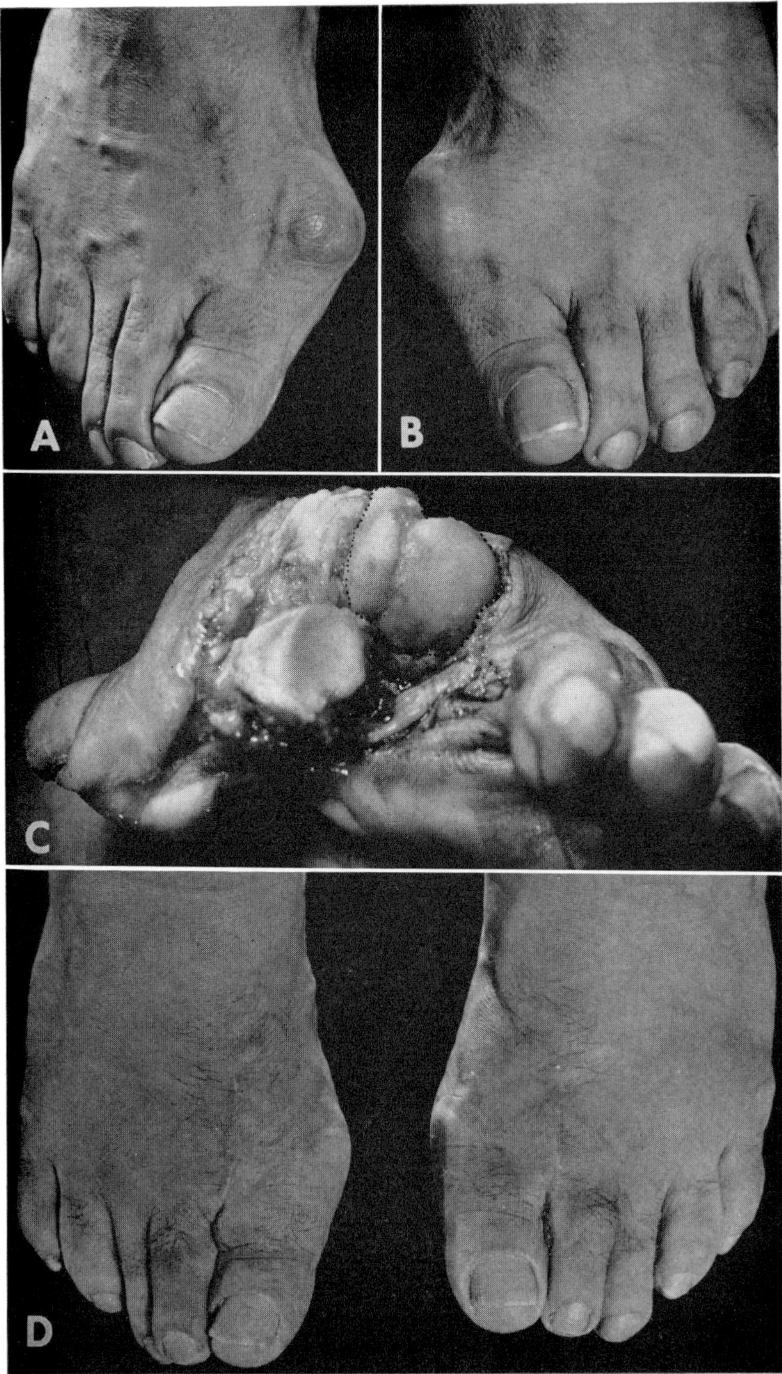

Figure 11–21. Woman, 48, with bilateral hallux valgus with limited, painful extension of the great toes, and varicose veins. Surgery: segmental resection of saphenous veins. Ten days later, a Keller resection through the interdigital approach and surgical syndactylia of first and second toes were performed. Forefeet prior to surgery (*A* and *B*); exposure of the left metatarsophalangeal joint—note the deep sagittal groove (*C*); forefeet after recovery (*D*). Patient was well pleased with the results and possesses good pressing-down power.

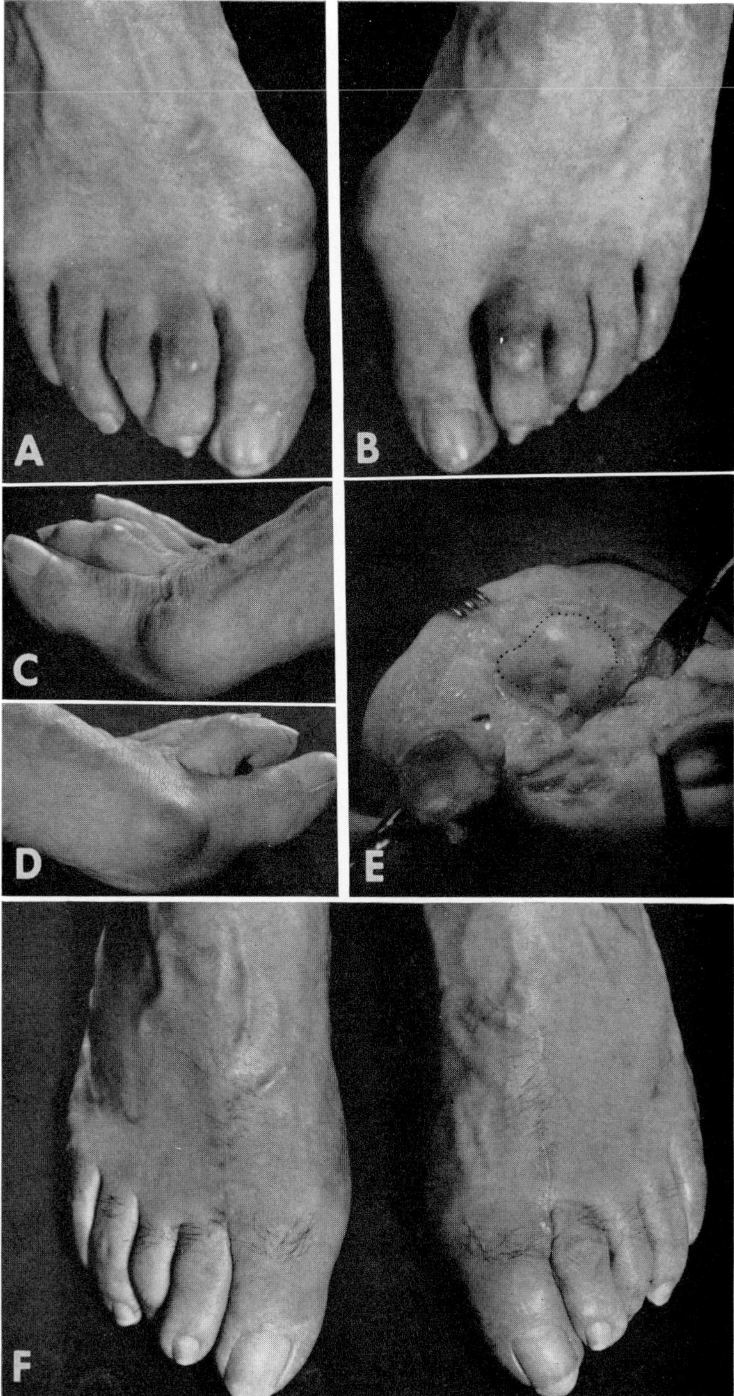

Figure 11–22. Woman, 57, with bilateral hallux valgus, arthritis of the first metatarsophalangeal joints, and hammered second toes. Surgery: Keller resection through interdigital approach, partial proximal phalangectomy of the second toes, and surgical syndactylia of the first and second digit: Dorsal view of both forefeet (*A* and *B*); profile views (*C* and *D*); surgical exposure of right metatarsophalangeal joint—note the central ulcer on the metatarsal head (*E*); after recovery (*F*). The patient was extremely happy with the outcome.

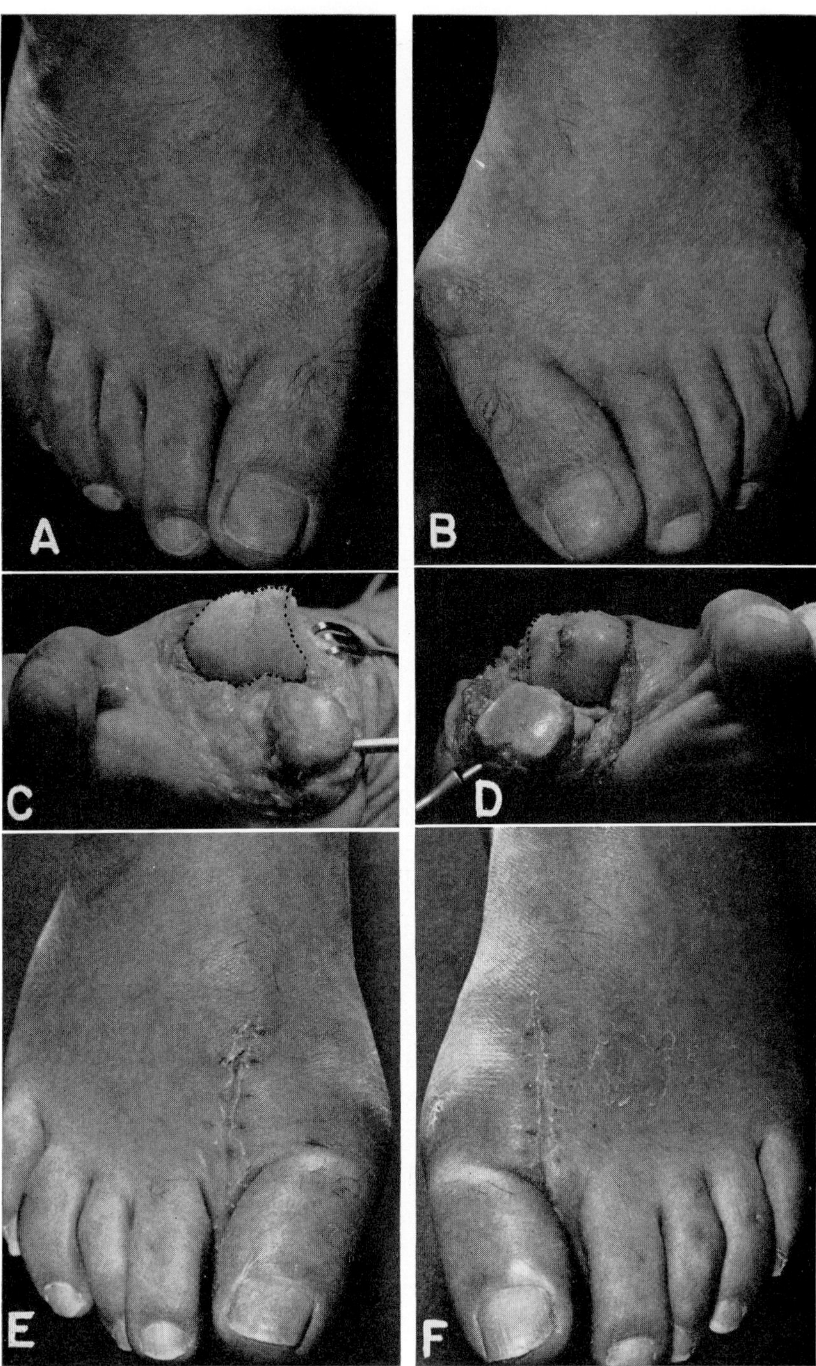

Figure 11–23. Woman, 59, with bilateral hallux valgus, arthritis of the first metatarsophalangeal joint. Surgery: Keller resection through interdigital approach without syndactylizing the first and second toes. Preoperative photographs (*A* and *B*); exposure of the first metatarsophalangeal joints on both sides (*C* and *D*); after recovery (*E* and *F*). The patient complains of "dangle toe" on the left side, which might have been avoided by surgical syndactylia of the first and second digits.

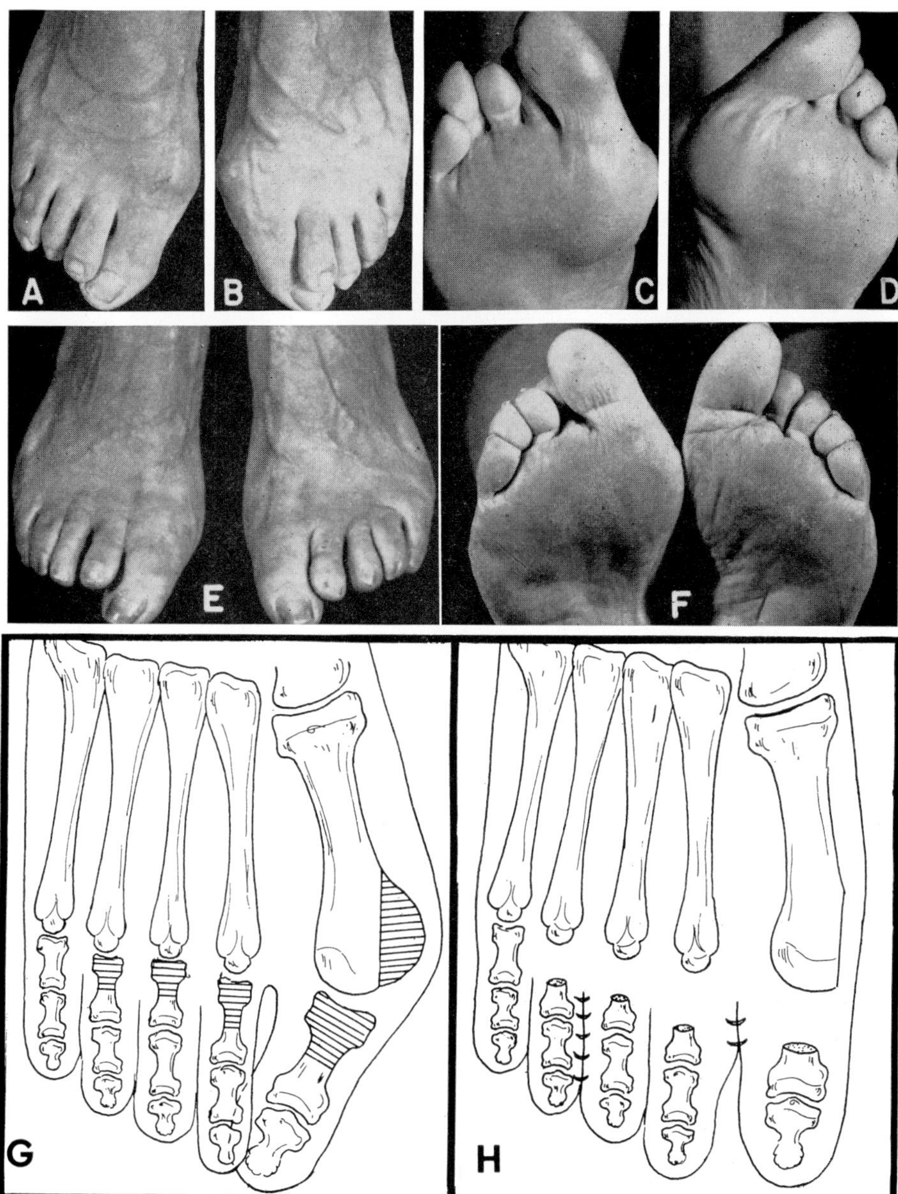

Figure 11–24. Woman, 49, with bilateral hallux valgus, overriding second toes, and resilient plantar bulge of the central metatarsal heads. Surgery: Keller resection through the interdigital approach, partial proximal phalangectomy of central toes, and surgical syndactylia of the first with second, and third with fourth digits. Dorsal view before surgery (*A* and *B*); plantar view before surgery (*C* and *D*); postoperative dorsal view of both feet—note the inadequate surgical syndactylia between the first and second toes on the right side (*E*); postoperative plantar view—note that the second toe on the right side has not come down to establish a fixed point (*F*); interpretative diagrams (*G* and *H*). The patient is relieved of discomfort due to hallux valgus and chafing by the shoe. The metatarsalgia persists.

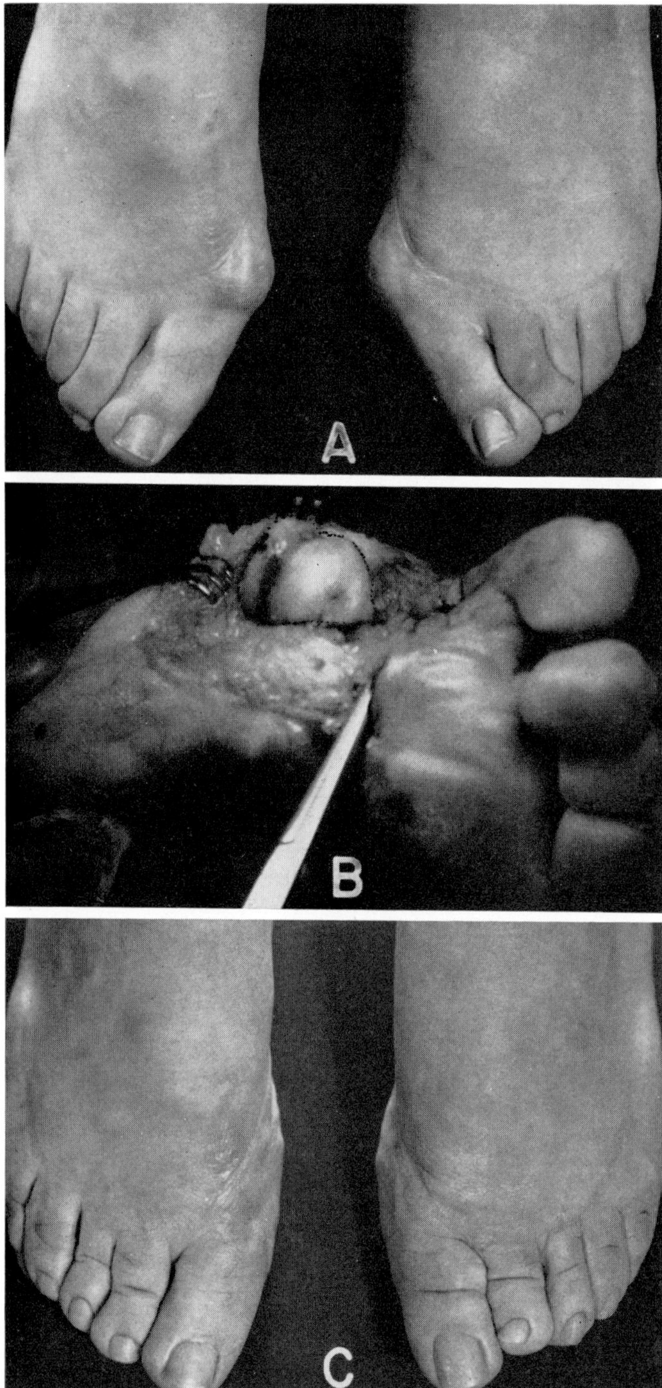

Figure 11–25. Woman, 50, with bilateral hallux valgus and hammered central toes. Surgery: Keller resection–right side through median incision and left by way of interdigital incision. Hammered lesser digits were subjected to partial proximal phalangectomy and surgical syndactylia. On the right side the second toe was connected to the third toe, and the fourth toe with the fifth toe. On the left side, the first and second toes were joined together and the third was connected with the fourth. Preoperative photographs of the right and left feet (*A*); interdigital exposure of left first metatarsophalangeal joint (*B*); after recovery (*C*). The patient reported satisfaction with the results. She has had no pain but of late has been experiencing a slight "burning sensation" when on her feet for long periods.

REFERENCES

Agnew, R. W.: Treatment of hallux valgus and rigidus. Brit. Med. J. *2*:557–558, 1936.

Anderson, R. L.: Hallux valgus: report of end results. South. Med. Surg. *91*:74–78, 1929.

Bankart, A. S. B.: The treatment of minor maladies of the foot. Lancet *1*:249–252, 1935.

Bentzon, P. G. K.: The treatment of hallux valgus by arthroplasty of the art. metatarso-phalangea I. Acta Orthop. Scand. *1*:96–99, 1930.

Bentzon, P. G. K.: After-examination of hallux valgus patients treated with arthroplastic resection of the head of the first metatarsal bone. Acta Orthop. Scand. *6*:195–206, 1935.

Bingham, R.: The Stone operation for hallux valgus. Clin. Orthop. *17*:366–370, 1960.

Blodgett, A. N.: Hallux valgus, with a report of two successful cases. Med. Rec. *18*:34–37, 1880.

Bonney, G., and Macnab, L.: Hallux valgus and hallux rigidus; a critical survey of operative results. J. Bone Joint Surg. *34*:366–385, 1952.

Brandes, M.: Zur operativen Therapie des Hallux valgus. Zbl. Chir. *56*:2434–2440, 1929.

Butcher: Excision of the metatarso-phalangeal articulation of the great toe; recovery, with perfect use of the foot. Dublin Quart. J. Med. Sci. *27*:48–50, 1859.

Campbell's *Operative Orthopaedics* (J. S. Speed and R. A. Knight, eds.). 3rd Ed. St. Louis, C. V. Mosby Co., 1956, Vol. 2, pp. 1948–1965.

Campbell's *Operative Orthopaedics* (A H. Crenshaw, ed.). 4th Ed., St. Louis, C. V. Mosby Co., 1963, Vol. 2, 1598–1613.

Clarke, J. J.: *Orthopaedic Surgery*. London, Cassell & Co., 1899, p. 127.

Cleveland, M., Willien, L. J., and Doran, P. C.: Surgical treatment of hallux valgus in troops in training at Fort Jackson during the year of 1942. J. Bone Joint Surg. *26*:531–534, 1944.

Cleveland, M., and Winant, E. M.: An end-result of the Keller operation. J. Bone Joint Surg. *32*:163–175, 1950.

Cornils, P.: *Ueber Gelenkresectionen bei Arthritis Deformans und Hallux valgus.* Inaugural-Dissertation. Jena, Von G. Neuenhahn, 1890, pp. 1–43.

Creer, W. S.: Correspondence. Brit. Med. J., *2*:558–559, 1936.

Davies-Colley, N.: Contractions of the metatarso-phalangeal joint of the great toe (hallux flexus). Brit. Med. J. *1*:728, 1887.

DeRacker, C.: La résection simple de l'exostose et de la première phalange dans le traitement de l'hallux valgus et de l'hallux rigidus; résultats eloignes. Acta Orthop. Belg. *17*:188–205, 1951.

Edenhuizen: Operation des Hallux valgus. Zbl. Chir. *40*:80, 1913. Also in Ztschr. Orthop. Chir. *31*:706, 1913.

Endler, F.: Zur Entwicklung einer kuenstlichen Arthroplastik des Grosszehengrundgelenkes und ihre bisherige Indikation. Ztschr. Orthop. *80*:480–487, 1951.

Fessler, J.: Die Operationen am Hallux valgus. Dtsch. Med. Wchnschr. *52*:2072–2074, 1926.

Fitzgerald, W.: Hallux valgus. J. Bone Joint Surg. *32*:139, 1950.

Fowler, G. R.: Partial resection of the head of the first metatarsal bone for hallux valgus. Med. Rec. *36*:253–255, 1889.

Fricke, J. L. G.: Exostosis of the ball of the foot. Dr. Fricke's report on the Hamburg Hospital for the First Quarter of 1836. Dublin J. Med. Sci. *11*:497–504, 1837.

Froriep, R.: *Commentatiuncula de Ossis Metatarsi Primi Exostosi*. Berolini: Joanni de Wiebel, 1834, pp. 1–8.

Galland, W. I., and Jordan, H.: Hallux valgus. Surg. Gyn. Obst. *66*:95–99, 1938.

Gilmore, G. H., and Bush, L. F.: Hallux valgus. Surg. Gyn. Obst. *104*:524–528, 1957.

Gottlieb, A.: Plastic orthopedics of the foot and lower extremity. Am. J. Surg. *8*:87–91, 1930.

Haggart, G. E., and Toomey, J. W.: Surgical correction of hallux valgus and dorsal medial exostosis. Surg. Clin. N. Amer. *19*:721–725, 1939.

Hallock, H.: The surgical treatment of common mechanical and functional disabilities of the feet. Am. Acad. Orthop. Surgeons *6*:160–173, 1949.

Halstead, A. E.: Hallux valgus. Ann. Surg. *43*:467–469, 1906.

Hamilton, F. H.: The use of warm and hot water in surgery. Med. Rec. *9*:249–252, 1874.

Harding, M. C.: Bunions: different types, different treatment. Southw. Med. *11*:360–362, 1927.

Heubach, F.: Ueber Hallux valgus und seine operative Behandlung nach Edm. Rose. Dtsch. Ztschr. Chir. *46*:210–275, 1897.

Heyfelder, O.: *Operationslehre und Statistik der Resectionen*. Vienna, W. Braumueller, 1861, pp. 203–205.

Hilton, J.: Resection of the metatarso-phalangeal joint of the great toe. Med. Tms. Gaz. *7*:141, 1853.

Hiss, J. M.: *Functional Foot Disorders*. Los Angeles University Press, 1937, p. 279.

Hiss, J. M.: *Functional Foot Disorders*. 3rd Ed., Los Angeles, Oxford Press, 1949, p. 565.

Hoffa, A.: *Lehrbuch der Orthopaedischen Chirurgie*. Stuttgart, F. Enke, 1894, pp. 739–744.

Holden, N. T.: The operative treatment of hallux valgus—a review of the Keller procedure. Guy's Hosp. Rep. *103*:274–278, 1954.

Hove, R. V.: A propos de la technique chirurgicale de l'hallux valgus. Acta Orthop. Belg. *17*:44–54, 1951.

Hueter, C.: Klinik der Gelenkkrankheiten. 1st Ed., Leipzig, F. C. W. Vogel, pp. 339–351, 1877.

Jones, E. A.: McBride operation for hallux valgus. Tr. New Engl. Surg. Soc. *23*:57–60, 1940.

Jones, R.: Discussion on the treatment of hallux valgus and rigidus. Brit. Med. J. *2*:651–656, 1924.

Joplin, R. J.: Sling procedure for correction of splay-foot, metatarsus primus varus, and hallux valgus. J. Bone Joint Surg. *32*:779–785, 1950.

Joplin, R. J.: Sling procedure for correction of splay-foot, metatarsus primus varus, and hallux valgus. J. Bone Joint Surg. *46*:690–693, 1964.

Jordan, H. H., and Brodsky, A. E.: Keller operation for hallux valgus and hallux rigidus. A.M.A. Arch. Surg. *62:*586–596, 1951.

Kaspar, M.: Die Resektion des Grundphalanx als Operation des Hallux valgus. Beitr. Klin. Chir. *157:*113–120, 1933.

Keller, W. L.: The surgical treatment of bunions and hallux valgus. New York Med. J. *80:*741–742, 1904.

Keller, W. L.: Further observations on the surgical treatment of hallux valgus and bunions. New York Med. J. *95:*696–698, 1912.

Kruimel, J. P.: Beitrag zu der operativen Behandlung des Hallux valgus. Zbl. Chir. *58:*8–11, 1931.

Lapidus, P. W.: The author's bunion operation from 1931 to 1959. Clin. Orthop. *16:*119–135, 1960.

Lexer, E.: Operation des Hallux valgus. Münch. Med. Wchnschr. *2:*1024, 1917.

Lloyd, E.: Hallux valgus: a comparison of results of two operations. Brit. J. Surg. *24:*241–245, 1936.

Lossen, H.: C. Hueter's *Grundiss der Chirurgie.* Leipzig, F. C. W. Vogel, 1884, pp. 325–328.

Lothrop, C. H.: Bunion. Boston Med. Surg. J. *88:*641–643, 1873.

McElvenny, R. T.: A study of hallux valgus: its cause and operative management. Part V. Keller procedure. Quart. Bull. Northw. Univ. Med. Sch. *21:*218–221, 1947.

McMurray, T. P.: Treatment of hallux valgus and rigidus. Brit. Med. J. *2:*218–221, 1936.

Manwaring, J. G. R.: Corns, hammer-toes and bunions. J. Michigan Med. Soc. *29:*497–499, 1930.

Mauclaire, P.: Greffes du cartilage. Presse Méd. *56:*545, 1920.

Mayo, C. H.: The surgical treatment of bunions. Ann. Surg. *48:*300–302, 1908.

Mayo, C. H.: The surgical treatment of bunions. Minnesota Med. J. *3:*326–331, 1920.

Milch, H.: Hallux valgus. J. Bone Joint Surg. *24:*486, 1942.

Morton, D. J.: *Human Locomotion and Body Form.* Baltimore, Williams & Wilkins Co., 1952, pp. 104–106.

Murphy, J. B.: Ankylosis; Arthroplasty, clinical and experimental. Trans. Am. Surg. Assoc. *22:*315–376, 1904.

Nelson, L. S., and Kaplan, E. B.: Hallux valgus. Survey of end results of various operative procedures for correction of hallux valgus performed at the hospital during the past ten years (1931–1940). Bull. Hosp. Joint Dis. *3:*17–25, 1942.

Olivecrona, H.: An operation for certain cases of hallux valgus. Acta Chir. Scand. *57:*396–402, 1924.

Pancoast, J.: *A Treatise on Operative Surgery.* Philadelphia, Carey & Hart, 1844, p. 133.

Perkins, G.: Removal of the metatarsal head for hallux valgus and hallux rigidus. Lancet *1:*540–541, 1927.

Perrot, A.: Pied plat transverse et hallux valgus, pathogénie et traitement. Schweiz. Med. Wchnschr. *76:*362–366, 1946.

Petersen, F.: Ueber Arthrectomie des ersten Mittelfuss-Zehen-Gelenkes. Arch. Klin. Chir. *37:* 677–678, and Fig. 6 at the end of the volume, 1888.

Pétrequin, J.: Bruchstuecke aus einer Reise in Italien; Musterung der Clinica. Ztschr. Ges. Med. *9:*274–288, 1838.

Platzgummer, H., and Jud, H.: Ergebnisse der Mayo-Plastik bei Hallux valgus. Chirurg *23:*391–392, 1952.

Pollosson, A.: De la métatarsalgie antérieure. Provence Méd. *6:*1–3, 1889. See Lancet *1:*436, 1889 and *1:*553, 1889.

Post, A. C.: Hallux valgus, with displacement of the smaller toes. Med. Rec. *22:*120–121, 1882.

Prignacchi, V., and Zanasi, R.: La tecnica di Hueter-Mayo nella cura chirurgical dell'alluce valgo. Chir. Org. Mov. *44:*234–242, 1957.

Radulesku, A., and Robnesku, N.: Arthroplasty with acrylic prothesis in the surgical treatment of arthritic hallux valgus (in Bulgarian). Khirurgiya *9:*776–782, 1956.

Rafarin, E.: *Un Nouveau Procédé pour le Traitement de l'Hallux Valgus.* Thesis. Paris, Vigot Frères, 1920, pp. 7–31.

Riedel: Zur operativen Behandlung des Hallux valgus. Cbl. Chir. *44:*753–755, 1886.

Rogers, W. A., and Joplin, R. J.: Hallux valgus, weak foot and the Keller operation: an end-result study. Surg. Clin. N. Amer. *27:*1295–1302, 1947.

Rose, A.: Resection considered as a remedy for abduction of the great toe—hallux valgus—and bunion. Med. Rec. *9:*200–201, 1874.

Royle, N. D.: Treatment of hallux valgus and hallux rigidus. Aust. N. Z. J. Surg. *1:*88–91, 1931.

Sayre, L. A.: *Lectures on Orthopedic Surgery.* New York, D. Appleton & Co., 1879, pp. 140–141.

Schanz, A.: Zur operativen des Hallux valgus. Zbl. Chir. *56:*209–210, 1929.

Schein, A. J.: The Keller operation—partial phalangectomy in hallux valgus and hallux rigidus. Surgery *7:*342–355, 1940.

Seiffert, J.: Nylon als Knorpelersatz bei der Hallux-valgus-Operation. Dtsch. Med. J. *4:* 414–415, 1952.

Singley, J. D.: The operative treatment of hallux valgus and bunion. J.A.M.A., *16:*1871–1872, 1913.

Soresi, A. L.: The radical cure of hallux valgus (bunion). Surg. Gyn. Obst. *52:*776–777, 1931.

Spiers, H. W.: End-result study of hallux valgus operations. J.A.M.A. *75:*306–307, 1920.

Starr, D.: The Keller operation. Bull. Vancouver Med. Assoc. *18:*301–330, 1942.

Steele, A. J.: Hallux valgus extremus. Tr. Am. Orthop. Assoc. *11:*17–21, 1898.

Syms, P.: Bunion: its aetiology, anatomy and operative treatment. New York Med. J. *66:* 448–451, 1897.

Thomas, F. B.: Keller's arthroplasty modified; a technique to insure post-operative distraction of the toe. J. Bone Joint Surg. *44:*356–365, 1962.

Veyrassat, J., and Patry, R.: La cure opératoire

de l'hallux valgus. Rev. Méd. Suisse Rom. *66*:608–613, 1946.

Wackerhagen, G.: Hallux valgus. Brooklyn Med. J. *9*:653–656, 1895.

Walsham, W. J., and Hughes, W. K.: *The Deformities of the Human Foot.* London, Baillière, Tindall & Cox, 1895, pp. 496–514.

Watson-Jones, R.: The treatment of hallux rigidus. Brit. Med. J. *1*:1165–1166, 1927.

Watson-Jones, R.: *Fractures and Joint Injuries.* 4th Ed., Baltimore, Williams & Wilkins Co., 1957, Vol. 1, pp. 345–347.

Weir, R. F.: The operative treatment of hallux valgus. Ann. Surg. *25*:444–453, 1897. See also discussion on pp. 480–485.

Chapter Twelve

ARTHRODESING OPERATIONS

Too often it is forgotten that the foot is designed primarily to sustain weight, and the stability of its joints takes precedence over movement. As a rule, a weight-bearing joint with complicated construction and greater range of motion deteriorates first and foremost; it may have to be eliminated surgically. Of the three joints of the hallucal ray, the middle—the metatarsophalangeal—possesses a bulbous articular bone and extensive capsular investment. It has a large sesamoid pad that is reinforced on either side by tendons. It allows considerable freedom of movement and bears the brunt of static stresses. It becomes disorganized most extensively and may necessitate surgical ankylosis. The aim of surgical effacement of the innermost cuneometatarsal joint is to redress the exaggerated varus position of the first metatarsal. Only indirectly does this operation contribute toward the correction of hallux valgus. The interphalangeal joint of the great toe is at times fused for paralytic states, but only rarely for static deformities.

Arthrodesis of the first metatarsophalangeal articulation. In Campbell's (1963) *Operative Orthopedics* we read: "Arthrodesis of the metatarsophalangeal joint of the great toe for hallux valgus was performed, according to Khoury, by Broca-Rose in 1895. Mauclaire also used the operation."

This statement necessitated an investigation as to its origination. Verbrugge (1933) published a set of diagrams illustrating various operations for hallux valgus. After No. 40, in the legend, he put Broca's and Rose's names and connected these two with a hyphen. In the text he wrote: "Broca-Rose (1895)—metatarsophalangeal arthrodesis. . . ." Khoury (1947) reproduced Verbrugge's sketches. Under No. 15 he inserted Broca's and Rose's names and hyphenated the two, as had Verbrugge. In the text he wrote: "In 1895 Broca-Rose performed arthrodesis and resected the sesamoids." McBride (1952) published a similar compilation, consisting of 57 sketches. In explanation of No. 42 he wrote: "Broca-Rose (1895): Does a resection arthrodesis of the first metatarsophalangeal joint and resects the sesamoids."

Hyphenation of two names is permissible. It is presumed that the authors whose names have been linked made their contribution about the same time. But by using singular "does" and "resects," McBride conveyed the erroneous impression that we are dealing with one person and not two. There were two

Brocas—Paul and August. Paul Broca (1852), who wrote about the deformity we now call hallux valgus, died in 1880. There were two surgeons named Rose who contributed toward the treatment of hallux valgus. A. Rose (1874) reported the first decapitation of the metatarsal of the great toe for uncomplicated hallux valgus; Edmond Rose's name is identified with the total resection of the first metatarsophalangeal joint. This operation was described by Heubach (1897), who made no mention of intentional arthrodesis.

Mauclaire (1910) described an operation that he called "oblique and conjugal osteotomy of the first metatarsal and the first phalanx." The line of resection of the metatarsal head started in the medial neck and ran distally toward the lateral edge of the articular surface. The line of resection of the phalangeal base began at the medial margin of the articular facet and took an oblique course toward the lateral shaft. The great toe was pushed back. Soft tissues attached to the lateral sesamoid were severed. Postoperatively the foot was immobilized for 2 weeks. The result, Mauclaire attested, was good. The toe was shortened, there was no pain, and there was some motion, which Mauclaire regarded a favorable sign at the time. Two decades later, commenting on this operation, Mauclaire (1933) wrote: "This is an ankylosing resection," which appears to be an afterthought. Had Mauclaire originally intended to fuse the joint, he would have immobilized the foot longer than 2 weeks and not boastfully reported movement after the operation. Joint stiffness appears to have developed insidiously, over a period of years.

Unintentional stiffness of the first metatarsophalangeal joint has been reported by numerous authors after many types of surgical procedures. The earliest hint of premeditated ankylosis for hallux valgus was given by Wyeth (1887). He resected a wedge shaped segment from the metatarsal and the phalanx, and advised holding these bones together "by silver wire suture" or "with small steel drills." Clutton (1894) was more explicit. He contended that, in hallux valgus, ankylosis of the joint in an "ideal" position would produce a most satisfactory and permanent result. Clutton denuded the hyaline coats of both metatarsal head and the base of the phalanx. He placed the two bones "in the position thought most desirable for ankylosis" and perforated them using a drill. He inserted an ivory peg into the drill hole to hold the two bones in apposition. Clutton fused seven joints in four patients by this method. The first operation was done in 1888, and the last in 1893. A picture shows one patient tiptoeing, after surgical ankylosis of the first metatarsophalangeal joint.

William Anderson (1897), who wielded considerable influence around the turn of the century, pronounced Clutton's fusion as "undoubtedly the best operation in the more severe procedures for hallux valgus. Involving obliteration of an important articulation," Anderson wrote, "it was feared that it might induce serious crippling, but the plan has been adopted with perfect success by Mr. Clutton, who, excising cartilaginous extremities of the bones and fixing the shaft in a suitable position by means of an ivory peg, has secured the best results."

Steele (1898) objected to the then popular decapitation of the first metatarsal. This was the way he worded it: "I disregard the advice usually given for relief of the deformity which is to remove the head of the metatarsal bone, for it seems to me that in such procedures the sustaining and propulsive power of the foot would be impaired... while not interfering with the bony structure of the metatarsal head, it is well to shave the cartilage . . . so that more prompt fibrous union takes place."

There appears to have been a lapse of interest in arthrodesis. Massart (1934) deplored the results of the Hueter resection and suggested lengthening the shortened first metatarsal by connecting it with the proximal phalanx. Treves (1937) mentioned fusion in passing. Thompson and McElvenny (1940) discussed arthrodesis of the first metatarsophalangeal joint in general. From a

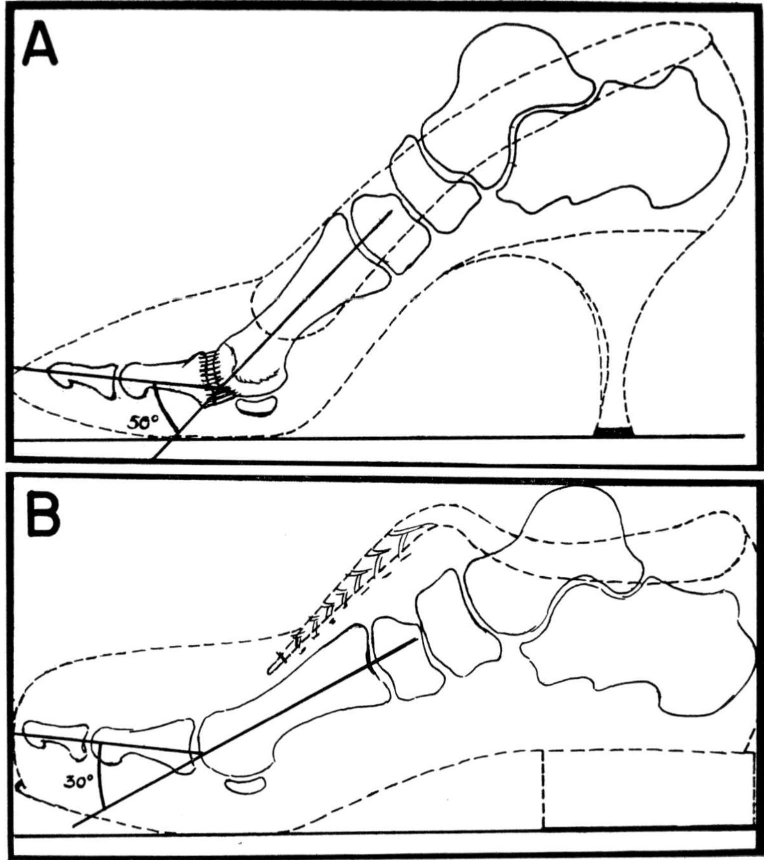

Figure 12–1. The degree of extension of fused great toe in women (*A*), and in men (*B*).

roentgenographic study of feet in shoes, they estimated that the great toe should be fixed in 15 degrees of extension from the plane of the ground. The plantar inclination of the first metatarsal was also taken into consideration. In women this bone formed an angle of about 35 degrees with the ground; in men this measurement did not exceed 15 degrees. If one had to judge by the angle formed between the extended axial lines of the first metatarsal and proximal phalanx, the optimum position of fusion in women would be 50 degrees—15 plus 35. In men it would range around 30—15 plus 15—degrees. The great toe should also be placed in a slight valgus position since the inner border of most prefabricated shoes tapers fibulaward as it approaches the toebox (Figs. 12–1 and 12–2).

Glissan (1946) saw a patient who had had an infection that resulted in ankylosis of the first metatarsophalangeal joint. The patient complained of no pain or discomfort referable to this joint. Glissan was impressed. He recommended surgical ankylosis of the joint for hallux valgus as well as hallux rigidus. In the former he combined arthrodesis with cuneiform osteotomy of the first metatarsal base. McKeever (1952) related a similar experience. He had operated on a patient with bilateral hallux valgus. One side became infected resulting in "rigid fibrous ankylosis" of the joint. When weight-bearing was resumed, it was noted that the varus deflection of the first metatarsal had diminished and the patient was relieved of pain. The obvious conclusion was that surgical fusion of the first metatarsophalangeal joint may be beneficial in some instances. McKeever devised a method of dovetailing the distal end of the first metatarsal into the base of the proximal phalanx and fixed the bones with a stainless steel screw. He advised 15 to 20 degrees of extension in men; in women 15 to 25, or even 35 degrees (Fig. 12–3).

There has been a recent surge of enthusiasm concerning surgical fusion of the first metatarsophalangeal joint. Smith (1952), Wishart (1953), MacDougall (1954), Hulbert (1955), J. Favreau and LaBelle (1957), Bingold (1958), Tupman (1958), Wilson (1958), Edelstein (1959), Zadik (1960), and others have spoken or written about this operation, which somehow has acquired the epithet "new." Some of these authors merely have reported successful results; others have described individual variations of surgical technique and of external or internal fixation. Harrison and Harvey (1963) indicated their preference for arthrodesis utilizing "a Charnley compression technique, not previously advocated for this joint." They seem to be unaware that Hulbert had described a similar method 8 years earlier (Fig. 12–4).

Clark (1953) made an attempt to stem the tide of enthusiasm for arthrodesis of the first metatarsophalangeal joint. He did not think "the new operation" had any "advantages to claim over conventional arthroplasties," which he thought had "the distinct recommendation that there was a fair chance of restoring the proper muscular control of the foot." Crymble (1956) also raised a voice of dissent. "The quality of the end results of arthrodesis of the metatarsophalangeal joint of the great toe," he wrote, "is not immeasurably better than that obtained by simple standard procedures to justify its routine use in hospital practice." But then he added: "Young patients with painful hallux rigidus, where operation is unavoidable, probably form a special group in which arthrodesis may be advantageous." Stamm (1957) conceded an occasional indication for arthrodesis of the first metatarsophalangeal joint: "When gross arthritic changes are present with marked limitation of movement or when the forefoot mechanism is unstable, it may be considered that no form of arthroplasty offers a reasonable chance of giving satisfactory results. In such cases arthrodesis of the joint in optimum functional position provides an

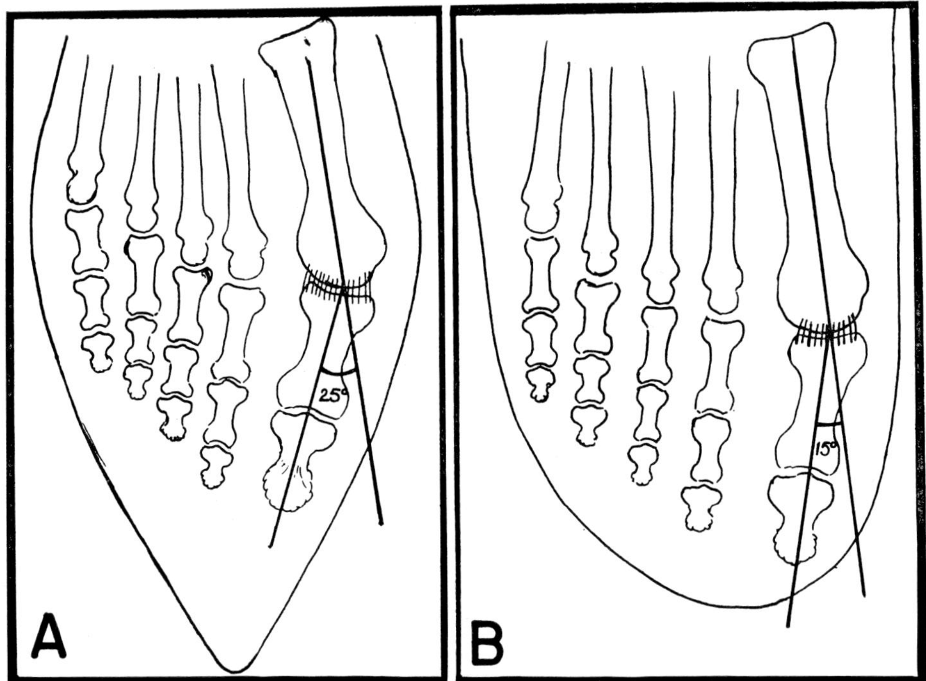

Figure 12–2. The degree of valgus of the great toe in women (*A*), and in men (*B*).

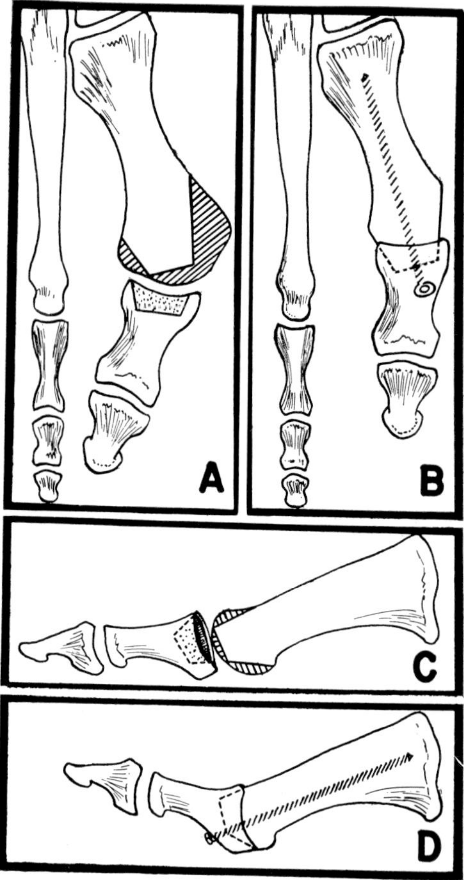

Figure 12–3. McKeever's method: reshaping the head of the first metatarsal and the base of the proximal phalanx (*A*); interlocking and transfixation with a screw (*B*); reshaped bones seen from the side (*C*); profile view of transfixed bones (*D*).

alternative solution to the problem." Bingold (1958) wrote: "A successful arthrodesis produces a strong great toe on which the weight is born and which plays its part in the final stages of propulsion . . . . Any tendency to metatarsalgia is therefore lessened." He recommended arthrodesis plus excision of the painful second metatarsal head in the presence of hallux valgus and severe metatarsalgia caused by dorsal dislocation of the second toe.

Tupman (1958) reported 42 fusions in 37 patients and gave the following as indications for arthrodesis of the first metatarsophalangeal joint: "(1) hallux valgus with splaying of the forefoot and short first metatarsal, (2) after unsuccessful Keller resection, (3) hallux rigidus, (4) rheumatoid arthritis with deformity and lateral deviation of the toes, and (5) poliomyelitis when flail joint makes it difficult for the patient to put on a shoe." Tupman reported three nonunions. In Zadik's series of 100 operations, in 72 patients, 24 had metatarsalgia before the operation and afterward all but six were relieved of this symptom. Zadik (1960) concluded: "Arthrodesis of the first metatarsophalangeal joint is a logical operation in hallux rigidus. It was often observed that when a hallux rigidus became completely stiff, the pain disappeared. It is also effective in hallux valgus, because it corrects defective weight distribution. . . ."

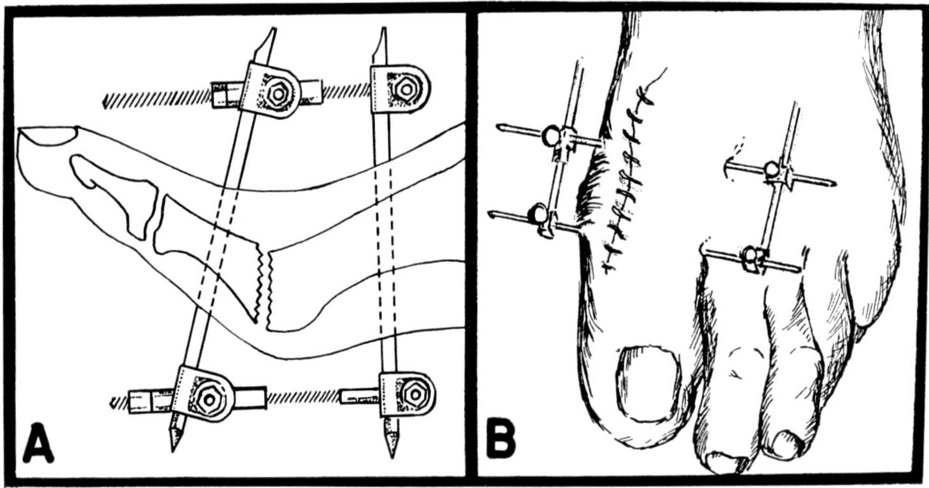

Figure 12–4. Compression clamps: Hulbert's (*A*) and Harrison and Harvey's (*B*).

Harrison and Harvey (1963) also noted "favorable effect of arthrodesis on metatarsalgia," which they ascribed to the preservation of the attachment of adductor hallucis to the base of the proximal phalanx. ". . . . For this reason," they concluded, "arthrodesis can be applied in the presence of splayed forepart of the foot or subluxated second toe without fear of aggravation or production of metatarsalgia. . . . Arthrodesis of the first metatarsophalangeal joint confers freedom from pain and high level of functional efficiency in a very high proportion of patients who suffer from hallux valgus and hallux rigidus."

Successful arthrodesis of the first metatarsophalangeal joint in optimum position of the great toe will amend the deformity of hallux valgus and dispose of the local pain; it may even alleviate generalized metatarsalgia. But it is not without any hazard. Nonunion has been reported by more than one author; others speak of discomfort on wearing shoes if the toe has not been placed in the desired position of extension and with moderate valgus deflection. Screws have been blamed for infection. We prefer to use an intramedullary Kirschner wire for fixation. This is passed through the tip of the big toe across the phalanges into the metatarsal, and then an attempt is made to place the hallux in optimum extension with a slight valgus deflection. The end of the pin juts out of the tip of the big toe. After the foot has been adequately immobilized in a cast, the pin can be removed without much difficulty (Fig. 12–5).

Arthrodesis of the first metatarsophalangeal joint has a definite place in the treatment of hallux valgus. After failure of more conservative operations—Schede's, Silver's, McBride's—one could still salvage the joint by a Keller resection. Arthrodesis of the first metatarsophalangeal joint combined with resection of the distal ends of the second—and sometimes also the third, fourth, and fifth metatarsals—offers one of the few solutions for severe hallux valgus with intractable metatarsalgia. The smaller toes are surgically syndactylized. The most legitimate indication for fusion of the first metatarsophalangeal joint is when the deformity of the great toe is of paralytic origin (Figs. 12–6 and 12–7).

Arthrodesis of the innermost cuneometatarsal joint—the Lapidus operation. Albrecht (1911) from Turner's clinic in St. Petersburg, now Leningrad, recommended resection and fusion of the first cuneometatarsal joint for hallux valgus. His article was written in Russian; abstracts of it appeared in French and German, but not in English. Truslow (1925)—who is generally credited as being the originator of wedge resection of the first cuneometatarsal joint—did not mention Albrecht in his article. Klein-

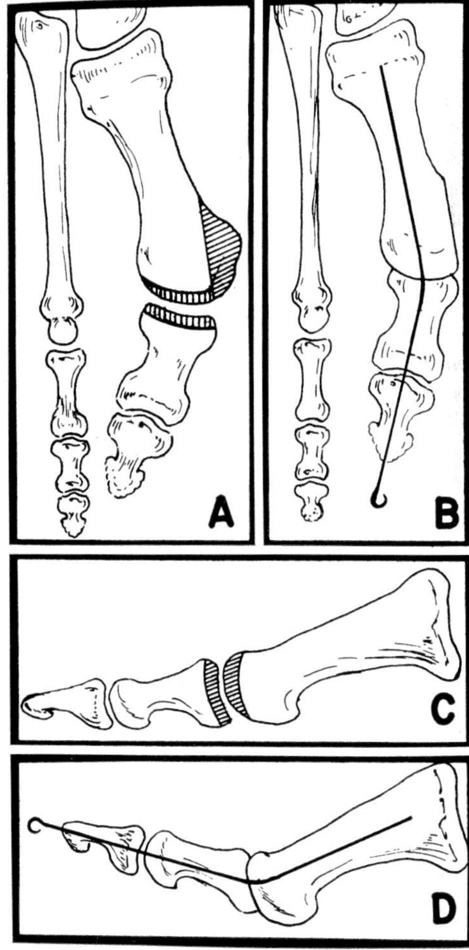

Figure 12–5. Intramedullary pin fixation after arthrodesis. Shaded areas indicate parts of skeletal elements to be resected (*A*). After the bones have been apposed and transfixed with intramedullary pin, the toe is pushed into the desired position of valgus (*B*). Bones seen from the side (*C*). Bending the intramedullary wire to obtain the desired degree of extension (*D*).

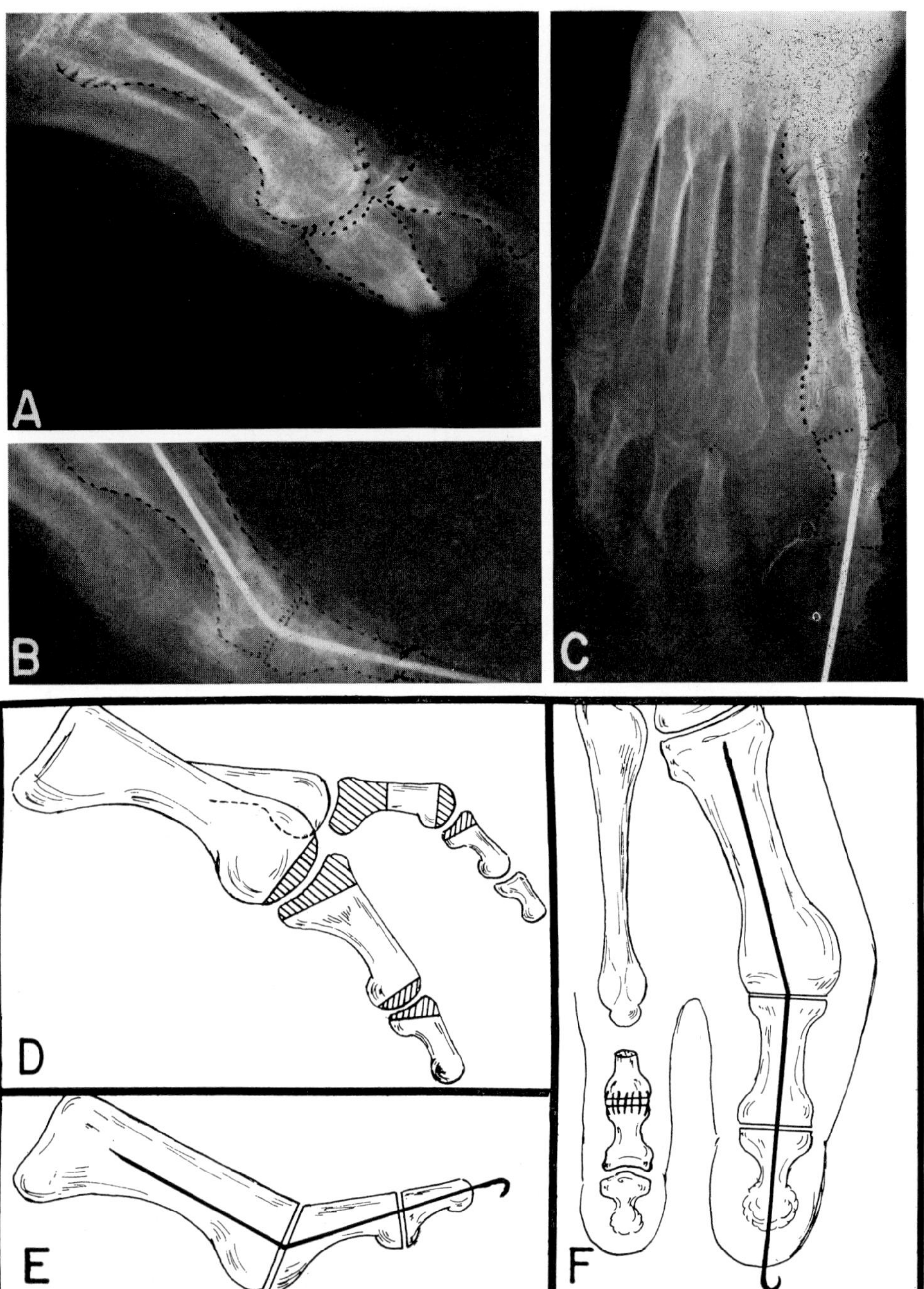

Figure 12–6. Woman, 54, with poliomyelitis in youth, hallux flexus and valgus, and hammered second toe. Surgery: fusion of the metatarsophalangeal and interphalangeal joints of the great toe, partial proximal phalangectomy of the second toe, and fusion of the proximal interphalangeal joint. Side view roentgenogram before surgery (*A*); after surgery (*B*); postoperative dorsoplantar view (*C*); interpretative diagrams (*D, E,* and *F*).

berg (1932) disclaimed any previous knowledge of the fact that the principle on which he based his operation had been enunciated by others; he described a method not unlike Albrecht's. As had Albrecht, Kleinberg supplemented the surgery at the cuneometatarsal joint with corrective work at the metatarsophalangeal articulation (Figs. 12–8 and 12–9).

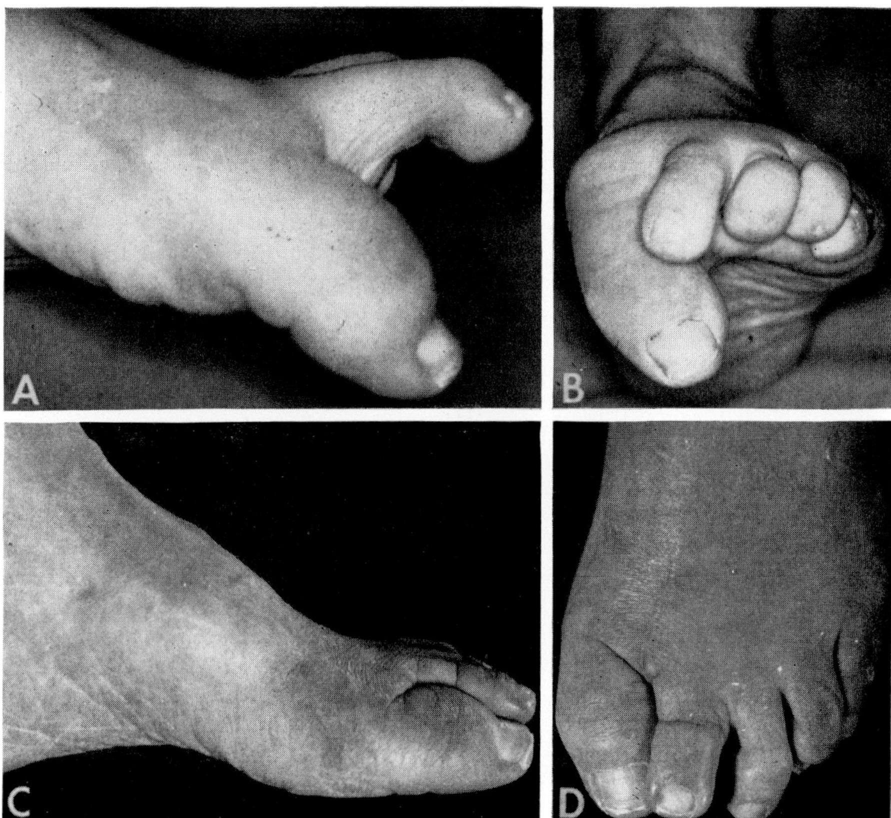

Figure 12–7. The same patient as in Figure 12–6. Forefoot seen from the side before surgery (*A*); frontal view (*B*); profile view after recovery (*C*); dorsal aspect after surgery (*D*). This patient now wears medium high heeled shoe with comfort.

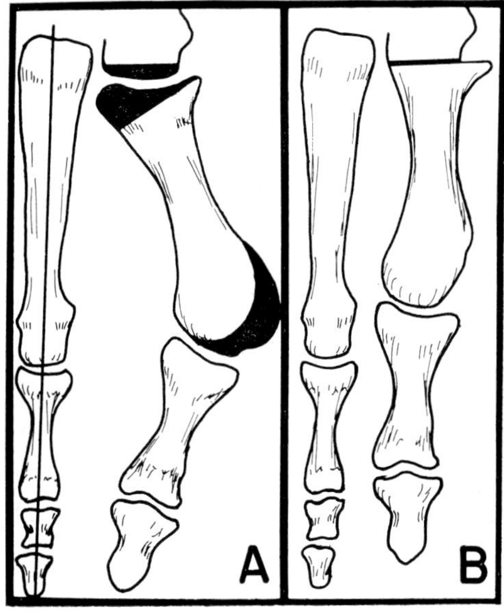

Figure 12–8. Albrecht's operation.

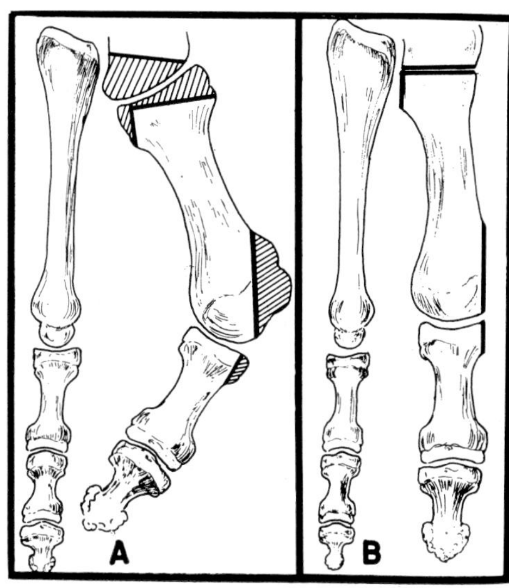

Figure 12–9. Kleinberg's method.

Lapidus (1934–1960) has been the most persistent advocate of cuneometatarsal fusion. For that reason, perhaps, his name is identified with this procedure. Lapidus received his medical education in Odessa, Russia. If he ever read Albrecht's article in the original, Lapidus made no mention of it when he published his first paper on hallux valgus. At the time, Lapidus was a junior member of the Hospital for Joint Diseases, where Kleinberg was a senior staffman. Preceding Lapidus by two years, Kleinberg had described almost the same procedure and called it "Author's Operation." Lapidus also labeled the method he described "Author's Operation" and let us know it was "the result of personal study." But then he added: "There is no priority to originality claimed by the writer, except for the details of the operation."

This same preamble recurs in almost every article Lapidus has penned about hallux valgus. "In my previous papers dealing with the correction of hallux valgus," Lapidus (1956) wrote, "I have stressed the fact that the operation described by me did not embody any new principles. Rather it combined a number of old ideas in such a way as to make it an effective therapeutic procedure." We pick up the last article by Lapidus (1960) and read: "Once more the author wishes to repeat that, except for the details of the operation, he does not claim priority or originality."

One tries to qualify the mood pervading these quotations, and conjecture at the motivation that compels Lapidus to repeat the same theme year after year. It is difficult to reconcile the urge to profess modesty with the unequivocal intent betrayed by the title of the more recent article by Lapidus: *The Author's Bunion Operation From 1931 to 1960.* The opening paragraph of this opus reads: "The author's bunion operation was first performed at the Hospital for Joint Diseases on April 18th, 1931, and thus far stood the test to time. The details of it were published as a preliminary communication in February, 1934."

In the preliminary communication referred to, Lapidus completely ignored Albrecht; Truslow's and Kleinberg's names appeared in the bibliography, but not in the text. Twenty-two years later Lapidus (1956) mentioned all three men. By then his own name had been firmly established as the uncontested originator of the procedure. It would have been simpler, and he need not have felt compelled to apologize each time, if at the beginning, Lapidus had said that he was about to propose a procedure that had been tried before, but that he was introducing some necessary modifications, even improvements, or that he was in a position to describe the operation in greater detail.

Reading successive articles put out by Lapidus in the past 30 years, one gets the impression that he is relying more on other procedures for correction of hallux valgus than on the one with which we have come to connect his name. Even when he attempted to fuse the innermost cuneometatarsal joint and establish a bony bridge between the bases of the first and second metatarsals, Lapidus supplemented this procedure with corrective surgery at the base of the great toe and utilized steps introduced by others. He resected the medial eminence, released the adductor tension, and transposed the abductor hallucis to a more dorsal position on the medial aspect of the first metatarsophalangeal joint. These steps cannot be considered integral parts of the Lapidus procedure. His operation is carried out at the cuneometatarsal junction and is primarily designed to correct metatarsus primus varus—or as he prefers to call it—metatarsus varus primus.

Lapidus approached the innermost cuneometatarsal joint through a longitudinal incision, measuring about 3¼ inches (9 cm.) along the dorsum of the first metatarsal and the adjoining cuneiform bone. The tendons of the long and short extensors were retracted medially. The space between the first and the second metatarsal bases was cleared. The cortex from the adjacent surfaces of the base of the first and the second metatarsals was removed, leaving the bone chips in situ. The first cuneometatarsal joint was opened from its dorsal aspect. The articular facets were denuded of their hyaline covering. A snug fitting of the resected surfaces was obtained. Number 0 chromic catgut was passed through a drill hole in the base of the first metatarsal and the strong dorsal ligamentous structure between the two medial cuneiform bones. The stitch was tied. Bone chips obtained from the resected medial eminence were packed in the space between the decorticated bases of the first and second metatarsals. The skin was closed (Fig. 12–10).

Lapidus (1956) stated that he had completely abandoned plaster of Paris immobilization; he considered the support afforded by the steel corset for 2 to 3 weeks sufficient. From a mechanical standpoint his procedure is as precarious, if not more, than Miller's (1927) or Hoke's (1931) arthrodesis for flatfoot. Circular casts are used after these operations and allowed to remain for at least 6 weeks. The aversion Lapidus holds for cast immobilization probably emanates from his zeal to prove that the length of disability after his operation is not much more than "in cases following the Keller-Brandes procedure." The worst thing a surgeon can do is to spite himself to prove a point.

After 30 years of ardent crusading, with ample interpolations from the works of embryologists and anthropologists, to corroborate his contention that "in a great majority of cases of hallux valgus there is metatarsus primus varus, which is primary underlying cause of the deformity, hallux valgus occurring secondarily"; that "no operative procedure is satisfactory, unless correction of the metatarsus varus primus is accomplished"; and that, following operations for hallux valgus, "a permanent result can be expected only when the first metatarsus varus is adequately corrected and this correction maintained"—after these similar pontifical pronouncements in the past, we find the ensuing more recent statements by Lapidus anticlimatic:

"In my further studies of hallux valgus, I have been convinced that the varus position of the first metatarsal is not always of prime importance and that in some cases it is unnecessary to complicate the simple correction of hallux valgus by fusing the first metatarsocuneiform joint as originally advocated by me. We must admit that with accumulation of the larger experience through many years, we have become more conservative and in a number of cases limited our procedure to a correc-

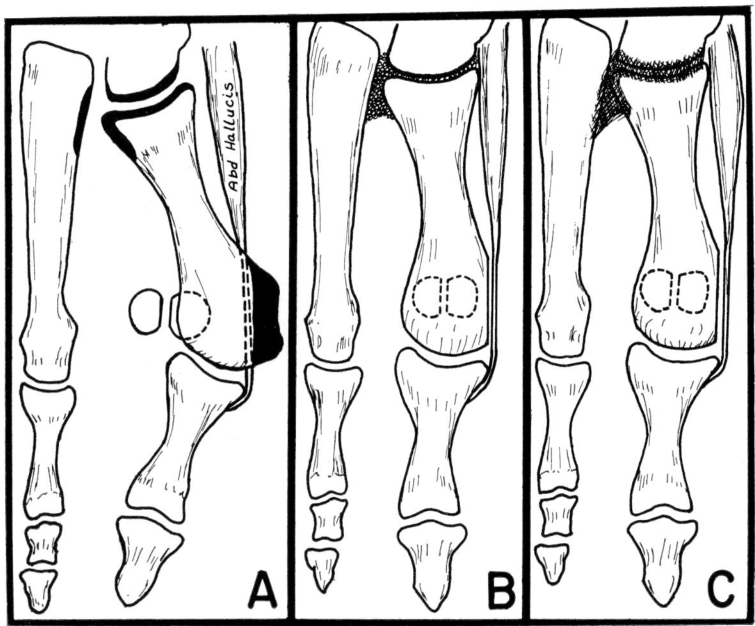

Figure 12–10. Lapidus' procedure.

tion of hallux valgus alone. It has been our observation that after satisfactory correction of hallux valgus, doing our modifications of the Silver procedure, the varus of the first metatarsal may diminish simultaneously, provided that there is adequate mobility of the first cuneiformo-metatarsal joint to allow the approximation of the first and second metatarsal heads."

Lapidus has given us no hint as to the mechanism whereby the dual desideratum—correction of hallux valgus and of metatarsus primus varus—can be obtained by Silver's operation, which is confined to the region of the first metatarsophalangeal joint, far distal from the primary "apex of angulation," which Lapidus has been insisting is located proximally at the first cuneometatarsal joint. It is on this basis that Lapidus leveled his charges against osteotomy of the first metatarsal for hallux valgus. "Osteotomy to correct an angulation of any long bones," he wrote, "is performed at the apex of the angulation and not distally or proximally to it; otherwise, a bayonet-shaped deformity is produced. An ankylosed knee joint with genu valgum or with flexion deformity is best corrected through the former line of the joint and not over the femur or the tibia. Therefore, it is the author's preference to correct metatarsus varus primus at the first cuneiformo-metatarsal joint; numerous osteotomies of the first metatarsal shaft and particularly so over the distal part never have seemed to the author to be mechanically sound. . . ."

The analogy of metatarsus varus with knockedknee is unfortunate. In genu valgum, supracondylar osteotomy is generally regarded as the operation of choice and no one would think of fusing the proximal joint—the hip. Lapidus stated that after osteotomy the fragments required a long time to consolidate, but following cuneometatarsal fusion they were usually solid at the end of 3 months. Practically all osteotomies consolidate by the end of 3 months, and some in even less time.

Stahl (1943) went on record with the following remark: "In connection herewith an account is given of a material of hallux valgus patients treated with arthrodesis of the tarsometatarsal joint and re-examined. The findings show that from a functional as well as from a morphological point of view, this method is not very suitable as a normal method in operative treatment of hallux valgus and pes transverse planus." According to Campbell's (1963) *Operative Orthopedics,* Lapidus' procedure "achieves an excellent correction, but weight bearing afterward must be delayed longer than after some other operations." Grannis, Meier, and Tanner (1956) wrote: "Lapidus reported a procedure in 1934 for the correction of metatarsus primus varus, the principle of which . . . is sound. The operation is relatively formidable . . . as remodeling and arthrodesis of the first metatarsocuneiform joint is required, and frequently in addition, it is necessary to do exostectomy and plastic procedure at the site of the bunion."

Lapidus specified that patients suitable for his operation must preferably be "young and robust," the varus deflection of the first metatarsal should be at least 15 degrees or more, and there must be a "fixed contracture" of the cuneometatarsal joint.

It is generally conceded that persons with hypermobile first metatarsal are prone to develop hallux valgus. Arthrodesis would be more justifiable when the innermost cuneometatarsal joint allows greater mobility. Under the body weight hypermobile first metatarsal tilts up and goes into varus deflection, both of which are undesirable. Lapidus, on the other hand, considered "lateral mobility at the cuneiformo-metatarsal joint" a contraindication to fusion of this articulation. In these instances, he preferred a modified Silver procedure at the first metatarsophalangeal joint.

Lapidus finally conceded that of late his indication for performing "a correction of metatarsus primus by resection of the cuneiform-metatarsal joint and of insertion of bone chips between the denuded surfaces of the bases of the first and second metatarsals" has been "less frequent than when it was first devised."

Lapidus deserves credit for having kept alive the concept of metatarsus primus varus. Many feel, however, that

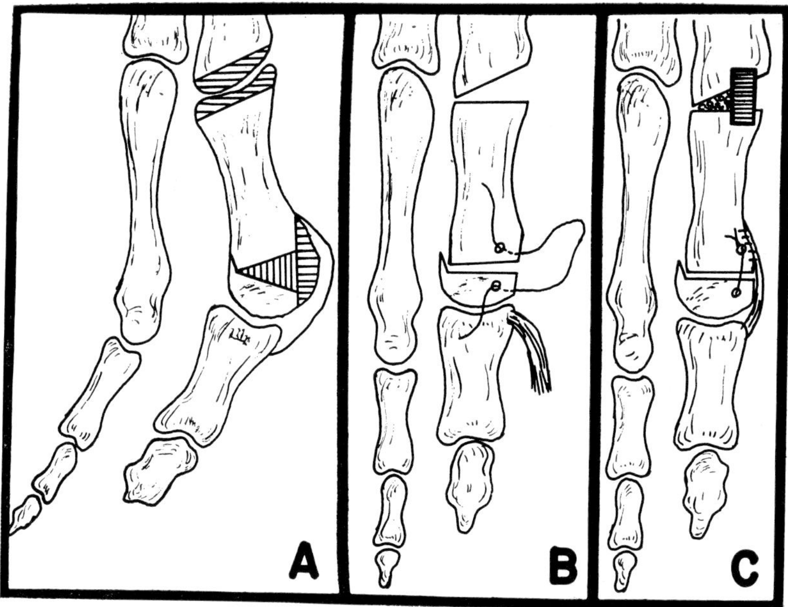

Figure 12–11. Durman's operation.

the exaggerated inward inclination of the first metatarsal can more expediently be corrected by osteotomy of this bone than by fusion of the cuneometatarsal joint. Union of the bones following osteotomy has greater chance of success than after arthrodesing operations, especially when the former is designed so as to provide a greater area of surface contact. Ironically, by incessantly stressing the importance of metatarsus primus varus in hallux valgus in order "to sell" his own operation, Lapidus has played into the hands of his competitors—the osteotomists—and reinforced their contention that such operations are sometimes needed.

Cuneometatarsal fusion has also been described by Armstrong (1937). Huc and Thyes (1938) fused this joint to correct the varus deformity, the torsion, and the dorsal tilt of the first metatarsal. They resected the proximal two-thirds of the basal phalanx to redress the valgus deflection of the great toe. Wissel (1952) corrected hallux valgus by resecting the proximal portion of the first phalanx. He fashioned a wedge out of the first phalanx and used it to fuse the innermost cuneometatarsal joint. Huc and Thyes, and Wissel, thus combined the Keller resection with arthrodesis of the proximal joint. Durman (1957) combined fusion of the innermost cuneometatarsal joint with a Peabody type of wedge osteotomy of the metatarsal head. He fused the proximal joint with a block of bone much like the one used in the (1931) Hoke operation for flatfoot (Fig. 12–11).

Fusion of the interphalangeal joint of the great toe. Glissan (1946) suggested surgical ankylosis of the interphalangeal joint for hallux valgus. He gave two indications after reconstructive work on the first metatarsophalangeal joint: (1) when the outward deviation of the distal phalanx persists or (2) the long extensor of the great toe remains and hinders adequate correction of hallux valgus. Rather than lengthen the extensor tendon, Glissan apparently preferred to sever it and fuse the interphalangeal joint. Occasionally, after a Keller resection, the great toe will knuckle at the interphalangeal joint; in such an instance, fusion of this articulation is indicated.

REFERENCES

Albrecht, G. H.: The pathology and treatment of hallux valgus (in Russian). Russ. Vrach. *10:* 14–19, 1911.

Anderson, W.: *The Deformities of Fingers and Toes.* London, J. & A. Churchill, 1897, p. 120.

Armstrong, W. P., Jr.: Treatment of hallux valgus (bunion). Am. J. Surg. *36:*332–338, 1937.

Bingold, A. C.: Arthrodesis of the great toe. Proc. Roy. Soc. Med. *51:*435–437, 1958.

Broca, P.: Des difformités de la partie antérieure du pied produite par l'action de la chaussure. Bull. Soc. Anat. *27:*60–67, 1852.

Campbell's *Operative Orthopaedics* (A. H. Crenshaw, ed.). 4th Ed. St. Louis, C. V. Mosby Co., 1963, Vol. 2, pp. 1598–1613.

Clark, J. M. P.: Operative treatment of hallux valgus and rigidus. Brit. Med. J. *1:*162, 1953.

Clutton, H. H.: The treatment of hallux valgus. St. Thomas Rep. *22:*1–12, 1894.

Crymble, B. T.: The results of arthrodesis of the great toe with special reference to hallux rigidus. Lancet *2:*1134–1136, 1956.

Durman, D. C.: Metatarsus primus varus and hallux valgus. A.M.A. Arch. Surg. *74:*128–135, 1957.

Edelstein, L. G.: Utilization of the proximal phalanx of the big toe for reconstruction of the first metatarsal bone following its extensive resection for hallux valgus (in Russian). Acta Travim. Tropez *20:*55–56, 1959.

Favreau, J. C., and LaBelle, P.: Hallux valgus and hallux rigidus. J. Bone Joint Surg. *39:*792–793, 1957.

Glissan, D. J.: Hallux valgus and hallux rigidus. Med. J. Aust. *2:*585–588, 1946.

Grannis, W. R., Meier, A. W., and Tanner, J. B.: Surgical treatment of bunions; distal metatarsal osteotomy. California Med. *85:*245–247, 1956.

Harrison, M. H. M., and Harvey, F. J.: Arthrodesis of the first metatarsophalangeal joint for hallux valgus and rigidus. J. Bone Joint Surg. *45:*471–480, 1963.

Heubach, F.: Ueber Hallux valgus und seine operative Behandlung nach Edm. Rose. Dtsch. Ztschr. Chir. *46:*210–275, 1897.

Hoke, M.: An operation for the correction of extremely relaxed flat feet. J. Bone Joint Surg. *13:*773–783, 1931.

Huc, G., and Thyes: Tactique opératoire dans l'hallux valgus. Rev. d'Orthop. Chir. *25:*720–721, 1938.

Hulbert, K. F.: Compression clamp for arthrodesis of the first metatarsophalangeal joint. Lancet *1:*597, 1955.

Khoury, C.: *Hallux Valgus.* Buenos Aires, Lopez & Etchegoyen, 1947.

Kleinberg, S.: Operative cure of hallux valgus and bunions. Am. J. Surg. *15:*75–81, 1932.

Lapidus, P. W.: The operative correction of the metatarsus varus primus in hallux valgus. Surg. Gyn. Obst. *58:*183–191, 1934.

Lapidus, P. W.: Discussion following McBride's paper. J.A.M.A. *105:*1068, 1935.

Lapidus, P. W.: A quarter of a century of experience with the operative correction of the metatarsus varus in hallux valgus. Bull. Hosp. Joint Dis. *17:*404–421, 1956.

Lapidus, P. W.: The author's bunion operation from 1931 to 1959. Clin. Orthop. *16:*119–135, 1960.

McBride, E. D.: Hallux valgus and bunion deformity. Am. Acad. Orthop. Surgeons *9:*334–346, 1952.

McKeever, D. C.: Arthrodesis of the first metatarsophalangeal joint for hallux valgus, hallux rigidus, and metatarsus primus varus. J. Bone Joint Surg. *34:*129–134, 1952.

MacDougall, A.: Hallux valgus. Brit. Med. J. *2:*231, 1954.

Massart, R.: Les résultats déplorables des opérations d'hallux valgus. Bull. Mém. Soc. Chir. *26:*669–674, 1934.

Mauclaire, P.: Ostéotomies obliques conjugées du 1ER métatarsien et de la 1RE phalange pour hallux valgus. Arch. Gén. Chir. *6:*41–45, 1910.

Mauclaire, P.: Traitement de l'hallux valgus grave par l'arthroplastie reconstitutive. Rev. Chir. *52:*661–674, 1933.

Miller, O. L.: A plastic flatfoot operation. J. Bone Joint Surg. *9:*84–91, 1927.

Rose, A.: Resection considered as a remedy for abduction of the great toe—hallux valgus—and bunion. Med. Rec. *9:*200–201, 1874.

Smith, N. R.: Hallux valgus and rigidus treated by arthrodesis of the metatarso-phalangeal joint. Brit. Med. J. *2:*1385–1387, 1952.

Stahl, F.: Zur Behandlung von Hallux valgus, des transeso-planus und Hallux rigidus durch ankylosiorende Operationen; eine Nachuntersuchung. Acta Orthop. Scand. *14:*97–126, 1943.

Stamm, T. T.: The surgical treatment of hallux valgus. Guy's Hosp. Rep. *106:*273–279, 1957.

Steele, A. J.: Hallux valgus extremus. Tr. Am. Orthop. Assoc. *11:*17–21, 1898.

Thompson, F. R., and McElvenny, R. T.: Arthrodesis of the first metatarso-phalangeal joint. J. Bone Joint Surg. *22:*555–558, 1940.

Treves, A.: Difformités du gros orteil. In *Traité de Chirurgie Orthopédique* (L. Ombrédanne and P. Mathieu, eds.). Paris, Masson et Cie., 1937, Vol. 5, pp. 4045–4061.

Truslow, W.: Metatarsus primus varus or hallux valgus? J. Bone Joint Surg. *7:*98–108, 1925.

Tupman, S.: Arthrodesis of first metatarso-phalangeal joint. J. Bone Joint Surg. *40:*826, 1958.

Verbrugge, J.: *Pathogénie et Traitement de l'Hallux Valgus.* Mém. Bull. Soc. Belge d'Orthop., pp. 3–40, 1933.

Wilson, C. L.: A method of fusion of the metatarsophalangeal joint of the great toe. J. Bone Joint Surg. *40:*384–385, 1958.

Wishart, J.: Arthrodesis of the first metatarsophalangeal joint for hallux valgus and rigidus. J. Bone Joint Surg. *35:*494, 1953.

Wissel, H.: Beitrag zur operativen Korrektur des Hallux valgus mit abnorm starker Abspreizstellung des I Metatarsale. Arch. Orthop. Unfall-Chir. *45:*100–104, 1952.

Wyeth, J. A.: *A Text-Book on Surgery.* New York, D. Appleton & Co., 1887, pp. 735–736.

Zadik, F. R.: Arthrodesis of the great toe. Brit. Med. J. *2:*1573–1574, 1960.

Chapter Thirteen

MISCELLANEOUS METHODS

A number of surgical procedures are seldom practiced at present in connection with hallux valgus and related forefoot deformities. They are presented here in their historical context; an unforeseen indication may arise for one of them. Also there are several relatively new operations that will require years for final assessment; they are recorded in the ensuing pages as they appear to us at present.

Amputation. In the report about Hilton's (1853) resection of the metatarsophalangeal joint of the great toe we read: "Although the importance of the great toe to safe and comfortable progression has long been fully acknowledged, yet it does not appear that much attention has hitherto been directed to avoiding of the amputation in cases usually submitted to that measure. A patient now under the care of Mr. Stanley, in St. Bartolomew's Hospital, affords us a good illustration of these remarks. He had had both great toes amputated, the one, on account of caries of the articular ends; the other, by reason of great distortion, attended with a very troublesome bunion. He is now under treatment for a bad fracture of the leg, met with in a fall, occasioned by the lameness consequent on the loss of his toe." Obviously neither the unnamed reporter, nor Hilton approved of amputation.

"If the joint becomes affected and the bone diseased," Annandale (1866) wrote, "amputation of the toe and the head of the metatarsal bone will be the only remedy." Lossen (1884) thought it was "wrong to exarticulate the great toe in hallux valgus," because this operation left a scar over the prominent metatarsal head and subjected it to pressure by the shoe. Walsham and Hughes (1895) conceded that "amputation of the great toe at the tarsometatarsal joint may be required in exceptional cases."

Even for fulminant infection, one would hesitate to amputate the great toe. There remain only a few indications for this drastic undertaking. Vascular insufficiency is one of them—the only valid one. Occlusive arterial disease is not an uncommon accompaniment of hallux valgus. Forefoot surgery should be avoided in arteriosclerotics. If operation is necessitated because of indolent infection or intractable pain, it should be carried out without tourniquet. When the hallux has already been disarticulated at the metatarsophalangeal joint and the surgical wound has healed with a tight, painful scar over

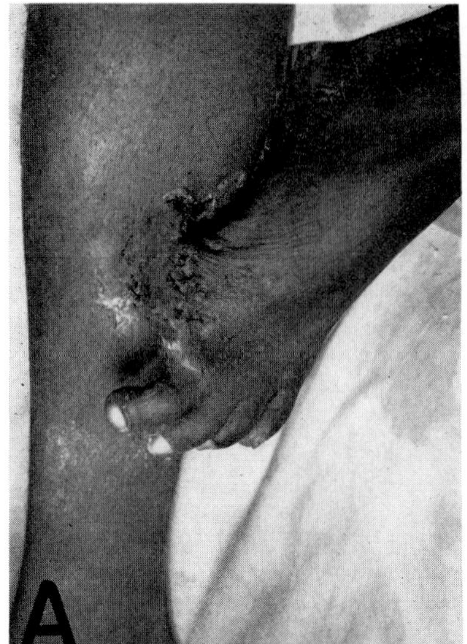

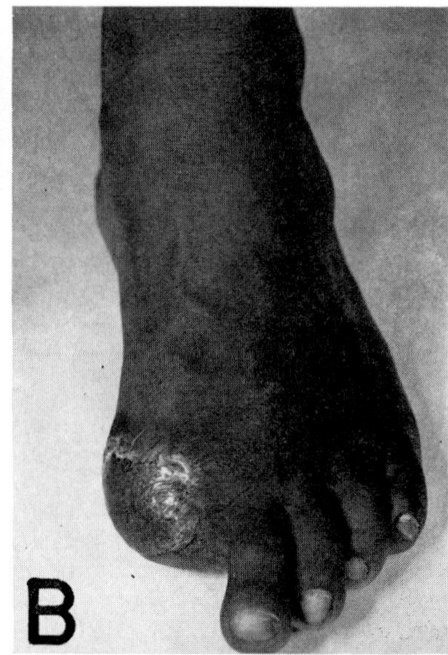

Figure 13–1. Amputated hallux, which healed with a painful scar: (*A*) cross-leg graft; (*B*) postoperative result.

the stump, rather than shorten the first metatarsal, padded skin may be provided by a pedicled graft from the opposite leg (Fig. 13–1).

Tenotomy of the extensors of the great toe. Nélaton (1859) recommended tenotomy of the long extensor of the great toe in comparatively young individuals with moderate hallux valgus. In conjunction with other procedures for hallux valgus, tenotomy of the extensor was advised by Reverdin (1881), Tubby (1912), and many others. Bankart (1913) sectioned both long and short extensors. Truslow (1925), Brooke (1941), and Mikhail (1960) also advised tenotomy of the short extensor.

Lengthening of the extensor of the great toe. Plastic elongation, in time, superseded tenotomy. "In six cases of beginning hallux valgus," Sheldon (1903) wrote, "I made an incision over the tendon of the extensor proprius hallucis and extensor brevis digitorum muscles a distance of one inch; divided one portion of each tendon at the upper end of the split and the remaining portion of the opposite end, thus dividing the tendons in such a manner that they could be lengthened two inches without complete separation of their fibers." In the ensuing decades Z-plasty of the long extensor of the great toe came into vogue. Stein (1938) recommended what he called "triple subtotal sections" of the tendon to allow it to be stretched (Fig. 13–2).

Transfer of the long tendons. In connection with hallux valgus, tendon transplantation came into vogue toward the termination of the last century. Ullmann (1894) disconnected the long extensor of the great toe from its insertion and reinserted it into the middle of the proximal phalanx; he also brought the long flexor to the medial side of the metatarsophalangeal joint and connected it to the extensor. Delbet (1896) left the extensor attached to the terminal phalanx but brought a loop of the tendon down to the medial side of the joint and sutured it to the capsule. Weir (1897) detached the extensor from its insertion and reimplanted it into the inner aspect of the proximal phalanx. Halstead (1906) fastened the extensor "well down on the inner side of the first phalanx without severing its attachment beyond." Albrecht (1911) dug a groove along the medial aspect of the first metatarsal and transplanted the extensor tendon into it. In some cases of hallux valgus, Bankart (1913) inserted the long extensor and flexor tendons into the head of the metatarsal bone in order to preserve their action. Keszly (1923) split the long

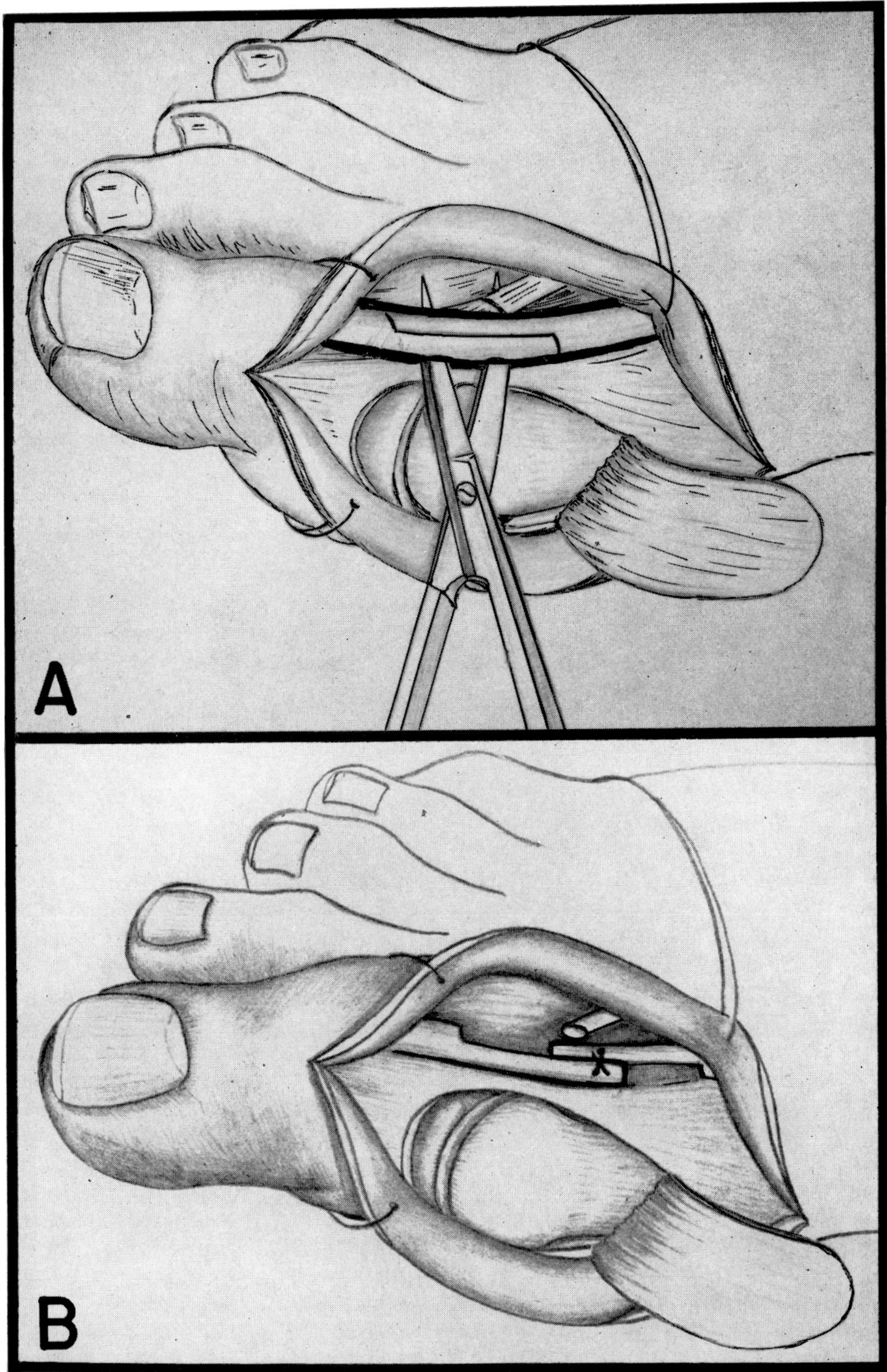

Figure 13–2. Tenotomy of the short extensor (*A*) and Z-plasty of the long extensor (*B*) of the great toe.

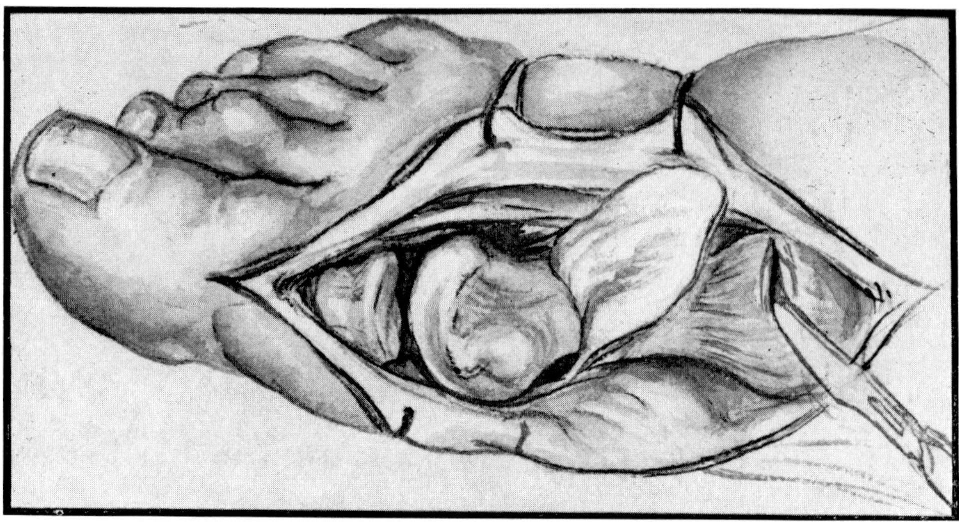

Figure 13—3. Medial capsulotomy of the innermost cuneometatarsal joint.

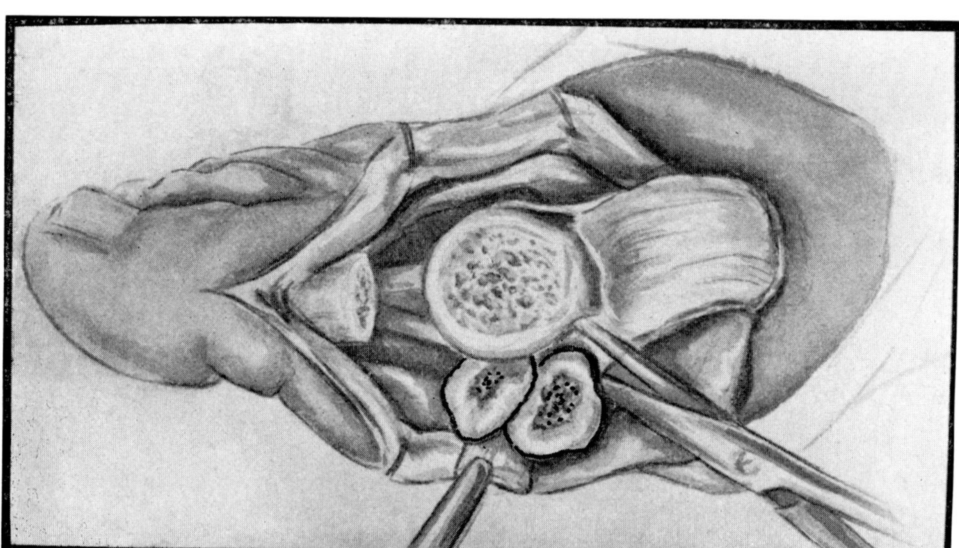

Figure 13—4. Sesamoidectomy.

extensor tendon longitudinally and connected the inner arm to the medial border of the basal phalanx. Mauclaire (1924) passed the severed end of the extensor of the great toe through an oblique tunnel into the head of the first metatarsal to make it serve as a suspensor and adductor of this bone.

Capsulotomy of the innermost cuneometatarsal joint. Matheis (1927) joined the chorus of those who insisted that the medial eminence of the first metatarsal head was not an exostosis but merely the displaced portion of the normal bone; therefore, it need not be removed. The basic disturbance in hallux valgus, Matheis contended, was inward inclination, *supination,* and dorsal tilt of the first metatarsal. To reverse these changes he detached the insertion of the tibialis anticus and released the capsule of the innermost cuneometatarsal articulation on its medial and dorsal aspects. The first metatarsal was then pushed plantarward close to the second metatarsal and *pronated.* The severed end of the anterior tibial tendon was reinserted further posteriorly on the tarsus. In addition, Matheis released the adductor tension on the lateral side of the first metatarsophalangeal joint and transposed the abductor hallucis to a more dorsal position on the medial side. We now occasionally carry out capsulotomy of the innermost cuneometatarsal joint in connection with a modified Silver procedure (Fig. 13–3).

Sesamoidectomy. Heubach (1897) considered removal of the sesamoids an important step in the Edmond Rose technique of resection of the first metatarsophalangeal joint. If left, he thought the sesamoids would continue to push the first metatarsal medially or press upon its resected edge. Weir (1897) and Tubby (1912) were among the many who removed the sesamoids in connection with other procedures. The most vociferous crusader of sesamoidectomy was Robinson (1918–1928). He even advocated extirpation of these small ossicles in the young as a preventive measure against hallux valgus; in an already established deformity, he considered the removal of these bones sufficient. In their discussion of the Keller operation, Jordan and Brodsky (1951) wrote: "If the sesamoid bones show enlargement and deformity or if they have been the site of localized pain, they can be removed easily after resection of the proximal phalanx but we have rarely found this necessary."

Sesamoids are now removed when inordinately enlarged, mushroomed and eroded on their articular aspect, or are painful. When wedged between the first and second metatarsal heads and correction of metatarsus primus varus is contemplated by osteotomy, the lateral sesamoid is extirpated. In shelling out the sesamoids, care must be taken not to injure the long flexor tendon of the great toe. Sesamoidectomy offers no difficulty when carried out in connection with a Keller resection (Fig. 13–4).

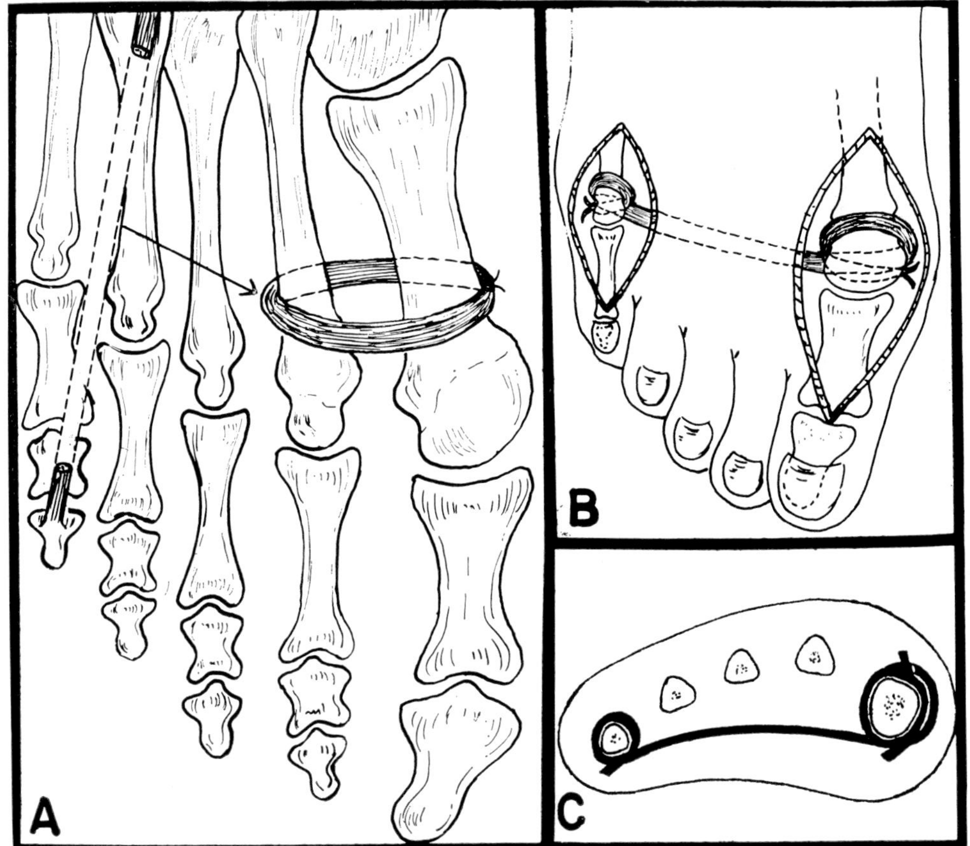

Figure 13–5. Circlage. (*A*) Lexer's method; (*B* and *C*) Goebell's method.

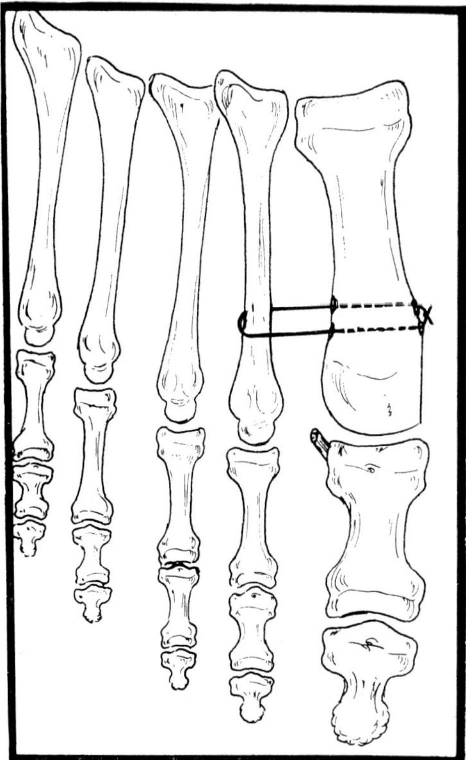

Figure 13–6. Lenggenhager's wire circlage.

Extirpation of os intermetatarseum. Just as some books are discussed more often than read, certain surgical procedures have been described time and again but seldom practiced. Young (1910)—the proponent of Dwight's accessory bone as a cause of hallux valgus—had this to say: "By means of x-ray the presence of supernumerary bone can be detected early; its removal should be followed by an arrest of the condition and a relief of all the symptoms. I have proposed this operation to a patient upon whom I first recognized this condition and have performed it upon the cadaver." Young recommended his operation—which he said was "original" and "new"—for hallux valgus in adolescents. He operated his first case on November 16, 1909. His report appeared 6 months later. This is too short a time to assess the result of any operation for hallux valgus. No one else appears to have practiced Young's operation, but it is mentioned in book after book and in numerous articles.

Epiphysiodesis. Unlike the four lateral metatarsals, the first one bears its epiphysis at its proximal end. This ossification center appears between the second and fourth years. In girls the epiphysis unites at about the fifteenth year and in boys two years later. In growing children and in adolescents with metatarsus primus varus, Ellis (1951) attempted partial arrest of growth by stapling the epiphysis to the metaphysis across the lateral portion of the plate. The growth center of the first metatarsal is thin; the promixal prong of the staple would penetrate the bone close to the cuneometatarsal joint and might even enter it. Moreover, one could not be certain how much correction would be obtained in time. Osteotomy is preferable.

Sling and circlage. Lexer (1919) tried to correct splaying of the forefoot by looping the extensor tendon of the fifth toe around the first and second metatarsals. Goebell (1927) described a method of approximation of the first and fifth metatarsals with a band of fascia. He ascribed this procedure to Martin Kirschner. Lenggenhager (1935) snugged the two medial metatarsals by a loop of wire. The wire encircled the second metatarsal; its ends were threaded through drill holes in the distal extremity of the first metatarsal and tied. In this way the wire was prevented from slipping backward on the narrower shaft and thereby losing its efficacy (Figs. 13–5 and 13–6).

McMurray (1936) had spoken of "stretched transverse metatarsal ligament" in hallux valgus. By way of comment, Cochrane (1936)—obviously unaware of what already had been practiced in Germany—asked: "Would it be feasible to manufacture a new set by a strip of fascia lata passed through or around the affected metatarsal bones?" Cochrane thought that a fascial circlage might prophylactically be utilized for early cases of hallux valgus and "weak" foot. Krida (1939) entitled his article *A New Operation for Metatarsalgia and Splay Foot* and described a procedure not unlike Goebell's (1927).

Petri's (1940) article featured several

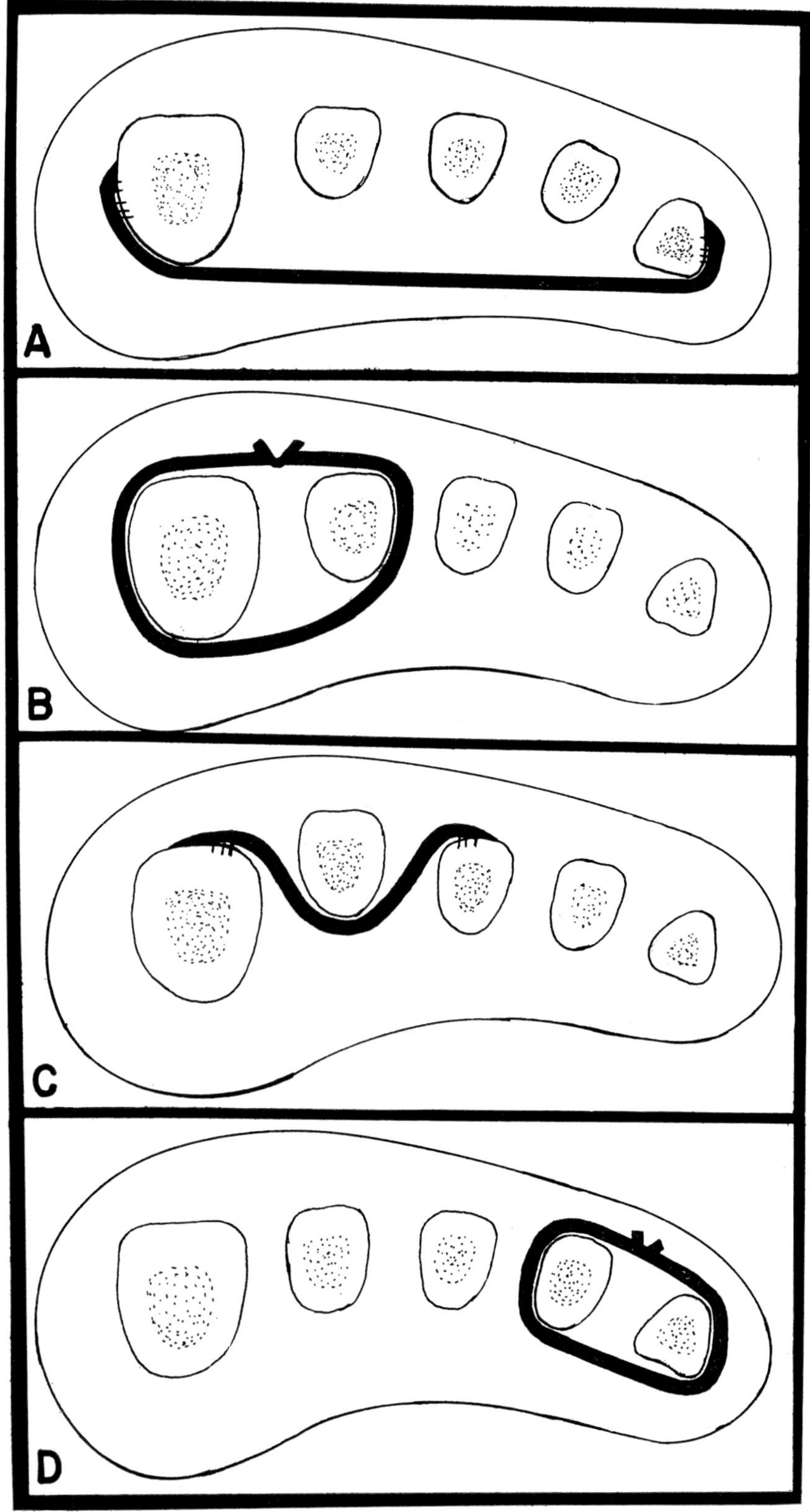

Figure 13–7. Petri's method.

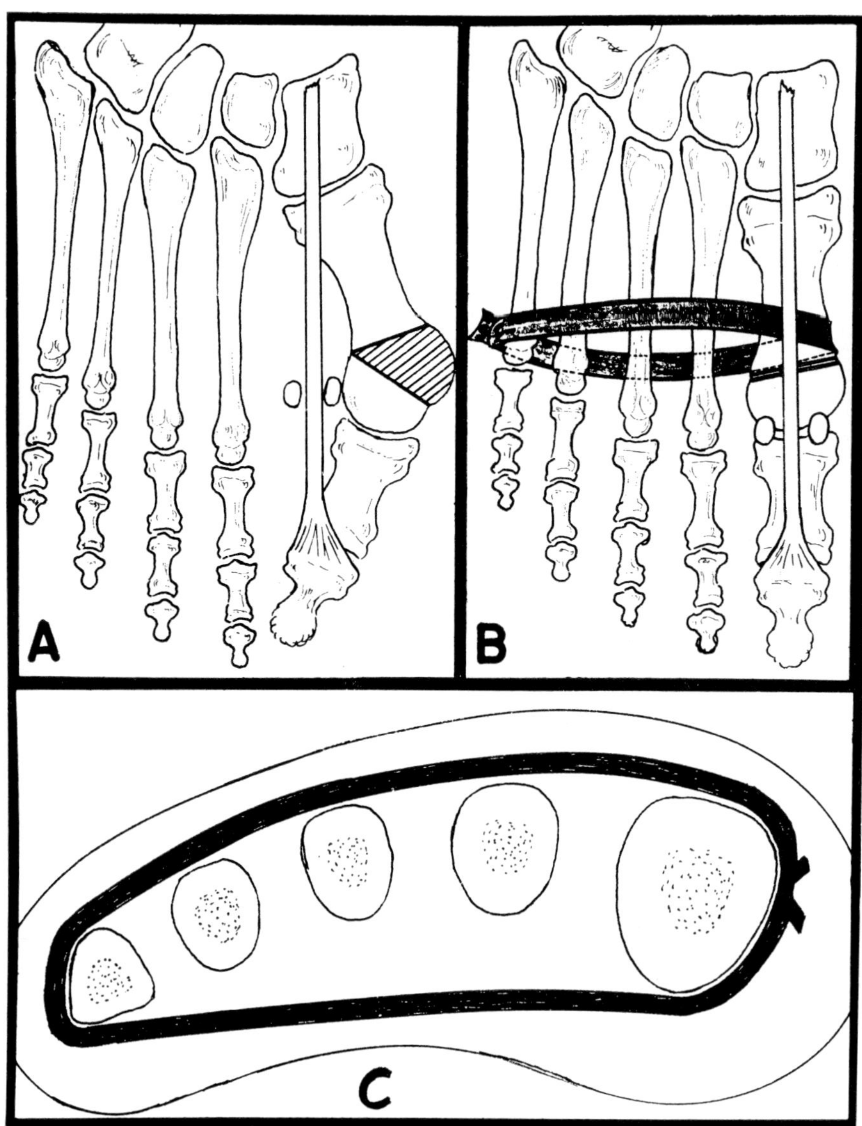

Figure 13–8. Massart's circlage.

methods of sling and circlage with the aid of free fascial strips. In one illustration, after osteotomy of the first metatarsal, the distal fragment is shown snugged closer to its fellow on the fibular side by an encircling band. In another diagram the fascial sling passes under all five metatarsals and is anchored to the marginal bones. Two illustrations show the second metatarsal supported by a sling, the ends of which are attached to the shafts of the flanking bones. A final pair of sketches shows the base of the proximal phalanx of the small toe excised, the lateral eminence of the fifth metatarsal sagittally resected, and the two fibular rays approximated by an encircling fascial band (Fig. 13–7).

French authors have made the distinction between total and partial circlage. Massart (1948) favored total circlage. He utilized two incisions: one along the medial and the other along the lateral border of the forefoot. For binding material he used kangaroo tendon. He introduced one end of the preserved tendon through the lateral skin cut, carried it across the dorsum of the forefoot close to the skeletal plane, delivered it out of the medial incision, threaded it back under the plantar aspect of the metatarsal bones, and then out of the lateral incision. The metatarsal bones were compressed together; the ends of the kangaroo tendon were tied under tension. Lelièvre (1952) recommended using a strip of the plantaris tendon for circlage. He also modified Massart's method; the tendon was looped around the first and fifth metatarsals and the central three bones were supported by a double band (Figs. 13–8 and 13–9).

Joplin (1950–1964) revived Lexer's operation; he used the long extensor tendon of the fifth toe. Joplin combined the sling procedure with his own modification of McBride's adductor transplant. More recently Joplin supplemented his technique with wedge osteotomy of the first cuneiform (Figs. 13–10 and 13–11).

Johnson (1958) encircled the first and the fifth metatarsals and supported the central rays with double bands. Wertheimer (1959) threaded the extensor tendon through the head of the fifth metatarsal, passed it under the necks of the central rays, threaded it through the head of the first, and sutured it to the abductor tendon, which had been detached from the base of the proximal phalanx. The adductor hallucis was

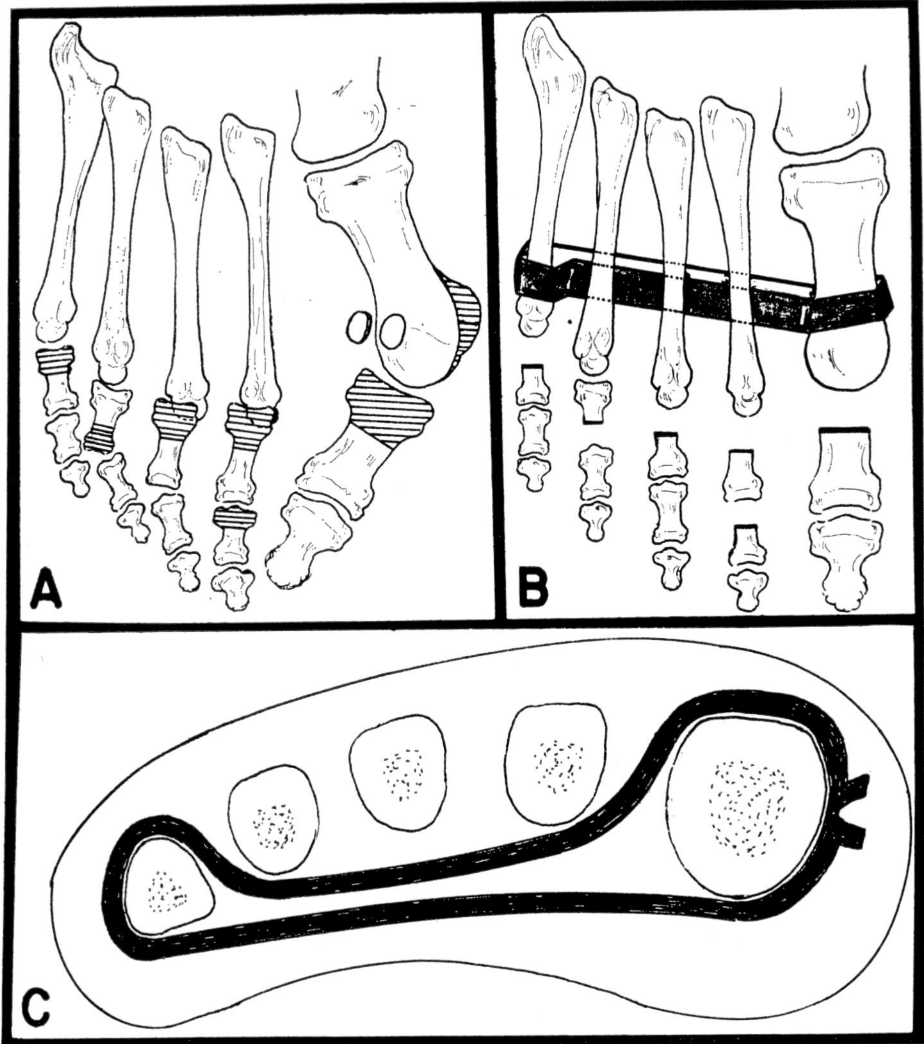

Figure 13–9. Lelièvre's sling.

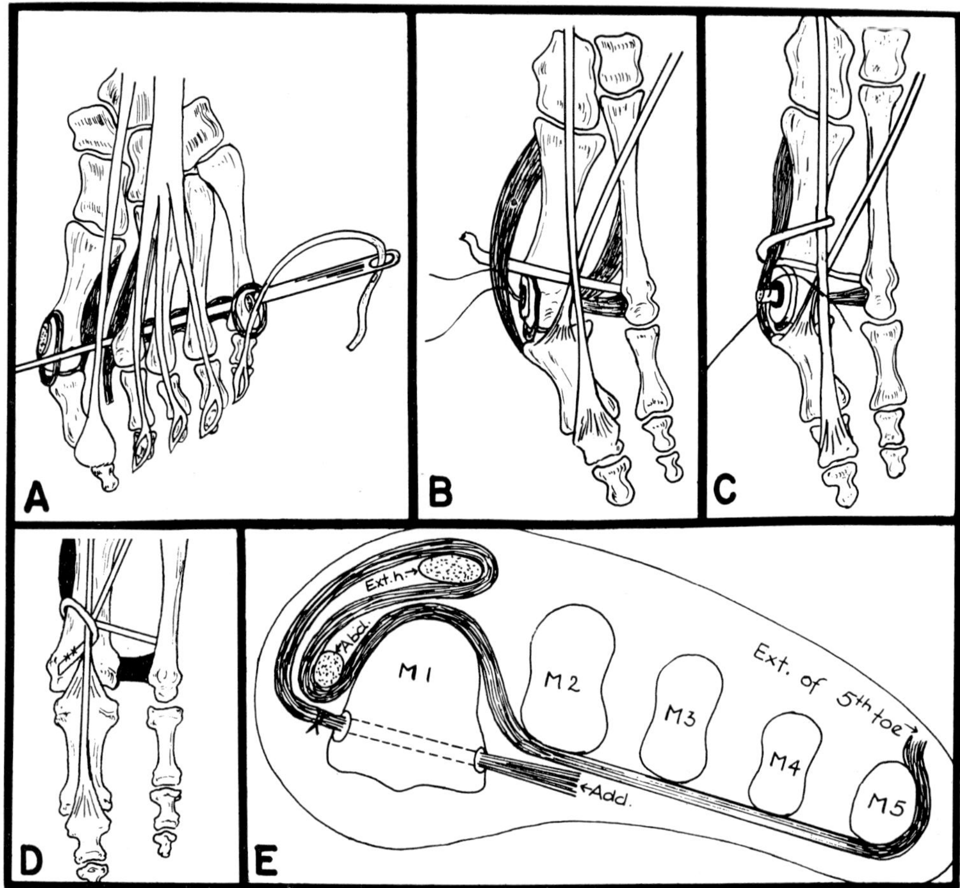

Figure 13–10. Joplin's sling.

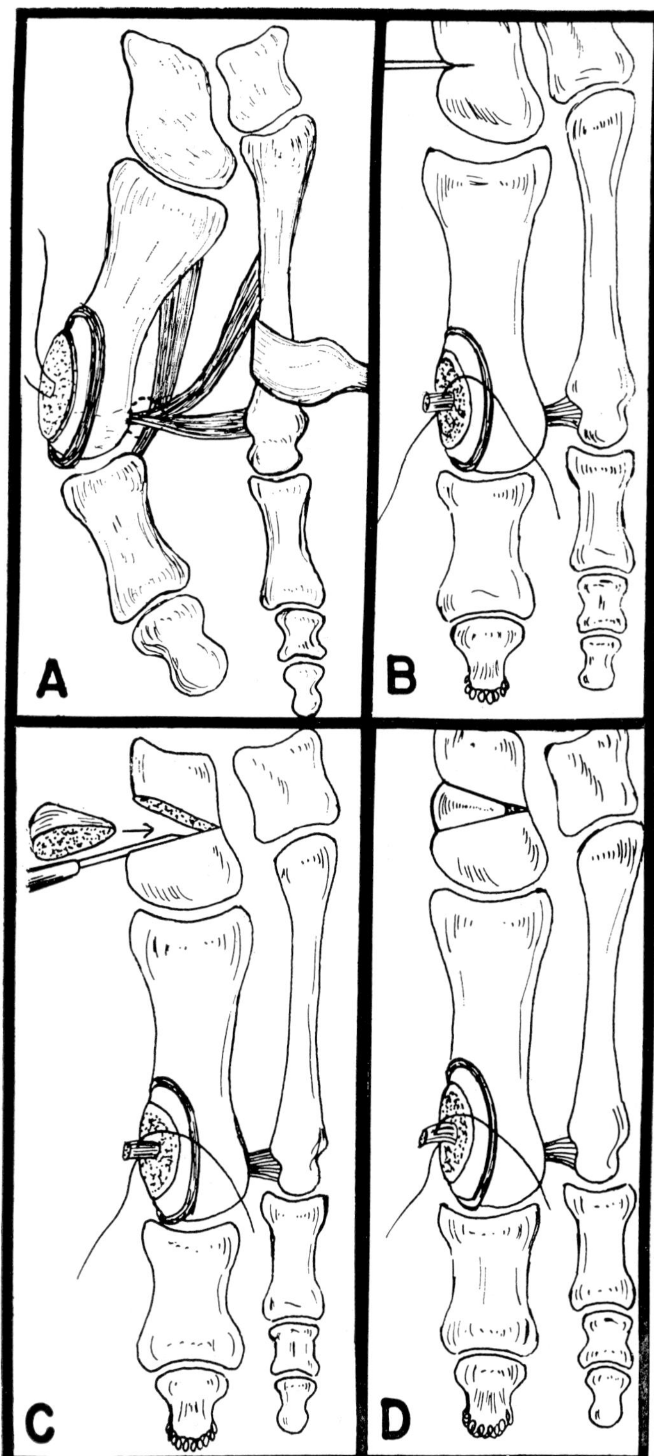

Figure 13–11. Joplin's osteotomy of innermost cuneiform and adductor transfer into the first metatarsal.

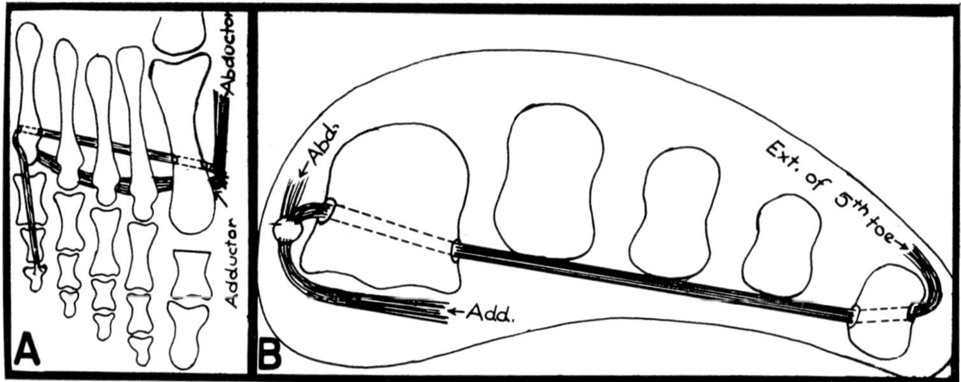

Figure 13–12. Wertheimer's sling.

similarly disconnected and reattached to the abductor on the medial side (Fig. 13–12).

Perhaps too much is being expected from sling and circlage procedures. It is not conceivable that a strip of fascia or tendon would resist stretching under the body weight. Circlage of the first and second metatarsals is a justifiable procedure when used in conjunction with osteotomy of the first metatarsal bone. We prefer to use stainless steel wire for this purpose and utilize Lenggenhager's (1935) technique.

Neurectomy. We learn from Joplin (1964) that, in the course of his sling procedure, he has of late been sectioning "the medial proper digital nerve," to ameliorate postoperative discomfort and procure smoother convalescence for the patient.

REFERENCES

Albrecht, G. A.: The pathology and treatment of hallux valgus (in Russian). Russ. Vrach. *10:*14–19, 1911.

Annandale, T.: *The Malformations, Diseases and Injuries of the Fingers and Toes.* Philadelphia, J. B. Lippincott and Co., 1866, pp. 110–123.

Bankart, A. S. B.: The pathology and treatment of hallux valgus. Med. Press Circ. *96:*33–35, 1913.

Brooke, R.: Treatment of hallux valgus deformity in soldiers. Brit. Med. J. *2:*605–606, 1941.

Cochrane, W. A.: Treatment of hallux valgus and rigidus. Brit. Med. J. *2:*651, 1936.

Delbet, P.: Hallux valgus bilatéral traité par résection semi-articulaire et la vaginoplastie artificielle. Rev. d'Orthop. *7:*221–227, 1896.

Ellis, V. H.: A method of correcting metatarsus primus varus. J. Bone Joint Surg. *33B:*415–417, 1951.

Goebell, R.: Über arthroplastische freie Fascien und Aponeurostransplantation nach Martin Kirschner. Arch. Klin. Chir. *146:*462–509, 1927.

Halstead, A. E.: Hallux valgus. Ann. Surg., *43:* 467–469, 1906.

Heubach, F.: Ueber Hallux valgus und seine operative Behandlung nach Edm. Rose. Dtsch. Ztschr. Chir. *46:*210–275, 1897.

Hilton, J.: Resection of the metatarso-phalangeal joint of the great toe. Med. Times Gaz. *7:*141, 1853.

Johnson, J. A.: Operation of hallux valgus by the sling procedure (in Norwegian). Nord. Med. *59:*103–105, 1958.

Joplin, R. J.: Sling procedure for correction of splay-foot, metatarsus primus varus, and hallux valgus. J. Bone Joint Surg. *32:*779–785, 1950.

Joplin, R. J.: Some common foot disorders amenable to surgery. Am. Acad. Orthopaed. Surg. Instructional Course Lect. *15:*144–158, 1958.

Joplin, R. J.: Sling procedure for correction of splay-foot, metatarsus primus varus, and hallux valgus. J. Bone Joint Surg., *46:*690–693, 1964.

Jordan, H. H., and Brodsky, A. E.: Keller operation for hallux valgus and hallux rigidus. A.M.A. Arch. Surg., *62:*586–596, 1951.

Keszly, S.: Eine neue Modifikation der operativen Behandlung des Hallux valgus. Zbl. Chir. *50:*91–94, 1923. Abstract in J. Bone Joint Surg. *5:*617, 1923.

Krida, A.: A new operation for metatarsalgia and splay-foot. Surg. Gyn. Obst. *69:*106–107, 1939.

Lelièvre, J.: *Pathologie du Pied.* Paris, Masson & Cie., 1952, pp. 755–756 and 766–767.

Lenggenhager, K.: Eine neue Operationsmethode zur Behandlung des Hallux valgus. Chirurg. *7:*689–692, 1935.

Lexer, E.: Die freien Transplantationen. *In Neue Dtsch. Chirurg.,* Stuttgart, F. Enke, 1919, pp. 398–402.

Lossen, H.: *In* C. Hueter's *Grundriss der Chir-*

urgie. Leipzig, F. C. W. Vogel, 1884, pp. 325–328.

McMurray, T. P.: Treatment of hallux valgus and rigidus. Brit. Med. J. *2:*218–221, 1936.

Massart, R.: Le relévement de l'arc interne du pied et la correction de l'élargissement de l'avant-pied, comme complément des opérations pour hallux valgus. Press. Med. *57* (Supplément 56: No. 23): 280, 1948.

Massart, R.: *Affections Médicales et Chirurgicales du Pied.* Paris, G. Doin & Co., 1948, pp. 76–82.

Matheis, H.: Die Entstehung und ursaechliche Behandlung des Hallux valgus. Ztschr. Orthop. Chir. *48:*1–21, 1927.

Mauclaire, P.: Ostéoplasties, arthroplasties et transplantations tendineuses combinées pour traiter l'hallux valgus. Rev. Orthop. *31:*305–313, 1924.

Mikhail, I. K.: Bunion, hallux valgus and metatarsus primus varus. Surg. Gyn. Obst. *111:* 637–646, 1960.

Nélaton, A.: *Elémens de Pathologie Chirurgicale.* Paris, G. Baillière, 1859, Vol. 5, pp. 969–971.

Petri, C.: Zur Behandlung von Vorfussdeformitaeten. Ztschr. Orthop. Grenzgb. *70:*343–349, 1940.

Reverdin, J.: De la déviation en dehors du gros orteil (hallux valgus, vulg. "oignon," "bunions," "Ballen") et de son traitement chirurgical. Trans. Internat. Med. Congr. *2:*408–412, 1881.

Robinson, H. A.: Bunion, its causes and cure. Surg. Gyn. Obst. *27:*343–345, 1918.

Robinson, H. A.: Bunion: its cause and cure. Internat. Clin. *2:*64–76, 1927.

Robinson, H. A.: The etiology of bunion. Mil. Surg. *62:*807–813, 1928.

Sheldon, J. G.: Hallux valgus. Med. Rec., New York, *64:*694–695, 1903.

Stein, H. C.: Hallux valgus. Surg. Gyn. Obst., *66:* 889–898, 1938.

Truslow, W.: Metatarsus primus varus or hallux valgus? J. Bone Joint Surg. *7:*98–108, 1925.

Tubby, A. H.: *Deformities Including Diseases of the Bones and Joints.* London, MacMillan & Co., 1912, Vol. 1, pp. 716–729.

Ullmann, E.: Die Behandlung des Hallux valgus mittels Sehnenplastik. Wiener Med. Wchnschr. *49:*2091–2092, 1894.

Walsham, W. J., and Hughes, W. K.: *The Deformities of the Human Foot.* London, Baillière, Tindall & Cox, 1895, pp. 496–514.

Weir, R. F.: The operative treatment of hallux valgus. Ann. Surg. *25:*444–452; see also discussion on pp. 480–485, 1897.

Wertheimer, V.: Our experience with functional stabilization of hallux valgus (in Serbian). Acta Chir. Jugosl. *6:*236–244, 1959.

Young, J. K.: A new operation for adolescent hallux valgus. Univ. Penn. Med. Bull. *23:* 459–468, 1910.

Chapter Fourteen

HALLUX RIGIDUS

No method of treatment for hallux valgus can be considered satisfactory unless commensurate attention is directed toward the accompanying deformities. These are varied and numerous–ingrown toenails, soft and hard corns, and so on. Not infrequently pain caused by an accompanying deformity overshadows discomfort due to hallux valgus. We consider the following as the most disabling: hallux rigidus, deformed smaller toes, and plantar incarceration of the central metatarsal heads. The tangled topic of hallux rigidus may perhaps be unraveled if we discuss it under the following headings: name, subgroups, causation, relation to other deformities, and treatment. After discussing these matters, we shall recapitulate what seems to us pertinent and essential.

Search for an appropriate name. In the literature one meets with a variety of terms used to denote incipient or established arthritis of the metatarsophalangeal joint of the great toe.

Davies-Colley (1887) of Guy's Hospital called attention to an affection of the great toe "of which he had been unable to find any description in surgical writing . . . . The disease," he said, "consisted simply of flexion of the first phalanx of the great toe through 30° to 60°, with extension of the second phalanx, and some swelling and stiffness of the metatarsophalangeal joint." Davies-Colley suggested that the deformity be called *hallux flexus.*

J. M. Cotterill (1888) described the same condition and singled out the following symptoms: "Apparent flexion of the first phalanx of the toe on its metatarsal bone," "inability to dorsiflex the toe," and "pain felt in efforts to dorsiflex the toe, as, for instance in the act of standing on tiptoe." "This pain," Cotterill said, "is usually felt over the dorsal aspect of the joint; at a later stage it may be most marked below the joint, or it may be absent throughout the whole course of the case." Cotterill used the term *hallux rigidus.*

Anderson (1891), preferred the term *hallux flexus,* which he said "may be defined as progressive diminution of the normal range of extension at the metatarsophalangeal, or more rarely, at the interphalangeal joint of the great toe . . . ."

Collier (1894) conceded that in hallux rigidus "the proximal phalanx is slightly flexed but never," he added, ". . . to such an extent as to warrant the application of the term hallux flexus." Commenting on Collier's paper, Cotterill (1894) said: "Strictly speaking, the great toe is not flexed on the metatarsal bone, but the metatarsal is, so to speak, flexed on the great toe; and therefore I objected to the term "hallux flexus," which was proposed by Mr. Davies-Colley, as misleading in pathology. This term should be restricted to those rare cases of pure plantar flexion of the hallux due to contraction of the muscles from spinal or other causes associated with flatfoot. . . ."

Davies-Colley joined the controversy. Referring to his original communication, Davies-Colley (1895) wrote: "I wrote a short account of one of the deformities of the great toe, to which I gave the name hallux flexus. Soon after reading this paper many articles and letters appeared on the subject of this and an allied deformity to which Mr. Cotterill has given the name hallux rigidus." Davies-Colley considered "the two affections . . . closely allied. The stiff great toe to which the term 'rigidus' has been applied," he wrote, "is a condition in which the first phalanx of the toe, while capable of complete flexion, cannot be extended beyond the straight line with the metatarsal bone. In the deformity called hallux flexus the first phalanx is flexed, and is often capable of still further flexion, but it cannot be extended even as far as the straight line with the first metatarsal bone. Both hallux flexus and hallux rigidus are alike in the fact that the first phalanx cannot be extended with anything like the normal range of movement; they differ only in the precise point at which the movement of extension is arrested. Hallux flexus may therefore be considered to be a more extreme form of hallux rigidus." Davies-Colley thus regarded the two conditions as being basically alike and differing only in the degree of dorsiflexion they did or did not permit.

Walsham and Hughes (1895) regarded *hallux flexus, hallux rigidus,* and *painful great toe* synonymous but preferred the term *hallux dolorosus.* Hiss (1937) favored the epithet *limitus.* Lambrinudi (1938) introduced the term *metatarsus primus elevatus* and suggested the possibility of its evolving into hallux rigidus later in life. Lapidus (1940) used the name *dorsal bunion.* More than one author has utilized the term *metatarsus nonextensus.* Inadequate as it is, *hallux rigidus* remains the most commonly accepted term designating degenerative arthritis of the first metatarsophalangeal joint.

Subgroups. Longuet (1904) distinguished several subgroups of hallux flexus and qualified them with the following adjectives: traumatic, neuroparalytic, dystrophic or senile, congenital, and adolescent. Nilsonne (1930) distinguished between primary and secondary hallux rigidus. He considered the latter an ordinary arthritis deformans caused by injury to the big toe and occurring mainly in older individuals; primary hallux rigidus manifested itself between the ages of twelve and fifteen years. Lelièvre (1952) separated hallux flexus completely from hallux rigidus. He ascribed the former mainly to paralytic and congenital causes and to severe flatfoot, and considered hallux rigidus an arthrosis of the metatarsophalangeal joint without any skeletal misalignment. Lelièvre further distinguished juvenile arthrosis from that occurring in adults and in the aged. The most commonly accepted classification is that given by Nilsonne: *primary* and *secondary* hallux rigidus, the latter being a sequel to longstanding valgus deformity of the great toe.

Causation. Davies-Colley (1887) considered two causes: injury to the joint followed by contraction similar to that observed in the knee joint; and the pressure of short rigid boots on an abnormally long great toe. He did not think flatfoot had much to do with the deformity. Cotterill (1888) thought hallux rigidus proper was "due to the invariable combination of flatfoot and boot pressure." Collier (1894) wrote: "The victims of this disorder are usually young persons at or about puberty. Males would appear to be more often affected than females (the same being true of flatfoot), no doubt due to the fact that young males are more frequently employed in arduous work, necessitating more standing and the carrying of heavier weights than in the case of young females."

Haward (1900) reported the case of "a boy aged 15 years who was admitted to the hospital on account of lameness due to the condition known as hallux rigidus. The patient is employed in the post office and has much standing," Haward wrote. He added: "There was a slight degree of flatfoot, and the right metatarsophalangeal joint was rigid, painful and incapable of voluntary movement. The position of the bones was not altered and there was no pain on moderate interarticular pressure, but any attempt to walk or to bear any weight on the foot gave severe pain."

"Hallux rigidus," Jansen (1921) wrote, "is due to extra strain upon the first metatarsophalangeal joint. It is apt to develop in people with slightly everted foot, in which the line of gravity in walking passes nearer the first metatarsal than normally. Hence in people with muscle weakness, especially those who have outgrown their strength, that is, the type of slight feebleness of growth. Their feet and hands are, as a rule, moist, blue and cold."

According to Nilsonne (1930), secondary hallux rigidus "is an ordinary arthritis deformans, quite common in elderly patients with deforming changes in some other small joints of the foot, or a local process arising from trauma of the great toe." Primary hallux rigidus, Nilsonne thought, usually manifests itself between the ages of 12 and 15 years in long, narrow feet with a marked falling down of the "metatarsal arch" and an unusually long first metatarsal bone. In the roentgenogram of a young girl, age 13, with symptoms of hallux flexus, Kingreen (1933) noticed evidences of fragmentation of the epiphysis of the proximal phalanx similar to the changes seen in Perthes'–Calvé's, or Kohler's–disease.

McMurray (1936) associated hallux rigidus with a long, narrow toe. Jack (1940) said the upward thrust of the first metatarsal head in the initial stage of the step injured the joint. "The cause of hallux rigidus," Bingold and Collins (1950) wrote, "is an abnormal gait developed either to protect an injured or inflamed joint from pressure of weight-bearing, or to stabilize a hypermobile first metatarsal. The effects of gait are to transfer most of the pressure from the flexor brevis tendon and the sesamoids to the base of the first phalanx. Excessive pressure on this joint predisposes to osteoarthritis."

Alt (1950) related hallux rigidus to "focal inflammatory affection" and chronic rheumatism. Breitenfelder (1951) saw a close relation between hallux rigidus and the "dorsal supination" of the anterior part of the foot, particularly of the heel in pes planus.

Kessel and Bonney (1958) studied ten adolescent and four adult patients with hallux rigidus. In two cases they noticed evidence of osteochondritis dissecans of the metatarsal head but did not think this was a common cause. Steinhauser (1959) examined two children, one aged 11 and another 13 years. Both had pain in the basal joint of the big toe. The roentgenograms were interpreted as showing growth disturbance of the epiphysis of the proximal phalanx. Steinhauser suspected avascular necrosis of this epiphysis and considered it a cause of hallux rigidus.

Relation to hallux valgus. Davies-Colley (1887) thought the condition he called hallux flexus, and others renamed hallux rigidus, would in time probably evolve into hallux valgus. The converse, however, is more true. Almost all cases of advanced hallux valgus are accompanied by osteoarthritis of the first metatarsophalangeal joint—in other words by secondary hallux rigidus.

Jansen (1921) pointed out that "hallux valgus, rigidus and malleus may occur separately but very often they are associated. Two principles make themselves felt in these conditions," he wrote, "disturbance of muscle balance which is most prominent in hallux valgus" and "joint wear, the arthritis deformans of text books . . . most prominent in hallux rigidus . . . ." Arthritis of the metatarsophalangeal joint was, he argued, accompanied by osteophytes: "the lipping causes pain from pressure in walking mostly on the plantar side, which contraction of the flexor brevis tries to forestall. The overexertion of this muscle leads to its permanent involuntary contracture. Thus, hallux malleus develops which, however, may also occur without primary hallux valgus by cramp of flexor brevis hallucis. The malleus position is apt to cause the abductor hallucis to slide downward and thus to strip it of its abduction power. When adductors prevail, hallux malleovalgus very frequently evolves . . . frequently hallux valgus is attended by hallux rigidus."

Speaking of hallux rigidus, hallux flexus, and hammer toe, Lake (1952) had this to say: "These conditions are quite commonly associated with hallux valgus, when they form but a part of the deformity of the foot as a whole, and so tend to be overshadowed. The terms are usually reserved for cases where there is little lateral deviation of the toe and where, therefore, they constitute the main deformity. Both conditions are essentially the same thing, the only difference being in the former the toe is held in extended position, or even slightly dorsiflexed, whereas in the latter it is rigidly plantarflexed."

Hallux rigidus and metatarsus elevatus. "The distortion of the foot," Collier (1894) wrote, speaking of hallux rigidus, "is characteristic and peculiar, and is due to the fact that any pressure between the head of the metatarsal bone and the sesamoid bones on the tendons of the short flexor cannot be tolerated. The metatarsal bone is flexed on the tarsus and is adducted to the midline from its fellows . . . ." Lambrinudi (1938) revived Collier's concept of the first metatarsal being "flexed on the tarsus," which according to the terminology of the period, would mean dorsiflexion. Lambrinudi coined a new term – *metatarsus primus elevatus* – and thought it likely "the condition may be responsible for a certain number of cases of hallux rigidus."

Lapidus (1940) considered hallux rigidus as one of the causes of "dorsal bunion"–the other three being paralytic deformities of the foot, congenital clubfoot, and severe congenital talipes planovalgus. "During the first stage of a step," Jack (1940) wrote, ". . . the upward thrust of the short flexors is unopposed, with the result that instead of rotating normally the head tends to ride forwards and upwards against the rim of the first phalanx constantly repeated with every step, this tendency of the first metatarsal head to push upwards, and forwards against the upper rim of the fixed phalanx is sufficient to strain the attachment of the dorsal capsular ligament, and to traumatize the articular cartilage of the joint, particularly on the phalangeal side where the epiphysis is not consolidated. The reaction to this trauma is a protective spasm of the short flexor in an attempt to fix the joint, but this merely increases the upward thrust under the metatarsal head, and so aggravates the trauma." He considered the metatarsal elevation primary and the joint disorder secondary.

Hallux rigidus and "winkle-picker's disease." Wilson (1960) described a condition of "tenosynovitis of the long extensor tendon of the hallux," which was said to be "usually associated with the dorsal osteophyte formation of hallux rigidus. The introduction of the new style of women's shoes, nicknamed winkle-picker, because of its sharp point," we are told, "has been responsible for the lesion becoming more prevalent. The shoe differs from its predecessors in that the proximal open rim of the toecap lies much more distally than previously, and therefore crosses the big toe joint beyond the metatarsophalangeal joint." Irritation from this rim is said to produce reactive tenosynovitis of the extensor tendon.

Treatment. Davies-Colley (1887) "excised the proximal half of the first phalanx, leaving the head of the metatarsal bone, with the sesamoid bones, and interfering as little as possible with the attachments of the muscles." Collier (1894) resected the head of the metatarsal bone. Watermann (1927) performed a cuneiform osteotomy of the head of the first metatarsal with the base of the wedge directed dorsalward. The osteotomy included the dorsal spur. Cochrane (1927) performed plantar capsul-

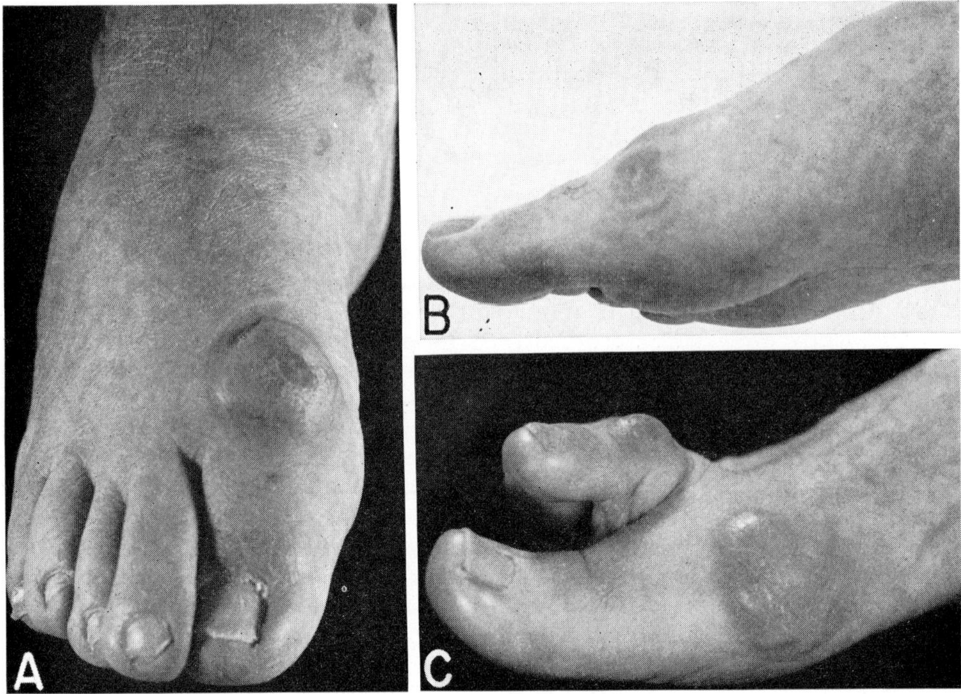

Figure 14–1. Gross appearance of hallux rigidus. Note the flexed position of the hallux in the photographs, which represent three different cases.

otomy of the first metatarsophalangeal joint and released the short flexor from the proximal phalanx. For incipient hallux rigidus Watson-Jones (1927) prescribed "correct size of boot"–that is, "three sizes larger than the number indicated on the measure-stick." In moderate cases he performed a "muscle slide" operation of the short flexor of the great toe. For what he called "the second stage of the traumatic type of hallux rigidus," he advised "manipulation under anaesthesia, followed by protection as above"–that is, corrective shoes. "In the final stage," he wrote, "where pathological changes have gone on from capsular contraction to cartilagenous erosion and osteophyte formation, a bone operation is clearly indicated, whether it takes the form of Mayo's operation, Kellar's (note the spelling, H.K.) operation, or a modified procedure." McMurray (1936) wrote: "The most satisfactory operation for the condition has been that of removal of the base of the phalanx. When this is carried out care should be taken to make certain that at least half of the phalanx is removed at the time of operation; if less than this is taken the usual result is painful fibrous ankylosis and the patient may even complain of more pain than previously." Severin (1947–1948) also favored resection of the proximal portion of the basal phalanx of the great toe.

McKeever (1952), Smith (1952), Bingold (1950), and many others have recommended fusion of the first metatarsophalangeal joint.

Kessel and Bonney (1958) carried out the same kind of osteotomy as had Watermann (1927), except that instead of removing the wedge of bone from the head of the first metatarsal, they removed it from the base of the proximal phalanx.

Recapitulation. Hallux flexus, rigidus dolorus, malleus, limitus nonextensus, and so on–synonymously used by various authors–merely describe one symptom or another: flexion deformity, rigidity, pain, hammering, limitation of motion and inhibition of extension. Metatarsus primus elevatus emphasizes the dorsal tilt of the first metatarsal head, and dorsal bunion refers to the spur on the top of it. The basic disturbance is the wear-and-tear type of arthritis of the big toe joint—osteoarthritis. Arthritis of the first metatarsophalangeal joint, without marked outward deviation of the great toe, is called hallux rigidus. Osteoarthritis of this joint often accompanies valgus deviation of the great toe. When the sesamoids are involved in the degenerative joint changes, the condition is called sesamoiditis or chondromalacia of the sesamoid bones. In these cases pain, disfunction, or disability may be due to arthritis. Arthritic spurs may become impinged upon and cause discomfort. In arthritis, forced movement beyond the limits allowed by interlocked articular surfaces is not tolerated. On the

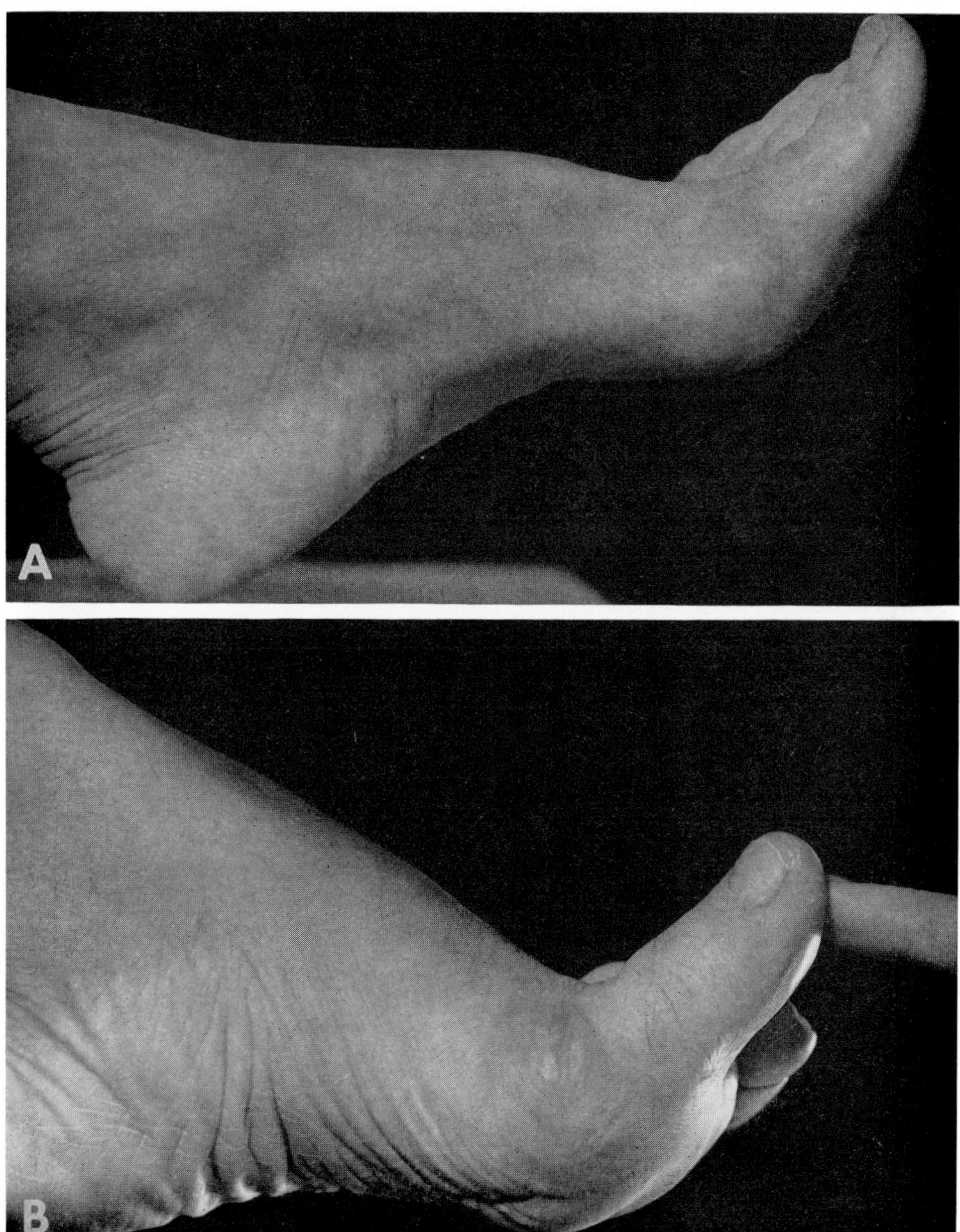

Figure 14–2. Normal range of active (*A*) and passive (*B*) entension of the great toe in a woman approximately 60 years of age.

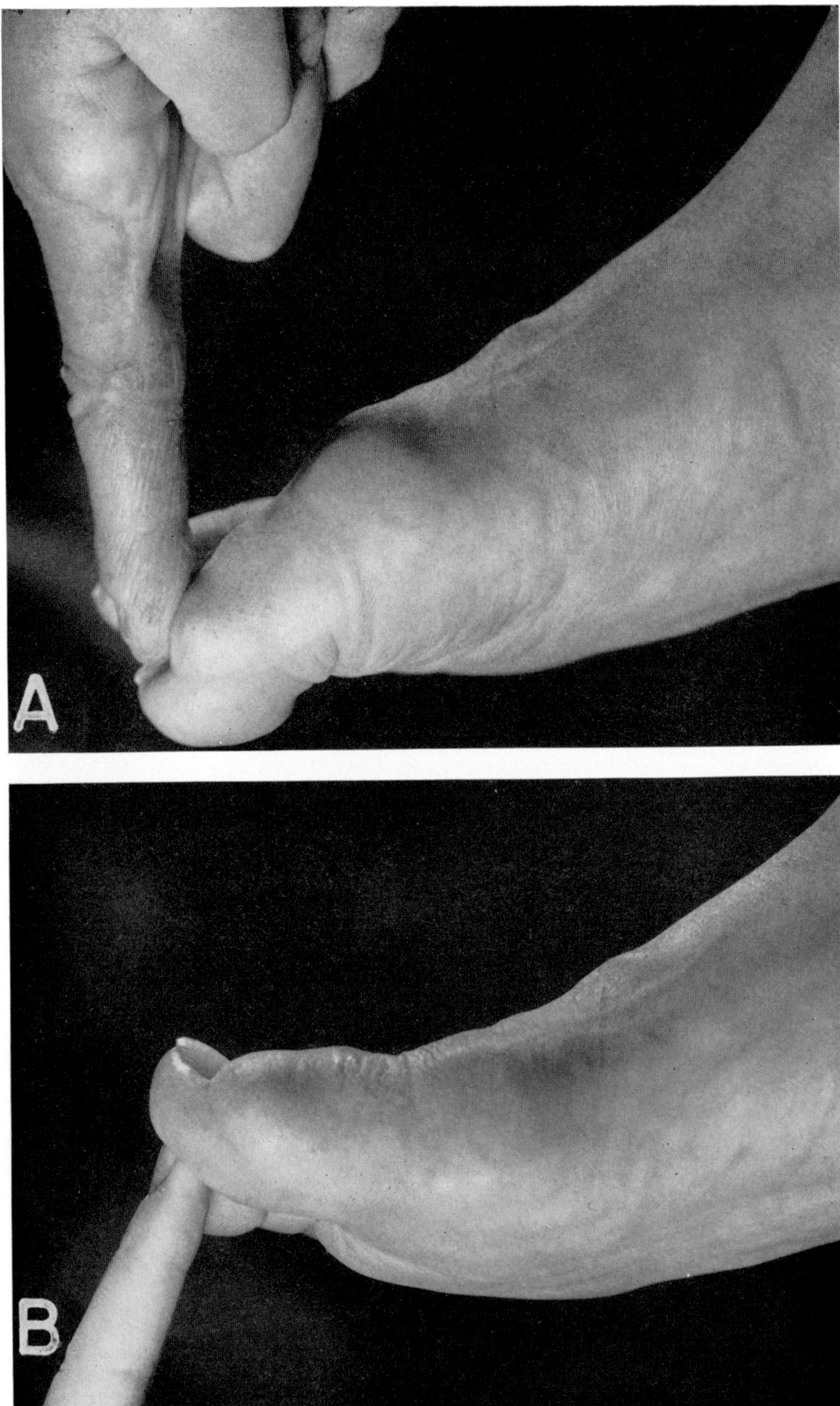

Figure 14–3. Limitation in passive range of flexion (*A*) and extension (*B*) of the great toe at the metatarsophalangeal joint of a young woman with hallux rigidus.

other hand, in the absence of arthritic changes at the joint, the pressure of footwear on the medially displaced metatarsal head—or laterally deviated great toe—also may cause discomfort. In uncomplicated hallux valgus, the pain is more severe when shoes are worn; in hallux rigidus without valgus deviation of the great toe or large dorsal spurs, shoes afford a measure of support and comfort, but prolonged weight-bearing will precipitate pain.

The main symptoms of hallux rigidus are pain in or around the first metatar-

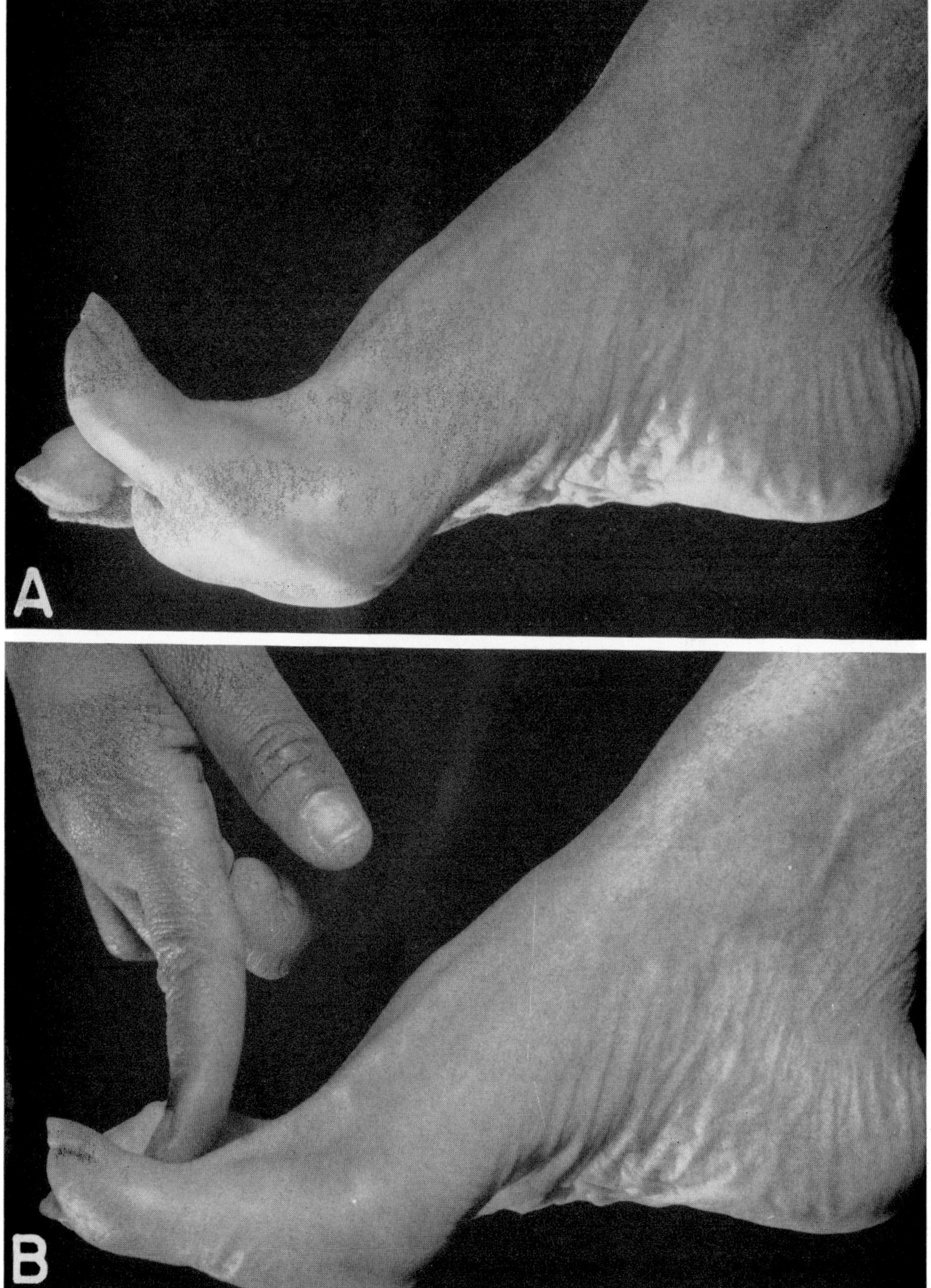

Figure 14–4. Hallux extensus (*A*). The great toe cannot be pushed plantarward (*B*).

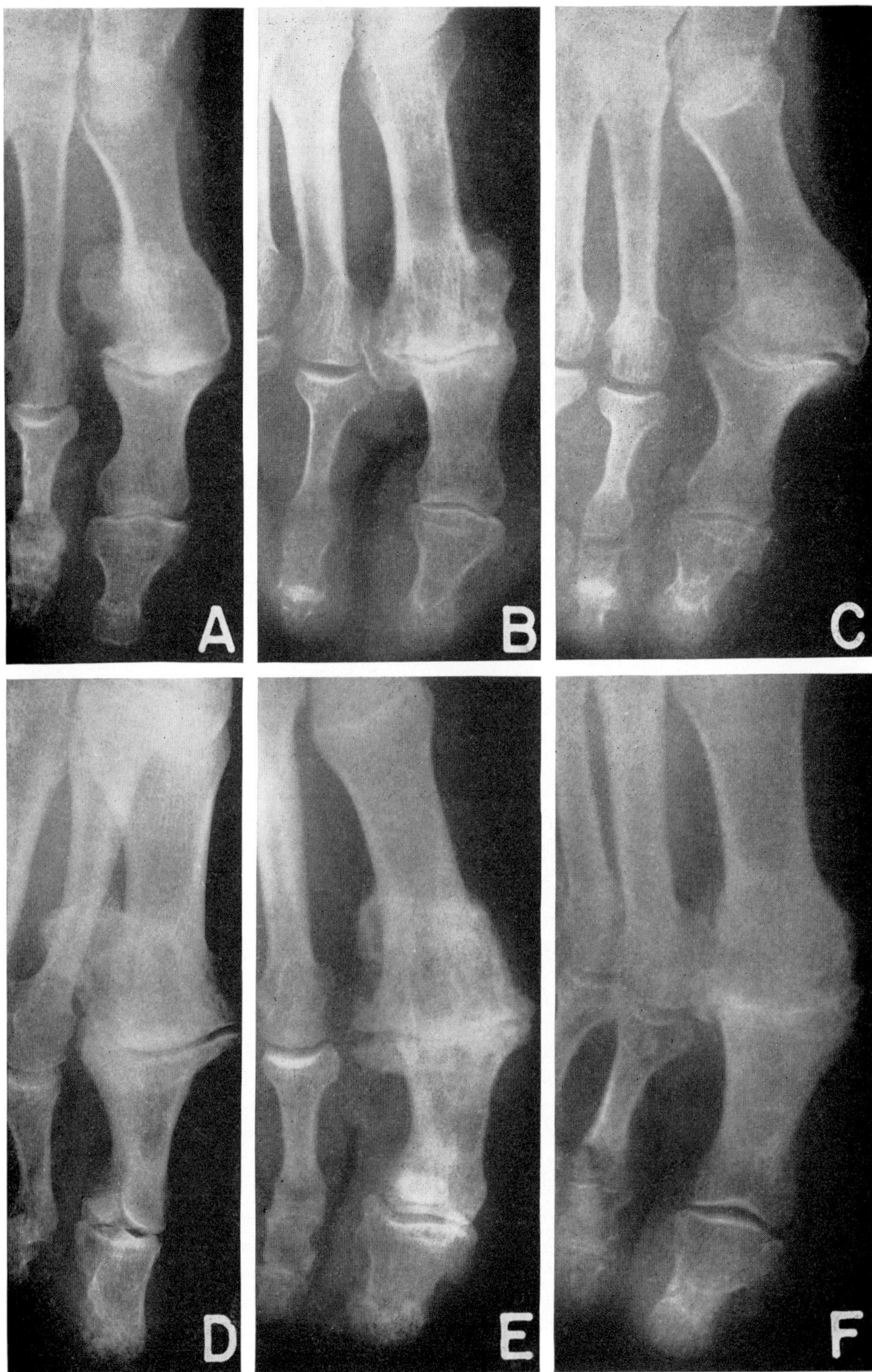

Figure 14–5. Roentgenographic manifestations of hallux rigidus.

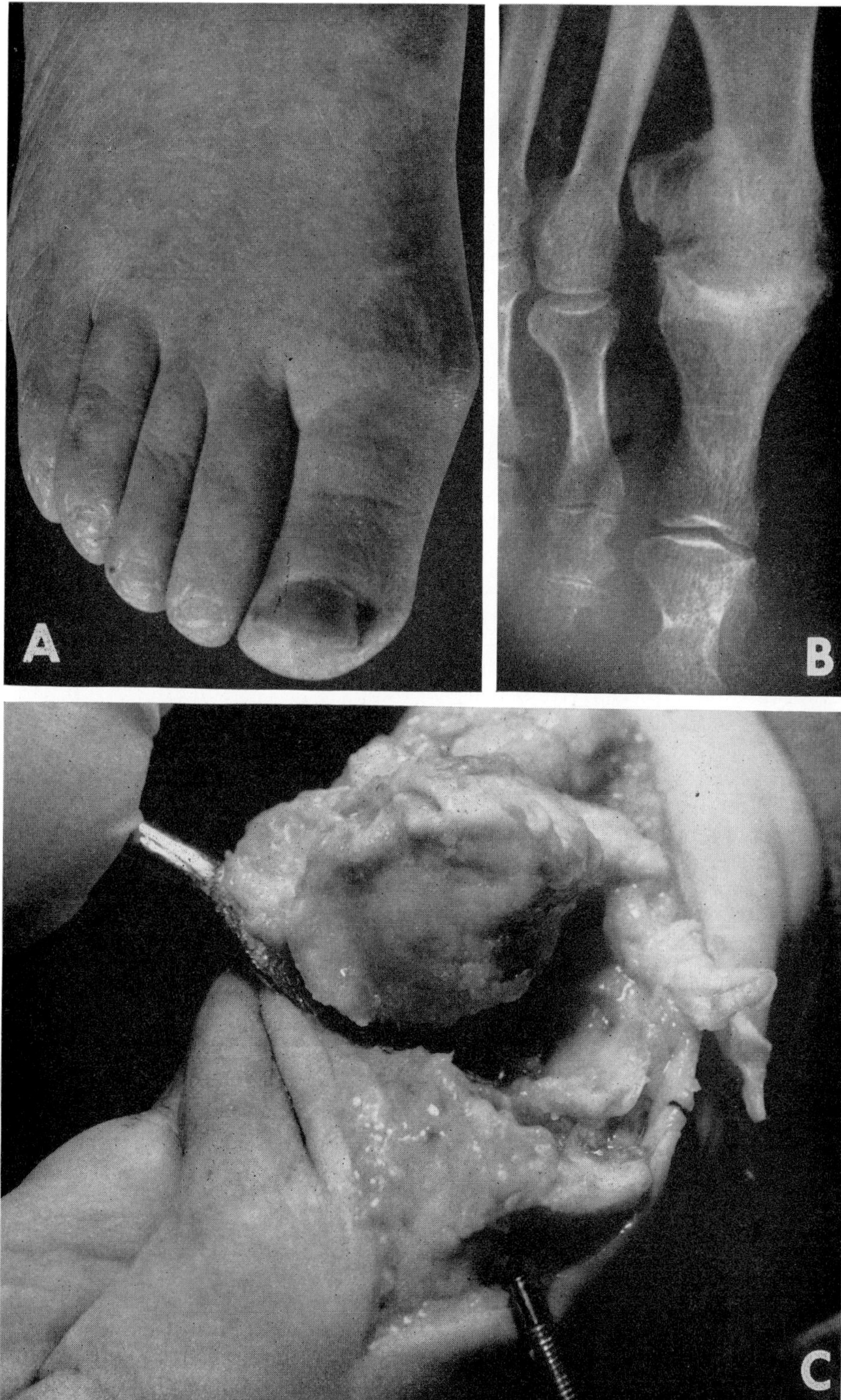

Figure 14–6. Primary hallux rigidus. Photograph of the forefoot (*A*). Roentgenogram (*B*). Surgically exposed first metatarsal head (*C*). Note the extensive central erosion of its hyaline surface and the proliferation of peripheral bone.

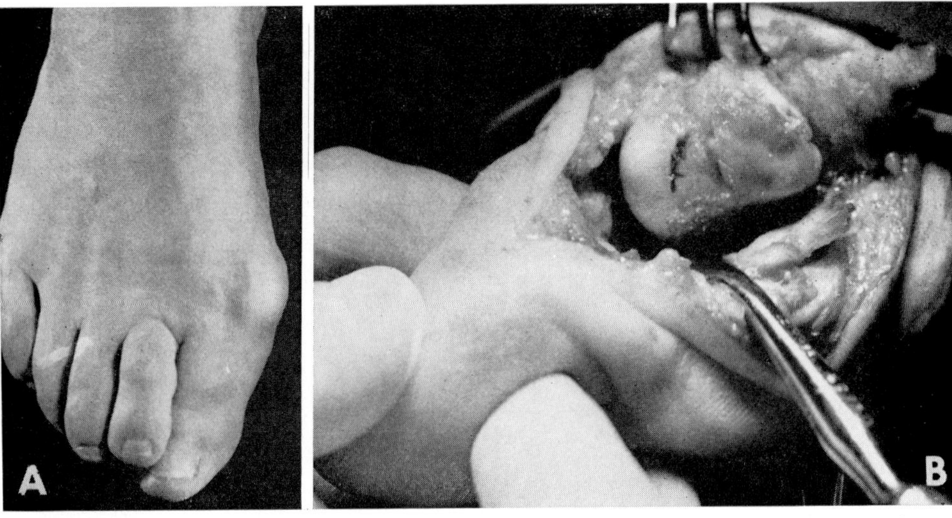

Figure 14–7. Secondary hallux rigidus associated with valgus deformity of the great toe. The surgically exposed first metatarsal head is not as extensively eroded as in Figure 14–6.

sophalangeal joint and limitation of motion. The pain is worse upon rising on the toes. The great toe is held in flexed position and cannot be pushed up. Less commonly, the converse is true; the great toe is fixed in extension and cannot be depressed. The last variety is spoken of as hallux extensus. One may palpate osteophytes occasionally. Roentgenograms may reveal narrowing or obliteration of the articular space and formation of marginal spurs. After surgical exposure the first metatarsal head is seen to bear a central ulcer with peripheral proliferation. Erosion of the hyaline surface is more extensive in primary hallux rigidus than in degenerative arthritis associated with valgus deformity of the great toe (Figs. 14–1 to 14–7).

Primary hallux rigidus–unassociated with hallux valgus and more generalized arthritis–is a disease of young adults; males are affected more commonly than females. It is said to favor tapered narrow feet with long first metatarsal or long hallux. In flatfoot the medial border of the foot gains in relative length, the first metatarsal is pushed forward, its base is depressed, and its head tilts up. This is another way of saying that the base of the proximal phalanx shifts plantarward, causing irritation and spasm of intrinsic muscles attached to it–the flexor hallucis brevis in particular. In the early stages, muscular spasm aggravates the flexion deformity of the toe until contractures and articular incongruities set in and the joint becomes interlocked in its final position. Trauma to the first metatarsophalangeal joint, caused by stubbing of the great toe, can result in degenerative arthritis. Senility is protracted trauma. Overweight and mechanical misalignments, such as pes planus and hallux valgus, cause untimely wear of the joint. Epiphysitis of the proximal phalanx of the great toe may occasionally be responsible for the development of hallux rigidus. Osteochondritis dissecans of the first metatarsal head is a rare cause (Fig. 14–8).

Not all cases of hallux rigidus require treatment. Mild grades occurring in young adults may be treated with rest and roomy shoe. One may have to prescribe a transverse bar or an insole; to counteract the inversion of the forefoot, an outer sole wedge may be added. Effacing the obstructing spurs around the margins of the metatarsal head benefit some cases of hallux rigidus. When degenerative joint changes are extensive and there is no associated metatarsalgia, the best treatment is the one Davies-Colley recommended almost three-quarters of a century ago–resection of the proximal half of the first phalanx of the great toe; if sesamoids are involved in the arthritic process, they should be removed. Fusion of the metatarsophalangeal joint is preferable when hallux rigidus is accompanied by metatarsalgia, in which instance the distal third of the second metatarsal is resected and its digit is syndactalized with the first or third toe (Figs. 14–9 to 14–14).

In growing children, the osteotomy of Watermann (1927) should be given a trial. Osteotomy described by Kessel and Bonney (1958) would involve the growth plate of the proximal phalanx (Fig. 14–15).

(References start on page 280.)

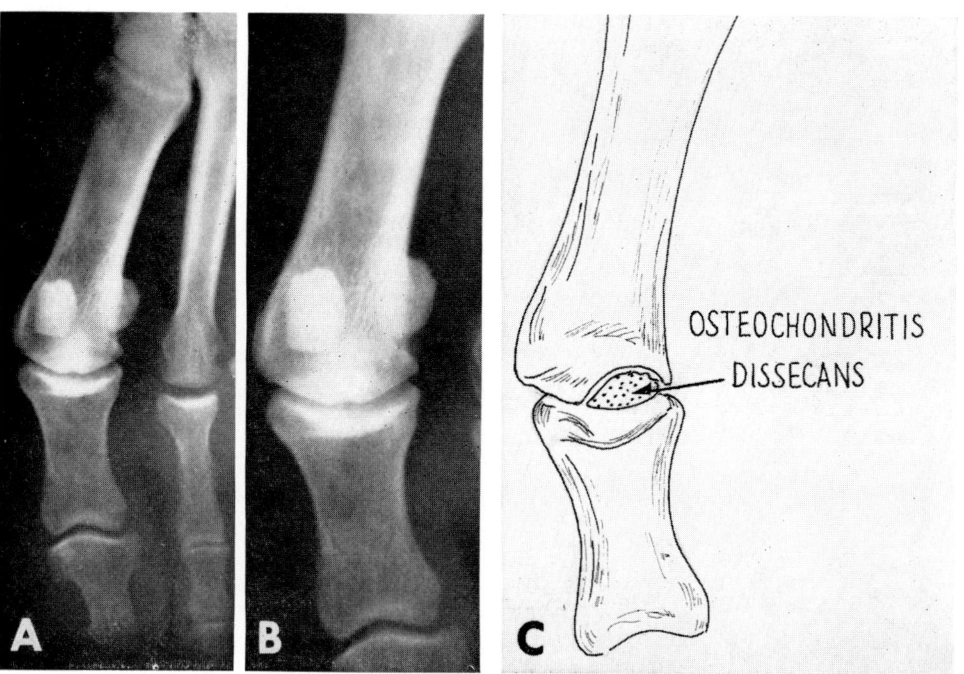

Figure 14–8. Osteochondritis dissecans.

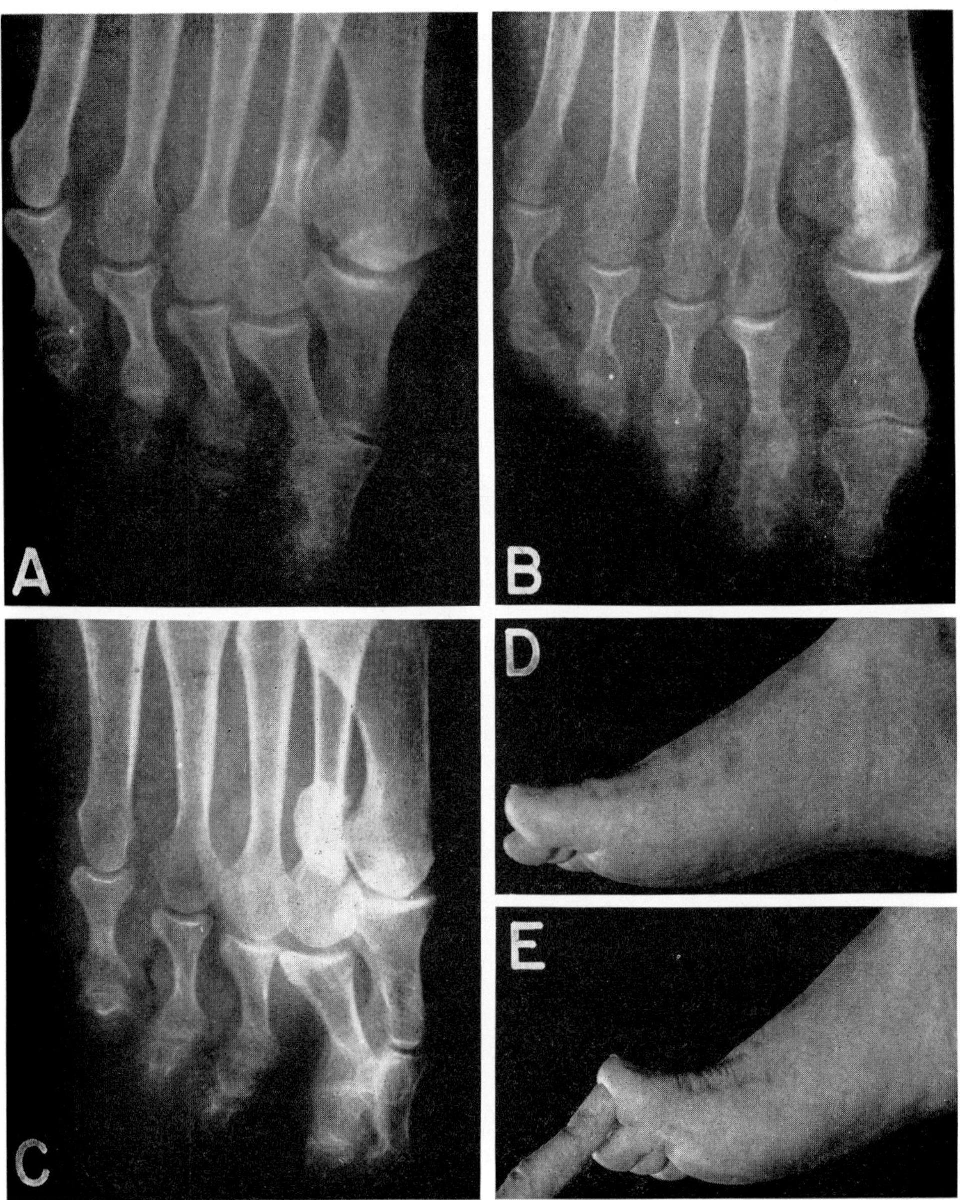

Figure 14–9. Woman with unilateral hallux rigidus. Surgery performed was the remodeling of the metatarsal head. Active extension after surgery (*D*); passive extension (*E*). The patient is satisfied. She can now wear high-heeled shoes with comfort.

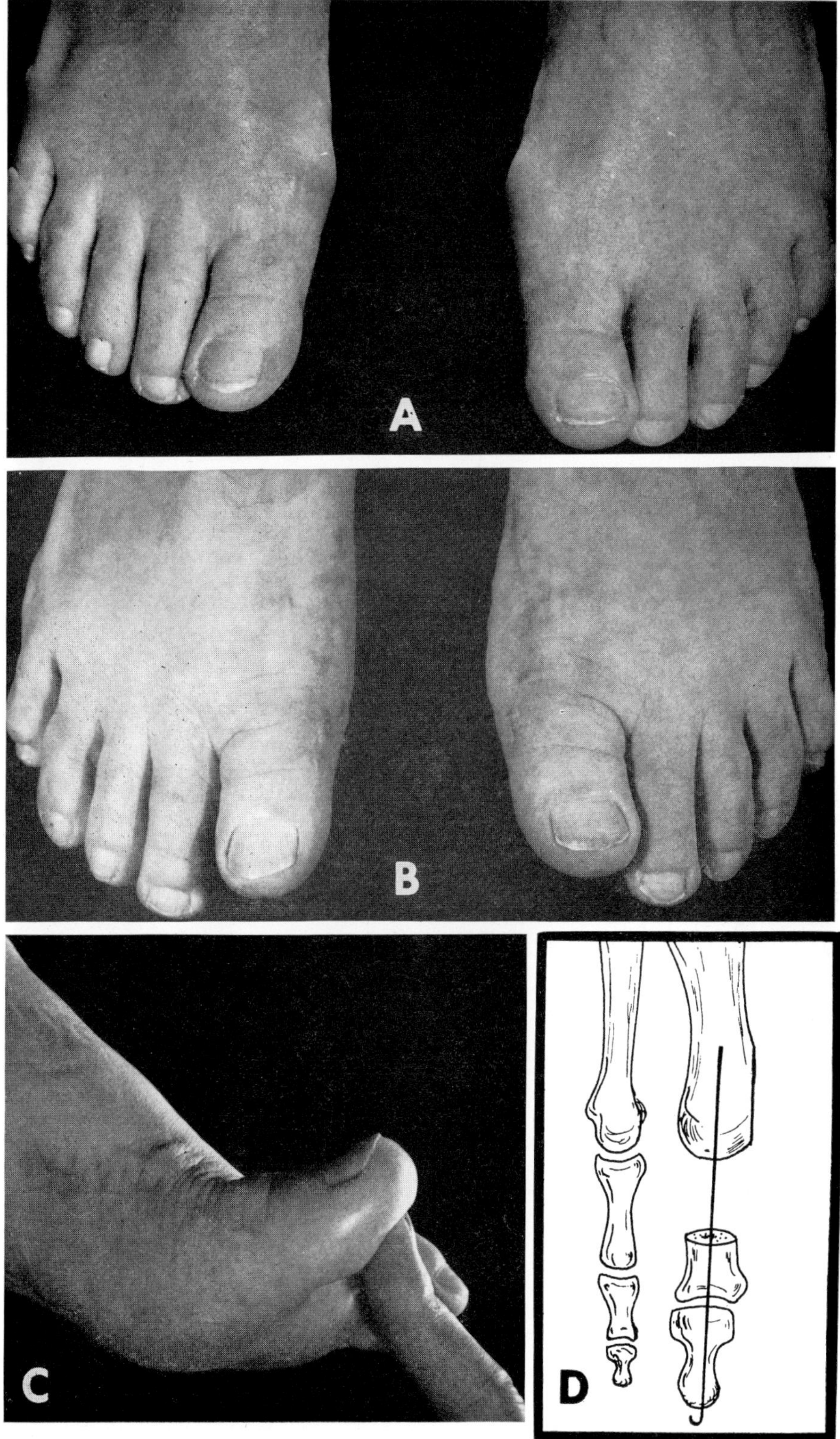

Figure 14–10. Woman with bilateral hallux rigidus. Preoperative photograph (*A*). Postoperative photograph (*B*). Passive extension of right great toe after recovery (*C*). Interpretative diagram (*D*).

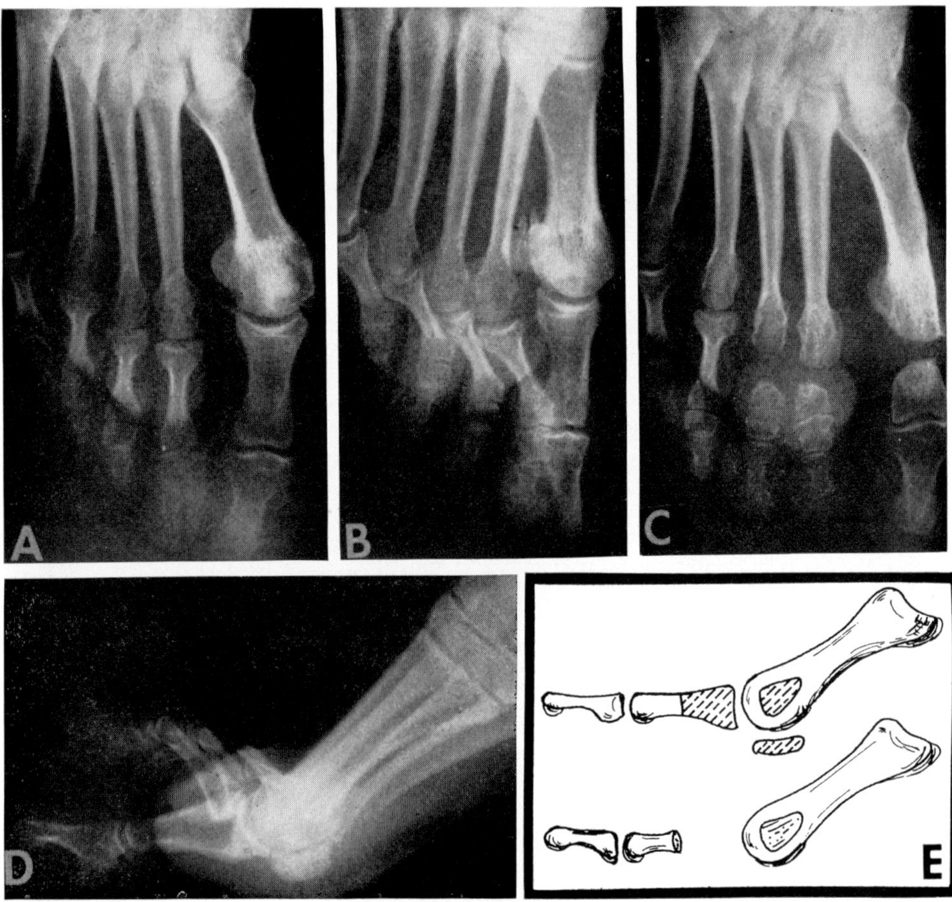

Figure 14–11. Woman with unilateral hallux rigidus and hammered second and third toe. Preoperative roentgenograms (*A, B,* and *D*). Postoperative roentgenogram (*C*). Interpretative diagram showing resection of the proximal half of the basal phalanx of the great toe and sagittal resection of the medial eminence of the first metatarsal head (*E*). The proximal phalanges of the second and third toes were partially resected and these two digits were surgically syndactylized.

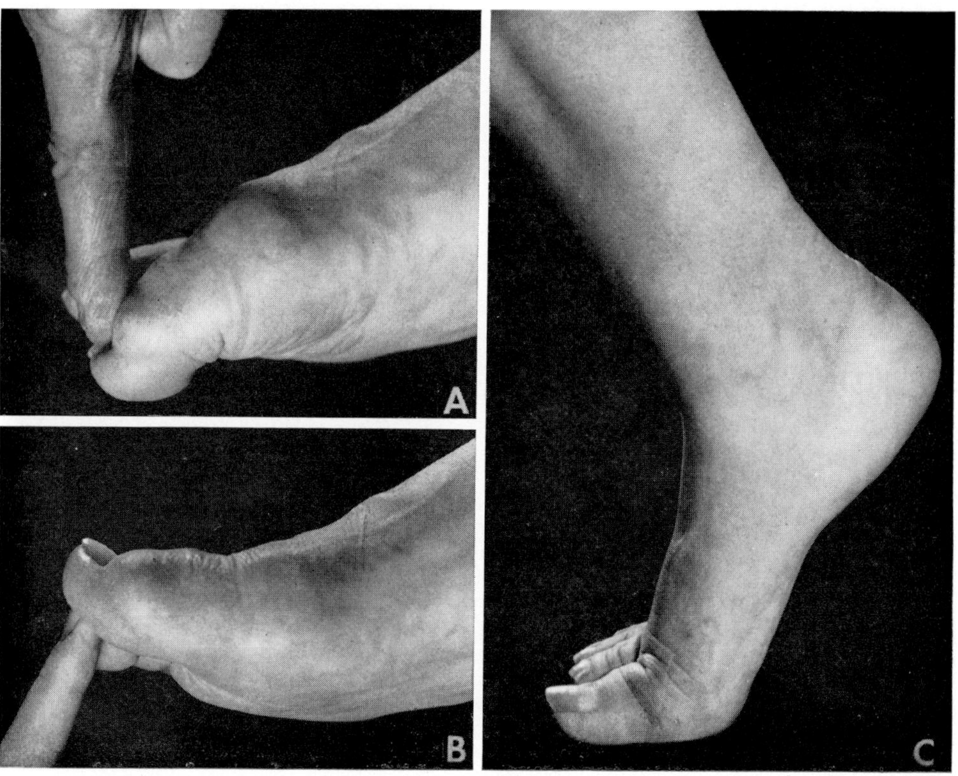

Figure 14–12. Same case as in Figure 14–11. Passive flexion before surgery (*A*). Passive extension (*B*). Patient tiptoeing–without pain (*C*).

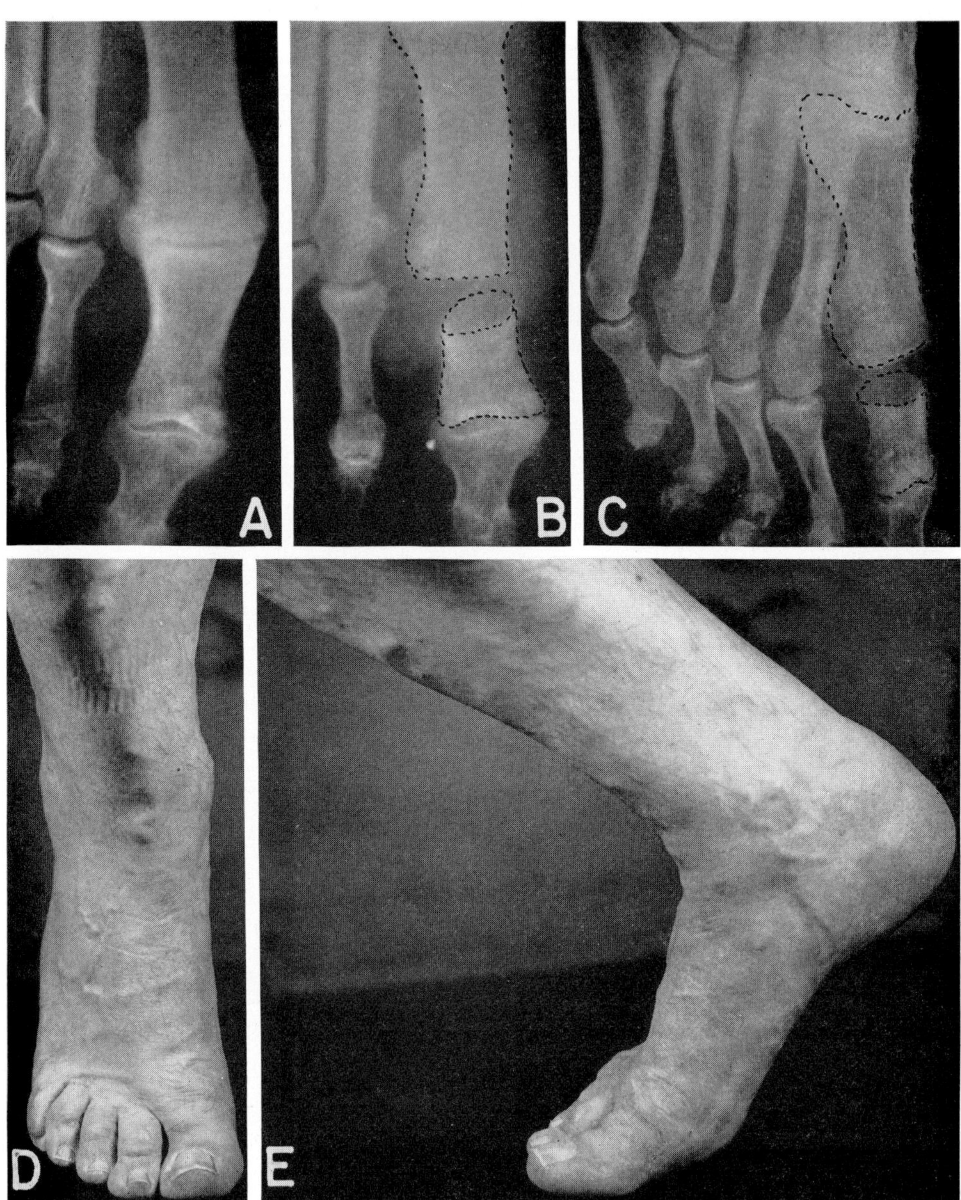

Figure 14–13. Man with unilateral hallux rigidus. Roentgenogram before surgery (*A*). Roentgenograms after surgery (*B* and *C*). Functional results—patient tiptoing without pain (*D* and *E*).

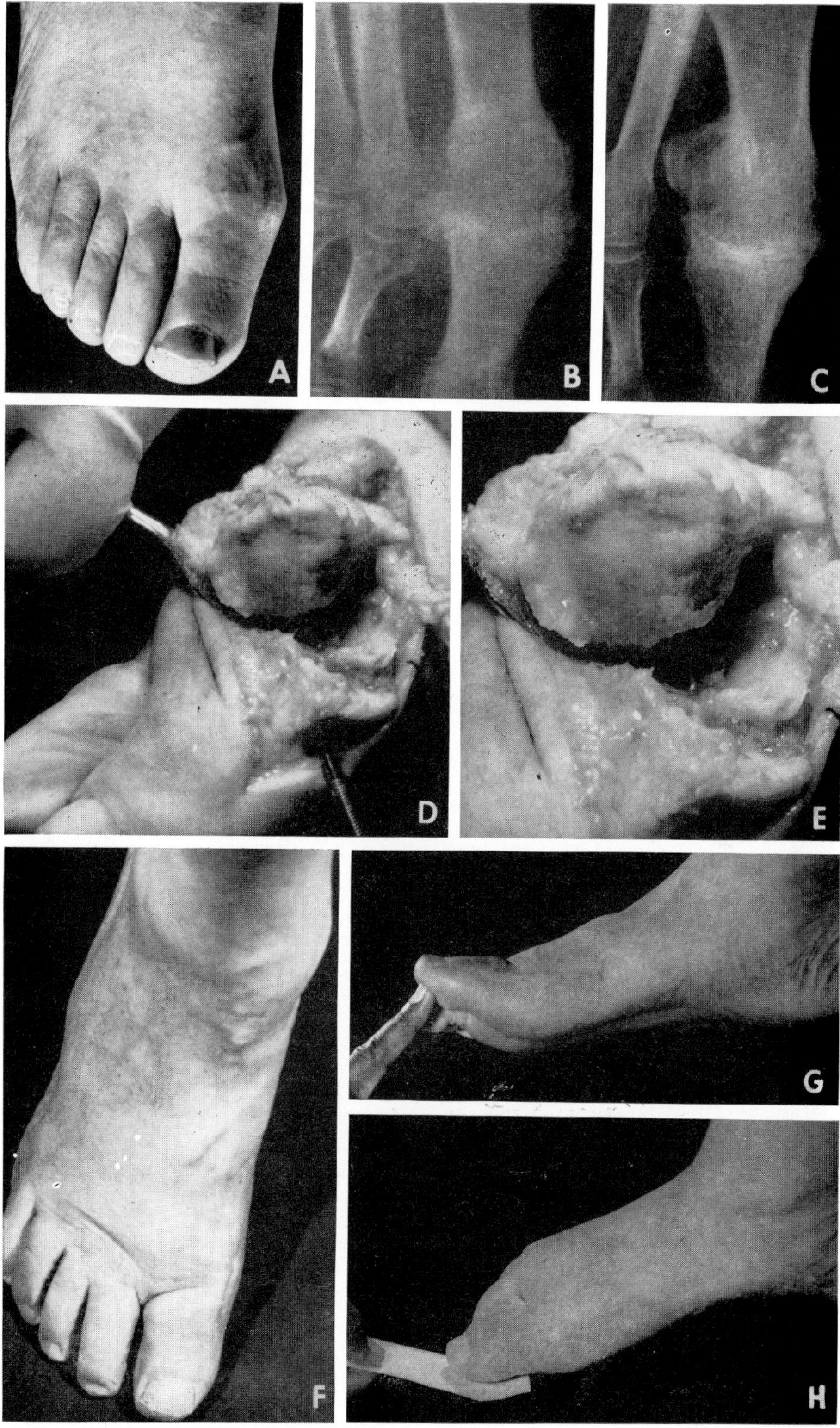

Figure 14–14. Man with unilateral hallux rigidus. Photograph before surgery (*A*). Preoperative roentgenogram (*B* and *C*). Surgical exposure of the metatarsal head (*D* and *E*). Surgery performed was resection of the proximal half of the first phalanx of the great toe. Tiptoing after surgery (*F*). Passive extension (*G*). Postoperative pressing-down action (*H*); a piece of paper pinned by the great toe could not be pulled away without tearing it.

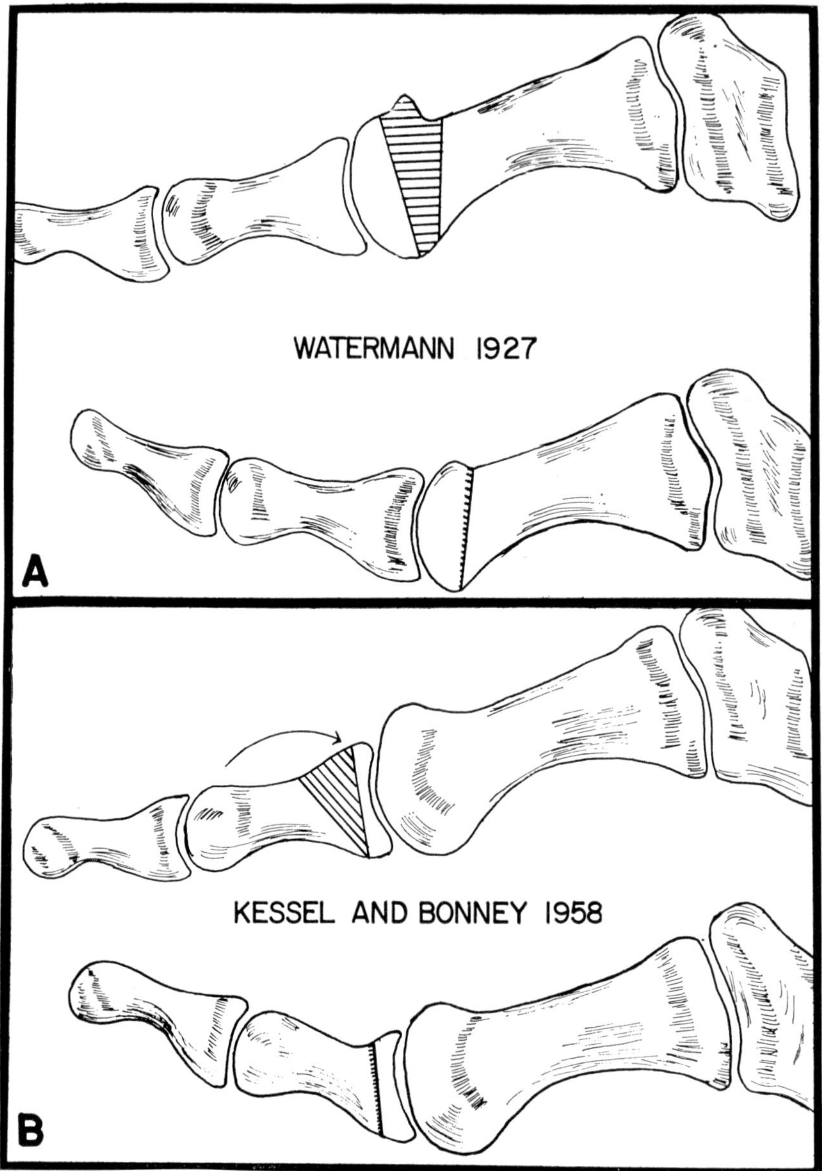

Figure 14–15. Watermann's osteotomy (*A*). Osteotomy described by Kessel and Bonney (*B*).

REFERENCES

Alt., W.: Unsere Ansicht über die Entstehung des Hallux rigidus. Med. Monattsschr. *4*:31–35, 1950.

Anderson, W.: Contractions of the fingers and toes; their varieties, pathology, and treatment. Lancet *2*:279–282, 1891.

Bingold, A. C., and Collins, D. H.: Hallux rigidus. J. Bone Joint Surg. *32*:214–222, 1950.

Breitenfelder, G.: Hallux rigidus Jugendlicher. Verh. Dtsch. Orthop. Ges. *80*:313–317, 1951.

Cochrane, W. A.: An operation for hallux rigidus. Brit. Med. J. *1*:1095–1096, 1927.

Collier, M.: Some cases of hallux rigidus: their symptoms, pathology, and treatment. Lancet *1*:1613–1614, 1894.

Cotterill, J. M.: Stiffness of the great toe in adolescents. Brit. Med. J. *1*:1158, 1888.

Cotterill, J. M.: See Collier's paper, (1894).

Davies-Colley, N.: Contraction of the metatarsophalangeal joint of the great toe (hallux flexus). Brit. Med. J. *1*:728, 1887.

Davies-Colley, N.: On hallux flexus, claw toe and pes cavus. Guy's Hosp. Rep. *52*:1–25, 1895.

Haward, W.: Hammer-toe and hallux valgus and rigidus. Lancet *2*:240–242, 1900.

Hiss, J. M.: *Functional Foot Disorders.* Los Angeles Univ. Press Co., 1937, pp. 251–259.

Jack, E. A.: The aetiology of hallux rigidus. Brit. J. Surg. *27*:492–497, 1940.

Jansen, M.: Hallux valgus, rigidus and malleus. J. Orthop. Surg. *3*:87–90, 1921.

Kessel, L., and Bonney, G.: Hallux rigidus in the adolescent. J. Bone Joint Surg. *40*:668–673, 1958.

Kingreen, O.: Zur Aetiologie des Hallux flexus. Zbl. Chir. *60*:2116–2118, 1933.

Lake, N. C.: *The Foot.* London, Baillière, Tindall & Cox, 1952, pp. 257–264.

Lambrinudi, C.: Metatarsus primus elevatus. Proc. Roy. Soc. Med. *31*:1273, 1938.

Lapidus, P. W.: "Dorsal bunion": its mechanics and operative correction. J. Bone Joint Surg. *22*:627–637, 1940.

Lelièvre, J.: *Pathologie du Pied.* Paris, Masson et Cie, 1952, pp. 331–333.

Longuet, L.: De l'hallux flexus. Rev. Orthop. *15*: 385–441, 1904.

McKeever, D. C.: Arthrodesis of the first metatarsophalangeal joint for hallux valgus, hallux rigidus, and metatarsus primus varus. J. Bone Joint Surg. *34*:129–134, 1952.

McMurray, T. P.: Treatment of hallux valgus and rigidus. Brit. Med. J. *2*:218–221, 1936.

Nilsonne, H.: Hallux rigidus and its treatment. Acta Orthop. Scand. *1*:295–303, 1930.

Severin, E.: Removal of the base of the proximal phalanx in hallux rigidus. Acta Orthop. Scand. *17–18*:77–87, 1947–1948.

Smith, N. R.: Hallux valgus and rigidus treated by arthrodesis of the metatarso-phalangeal joint. Brit. Med. J. *2*:1385–1387, 1952.

Steinhauser, W.: Osteochondrose der basalen Epiphyse der Grundphalanx, Grosszehe und Hallux rigidus. Beit. Ges. Arbeit. Orthop. *6*:177–182, 1959.

Walsham, W. J., and Hughes, W. K.: *The Deformities of the Human Foot.* London, Baillière, Tindall and Cox, 1895, pp. 512–514.

Watermann, H.: Die Arthritis deformans Grosszehengrundgelenkes. Ztschr. Orthop. Chir. *48*: 346–355, 1927.

Watson-Jones, R.: Treatment of hallux rigidus. Brit. Med. J. *1*:1165–1166, 1927.

Wilson, J. N.: "Winkle-picker's" disease. Brit. Med. J. *2*:944, 1960.

Chapter Fifteen

DEFORMITIES OF THE LESSER TOES

As in the case of hallux valgus or rigidus, lack of historical perspective is evident by most authors writing about the deformities of the smaller toes. Here again the dominant tendency is to view sundry malformations as independent entities; interrelations are insufficiently stressed. In most instances no attempt is made to correlate the deformity of the toe with the general derangement of the forefoot or the foot. There is considerable confusion concerning the nature of various deformities.

Malformations of the lesser toes are varied and numerous. When deformed digits of one foot are correspondingly mirrored by the other, one must suspect congenital origin; some of these appear in more than one member of the same family. With a few exceptions, unilateral or asymmetrical deformities are acquired; they often accompany hallux valgus. This is especially true of the second toe, which may ride or lie under the outwardly deviated hallux. More often the second toe is hammered. The second toe is also the favored seat of digital gigantism, which is of congenital origin even though unilateral. The second interdigital space is the one most commonly obliterated by congenital syndactylia. The second and third toes are sometimes seen to diverge from one another; this deformity may be congenital or acquired. Congenital curling has a predilection for the third toe and microdactylia for the third and fourth toes, more often the latter. Soft corn is acquired; it is located almost exclusively in the web between the fourth and fifth toes. At birth the fifth toe is sometimes seen to assume an extended position; in time it inclines medially and mounts over the base of the fourth toe. Supernumerary digits and duplicated or concealed phalanges occur along the free borders of the marginal toes, most commonly on the side of the fifth (Figs. 15–1 to 15–11).

From a clinical point of view the most significant deformities of the lesser digits are: hammertoe, clawtoes, and digitus minimus varus. The others are either rare or rarely require surgical correction.

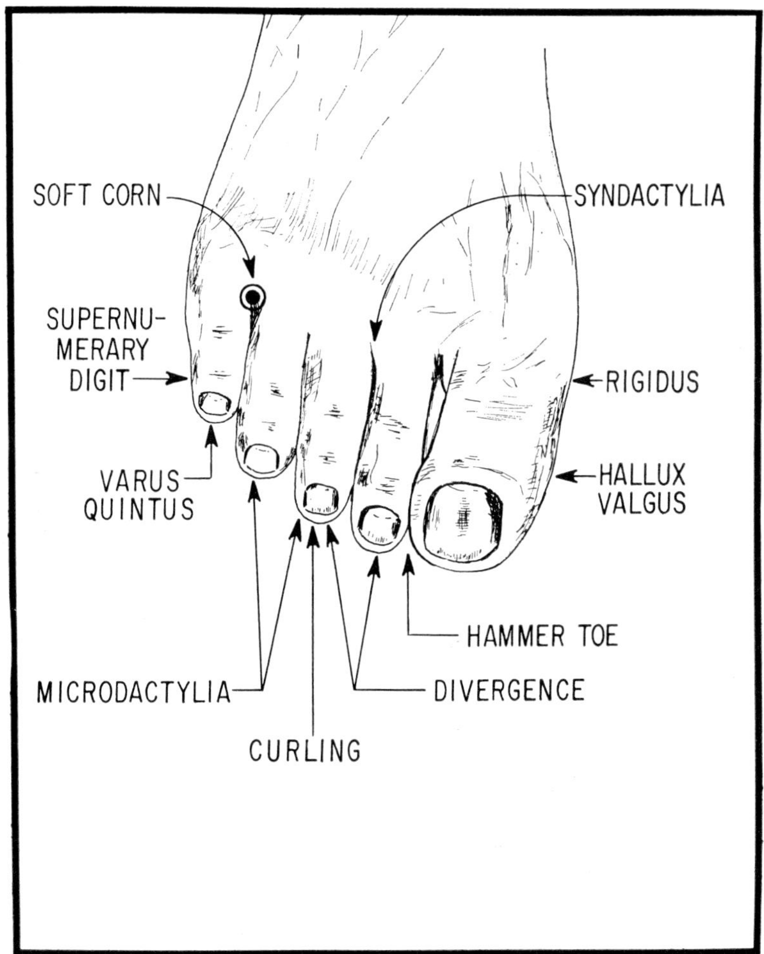

Figure 15–1. Favored sites of various deformities of the toes.

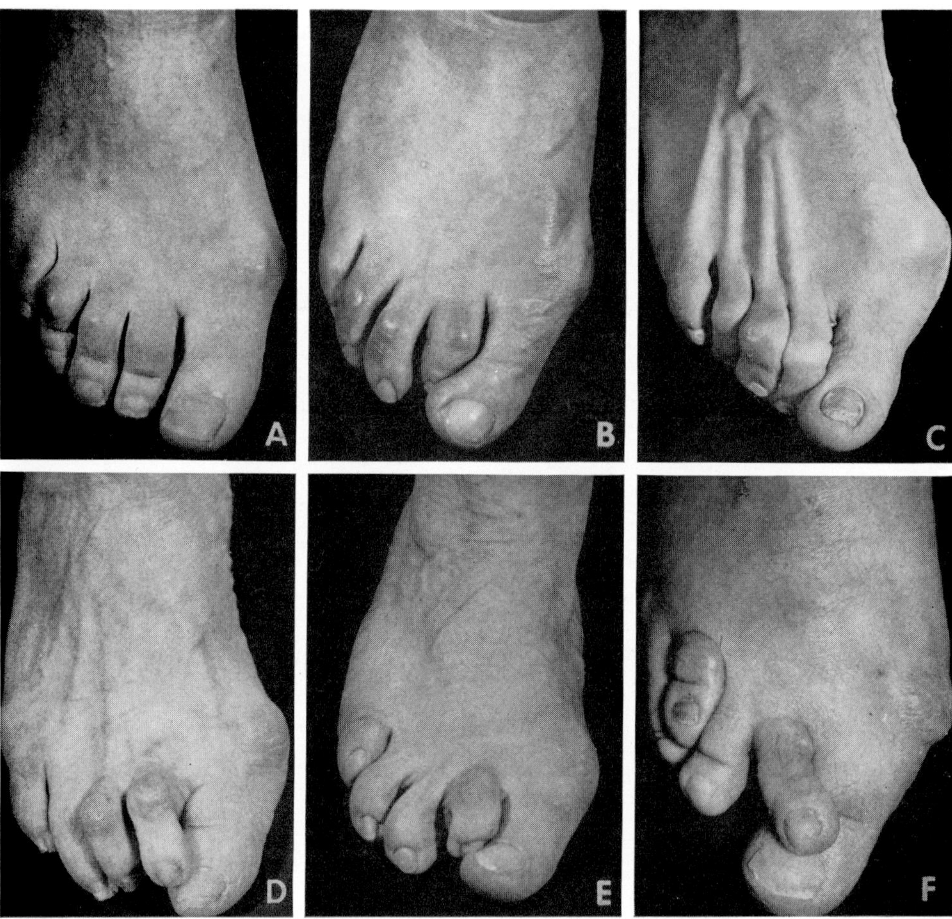

Figure 15–2. Deformities of the lesser toes associated with hallux valgus.

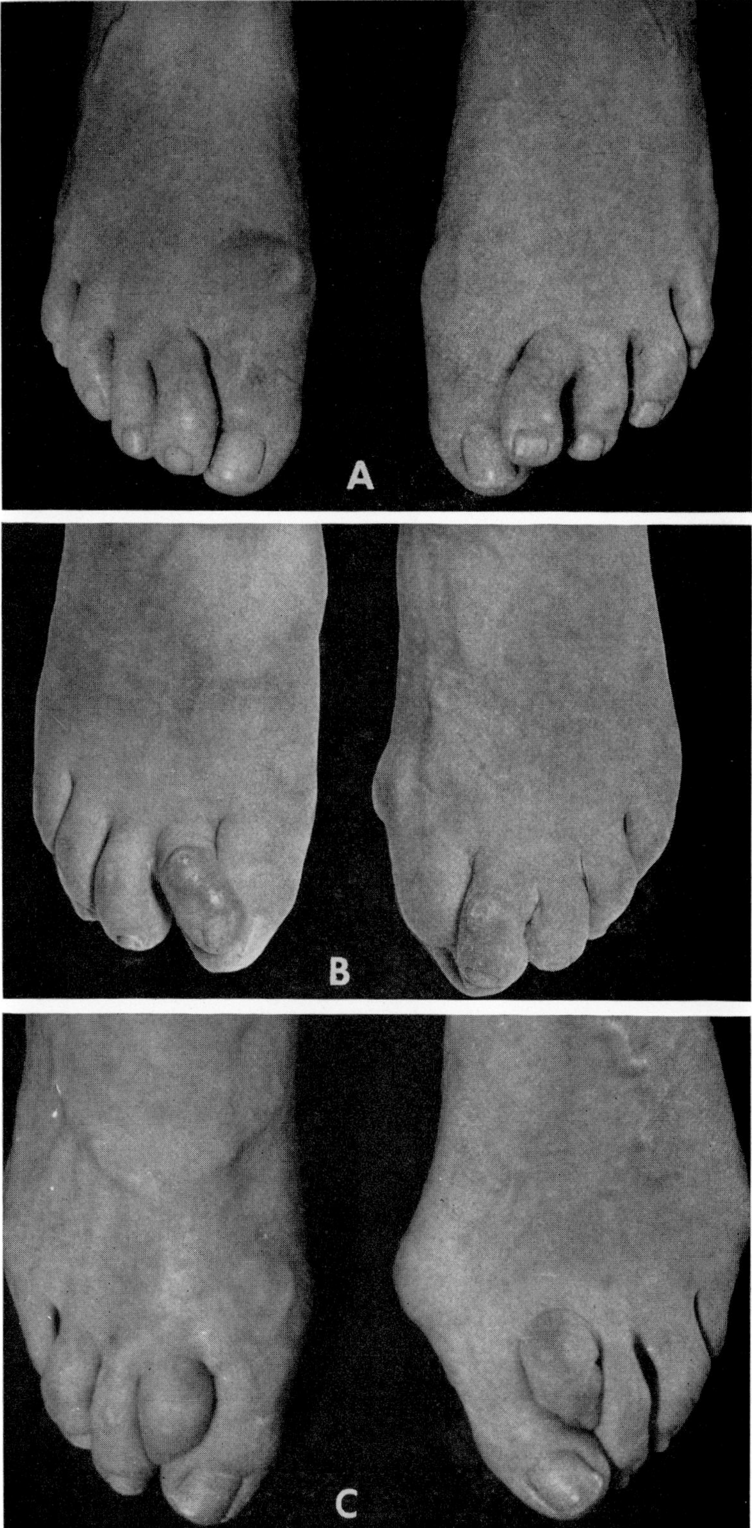

Figure 15–3. Bilateral, symmetrical congenital deformities of the second toe. Interphalangeal valgus deformity of the second toes (*A*). Overriding second toes (*B*). Hammered second toes (*C*).

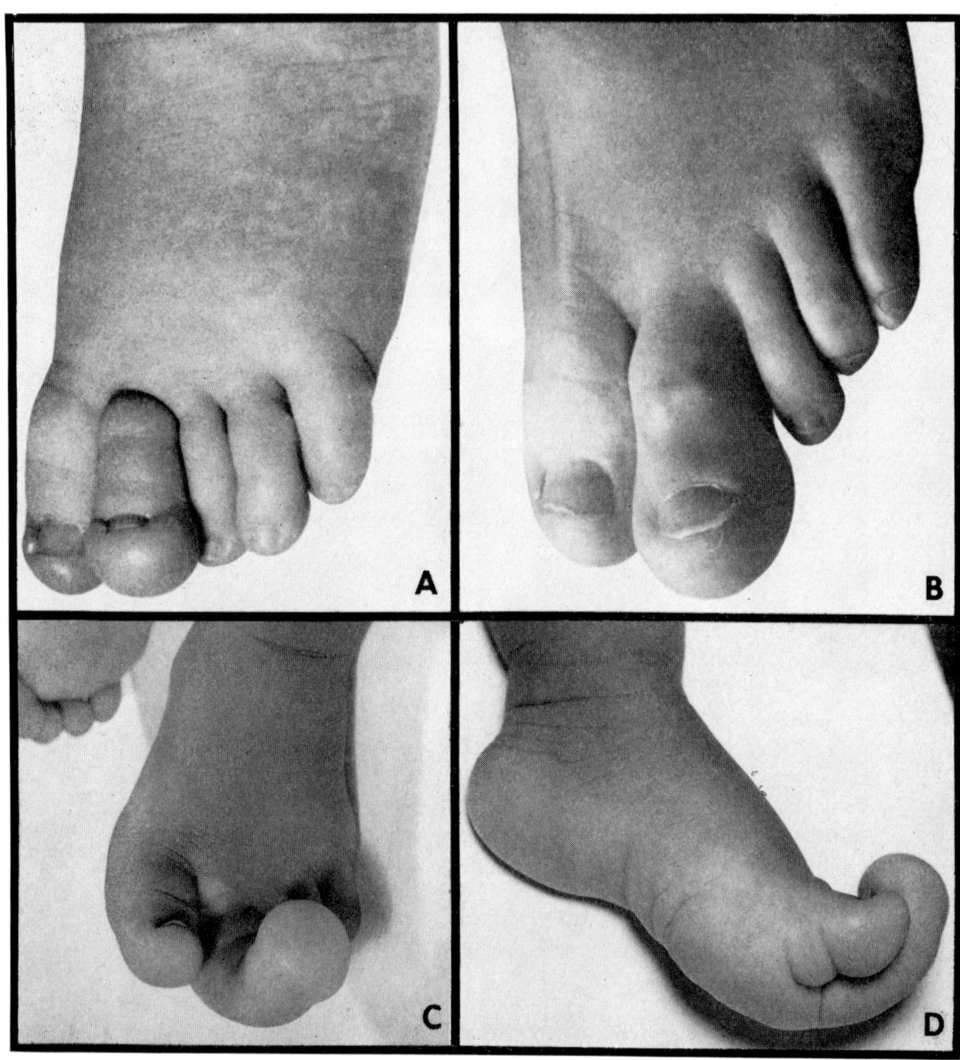

Figure 15–4. Unilateral digital gigantism. Patients in (*A*) and (*B*) were white children. Patient in (*C*) is a colored child; viewed from the medial side (*D*). All these children were females.

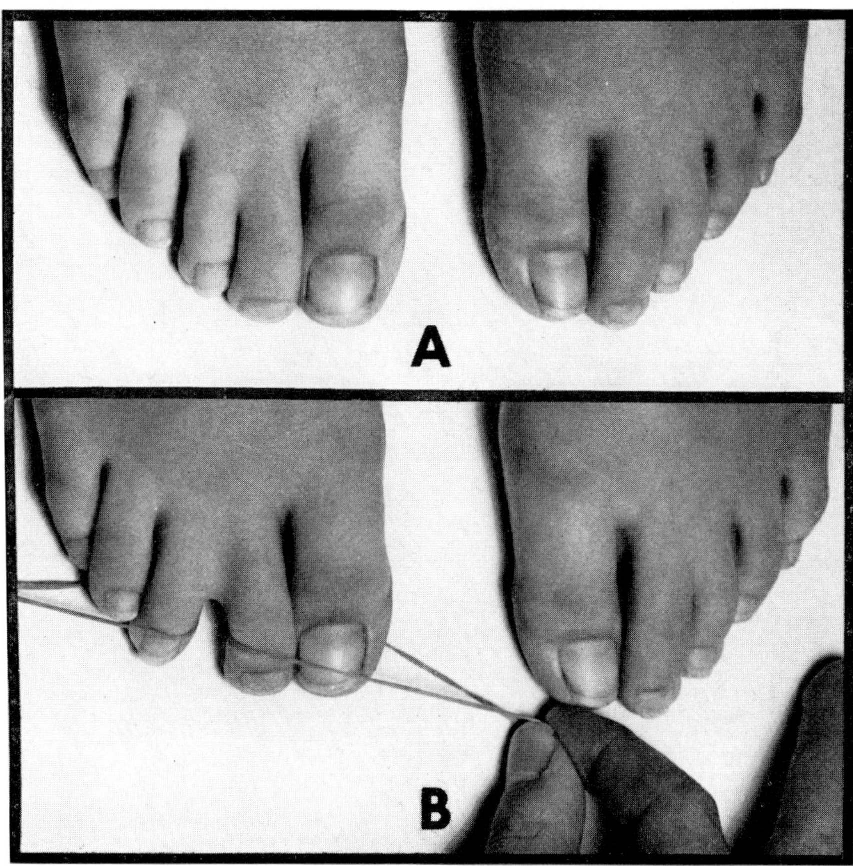

Figure 15–5. Congenital syndactylia of the toes.

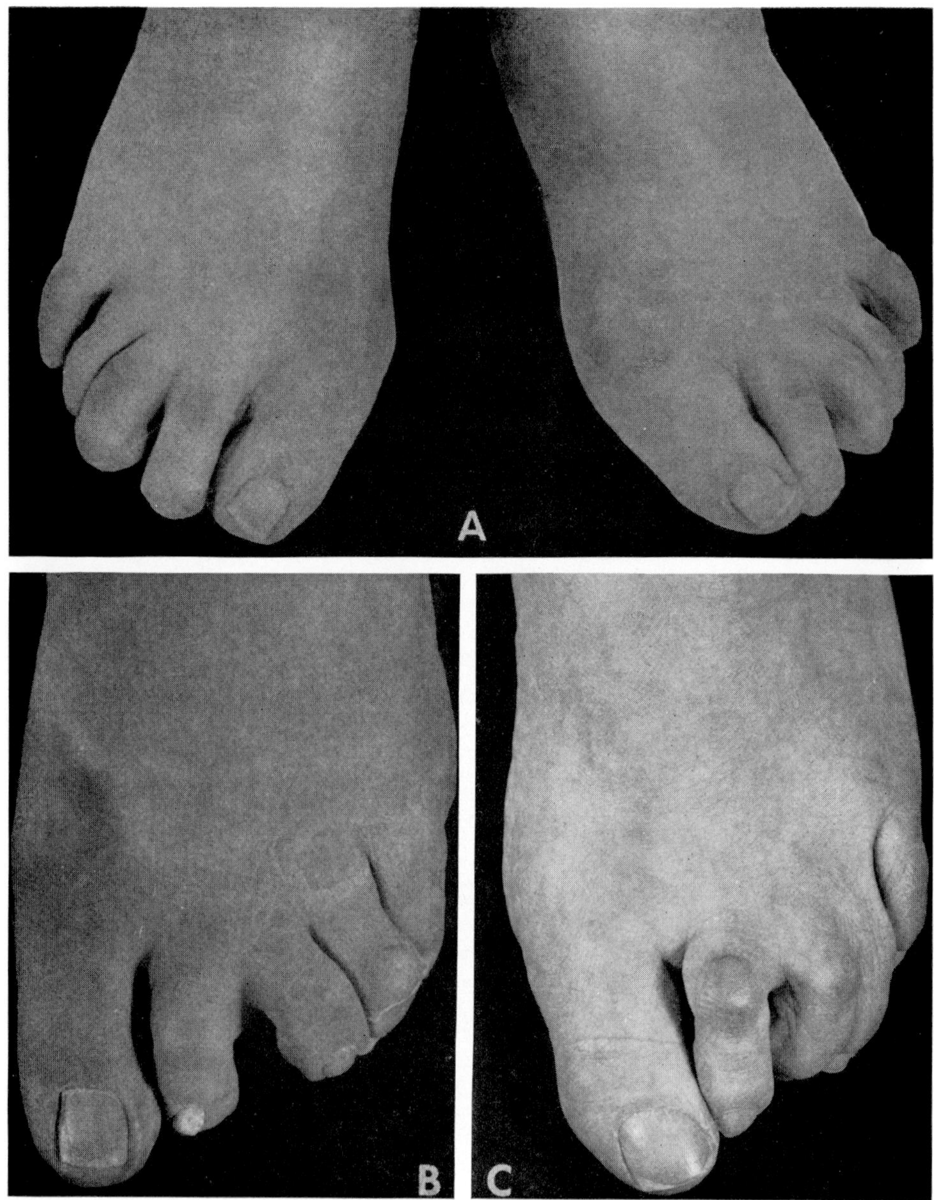

Figure 15–6. Diverging toes. Bilateral congenital (*A*). Unilateral congenital (*B*). Unilateral acquired (*C*).

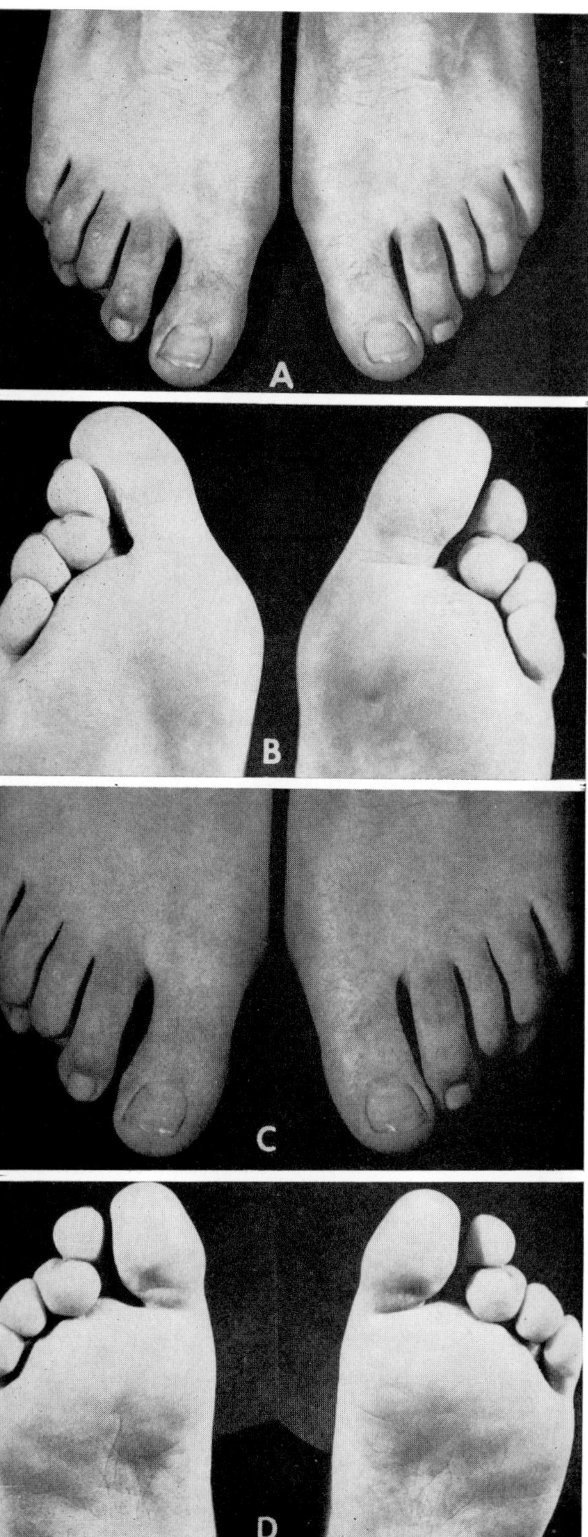

Figure 15–7. Curling third toes, bilateral congenital. Dorsal and plantar view of the forefoot of a boy aged twenty (*A* and *B*). Similar views of a girl about seven (*C* and *D*). Both are symptomatic.

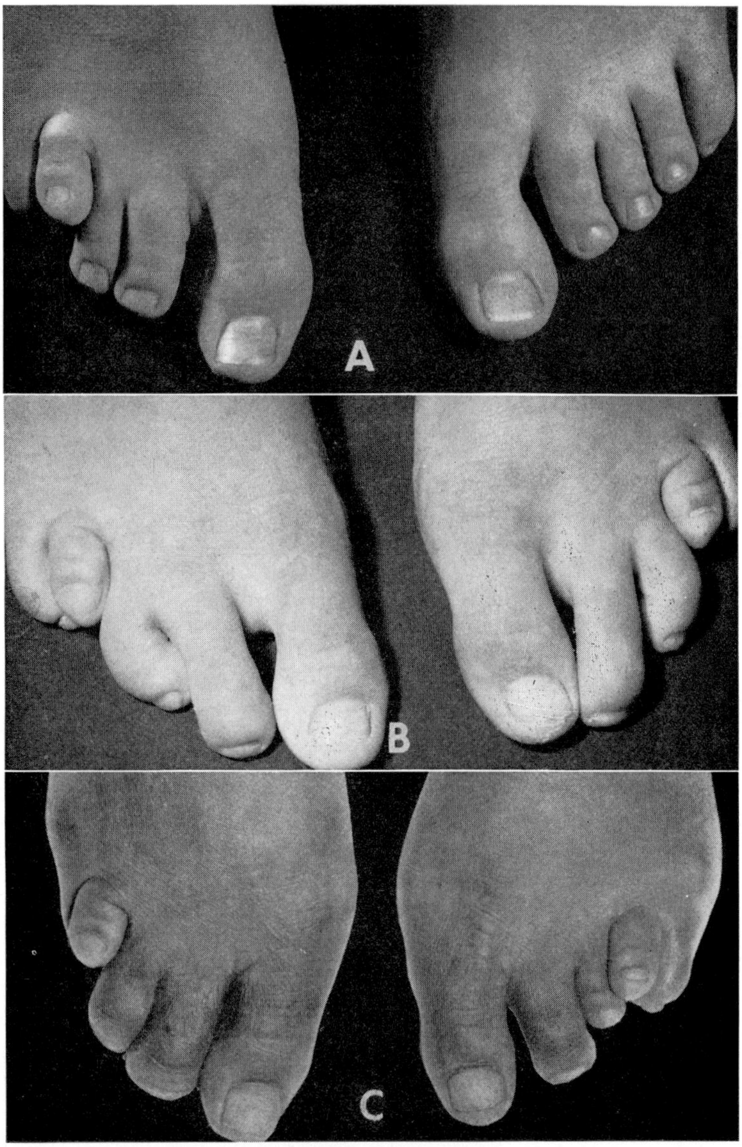

Figure 15–8. Microdactylia.

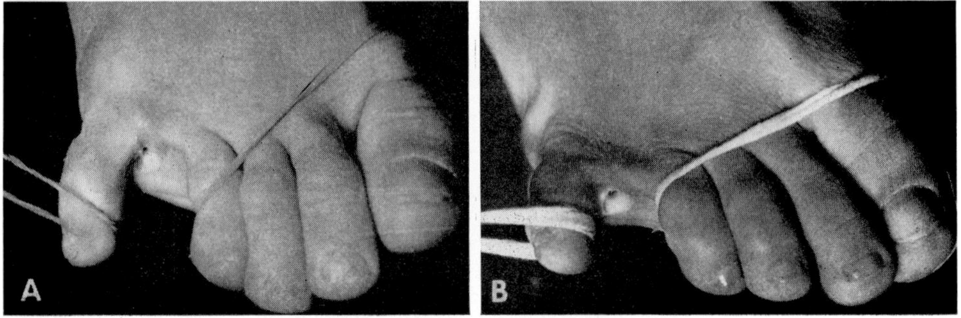

Figure 15–9. Two cases of interdigital soft corn.

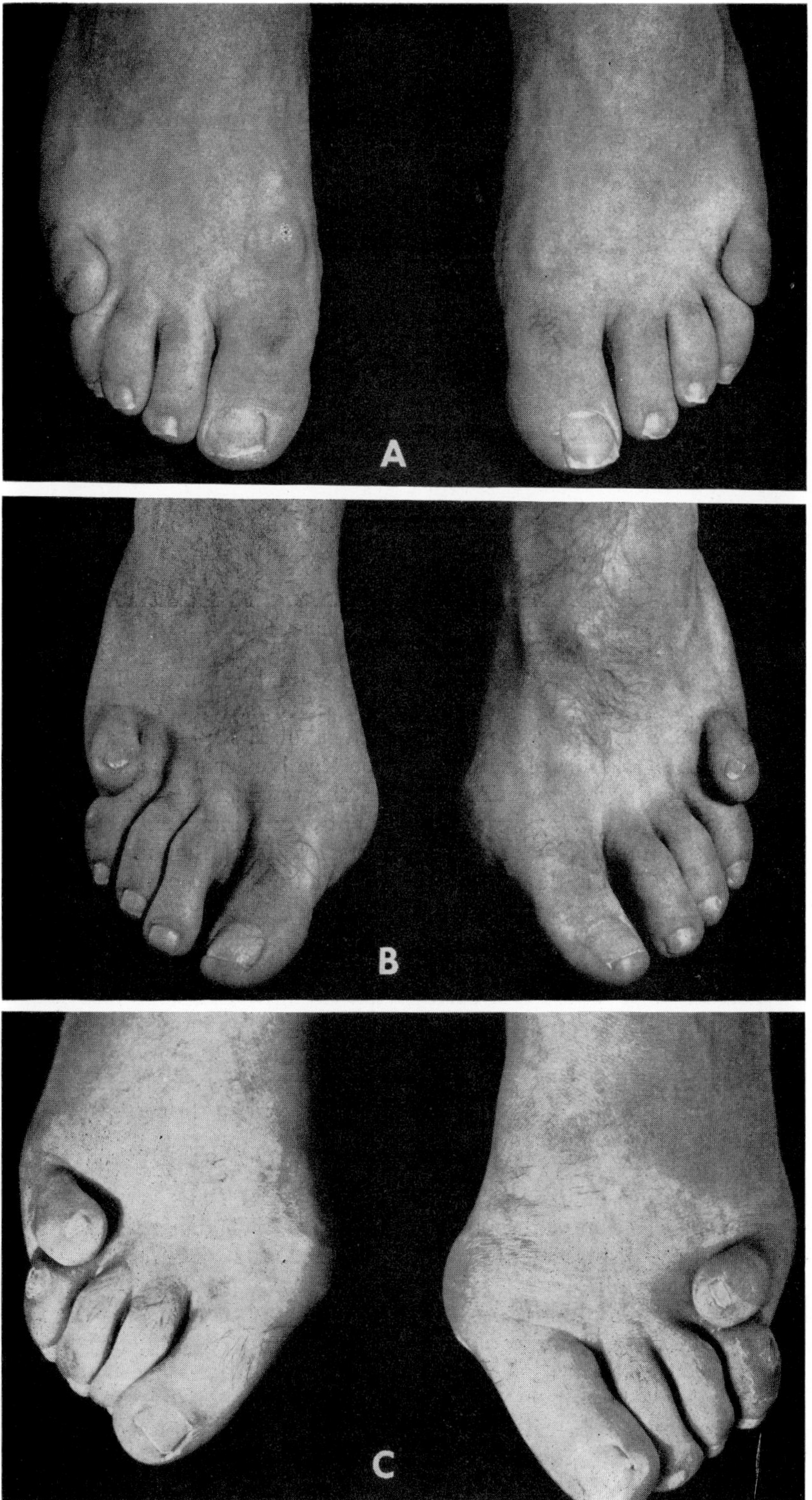

Figure 15—10. Three cases of digitus minimus varus. They are bilateral, congenital, and familial.

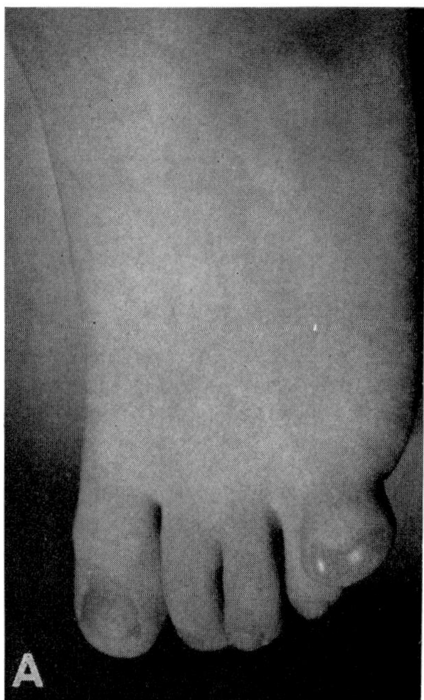

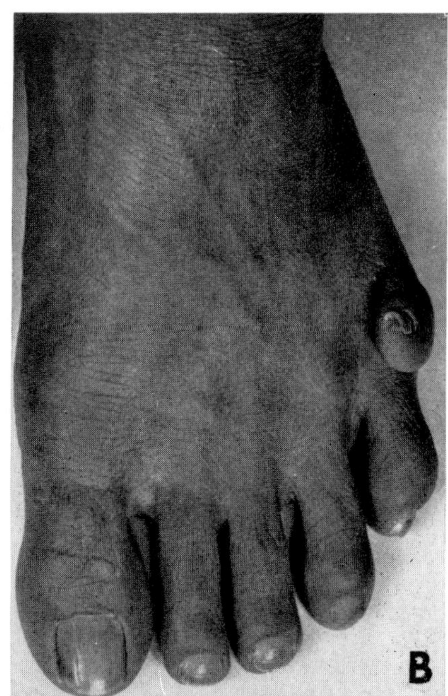

Figure 15–11. Duplicated supernumerary fifth toe.

HAMMERTOE

Blum (1883) defined hammertoe as a deviation in the dorsoplantar plane with the digit simulating the configuration of a swan's neck. Shattock (1886) dissected two hammertoes obtained by amputation. He gave the following description: "The joint between the first and second phalanges is flexed to a right angle; that between the second and third is very slightly hyperextended. There is a corn over the summit of the convexity, and beneath the corn is a well defined pressure bursa." Because the specimens he examined had been secured by disarticulation through the metatarsophalangeal joint, Shattock failed to record the most important feature of hammertoe—the hyperextended position of the proximal phalanx and the displacement of its base at the metatarsophalangeal joint.

In a typical hammertoe the proximal phalanx is extended, the middle one is bent plantarward, and the distal segment is usually flexed but may maintain a neutral stance or tilt up. The knuckled proximal interphalangeal joint bears a dorsal corn. Between the indurated skin and the underlying bone is a bursa that sometimes becomes inflamed and results in regional cellulitis. The pulp of the terminal phalanx may also possess a clavus on its plantar aspect or along the free border of the nail. Less obvious to the naked eye are skeletal misalignments, capsular contractures, and the dorsal shift of the interosseous tendons in relation to the flanking metatarsal heads. The extended position of the proximal phalanx and the dorsal shift of its base are to be regarded as cardinal changes. Less commonly the base of the proximal phalanx is displaced sideways. In long-standing hammertoe, hyaline surfaces of the bones entering into the metatarsophalangeal joint are eroded and surrounding soft tissues have undergone contracture.

Causation. The causes of hammertoe have been debated. LaForest (1782) regarded the deformity as a familial trait. During the discussion that followed the paper by Adams (1888), Pye referred to the very strong hereditary tendency. Brown asked whether heredity might not be in the shoemakers rather than in patients; in those days bootmaking was a family business—the father taught his son how to make the shoe appear trim, fashionable. Shattock spoke of the analogy to the clawhand of Duchenne's paralysis and suggested the possibility of defective activity by pedal interossei in causing hammertoe.

Thus far no one has demonstrated any paralysis of pedal interossei in hammertoes. Short, tapered, tilted shoes undoubtedly constitute a major cause. But one cannot overlook the fact that the second toe is sometimes seen to curl plantarward before the child has worn shoes, that this deformity is often bilateral and symmetrical, and that it manifests itself in more than one member of the same family. There is also the factor of the long second—sometimes also the third—toe, which is inherited. The second toe gains in relative length in marked deviations of the hallux and when the hallux has been shortened surgically. Discrepancy in the relative lengths of neighboring toes must be regarded a predisposing factor in the production of hammertoe; cramping shoes are considered the exciting cause. An outjutting toe is pushed back by the tip of the shoe forcing it to bend on itself.

Treatment. The treatment of hammertoe has also been the subject of controversy.

Palliative methods. These are practiced mainly to alleviate pain. Pads and props have been prescribed from time immemorial. Not long ago McFadyean (1942) advised patients with "hammertoe and bursitis" to procure "standard well fitting" footwear 3 months before wearing it. During this interval the shoe is stretched with a small metal "dome of silence" and accurately centered on the wooden "tree" to establish a stall for the knuckled joint. Milgram (1964) spoke of strapping the toes, using an "under-and-over" strip of adhesive tape. For prompt relief from pain he recommended "a crescentic transverse incision through the dorsum of the shoe."

There is no denying that protective pads alleviate discomfort due to chafing by the shoe. The success of commercial firms dispensing these items attests to the efficacy of their products in procuring a measure of comfort, but they do not correct the deformity; they merely palliate pain. There is a prop that is placed on the flexor aspect of the hammered toes; it is held in place with an elastic strap. The prop functions as a platform on which the toe can press, establish a fixed point, enlarge the tread, and save the corresponding metatarsal from excessive stress. For cases deemed unsuitable for surgery, such a "grip" prop may well be recommended. One may also use this prop in conjunction with a dorsal pad to protect the corn from pressure (Fig. 15–12).

Mechanical contrivances. In wading through the literature, one is appalled by the number of mechanical contrivances that supposedly correct hammertoe deformity. The sandal devised by Bigg (1865) was featured in textbook after textbook as a panacea for hammertoes. For incipient hammertoe, Anderson (1897) recommended "extension splints." Trethowan (1925) advised "daily manipulations to correct the deformity passively, with retentive splints to hold toes straight by day and night." Neither Anderson nor Trethowan spoke with much conviction; they indicated that ultimately one had to resort to surgery to correct hammertoes (Fig. 15–13).

Amputation. In the past amputation featured prominently as an expeditious method of getting rid of the painful deformed digits. Anderson (1897), Merrill (1912), and Robert Jones (1917) warned against this practice. Their main objection to amputating the second toe was that it would deprive the great toe of its lateral buttress and pave the way for hallux valgus. Ely (1926) questioned the validity of this contention. He considered amputation as the most satisfactory treatment for hammertoe.

There may be an occasional indication for amputating the terminal phalanx: when the nail is thick or horny, the distal phalanx is bent plantarward and there is a painful corn at the tip of the toe. No toe needs to be excised in its entirety unless severely infected or gangrenous. The smaller toes afford a measure of support for their neighbors and prevent them from deviating to one side or another. They also broaden the

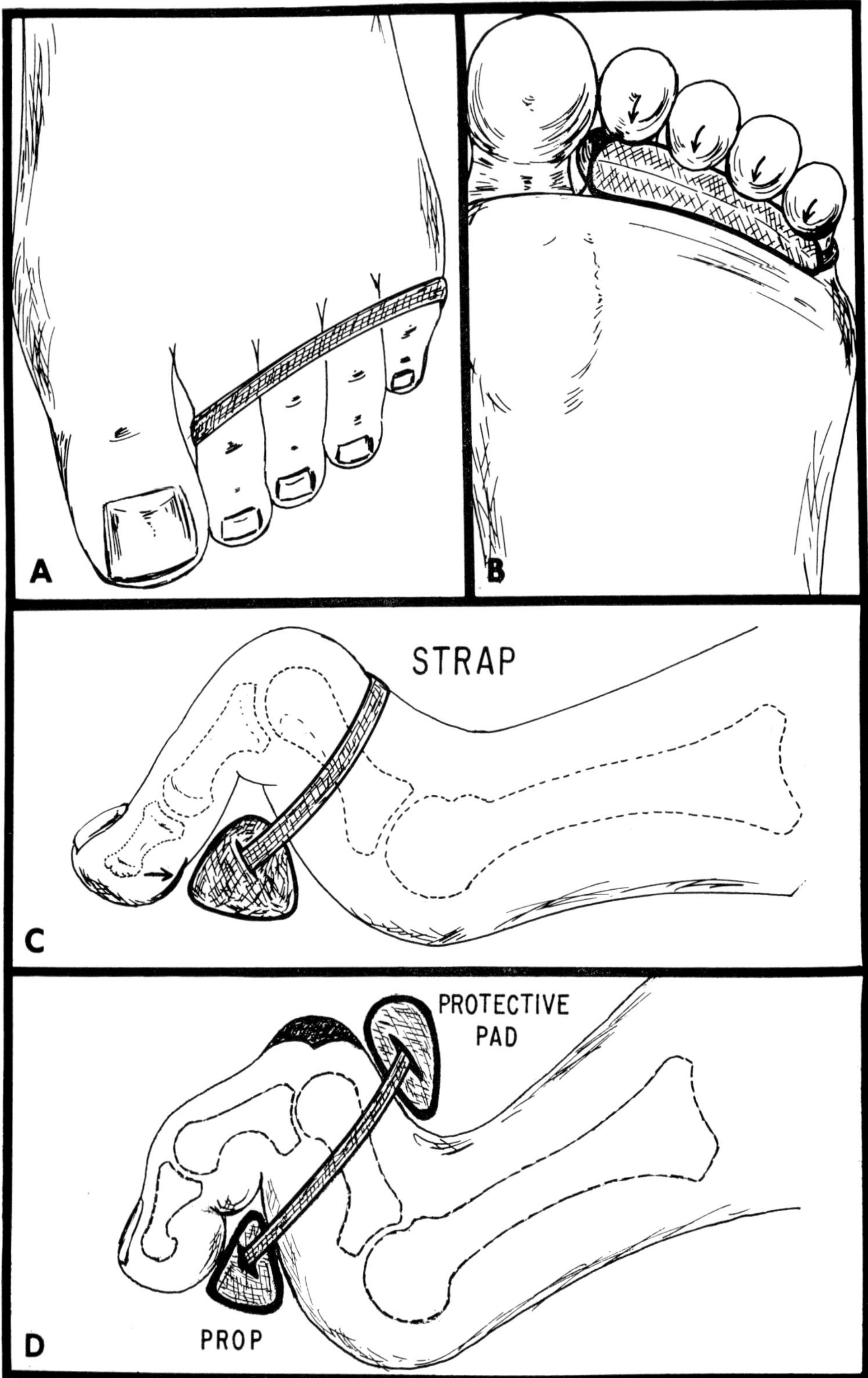

Figure 15–12. Grip prop and protective pad.

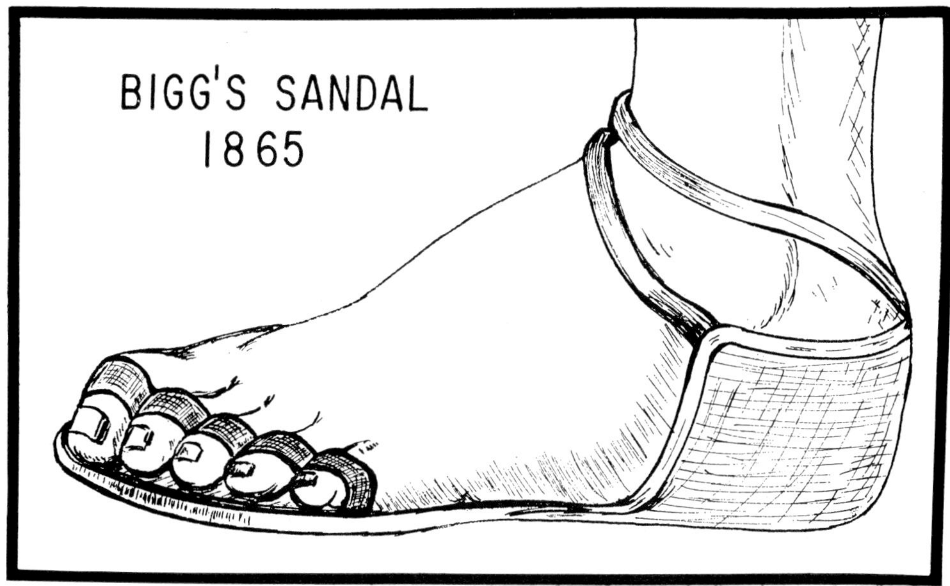

Figure 15–13. Bigg's sandal.

tread and relieve the heads of their respective metatarsals from excessive stress—thus relieving metatarsalgia.

Soft tissue surgery. This procedure was initiated by Boyer (1816); he resected a segment of the long extensor tendon. Mellet (1835) sectioned both the flexors and extensors. Tamplin (1846) divided the flexors. Adams (1888) advised subcutaneous division of collateral ligaments of the knuckled joint. Merrill (1912) shifted the insertion of the long flexor to the base of the proximal phalanx and transferred the extensor tendon to the metatarsal head. Schlaepfer (1918) approached the first interphalangeal joint through a plantar incision; he released the capsule and the collateral ligaments and lengthened the flexor tendon by Z-plasty. Lenggenhager (1935) performed dorsal capsulotomy of the metatarsophalangeal joint and plantar capsulotomy of the first interphalangeal articulation. He sectioned both long and short extensors and inserted the long extensors into the dorsum of the distal phalanx. Lapidus (1939) released the dorsal capsule of the metatarsophalangeal joint and the plantar capsules of the interphalangeal articulations. He also tenotomized the long flexor.

Extensor tenotomy and dorsal capsulotomy of the metatarsophalangeal joint are at times indicated. One cannot too strongly condemn tenotomy of the toe flexors. The smaller toes are useless if their tips cannot exert pressure on the proffered surface and establish a fixed point. This grip mechanism depends mainly on the integrity of the flexors, especially the long one. On the whole, for correction of hammertoes, the results of soft tissue surgery have been extremely disappointing—unless combined with attempts to redress the skeletal deformities.

Surgery on bones and joints. This procedure came into vogue toward the end of the last century. To correct "displacement of the smaller toes," Post (1882) "excised the distal extremity" of the proximal phalanges. Anderson (1887, 1897) specifically recommended decapitation of the proximal phalanx for hammertoe. Terrier (1888) thought the base of the middle phalanx should also be excised. O'Neill (1911) remodeled the resected ends of the bones and interposed fatty or fibrous tissue. Tierny (1926) carried out transcervical osteotomy of the first phalanx, straightened the toe, and invaginated the spiked end of the proximal fragment into a hole on the dorsum of the capital piece. Bragard (1926) shortened the first pha-

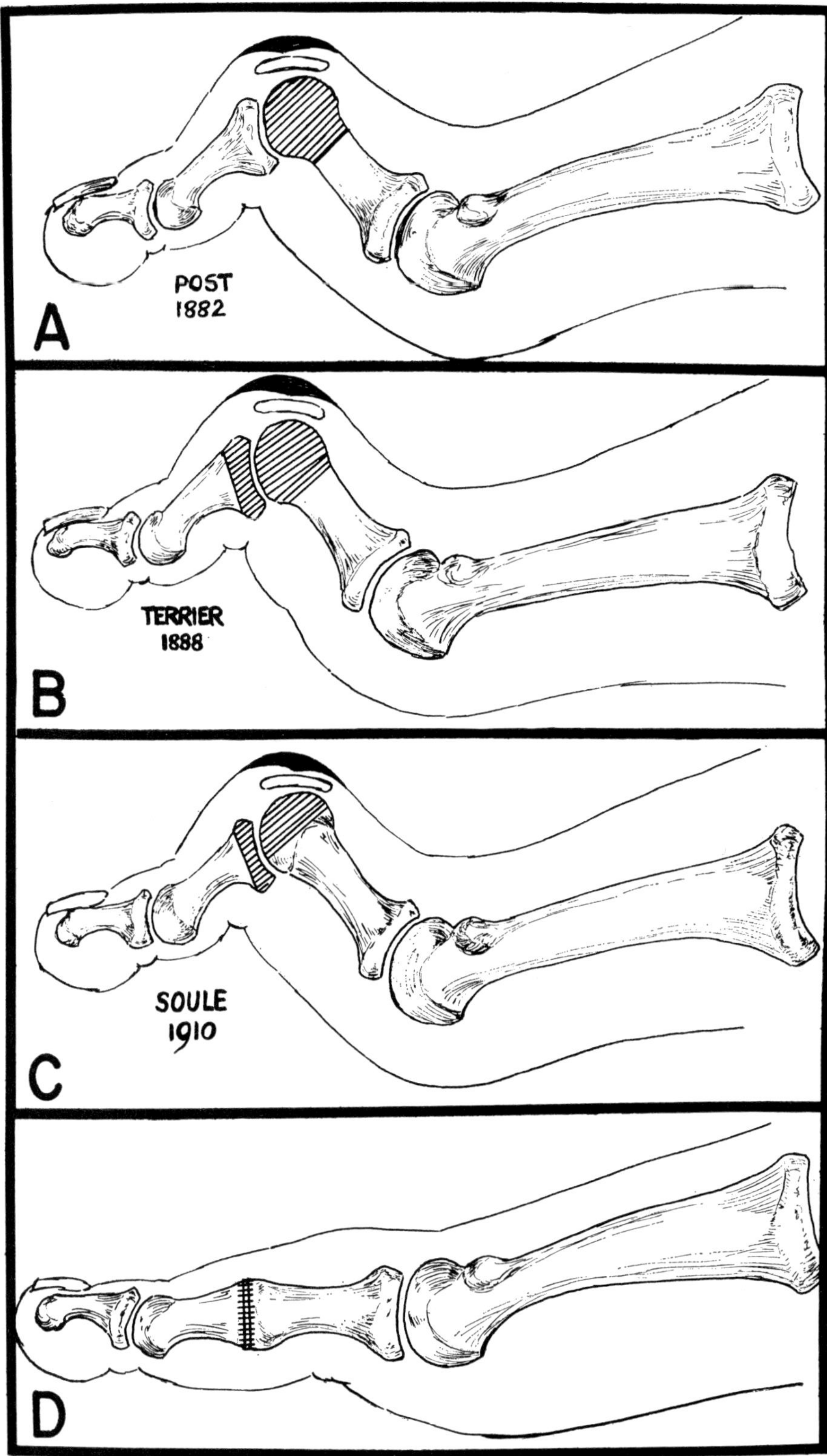

Figure 15–14. Resection of articular bones of the proximal interphalangeal joint (*A* and *B*); arthrodesis (*C* and *D*).

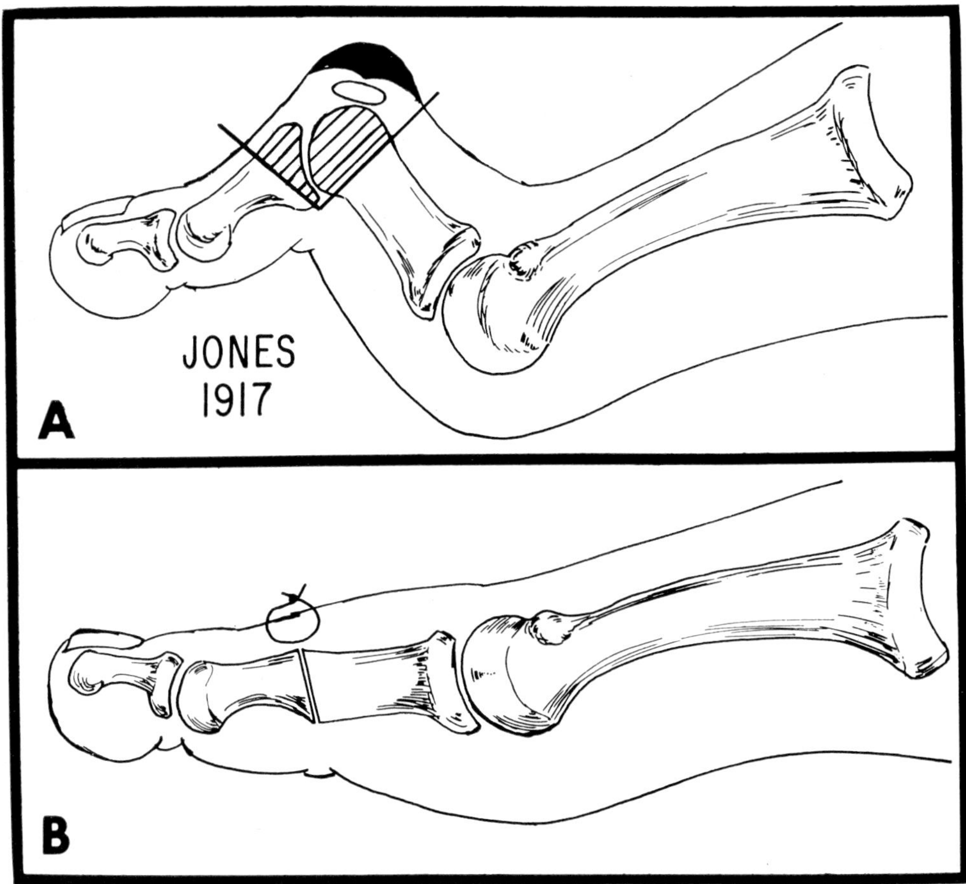

Figure 15–15. Jones wedge resection and fusion of the first interphalangeal joint.

lanx by resecting a segment from the midshaft. Wallet (1937) performed multiple arthroplasties of the central three toes. Arthroplasty was also recommended by Decoppet (1947). Borg (1950) described what he called "Sjovall's operation method," which was not unlike the original resection of Terrier.

Resection of both articular bones yielded a satisfactory result if followed by stiffness of the joint. *Intentional arthrodesis* of the proximal interphalangeal joint was first described by Soule (1910). Sir Robert Jones (1917) merely popularized this operation, but somehow his name became tagged onto it. Higgs (1931) denuded articular ends of bones and dovetailed them by a spike-and-hole method somewhat similar to Tierny's. Young (1938) converted the head of the proximal phalanx into a truncated cone; after appropriately excavating the base of the middle phalanx, the two bones were locked. Taylor (1940) recommended the use of a Kirschner wire for intramedullary fixation. Selig (1941) described the same technique but called it *a new procedure.* The only novel feature of Selig's operation was the bending of the extruded end of the fixation wire (Figs. 15–14 to 15–17).

A common objection to fusion of the first interphalangeal joint is that it takes a long time—sometimes 8 weeks or more —for the bones to consolidate. In most instances, there is fixed contracture around the metatarsophalangeal joint, erosion of articular surfaces, and a variable degree of subluxation or even dislocation of the bones. In these cases fusion of the interphalangeal joint results in a straight toe that sticks up. Tenotomy of the extensor tendons and dorsal capsulotomy of the metatarsophalangeal joint may permit the toe to

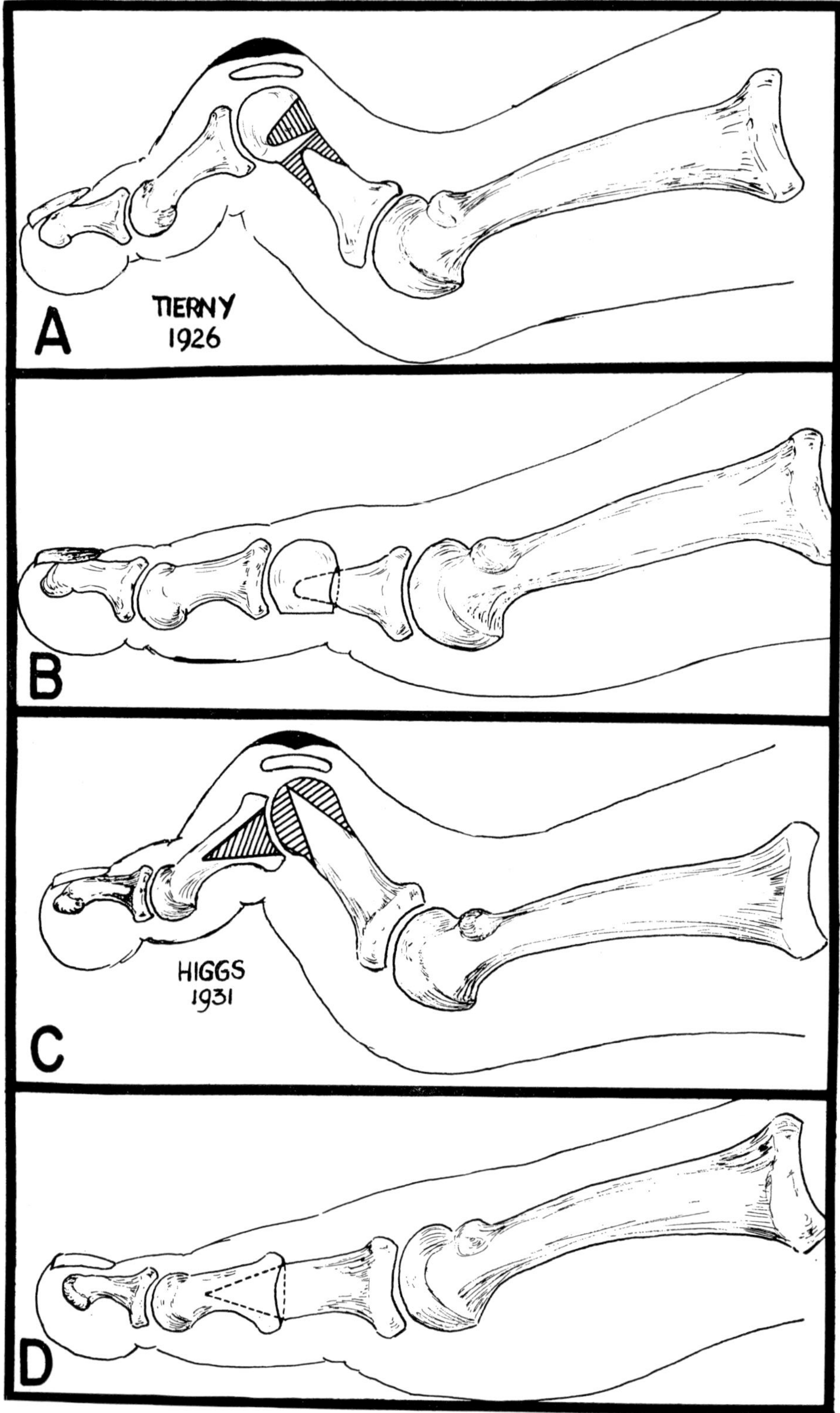

Figure 15–16. Invagination methods: Tierny's osteotomy (*A* and *B*); Higg's fusion (*C* and *D*).

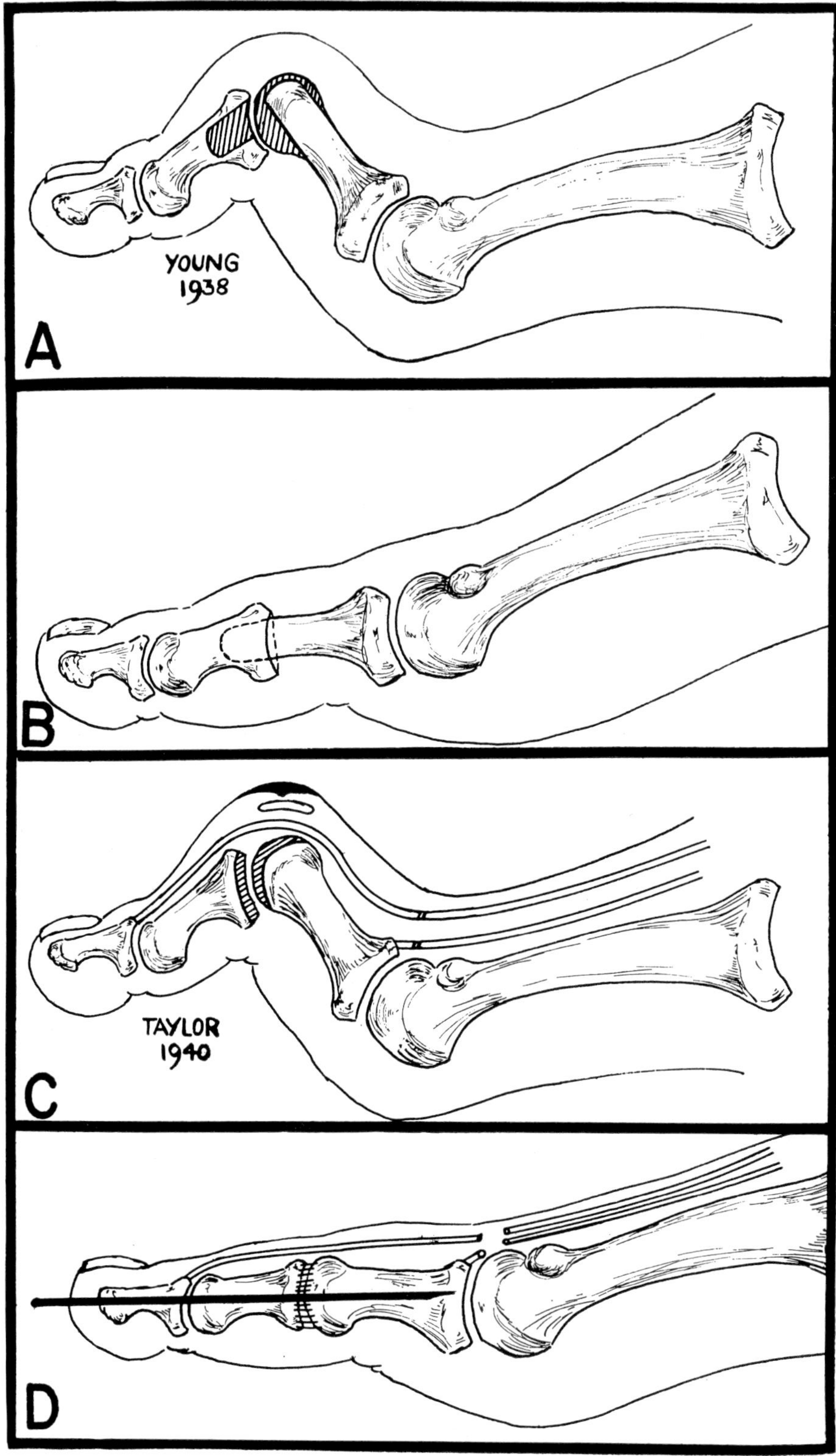

Figure 15–17. More refined invagination: Young's (*A* and *B*); Taylor's (*C* and *D*).

be pushed plantarward, but subluxation of the bones often remains unreduced. DuVries (1959) recommended open reduction of dislocation of the first phalanx at the metatarsophalangeal joint; it is questionable if the toe will regain its flexibility afterwards.

Resection of the proximal portion of the first phalanx is a more rational method of reducing dislocations at the metatarsophalangeal joints. This operation has been linked with Keller's name. Keller did not describe any procedure for hammertoe. Kreuz (1923) from Gocht's clinic spoke about partial proximal phalangectomy. Gocht was said to have practiced resection of the proximal half of the basal phalanges of the central toes through a transverse plantar incision. Gocht and Debrunner (1925) again described this operation. Subsequently Kuhns (1937); Michele and Krueger (1948); Le Cocq (1949); and Glassman, Wallin, and Sideman (1949) came out with glowing reports following proximal phalangectomy.

Partial proximal phalangectomy promotes motion at the metatarsophalangeal joint, where mobility is most needed. If only the base of the phalanx is resected, the toe in time retracts and stiffens, and cannot bend at the metatarsophalangeal joint. Excision of a sizable segment of bone deprives the toe of a stable foundation; it becomes flail and dangles. Even if the toe touches the proffered surface, it cannot press down on it with sufficient force to obtain purchase. To obviate these hazards surgical syndactylia of the adjacent toes has been proposed.

Combined bone resection and surgical syndactylia of toes. Phelps (1894) made use of surgical syndactylia of the toes in the treatment of soft corns. In Petri's (1940) article on forefoot deformities, he included a diagram that showed the two medial toes sutured together. Ramstedt (1947) utilized surgical syndactylia for hallux valgus and hammertoes. Kelikian, Clayton, and Loseff (1961) treated numerous toe deformities—congenital as well as acquired—with surgical syndactylia. They described in some detail the technique devised by the senior author and recommended dovetailing skinplasty with proximal phalangectomy. The foot is prepared in the usual manner; hemostasis is secured with the aid of a pneumatic tourniquet. A silk thread is passed through each pulp of the two neighboring toes; the strands of the thread are brought together and clamped with a hemostat. The assistant puts traction on these forceps to straighten the toes and pulls them apart to bring the webspace into full view. The area is now delineated by three sets of incisions: a web-bisecting incision, a pair of paradigital incisions, and a pair of connecting, or what we like to call, "sartorial" skin cuts.

The web-bisecting incision starts on the dorsum of the forefoot in the selected intermetatarsal groove; it passes distally, dips plantarward and bisects the web. The incision ends at about the same point posteriorly on the plantar aspect of the forefoot as it does on the dorsum. The two *paradigital incisions,* one for each toe, fork out from the point where the web-bisecting cut begins to dip in a plantar direction. These incisions are extended lengthwise along the adjacent side of each toe; they terminate on the side of the distal phalanx at a point below and just proximal to the base of the nail. When one toe is short, as is the case of the fifth, the incision on the side of its neighbor is of commensurate length. By placing the paradigital incision slightly closer—but not too close—to the plantar border of the toe, one can ensure a semblance of interdigital groove after surgical syndactylia. The *sartorial cut* connects the terminal point of the paradigital incision on either side with the plantar end of the web-bisecting incision. The intervening triangular patch of skin is dissected and discarded. In undermining the skin in this area, care is taken not to puncture the plexus of veins that is ordinarily present.

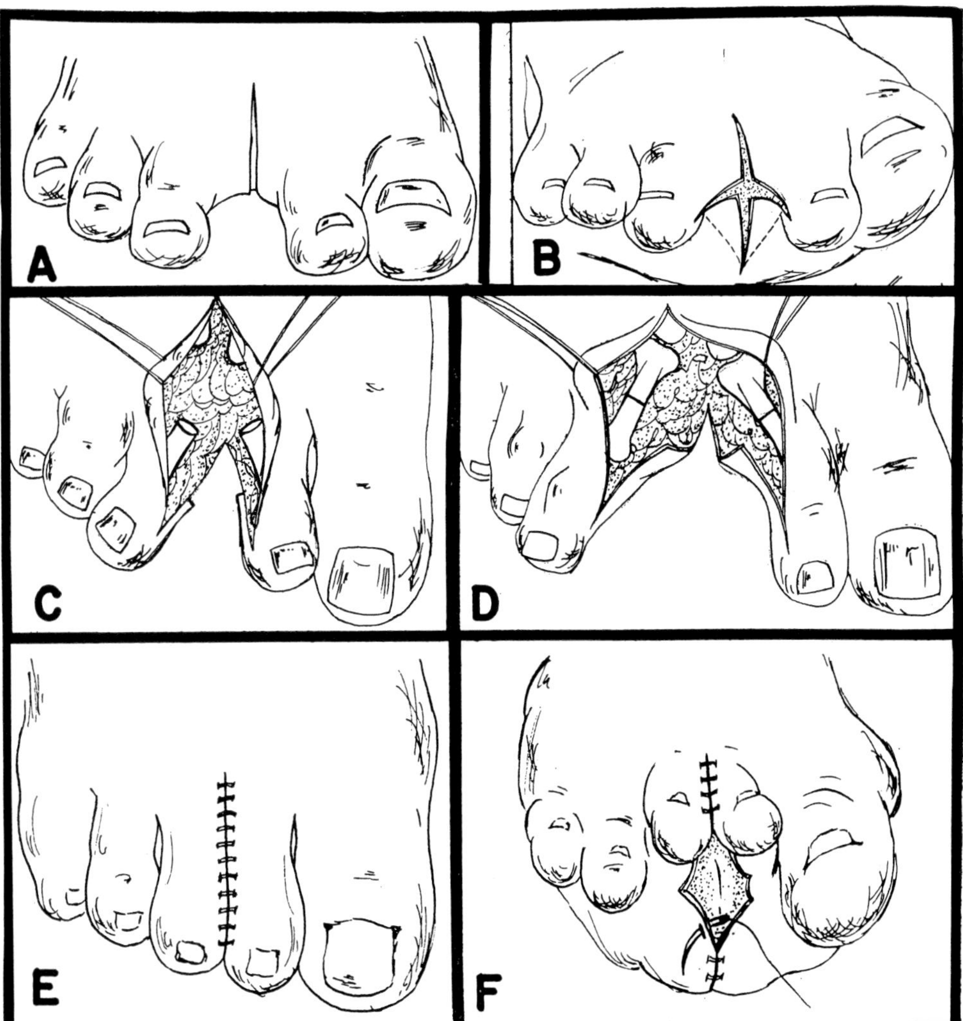

Figure 15–18. Technique of partial proximal phalangectomy and surgical syndactylia of the adjacent toes.

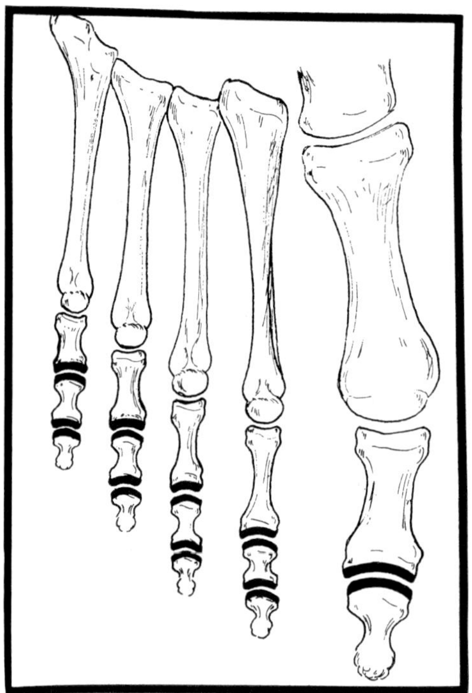

Figure 15–19. Stepladder position of the interphalangeal joints.

The partial or total resection of the proximal phalanx is effected through the paradigital incision. The shaft of the phalanx is sought, and a small retractor is passed dorsally to protect the extensor tendon. The long flexor on the plantar aspect is enclosed in a fibrous sheath that blends with the periosteum on either side. The toe is rotated until the junction of the fibrous sheath and the bone is seen. The point scalpel penetrates the sheath, and hugging the inferior surface of the phalanx, it sweeps toward the metatarsophalangeal joint. After the fibrous sheath is severed, another small retractor is introduced to protect the plantar soft tissues. The phalanx is divided at the desired level. A small paddle screw is inserted into the medullary cavity of the proximal fragment. The transfixation screw is used as a lever to lift the bone out of the wound. The proximal fragment is dissected free and discarded. Rarely, the entire phalanx is enucleated. As a rule the proximal half or two-thirds is removed.

After bone resection, the surgical wound is packed with a moist sponge and the pneumatic tourniquet is deflated. It is advisable to wait a few minutes until post-tourniquet hyperemia subsides; the bleeders are clamped and ligated. The terminal points of the paradigital incisions are approximated by a No. 34 stainless steel wire suture. The strands of the wire are temporarily twisted, the two toes are brought together, and the level of the nails is scrutinized. Eversion and inversion of the toes are avoided; if necessary the wire suture is removed and reapplied. We usually approximate the dorsal skin edges with fine silk or nylon and use four O plain catgut to bring the plantar margins together (Fig. 15–18).

To quote a favorite aphorism of ours: "Two dangling digits dangle less when they dangle together." Resection of bone enhances the mobility at the metatarsophalangeal joint. Surgical syndactylia stabilizes the toes and augments their pressing-down power. Two toes thus connected can bear pressure and establish a fixed point more effectively than a single dangling digit. Because the interphalangeal joints of neighboring toes are not in the same coronal plane, the phalanx of one digit stabilizes the joint of the other. The combined action of the long flexors is transferred to the metatarsophalangeal junction, where flexion is indispensable (Figs. 15–19 to 15–21).

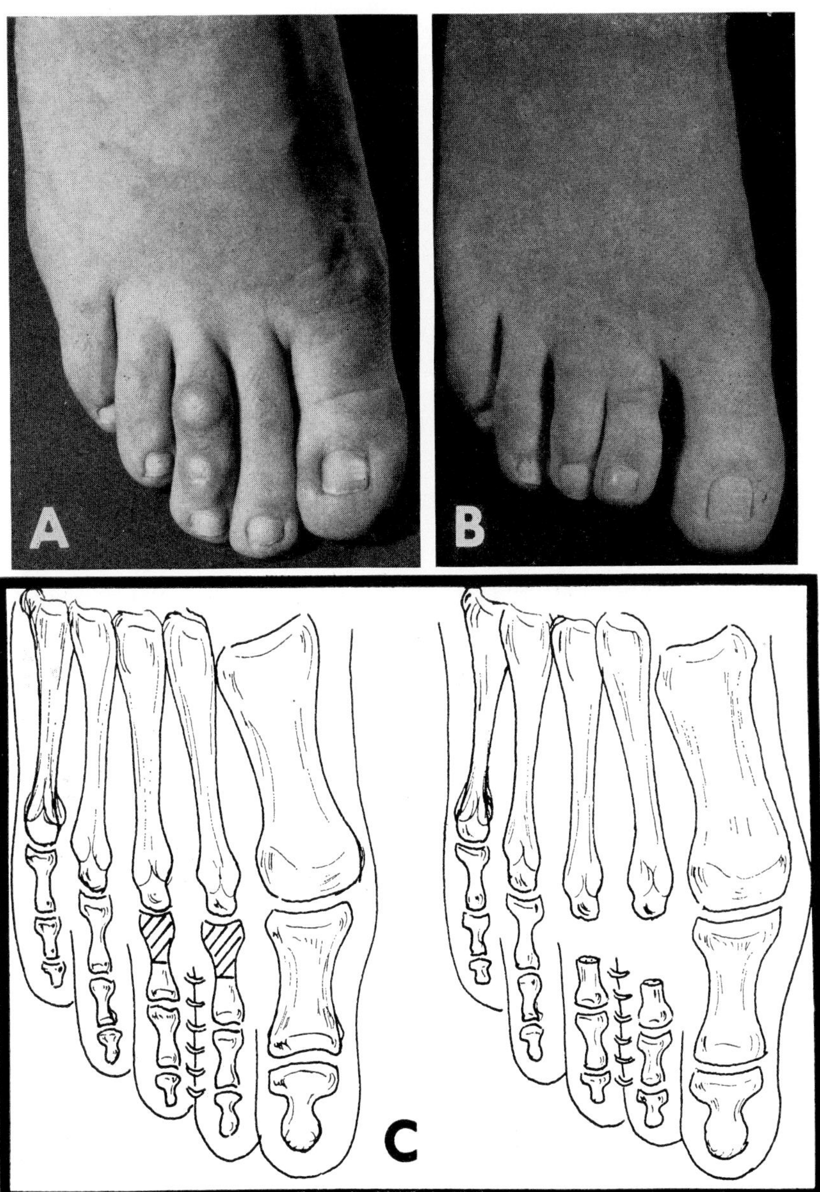

Figure 15–20. Young woman with unilateral hammered third toe and long second toe. Surgery performed was partial proximal phalangectomy and surgical syndactylia of the second and third toes. Photograph before surgery (*A*). After surgery (B); note the interdigital crease between the two syndactylized toes. Interpretative diagram (*C*). Patient is satisfied.

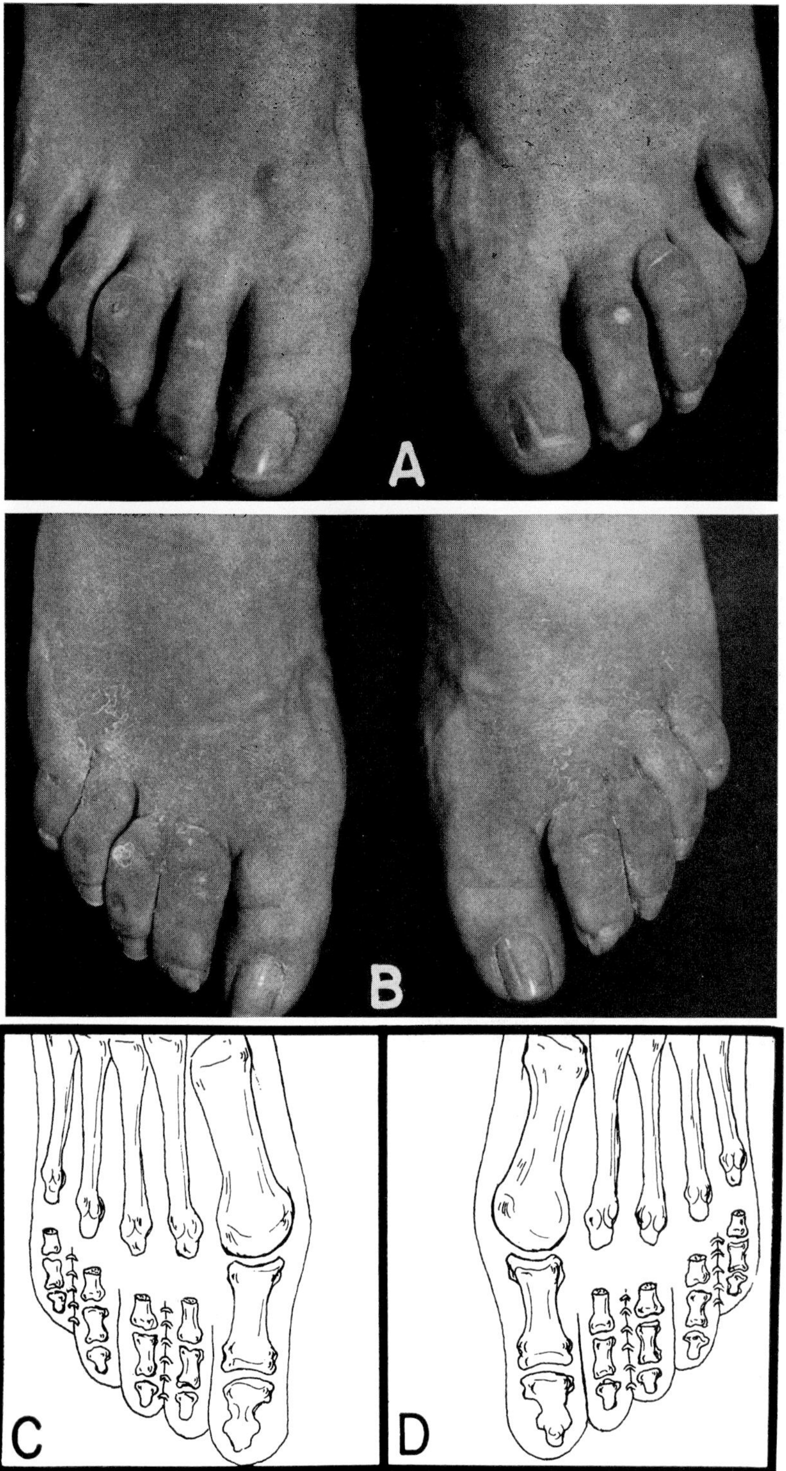

Figure 15–21. Woman with multiple, bilateral hammertoes almost merging in claw deformity. Surgery performed was partial proximal phalangectomy and surgical syndactylia of adjacent digits. Preoperative photograph (*A*). Postoperative photograph (*B*). Interpretative diagrams (*C* and *D*). Patient is satisfied.

CLAWTOES

In the course of the discussion following the paper by Adams (1888), when Shattock evoked Duchenne's name, he could not have imagined the confusion that would result from his casual remark about something possibly being amiss with the pedal interossei in hammertoe. Duchenne (1867) had described a deformity—which he called *claw cavus foot*—and ascribed it to the inactivity of pedal interossei due to lateral plantar nerve palsy. Because of the loss of "the moderating action of interossei," Duchenne argued, unopposed toe flexors bent the middle and terminal phalanges plantarward; clawing of the toes set in and gradually increased; the bases of the hyperextended proximal phalanges bore down on the metatarsal heads and caused them to become depressed; the longitudinal arch of the foot gained height; and cavus foot developed. "It may be noticed that," Duchenne deduced, "the mechanism of clawing is absolutely the same as in the hand, where the heads of the medial four metacarpals are equally pushed by the proximal phalanges of the fingers, resulting in a form of cavus of the palm and of the hand."

On the surface, Duchenne's analogy is convincing. In clawhand the fingers are extended at the metacarpophalangeal articulation and flexed at the interphalangeal joints. Because of atrophy of volar intrinsic muscles, the palm assumes a hollow appearance, which is accentuated by the prominence of the unpadded metacarpal heads. In cavus foot the sole under the midfoot appears hollow, the metatarsal heads bulge prominently under the unpadded plantar skin, and the toes are retracted dorsally at the metatarsophalangeal articulations and bent plantarward at the phalangeal joints. But here the resemblance ends. Unlike the similarly named muscles in the hand, pedal interossei insert mainly into the bases of the proximal phalanges; they do not connect with the terminal two segments. One cannot speak of "the moderating action of interossei" on the middle and distal phalanges in preventing flexion at the interphalangeal joints. But who could question Duchenne's overwhelming authority?

By way of analogy with Duchenne's *main en griffe,* the unfortunate term *clawfoot* appeared in the literature, and the epithets *hammered* and *clawed* began to be used interchangeably. The same year that Shattock raised the question of interosseous inactivity in hammertoe, Fisher (1888) defined hammertoe as "contraction of one or more toes into a clawlike position." G. K. Young (1906) complained that some surgeons tried to draw a distinction between "hammer-toe and claw-shaped toes." Hoffmann (1911) spoke of clawtoes as multiple hammertoe. Trethowan (1923) considered the condition of the toes in cavus foot "comparable with the *main-en-griffe* deformity of the hand in ulnar and median paralysis." Schnepp (1937) described clawfoot as "a deformity characterized by high arch, lowered forefoot, contracted plantar structures, and multiple hammertoes." According to C. S. Young (1938), hammertoe commonly occurred singly in one or both feet, the second toe being most frequently affected; clawtoe, he said, was usually bilateral and involved all the digits.

It is perhaps safe to say that clawtoes constitute a multiple, exaggerated form of hammertoe. In clawtoes, retraction at the metatarsophalangeal junction is more marked; the joints are stiff, unbending; and the toes stand cocked. In more advanced forms of the deformity, upward thrust against the metatarsal head fails to straighten the corresponding toe or bring the pulp of the distal phalanx down to the level of the metatarsal heads. By the same token, hammertoes complicated with fixed incarceration of the metatarsal heads may be said to have become clawed (Fig. 15–22).

Clawtoes usually accompany pes cavus, but they also occur independently. Clawtoes are sometimes seen in association with rheumatoid arthritis, Sudeck's atrophy, immersion feet, or frostbite. One often sees fixed contracture of the toes in Friedreich's ataxia, Little's disease, muscular dystrophies, and other disorders of neuromuscular systems. The

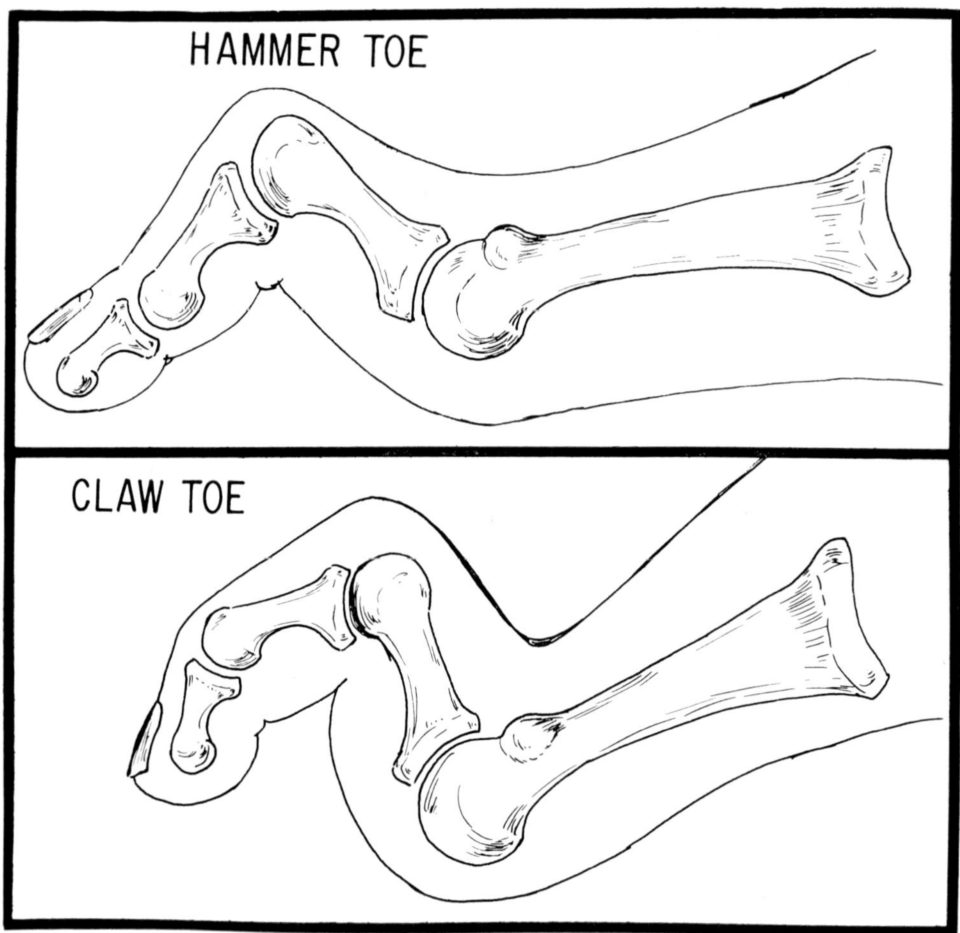

Figure 15–22. Diagram of a hammertoe (*A*). Diagram of a clawtoes (*B*).

frequency of clawtoes in patients with spina bifida occulta was recorded by Hackenbroch (1924). According to Goff (1926), pes cavus with its characteristic "pseudohammer toes" constitutes a stigma of congenital syphilis. A common cause of clawtoes is chronic dependent edema, especially after the foot has been encased in a cast for a protracted length of time. The cause of clawtoes may thus be regional or remote. Hammertoe is a regional disturbance.

Clawtoes are seen in connection with many conditions other than cavus foot, and only a comparatively small number of cavus foot can be traced to paralytic causes, least of all to the selective paralysis of muscles innervated by the lateral plantar nerve. But based on the supposition that in clawtoes pedal interossei are paralyzed, numerous surgical procedures have been proposed to restore muscle balance. These operations have been patterned after procedures that had been beneficially utilized in the hand. When these procedures were transposed to the foot, it was hoped that they would yield commensurate benefit. In most instances not much was accomplished. In some cases the existing deformity or dysfunction was aggravated, proof once again that the hand and the foot are two different organs and cannot be treated the same way.

Treatment. The treatment of clawtoes depends on many factors, but mainly on the flexibility of the metatarsophalangeal joint and the resilience of the foot as a whole. When contracted toes are not associated with cavus foot, they may be treated in the same manner outlined for hammertoes. As for combined deformities, some claim that the cavus of the foot will disappear when the toes are straightened; others contend exactly the opposite—that clawing of the toes will vanish once the cavus is corrected. Both groups overstate their points. In more resilient feet, clawing of the toes may be rectified independently. In rigid cavus, correction of digital deformities may dispose of the dorsal corns on the toes, but it leaves the patient with the more disabling plantar keratoses due to incarcerated metatarsal heads. Such cases require simultaneous attention to both segments of the foot.

Conservative methods have been proposed from time to time. For what he graded as first degree clawing, Sir Robert Jones (1917) advised stretching the Achilles tendon and the contracted structures on the plantar aspect of the foot. The patient was then prescribed roomy shoes with no heel. The shoe was provided with a half-inch transverse bar to relieve stress on the metatarsal heads. Rocyn Jones (1927) recommended manipulation of the toes and flexion and extension exercises. At night a rectangular slotted metal splint was worn, with tapes binding the toes to it. A roomy shoe was prescribed; when the patient tended to develop plantar callosities, a transverse bar was added to the shoe (Fig. 15–23).

Mechanical methods, such as *redressement forcé*—with the aid of the Thomas wrench or Redard's (1896) "tarsoclaste"—had their vogue. Willens (1908) voiced what must have been a fairly universal disappointment with these "bloodless" methods.

Surgical release of the soft tissues attached to the plantar aspect of the os calcis was practiced by Gross (1864), Phelps (1881), Fisher (1888), Kellock (1895), Barwell (1898), Muirhead Little (1903), and many others long before Steindler (1917) spoke about it and the euphonious term *Steindler stripping* achieved the contagion of a catch phrase. In a later communication Steindler (1920) warned against simultaneous tenoplasty of the tendo achillis. According to him the tension of the intact tendo achillis was necessary for correcting the cavus deformity. Rugh (1927) quoted the shopworn cliché: "What is new is not true and what is true is not new." He then went ahead to prove that by "new application of fundamental principles" one is justified in claiming originality for a procedure. Rugh resected the plantar fascia and inserted a piece of fat in the interval. Rugh subtitled his article *A New Operation,* and so on. After disconnecting the plantar

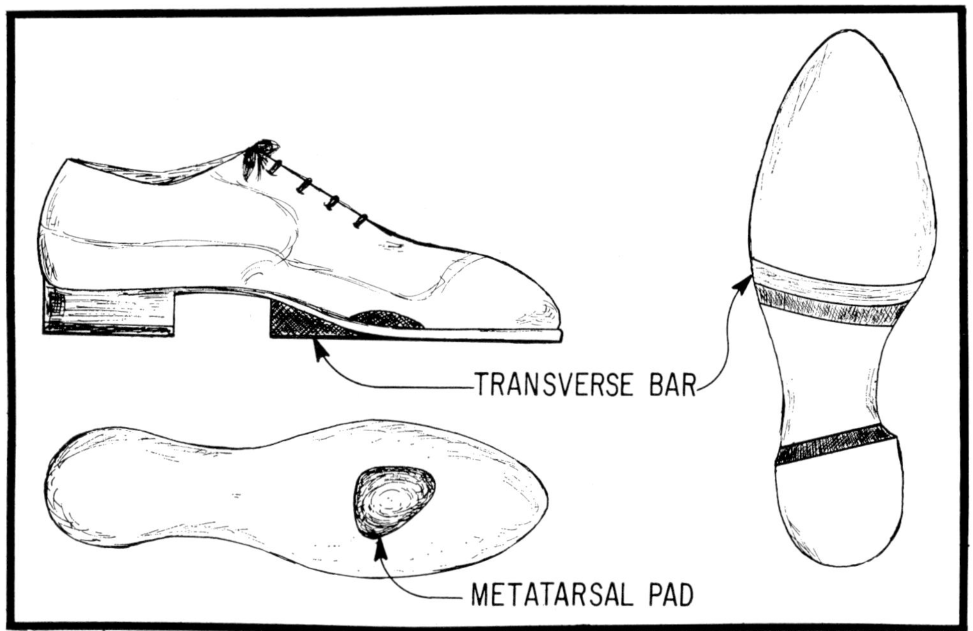

Figure 15–23. Shoe with transverse bar and metatarsal pad.

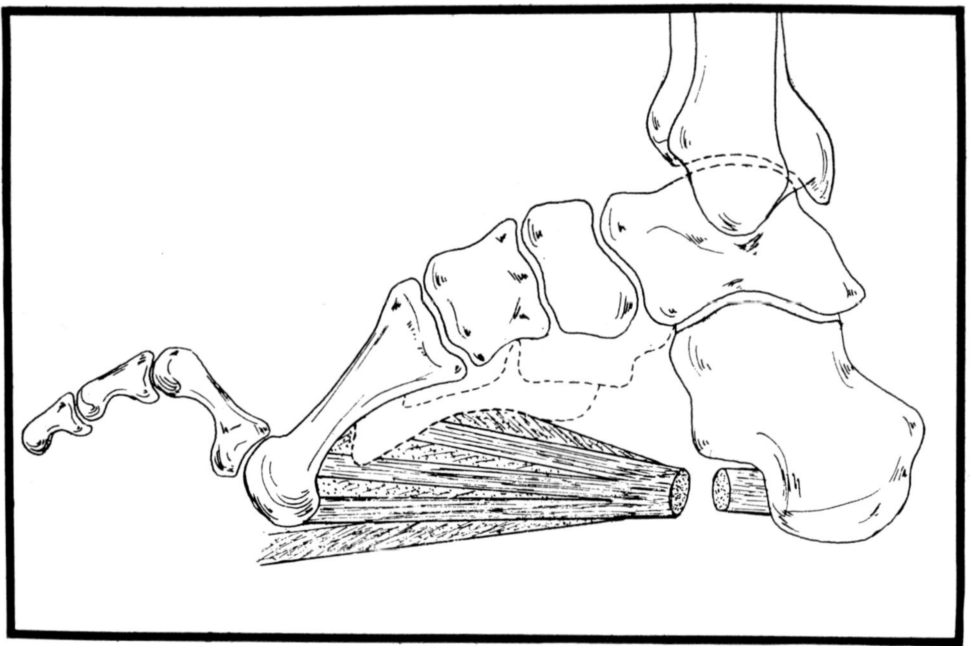

Figure 15–24. Detachment of tissues from the underaspect of the os calcis.

fascia and flexor brevis muscle from the os calcis, Spitzy (1927) stripped the calcaneonavicular and calcaneocuboid ligaments (Fig. 15–24).

Surgeons in the preceding two centuries did not make a clear distinction between pes cavus and clubfoot in general. *Tenotomy* of the heelcord was a favorite operation for almost all forms of resistent talipes. It is not definitely known who first carried out tenoplasty of the Achilles tendon. Nor did earlier surgeons differentiate clawtoes from hammertoes. As for the hammertoes, some surgeons divided the digital extensors; others severed the flexors, and there were those who tenotomized both sets.

At the beginning of the present century, Sherman (1905) introduced what was considered a new concept at the time–*tendon transplantation*. He detached the long extensors from their insertion into the toes and connected them to the metatarsal bones just behind their heads. Ducroquet (1910) shifted the insertion of the extensor hallucis longus to the distal end of the first metatarsal. Forbes (1910, 1913) repeated Sherman's extensor transfer but called it "my procedure." For the suspension operation associated with his name, Sir Robert Jones (1917) accorded Ducroquet the same oversight as Forbes had bestowed on Sherman. Hibbs (1919) transferred the common extensors into the midtarsus.

Trethowan (1925) had already spoken of dorsal capsulotomy of the metatarsophalangeal joints as the "older method" when Heyman (1932) came along claiming originality for this additional step to the operation described by Sherman and Forbes. Heyman interpolated the stock *apologia* of all those who revive antiquated procedures and try to convey the impression that they had contributed something new, be it a minor detail. "At the time these operations were done," Heyman wrote, "the writer was not familiar with the work of Sherman and Forbes published a number of years ago, and can, therefore, claim no originality for the method except for a very important detail not mentioned by either of these writers, and to his knowledge not mentioned elsewhere–namely, capsulotomy of the metatarsophalangeal joint." The desire to seem unique, original, is human. The zeal for originality in the face of avowed ignorance of what has been done before appears to be a peculiarity of orthopedic surgeons. Heyman's–as well as Rugh's–preamble has appeared in numerous opening paragraphs.

For correction of what they called "mild clawfoot," Dickson and Diveley (1926) advised the transfer of "extensor proprius hallucis" into the flexor hallucis longus. In the discussion that followed, the pundits of the period—Campbell, Meyerding, Lowman, and Steindler—expressed their exalted approval. To correct the same deformity, Forrester-Brown (1938) recommended transplantation of the long flexor into the extensor hallucis longus—exactly the reverse of the operation described by Dickson and Diveley. Taylor (1951) extended Forrester-Brown's operation to the lesser toes.

Notwithstanding the high praise it received at the time, the procedure described by Dickson and Diveley was soon forgotten. The operations of Forrester-Brown and Taylor exemplify procedures that were transposed from the hand to the foot. Forrester-Brown admitted that the operation he described was based on the principle suggested by Sir Harold Stiles (1922) for the treatment of claw-hand due to ulnar nerve palsy. Stiles transferred the sublimis tendon into the extensor expansion of the finger, so that it would cause flexion at the metacarpophalangeal articulation and extension at the interphalangeal joint. In the foot, the analogous muscle to sublimis is the flexor digitorum brevis. The individual tendons of this muscle are puny; they are difficult to dissect free and even harder to transfer. Forrester-Brown avoided tackling them. He transferred flexor hallucis longus into the long extensor of the great toe. A muscle that plays a paramount role in the all-important pressing-down action of the big toe was thus sacrificed in favor of the dubious benefit of enhancing extension of the distal phalanx. The same criticism may well be leveled against Taylor's "flexor-extensor" transfer. In his turn Taylor confessed having benefited from the principle first formulated by Stiles and later transposed from the hand to the foot by Forrester-Brown.

In his presidential address before the Orthopedic Section of Royal Society of Medicine, Todd (1934) vehemently attacked the alleged "anology between pes cavus and ulnar claw-hand." He dismissed the concept of interosseous insufficiency in the causation of cavus foot as mere fiction and advised that it be dropped, once and for all, "the sooner the better." But it was not. It had had too many authoritative adherents—Sherman (1905), Hibbs (1919), Mills (1924), Lambrinudi (1927–1942), and Stamm (1948). More recently Garceau and Brahms (1956), leaned heavily on what Todd called fiction to justify *denervation* of muscles supplied by the medial plantar nerve—namely, the abductor hallucis, flexor digitorum brevis, and quadratus plantae. They have not followed their preliminary report with a definitive one. They probably will not.

When Sir Robert Jones (1917) described the transfer of extensor hallucis longus into the first metatarsal, he said nothing about *arthrodesing* the interphalangeal joint of the great toe, which procedure is now regarded as an essential step of the suspension operation. This suggestion first appeared in an article by Stuart (1924). O'Donoghue and Stauffer (1943) described what they called "an improved operative method for obtaining bony fusion of the great toe." The improvement consisted of intramedullary wire fixation of the phalanges—a procedure already described by Taylor (1940), and Selig (1941), in connection with arthrodesis of the first interphalangeal joint of one of the smaller toes.

The theory of interosseous insufficiency was also evoked in defense of what has come to be known as *Lambrinudi's operation* for clawtoes. Lambrinudi (1927–1942) considered clawing of the toe primary and cavus foot secondary. He fused both interphalangeal joints and tenotomized the extensor tendon. By eliminating the interphalangeal joints, he converted the segmented toe into a single rod; the action of the long flexor was thereby transferred from the distal to the proximal phalanx. This operation has been endorsed by Stamm

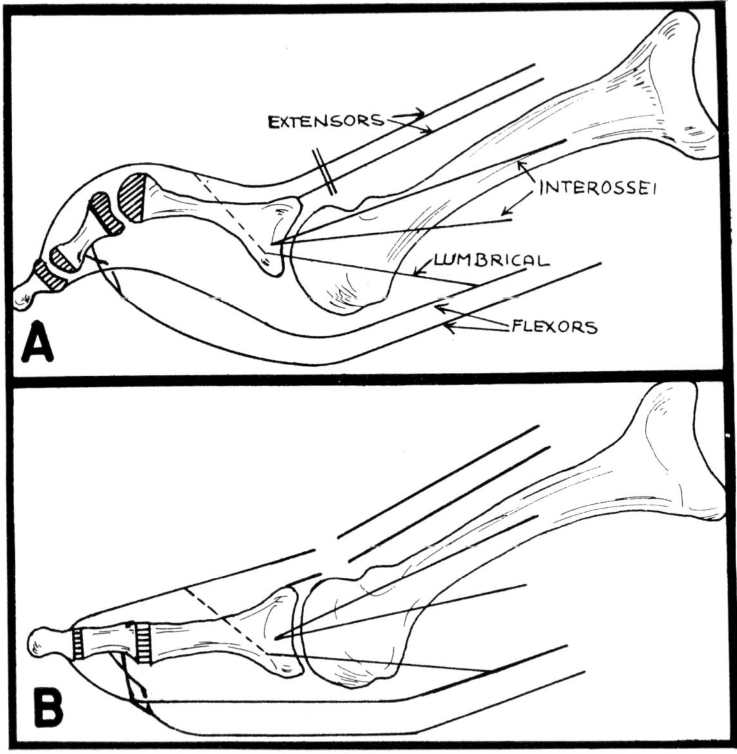

Figure 15–25. Lambrinudi's operation for clawtoes.

(1943–1948), Nissen (1957), Perkins (1961), and others (Fig. 15–25).

Decapitation of all five metatarsals was advocated by Hoffmann (1911) for severe grades of rigid clawtoes. In some instances he also removed "parts of the necks of the metatarsal bones." *Osteotomy of the first metatarsal* was first recommended by Scherb (1924) and later by Hackenbroch (1924), Rosenzweig (1934), and Farkas (1935). McElvenny and Caldwell (1958) *elevated and derotated*—"supinated"—the first metatarsal and maintained this position by fusion of the first cuneometatarsal joint.

For the correction of fixed cavus, with established skeletal deformities, Steindler (1921) advised *cuneiform tarsectomy.* The wedge of bone resected had a dorsal base that spanned the neck of the talus; its apex was directed plantarward and reached the inferior cortex of the cuboid bone. For correction of dropped forefoot following Whitman astragalectomy, Stephens (1923) removed a wedge of bone with the base up and apex down; it included the proximal parts of the metatarsals and the distal portions of the tarsal bones. Foley (1924) reported successful correction of cavus foot by wedge resection of the anterior tarsal bones. Stuart (1924) advised *triple arthrodesis* for advanced skeletal deformities. *Wedge osteotomy of os calcis* has been recommended by Dwyer (1955, 1959) to correct cavus foot complicated by varus of the heel.

Astragalectomy and amputation of all the toes was advised by Sir Robert Jones (1917) for what he called fifth degree clawfoot, with equinovarus and intractable callosities, Perkins (1961) amputated the forefoot through metatarsal necks in severe hallux valgus with clawing of the toes (Figs. 15–26 to 15–28).

We may perhaps bring the management of clawtoes into proper focus by restating what we have said before: the main function of the toes is to contact the proffered surface and exert strong enough pressure on it to obtain purchase, a fixed point, from which the body can be propelled. Toes that fail to touch the surface under them and press down with sufficient vigor constitute the most common cause of meta-

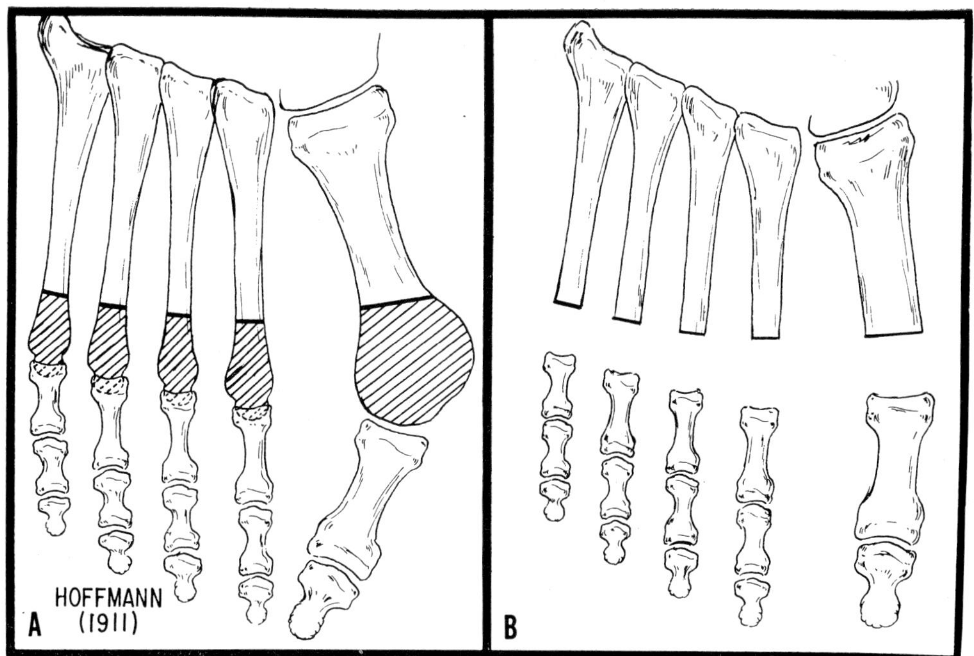

Figure 15–26. Decapitation of metatarsal bones.

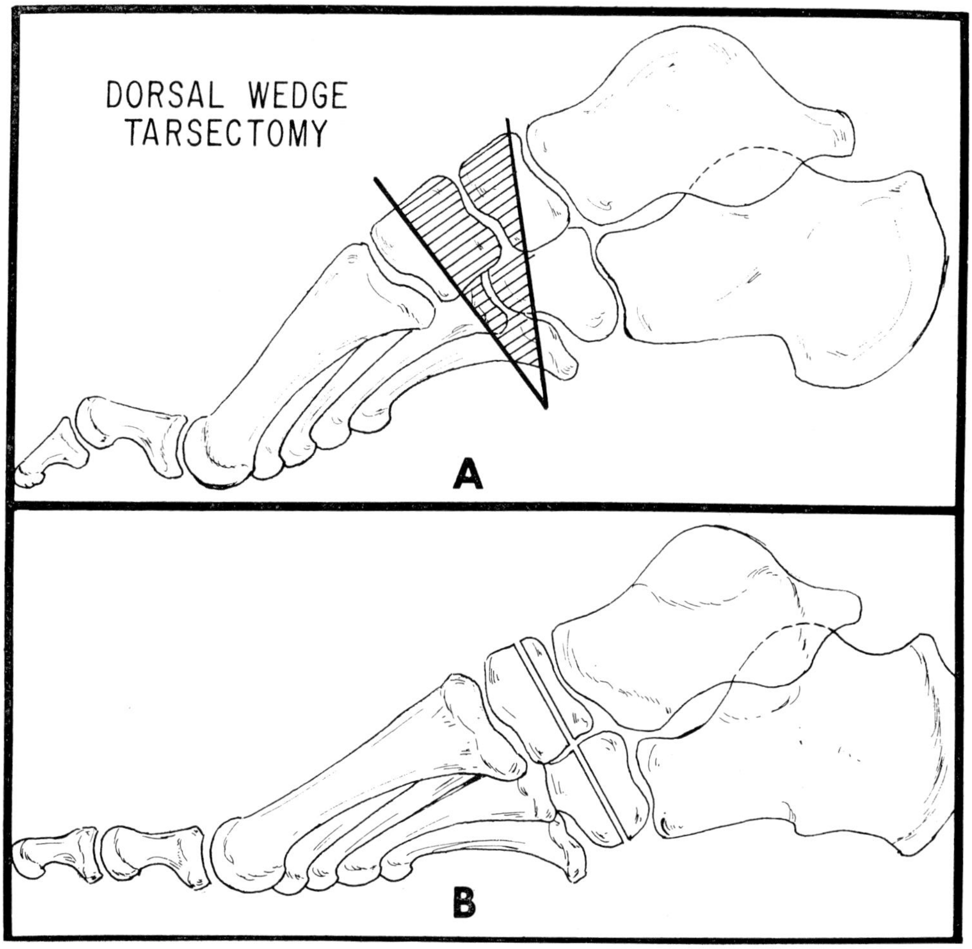

DORSAL WEDGE TARSECTOMY

Figure 15–27. Cuneiform tarsectomy.

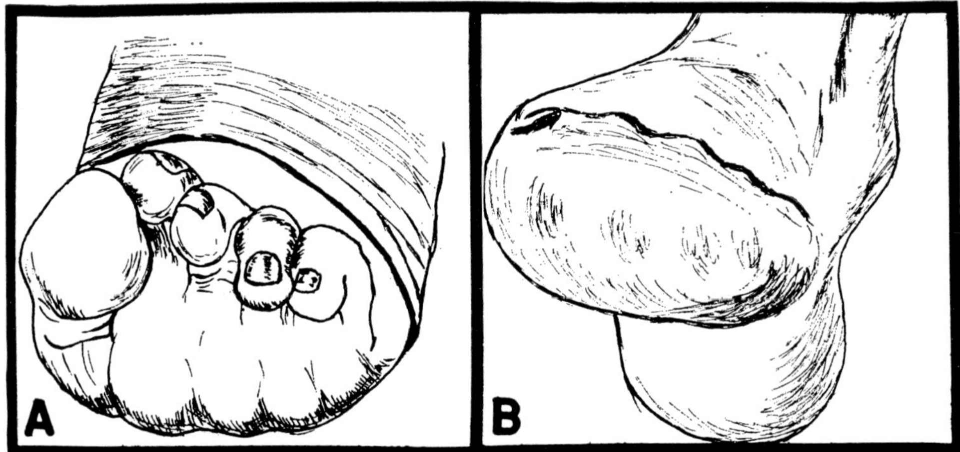

Figure 15–28. Amputation of the clawed toes.

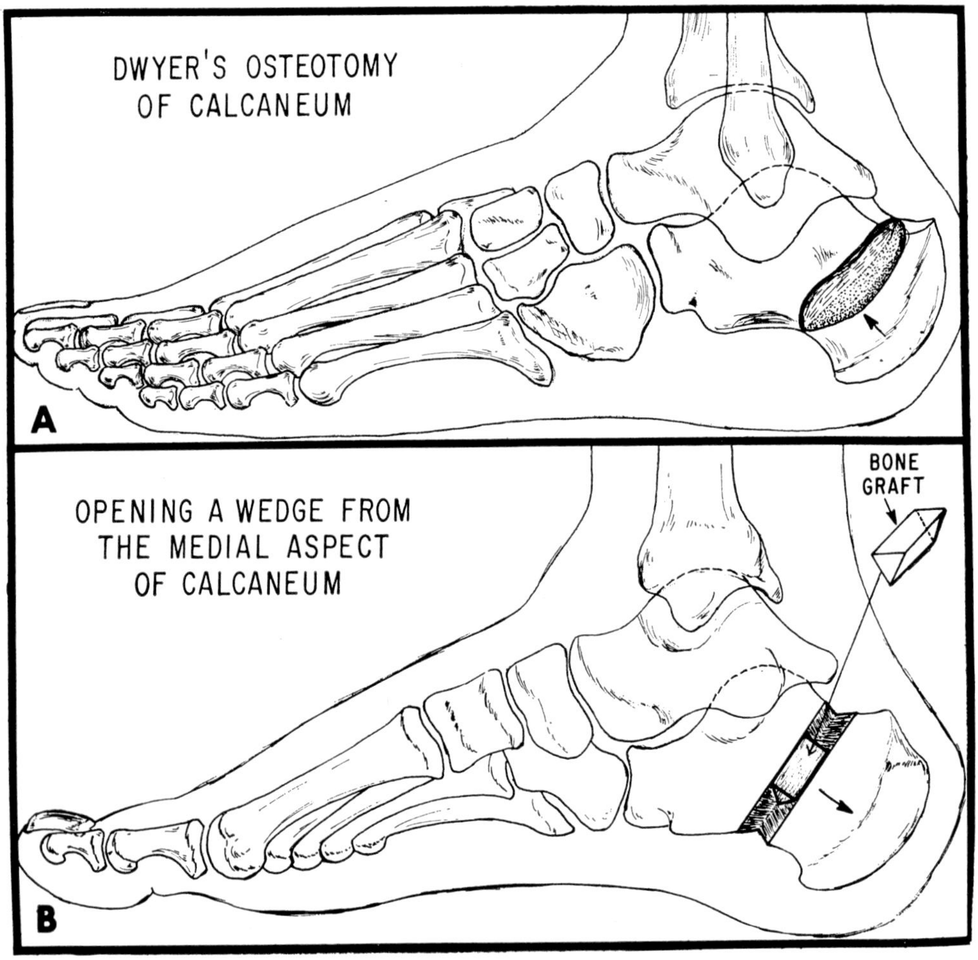

DWYER'S OSTEOTOMY
OF CALCANEUM

A

OPENING A WEDGE FROM
THE MEDIAL ASPECT
OF CALCANEUM

BONE
GRAFT

B

Figure 15–29. Osteotomy of calcaneum.

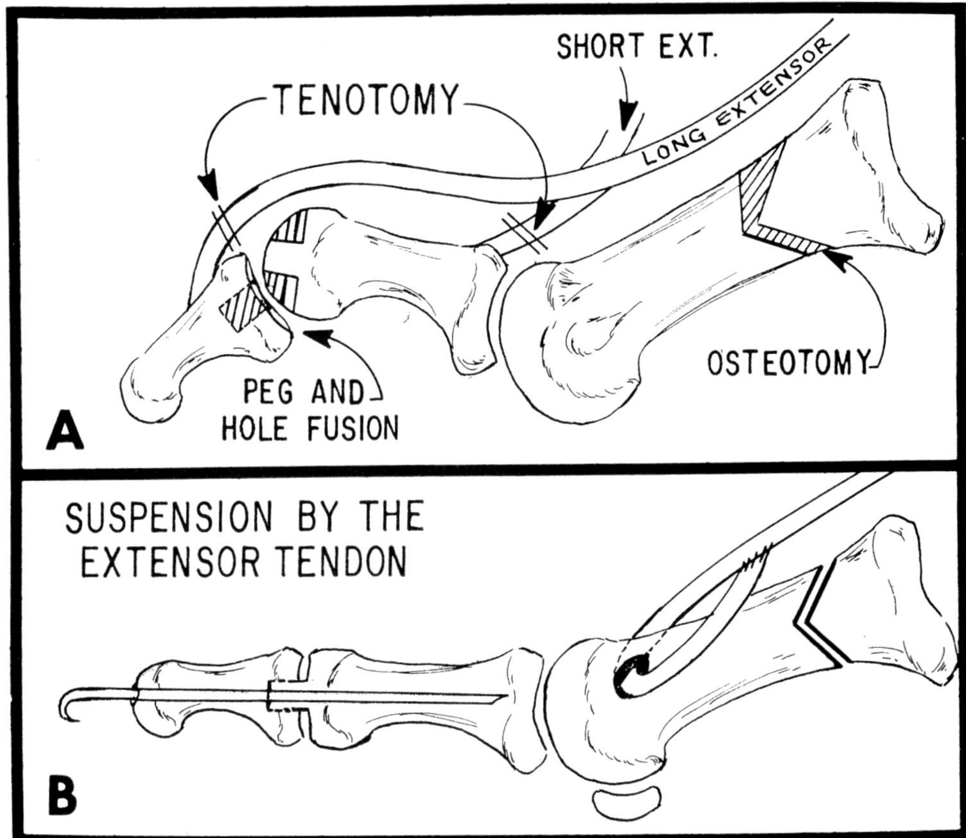

Figure 15–30. Osteotomy of the first metatarsal and the Jones suspension operation.

tarsalgia. In the combined deformity of clawtoes and cavus foot the bearing surface of the sole is considerably curtailed. The aim of surgery is to expand this surface, enlarge the tread, and restore the pressing-down action of the toes.

Early cavus foot and clawing of the toes in children should be given a trial of manipulation and periodic application of corrective casts as is ordinarily practiced for clubfoot. The cast holds the foot dorsiflexed at the ankle, with the heel in valgus and the metatarsal heads lifted. In growing children, bone resection and joint fusion are avoided. Capsulotomies and tenotomy of the extensors are permissible; one may have to lengthen the Achilles tendon. Tenoplasty of the heelcord should not be carried out simultaneously with detachment of the soft tissues from the underaspect of os calcis. Steindler stripping should be given a trial before the age of ten, provided there is no varus of the heel, nor as yet fixed skeletal changes. In the presence of definite varus of the heel, Dwyer's osteotomy is indicated. We have modified this operation somewhat: instead of removing a cuneiform piece from the lateral side, we open a wedge on the medial aspect of the calcaneum and plug the gap with bone graft. When there is also sharp plantar inclination of the first metatarsal, we osteotomize this bone near its base, tilt the distal fragment, and hold it up with the aid of a Jones suspension (Figs. 15–29 and 15–30).

Established cavus with fixed skeletal deformity necessitates either dorsal wedge resection of anterior tarsal bones or triple arthrodesis. The choice depends on the point from which the forepart of the foot drops. Tarsectomy is indicated if the heel is not in varus and the point from which the forefoot drops is distal to the naviculocuneiform joint. If the wedge of bone is to include the navicular bone and the neck of the talus, triple arthrodesis is preferred. In

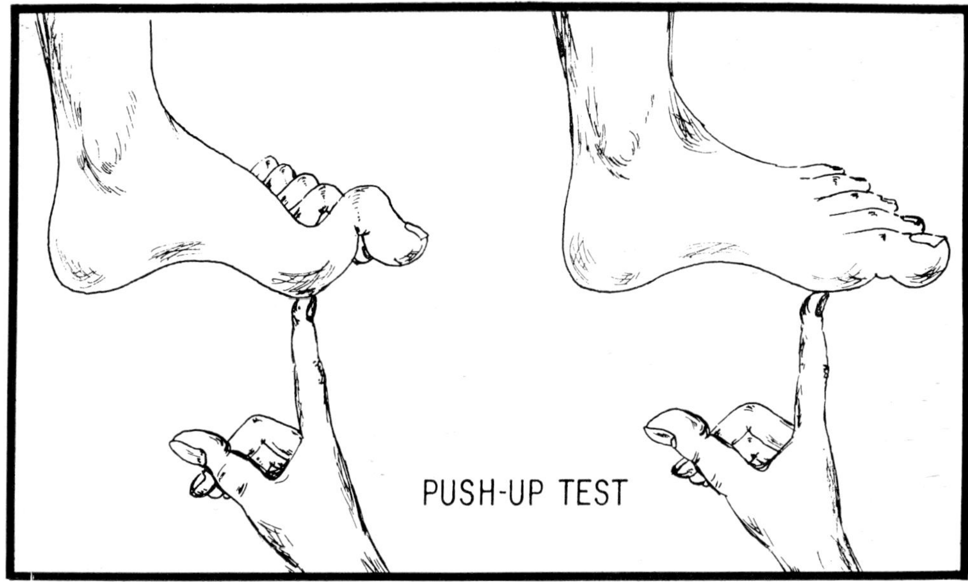

Figure 15–31. Push-up test.

adults, fixed varus of the heel is best corrected by triple arthrodesis rather than by combined cuneiform tarsectomy and wedge osteotomy of the calcaneum.

Correction of cavus deformity results in straightening the toes, provided these have remained pliable—when the push-up test against the metatarsal heads brings the terminal phalanges down to the level of the metatarsal heads. Interphalangeal fusion is in order when upward thrust on the metatarsal heads causes flexion at the metatarsophalangeal articulations, and the tips of the toes remain in midair because of fixed knuckling of the digital joints. We have never needed to fuse both interphalangeal joints as recommended by Lambrinudi; we carry out arthrodesis of the first articulation only (Fig. 15–31).

Interphalangeal fusion is ill advised in children, because it stunts growth of the toe. It should also be avoided in fixed incarceration of the metatarsal heads, dislocation of the bones entering into the metatarsophalangeal joints, or interlocking due to arthritis. These cases require resection of one of the articular bones—either the base of the proximal phalanx or the distal extremity of the metatarsal bone. One may have to combine fusion of the first interphalangeal joint with resection of the proximal portion of the basal phalanx of the toe. Partial proximal phalangectomy and surgical syndactylia of adjacent toes is another method that may be utilized beneficially (Figs. 15–32 to 15–35).

Flexibility of the metatarsophalangeal joints provides the key to treatment of plantar bulge of the metatarsal heads and the underlying painful keratoses. In clawtoes due to rheumatoid arthritis, the proximal portion of the basal phalanx and the distal segment of the metatarsal of the same ray may have to be resected to bring the toes down. In ordinary fixed incarceration of the central heads, we prefer to resect the distal third of the offending metatarsal bone. This portion of the bone is sought through the extended dorsal limb of the web-bisecting incision described in connection with surgical syndactylia of the toes at the end of the preceding section. The periosteum is split lengthwise and stripped, and two retractors are passed around the metatarsal shaft. The bone is divided at the desired level. The distal fragment is lifted out of the wound. A paddle screw transfixes the distal fragment and is carried out through an arc toward the toe; this maneuver greatly facilitates the delivery of the distal fragment. The cut surface of the proximal fragment is then rendered smooth and round.

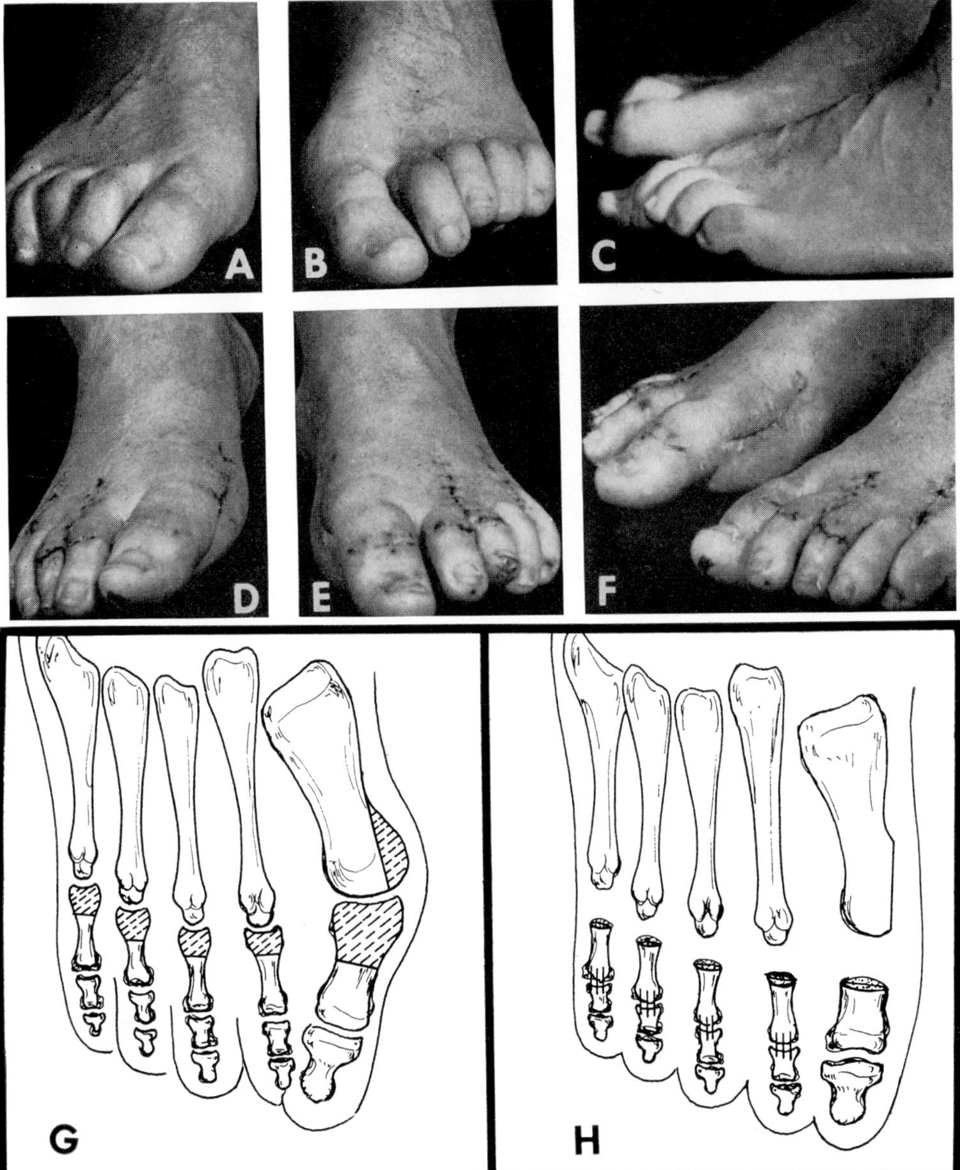

Figure 15—32. Man with bilateral clawtoes. Surgery performed was partial proximal phalangectomy of all toes, and fusion of the proximal interphalangeal joints of lesser toes. Preoperative photographs (*A, B,* and *C*). Postoperative photographs (*D, E,* and *F*). Interpretative diagrams (*G* and *H*). Patient now wears shoes in comfort and is satisfied.

When the distal segments of all three central metatarsals are to be resected, two incisions are used: one between the second and third, and another between the fourth and fifth, metatarsals. The distal half or more of the fifth metatarsal is resected in marked splaying of this ray. The plane of resection of this bone should be oblique and beveled, looking laterally and forward. Passing from the tibial of the fibular border, the plane of resection of each central metatarsal shifts closer to the tarsus; more bone is resected from the fourth metatarsal than from the third, and more from the latter than from the second. When the head of the first metatarsal is resected, it is advisable to ex-

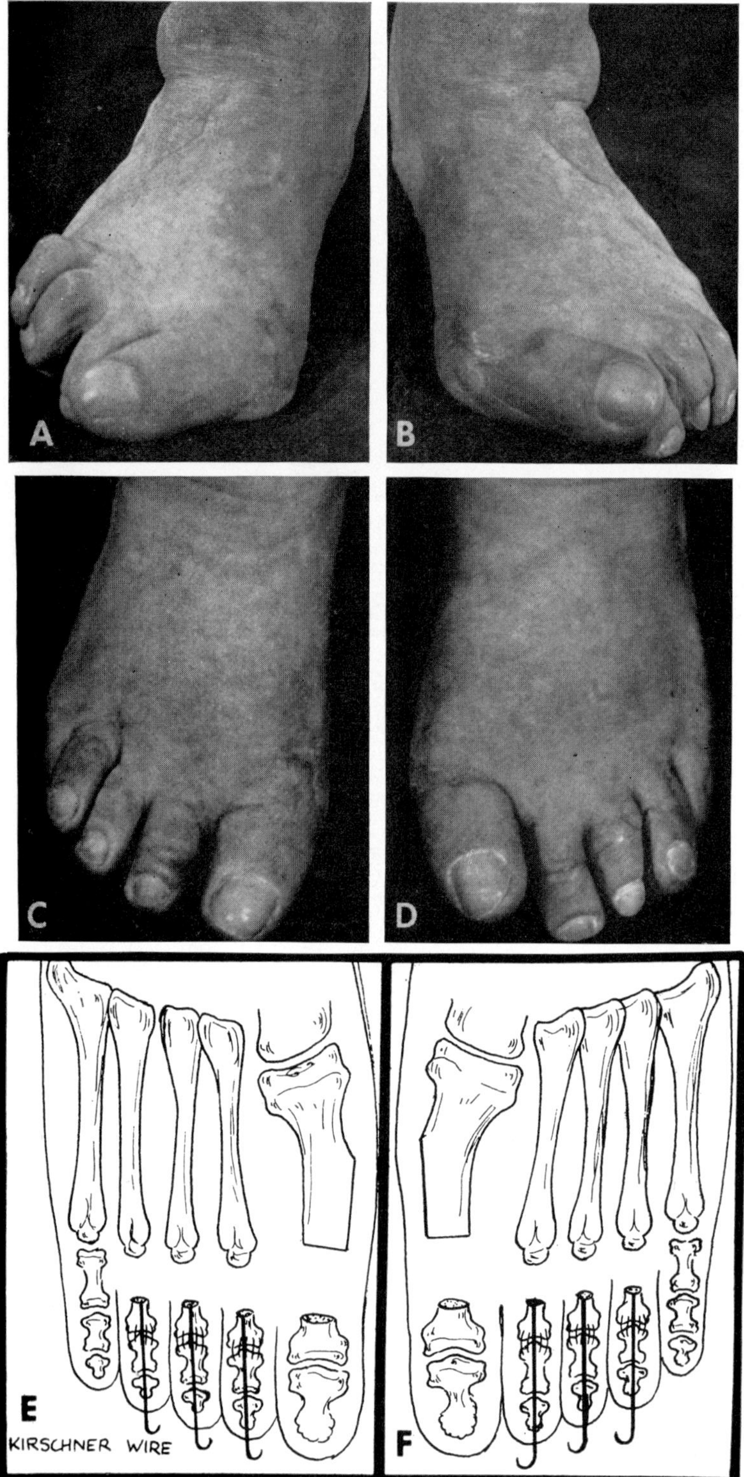

Figure 15–33. Woman with bilateral hallux valgus and hammertoes that had become clawed owing to fixed contracture of the joints. Surgery performed was Keller resection for the great toes, and partial proximal phalangectomy and fusion of the first interphalangeal joints of the three central toes on both sides. Preoperative photographs (*A* and *B*). Postoperative photographs (*C* and *D*). Interpretative diagrams (*E* and *F*). Patient is satisfied.

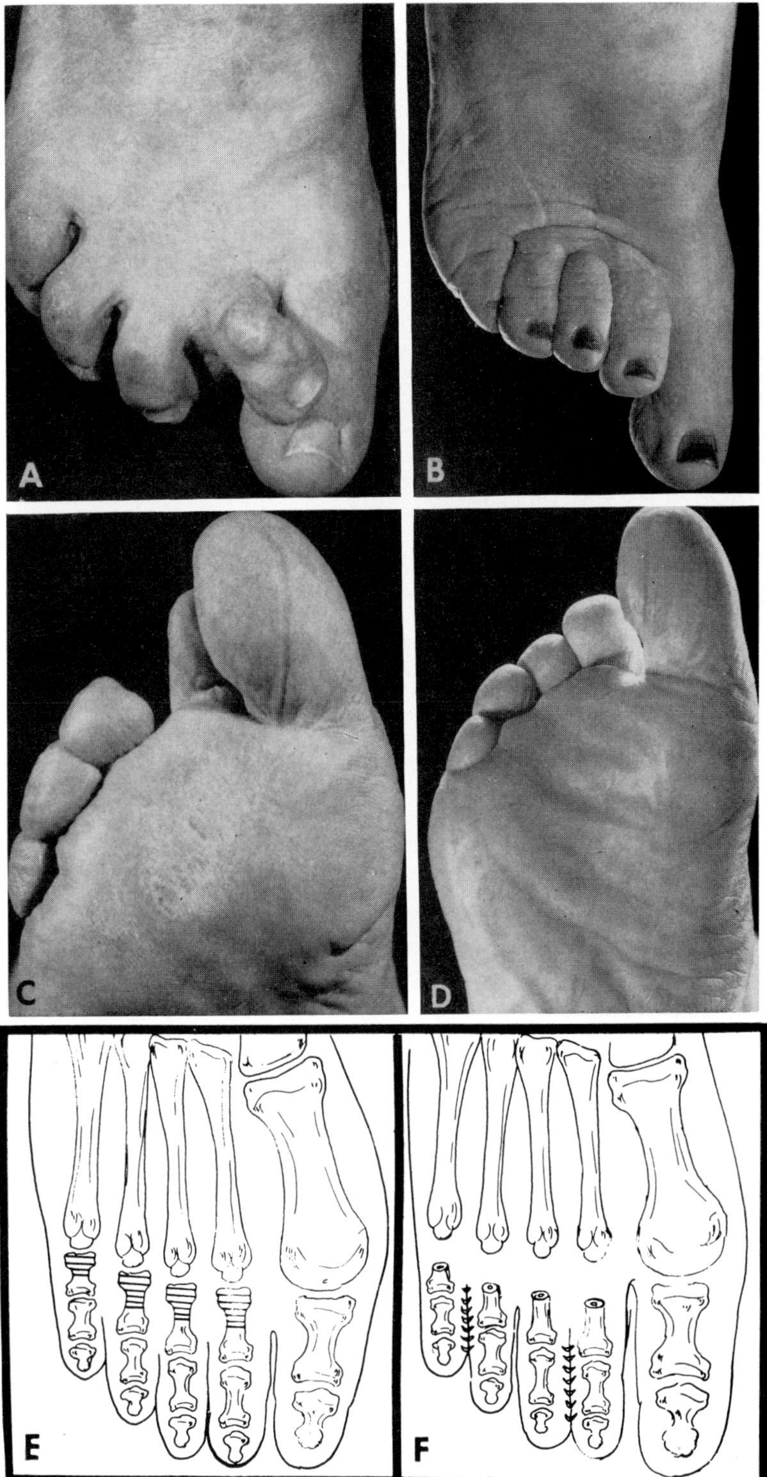

Figure 15–34. Woman with unilateral clawed lateral three toes and overlapping second toe. Surgery performed was partial proximal phalangectomy of the lesser toes and surgical syndactylia of each pair. Preoperative dorsal view photograph (*A*). Postoperative dorsal view photograph (*B*). Preoperative plantar view photograph (*C*). Postoperative plantar view photograph (*D*). Interpretative diagrams (*E* and *F*). Patient is satisfied.

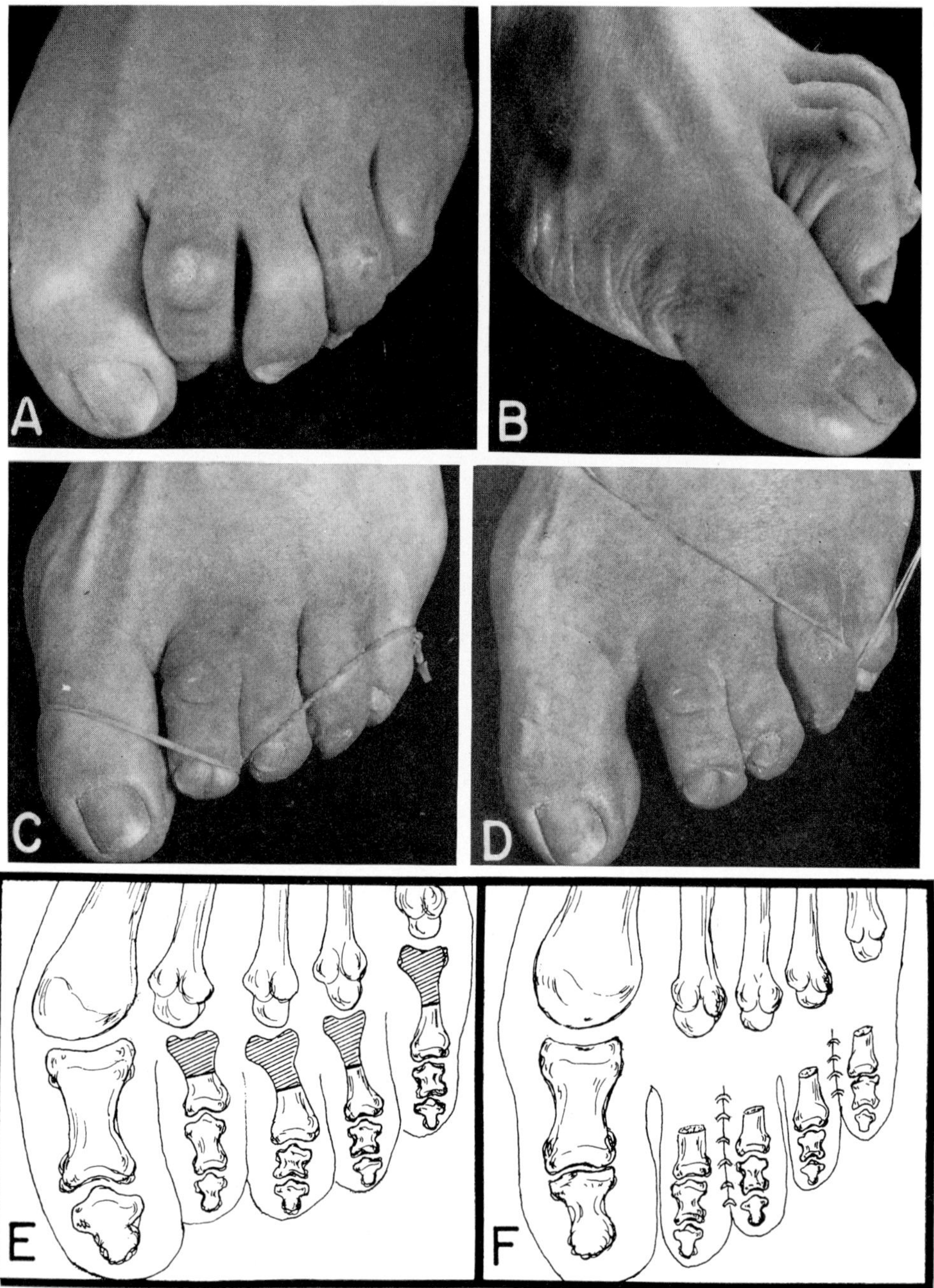

Figure 15–35. Woman with unilateral clawed lesser toes. Surgery performed was partial proximal phalangectomy of lesser toes, and surgical syndactylia of each pair of adjacent toes. Preoperative photographs (*A* and *B*). Postoperative photographs (*C* and *D*). Interpretative diagrams (*E* and *F*). The patient serves full duty as a nurse and wears shoes in comfort.

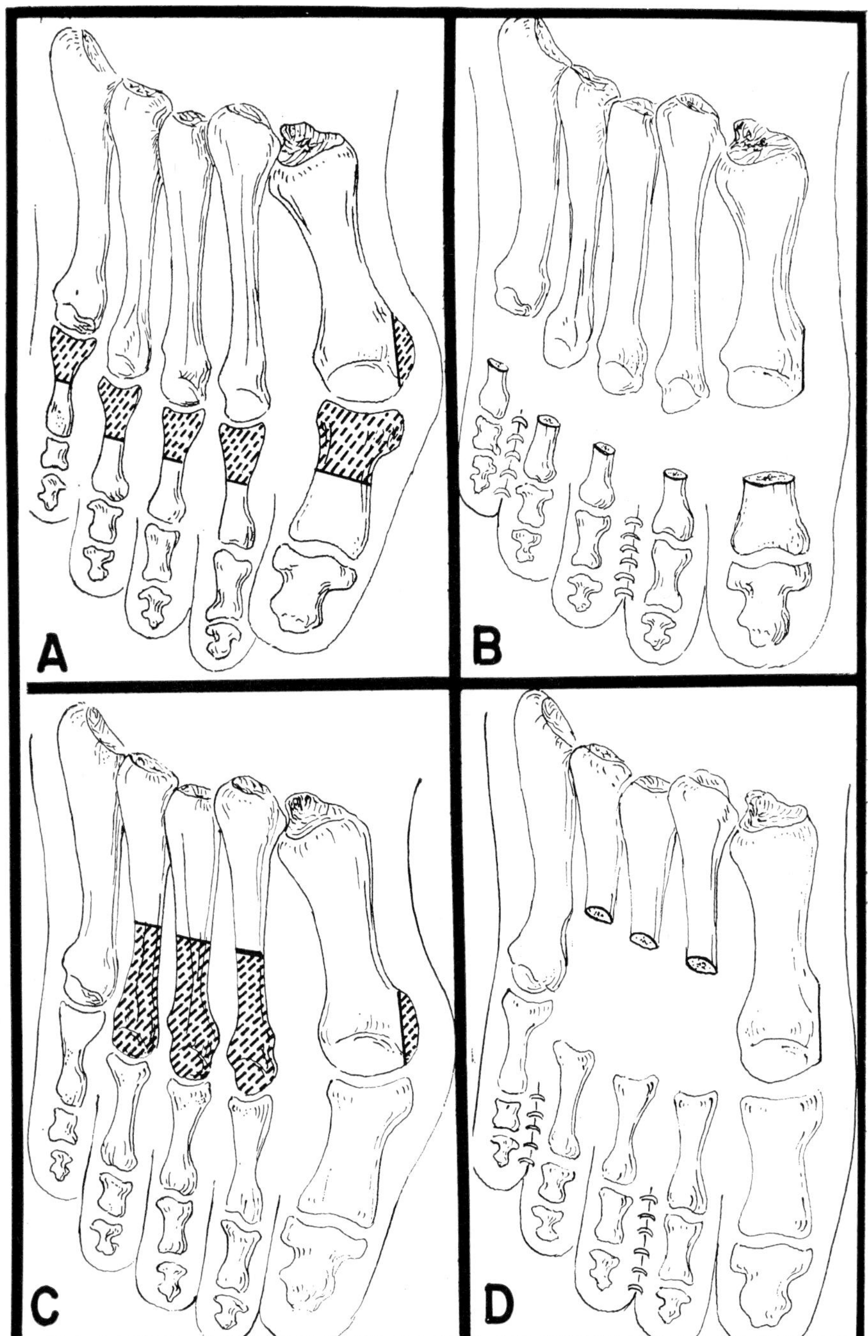

Figure 15–36. Patterns of bone resection.

cise the distal one-fourth of the second and sometimes of the third metatarsal. Resection of the distal portions of the metatarsals leaves the corresponding toes without foundation; they become flail and dangle. They are stabilized by surgical syndactylia (Figs. 15–36 to 15–43).

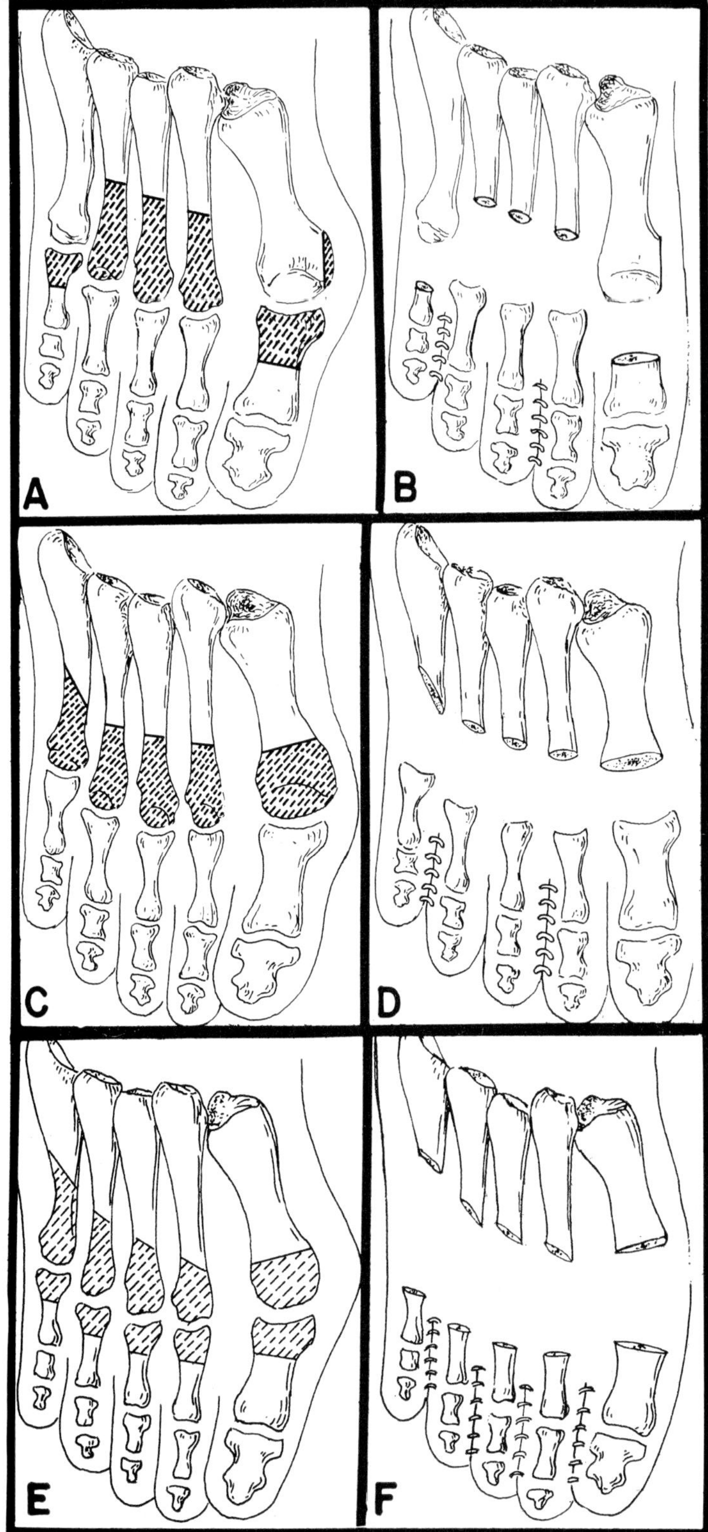

Figure 15–37. Patterns of bone resection.

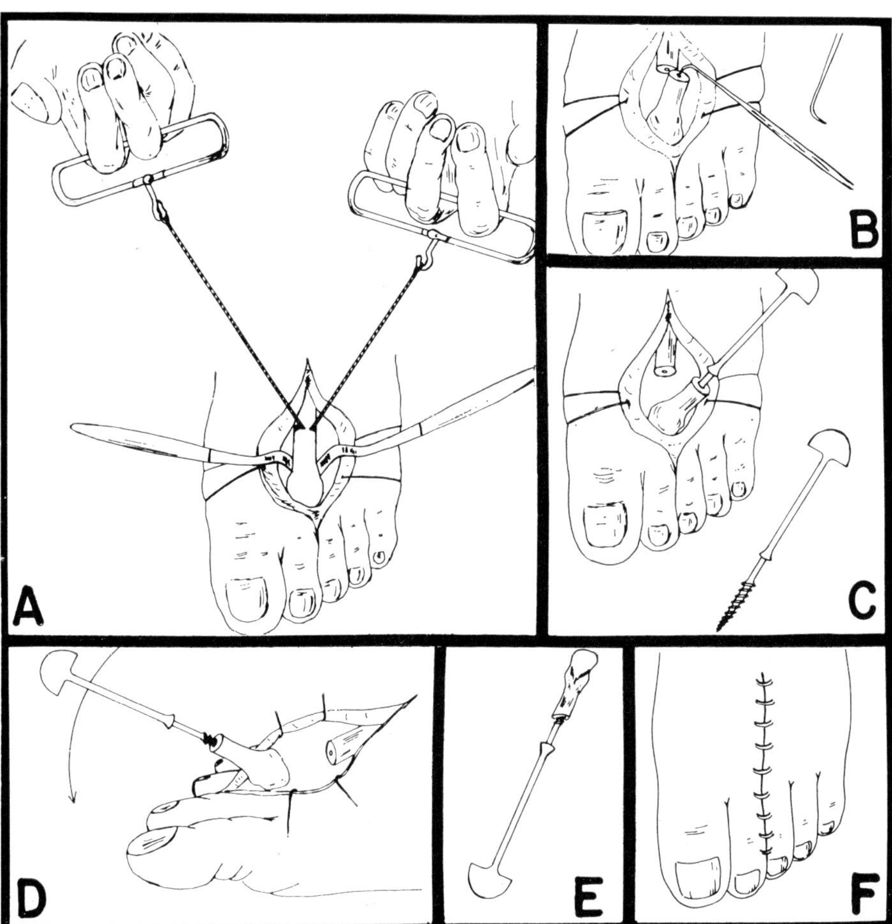

Figure 15–38. Technique of resection of distal third of the metatarsal bone and syndactylia of adjacent toes.

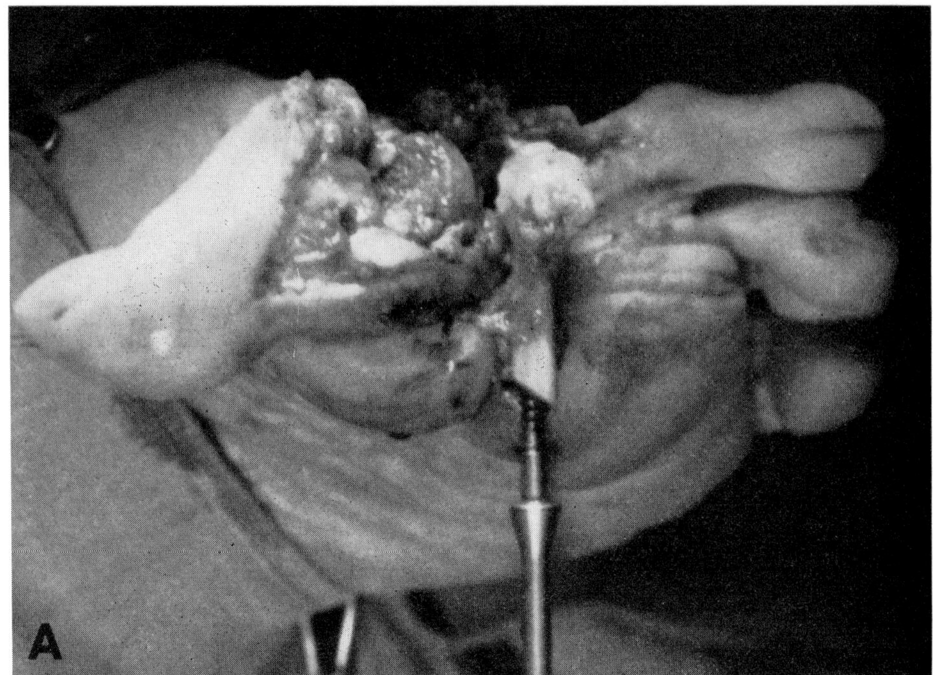

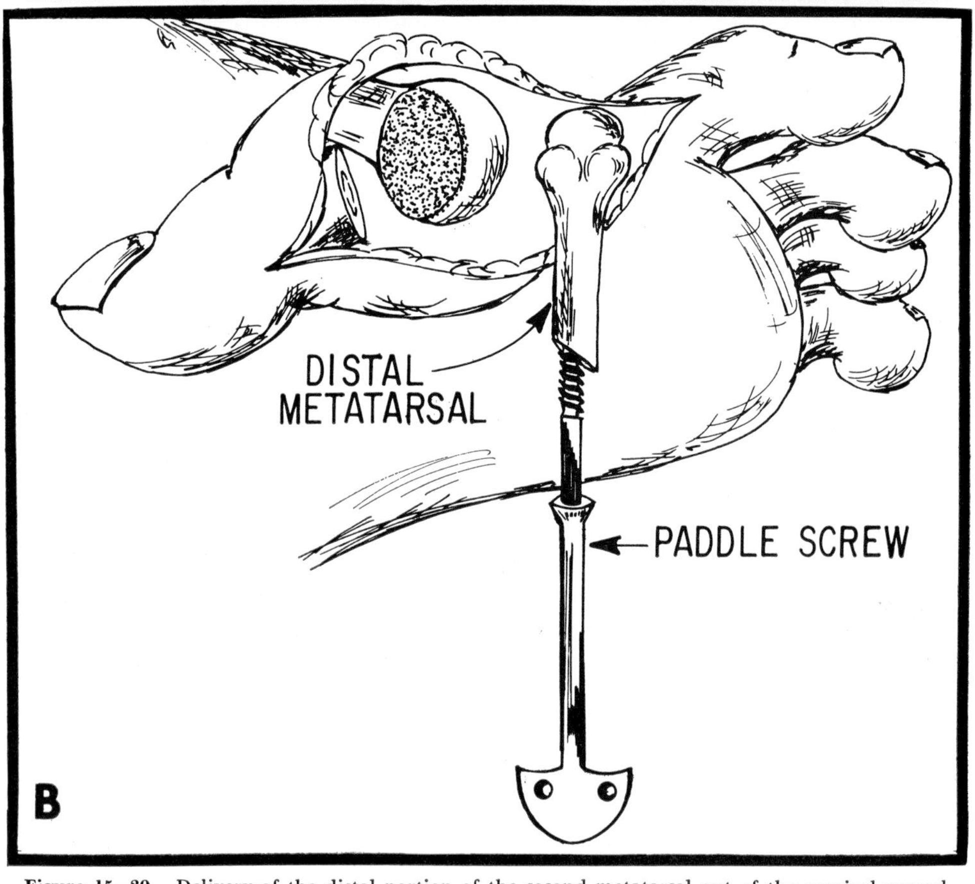

Figure 15–39. Delivery of the distal portion of the second metatarsal out of the surgical wound.

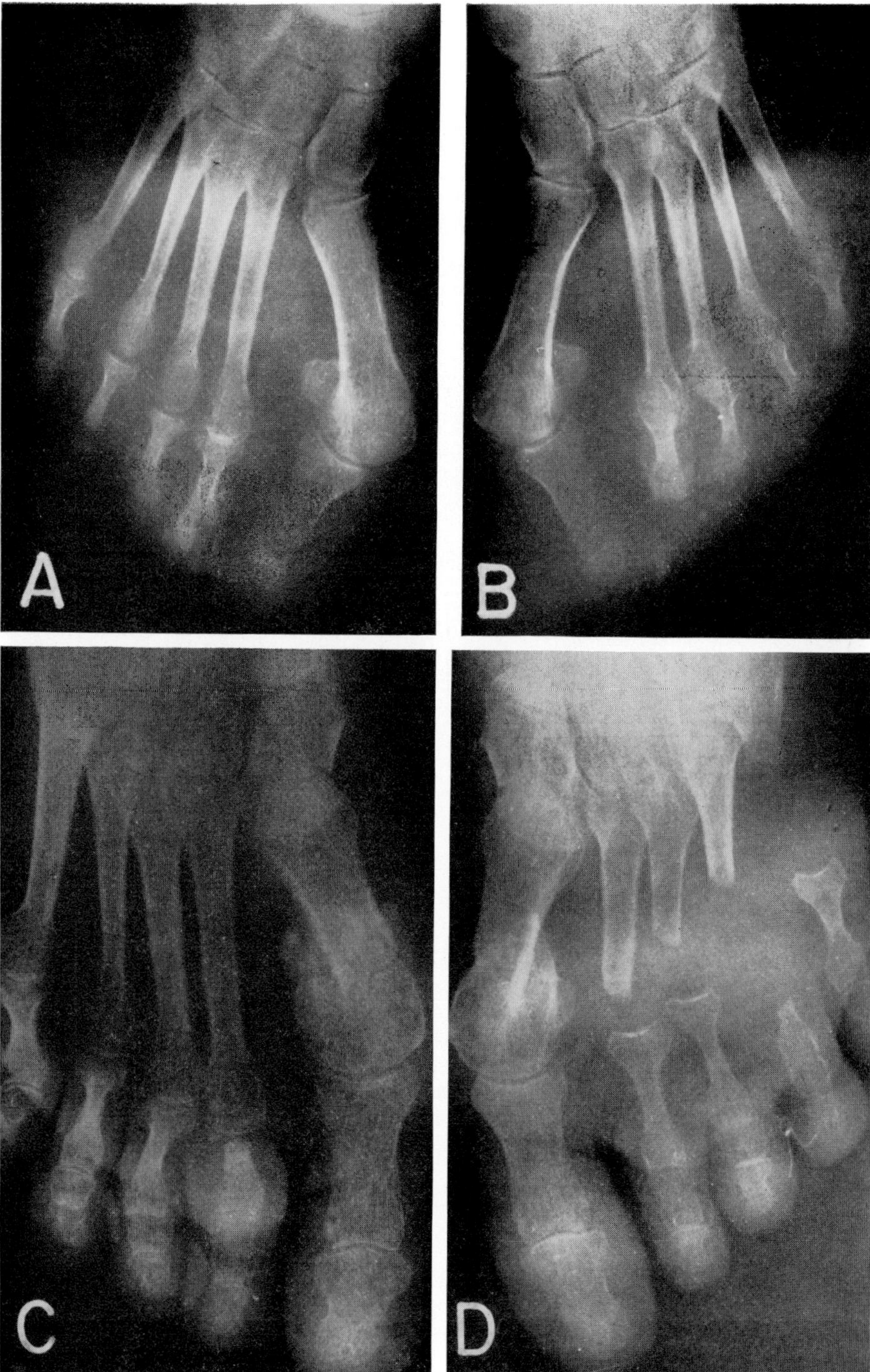

Figure 15–40. Woman with bilateral hallux valgus; hammered second toe on the right side; and clawed lesser toes on the left, which would not budge following upward thrust on the metatarsal heads. Surgery performed was Thomasen *peg-and-hole* osteotomy for correction of hallux valgus on both sides, partial proximal phalangectomy of right second toe and surgical syndactylia of this digit with the third, and resection of distal portions of all lateral four metatarsals on the left side. In addition the fourth proximal was resected and each pair of adjacent toes were syndactylized.

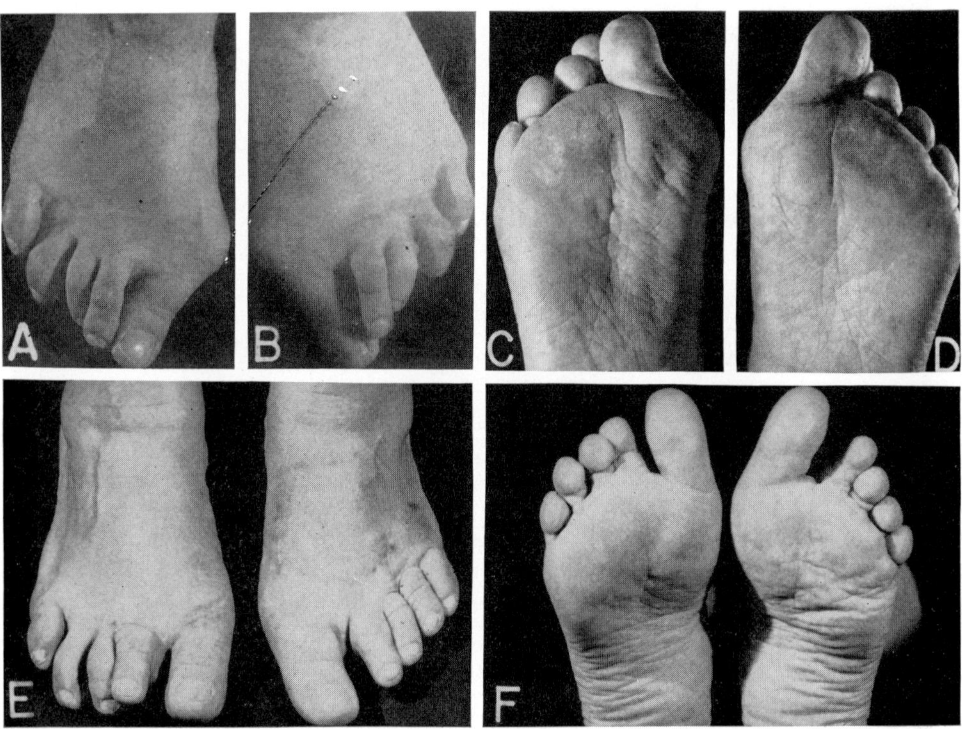

Figure 15–41. The same case as in Figure 15–40. Preoperative dorsal view photographs (*A* and *B*). Preoperative plantar views (*C* and *D*). Postoperative dorsal view (*E*). Postoperative plantar view (*F*). Patient is satisfied.

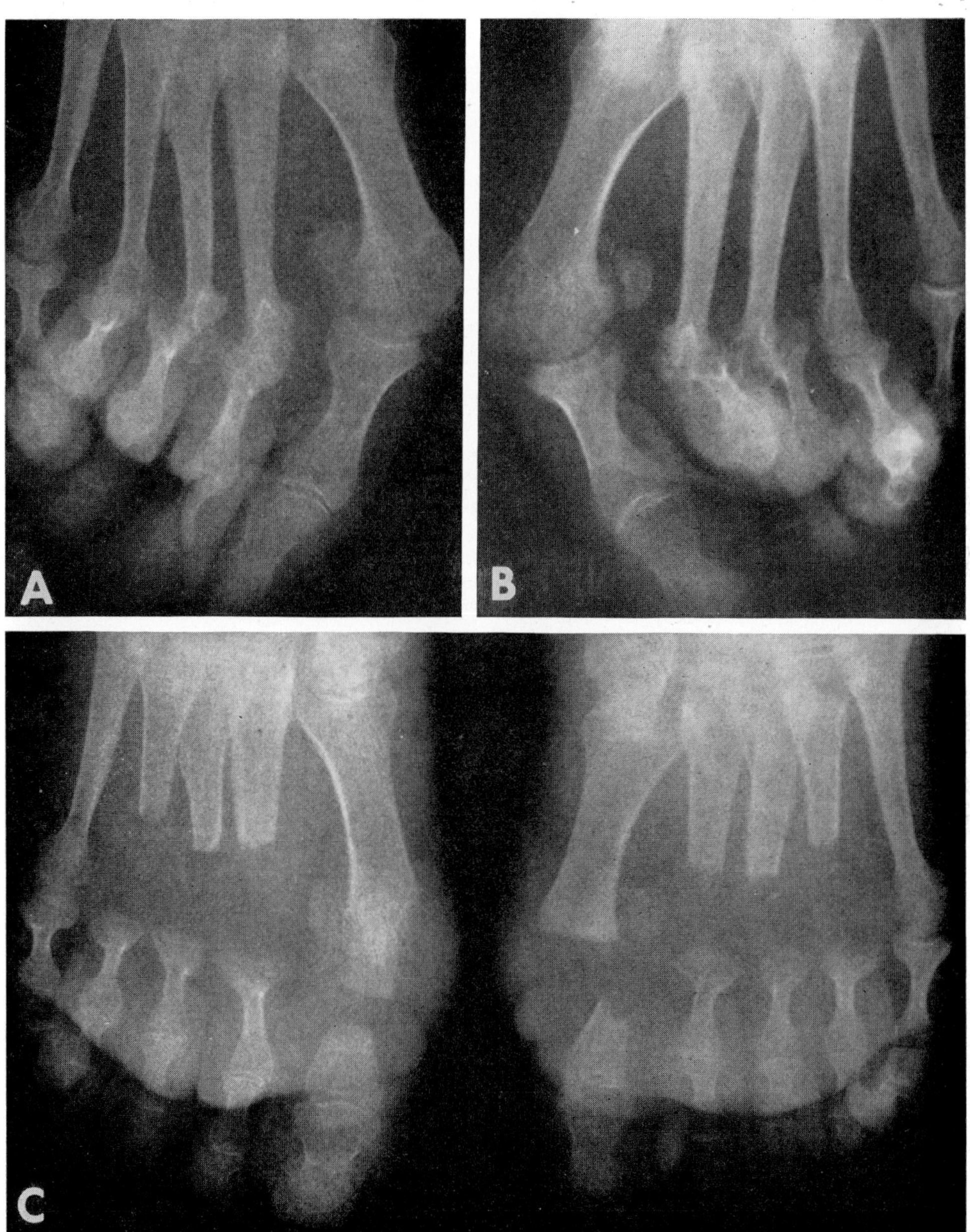

Figure 15–42. Woman with bilateral hallux valgus and clawtoes due to rheumatoid arthritis. Surgery performed was resection of first metatarsophalangeal joints on both sides. In addition, on the right the medial eminence was sagittally resected. The distal halves of central three metatarsal bones were resected on both sides, and on both sides the first and second toes were syndactylized together and the third toe was connected with the fourth.

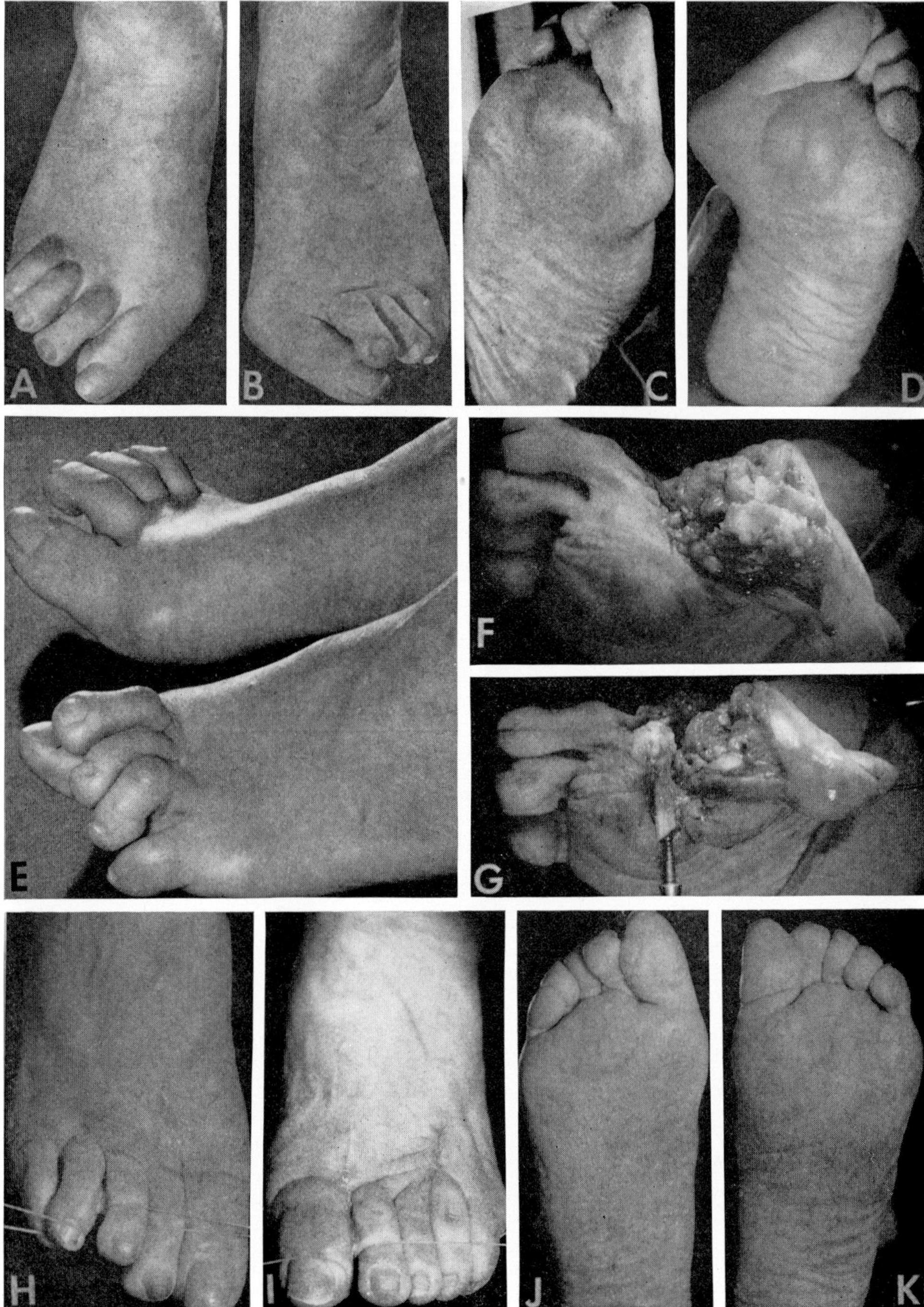

Figure 15–43. The same case as in Figure 15–42. Preoperative dorsal view photographs (*A* and *B*). Preoperative plantar views (*C* and *D*). Side view photograph (*E*). Surgically exposed right first metatarsophalangeal joint (*F*). Delivery of the distal segment of the second metatarsal (*G*). Postoperative photographs (*H* to *K*). Patient is satisfied but complains of pain under the fifth metatarsal head. Probably this bone should also have been resected.

DIGITUS MINIMUS VARUS

In the literature the epithets *varus, elevated, overlapping,* and *contracted* are indiscriminately used to describe the deformities of the small toe. Varus deflection of the fifth toe may be congenital or acquired. The *congenital variety* is, as a rule, bilateral and it appears in more than one member of the same family. Its earliest indication is dorsal tilt of the proximal phalanx. The small toe then insidiously inclines medially and straddles the base of the fourth digit. In full-fledged deformity, the fifth toe also undergoes rotation around its own longitudinal axis; its pulp points toward the midsagittal plane and its nail slants laterally.

Numerous surgical procedures have been proposed for digitus quintus varus. Amputation was a common practice at one time. Soft tissue surgery has been recommended by Lantzounis (1940), Lapidus (1942), Goodwin and Swisher (1943), Stamm (1948), Wilson (1953), and DuVries (1959). Lantzounis detached the extensor of the small toe from its insertion; he threaded the severed tendon through a drill hole behind the fifth metatarsal head and sutured it to itself. Lapidus divided the extensor tendon over the middle of the fifth metatarsal, passed the distal portion through a drill hole in the proximal phalanx from the medial side, brought it out laterally, and sutured it to the abductor of the small toe. Goodwin and Swisher combined plastic elongation of the extensor tendon with capsulotomy of the fifth metatarsophalangeal joint and Y advancement of dorsal skin. Stamm and Wilson tenotomized the extensor, released the dorsal capsule and utilized the principle of V-plasty to relieve the tension of the skin. DuVries performed extensor tenotomy and dorsal capsulotomy, and released the skin contracture by a complicated incision in the fourth interdigital space. These plastic soft tissue procedures do not yield lasting results.

Surgery on the skeletal elements has also been diversified—but not as much. Gocht and Debrunner (1925) enucleated the proximal phalanx through an incision on the lateral aspect of the small toe. According to Straub (1951), Ruiz-Mora removed the proximal phalanx through a pair of elliptical skin cuts on the plantar aspect of the toe. It was hoped that the resulting surgical scar would hold the toe in correct position. McFarland (1950) and Scrase (1954) excised the proximal phalanx and syndactylized the fourth and fifth toes together. Scrase also divided the extensor tendon (Fig. 15–44).

In children we tenotomize the extensor tendon, release the capsule on the dorsal and medial aspect of the fifth metatarsophalangeal joint, and syndactylize the fourth and fifth toes together. In adults we, in addition, excise the proximal phalanx of the fifth toe in part or completely (Fig. 15–45).

Acquired varus of the fifth toe is usually unilateral. It often accompanies hallux valgus and should be regarded as the local manifestation of forefoot splaying. The fifth metatarsal is either hypermobile or in a fixed valgus position.

"A bunionette," Horace Davies (1949) wrote, "is it not uncommonly seen in combination with pes and hallux valgus and general splaying of the forefoot, and is . . . regarded as a secondary deformity in these cases. Chronic irritation due to pressure upon the lateral surface of the foot in cross legged or sartorial position is also considered as a causative factor, for it was this that gave rise to the name 'tailor's bunion.' " Davies then related the case of a nine year old girl with bilateral bunionette, which he regarded "as a primary and independent deformity." He called the latter variety *metatarsus quintus valgus* and ascribed it to the persistence of "the embryonic splaying of the fifth metatarsal due to incomplete or imperfect development of the transverse metatarsal ligament."

Bunionette consists of the outwardly protruding portion of the fifth metatarsal head. It is analogous to the medial eminence of the first metatarsal head in hallux valgus. "Rarely do these cases require active treatment other than provision of well-fitting shoes," Davies

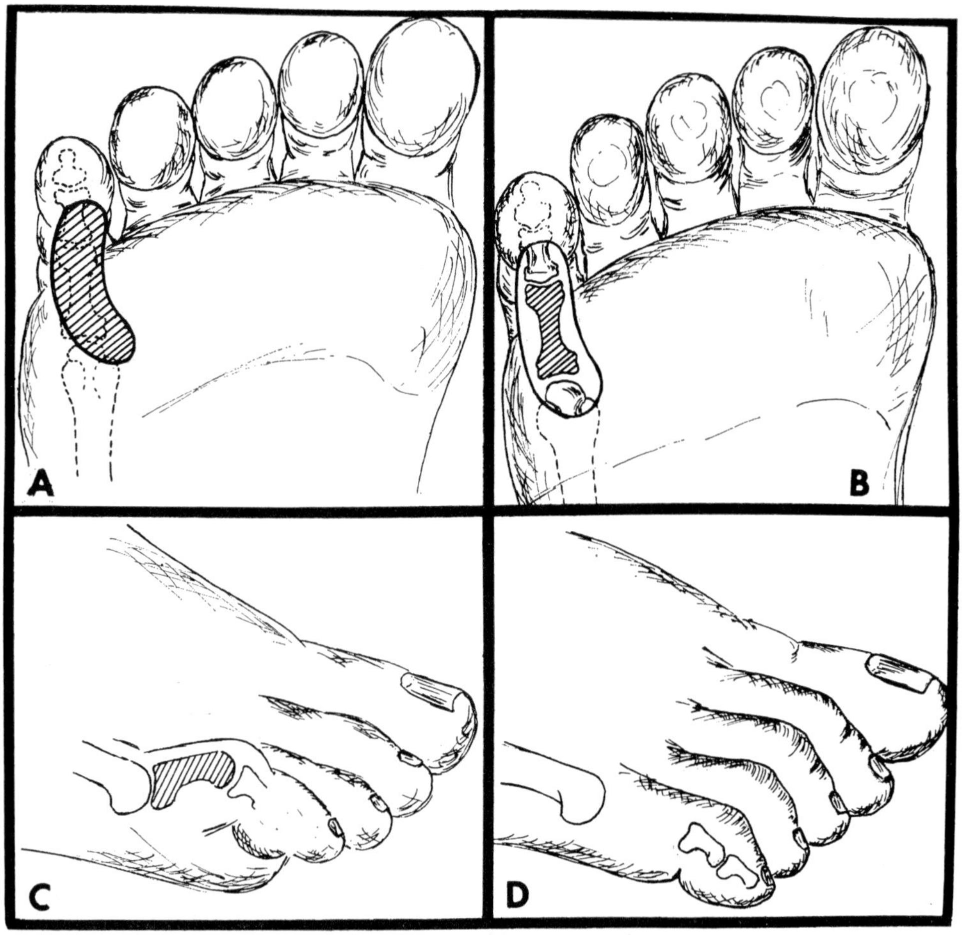

Figure 15–44. Ruiz-Mora operation.

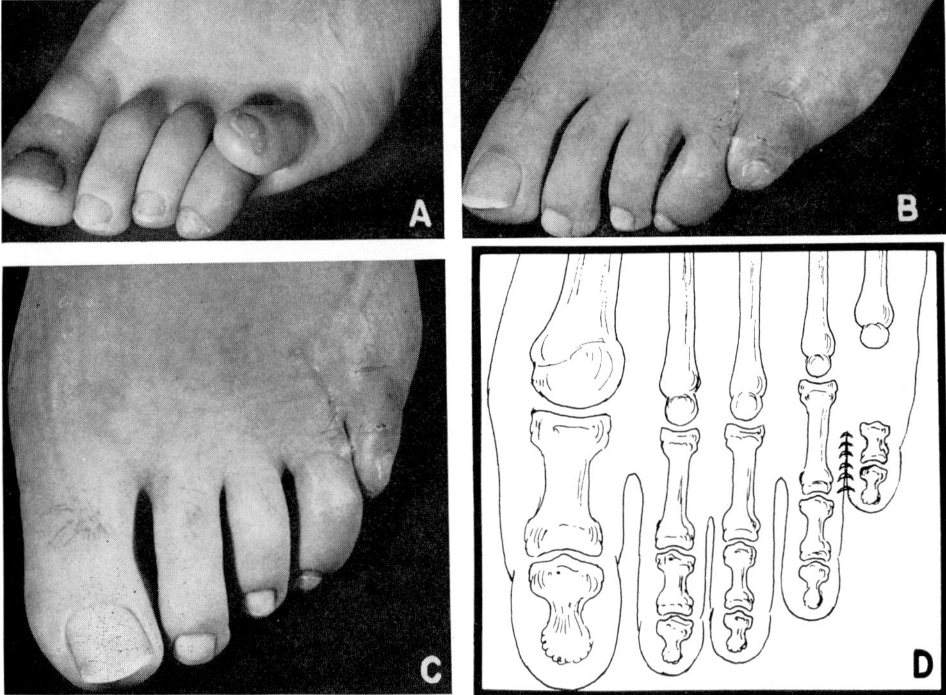

Figure 15–45. Woman with left digitus minimus varus. Surgery performed was resection of the proximal phalanx of the small toe and surgical syndactylia of this digit with its neighbor on the medial side. Preoperative photograph (*A*). Postoperative photographs (*B* and *C*). Interpretative diagram (*D*).

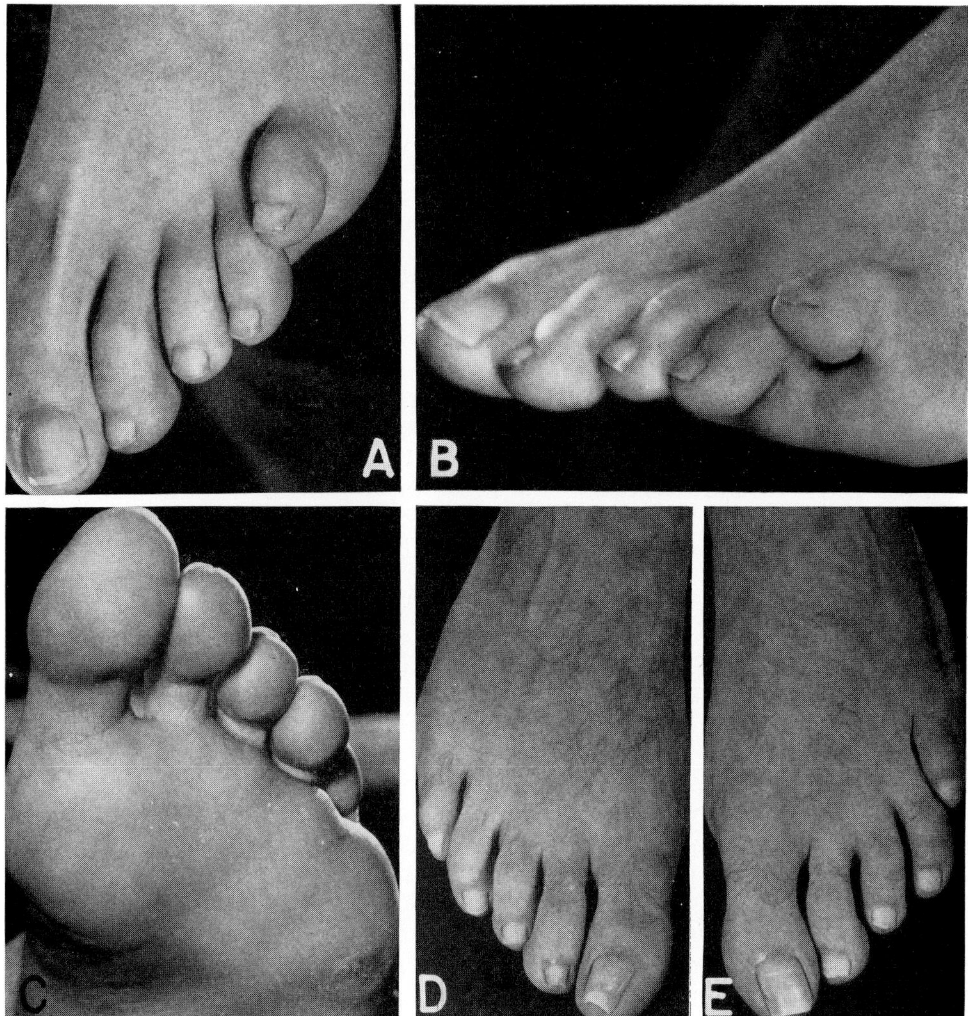

Figure 15–46. Man with dorsally displaced, clawed, contracted left small toe and plantar incarceration of fifth metatarsal head. Surgery performed was beveled resection of distal third of the fifth metatarsal and surgical syndactylia of the fourth and fifth toes. Preoperative photographs of the left forefoot (*A, B,* and *C*). Photograph of right forefoot, shown here for comparison (*D*). Postoperative photograph of left forefoot (*E*).

wrote. "Bunionectomy of the metatarsal head may be necessary in pronounced cases with clinical symptoms. If the primary factor is the abduction of the first metatarsal shaft, osteotomy should theoretically be the treatment of choice, but in practice, as for metatarsus primus varus, the procedure is in both unnecessary and often unsatisfactory."

Not many would agree that osteotomy is unnecessary and often unsatisfactory for metatarsus primus varus. Fifth metatarsal osteotomy is another matter. This bone is closer to the ground. We know from our experience with fractures that angulation and callus formation is not well tolerated in this region. Hohmann (1951) advised osteotomy through the neck of the bone and pushed the capital fragment closer to the fourth metatarsal. No one else appears to have adopted this procedure. Sagittal resection of the lateral eminence is practiced more frequently. At best it is a temporizing measure like simple exostectomy on the medial side of the foot; in time the deformity will recur. Resection of the fifth metatarsal head has also been practiced; it is often followed by formation of painful spurs.

"Having tried all these things and having had them fail occasionally," McKeever (1959) wrote, "I began to resect more and more of the fifth metatarsal in conjunction with amputation of the fifth toe, finally arriving at a beveled-off osteotomy slightly proximal to the middle of the fifth metatarsal with removal of all the metatarsal distal to this. . . . This resection amounts to between one-half and two-thirds of the distal portion of the metatarsal. I then began to remove the metatarsal without amputation of the toe."

Brown (1959) advised resection of the entire fifth ray—including the small toe —for splayfoot. This operation seems too drastic. The base of the fifth metatarsal provides an anchorage for the short peroneal muscle and serves as a pulley for the tendon of the long peroneal muscle; it is also an important weight-sustaining pillar. The small toe is needlessly sacrificed. It can be saved. If in varus deflection, it may be brought parallel to the fourth toe and syndactylized with it. Surgical syndactylia prevents the toe from retracting (Figs. 15–46 and 15–47).

Less common deformities of the lesser toes. In the past *macrodactylic second toe* was treated by amputation. This led to the valgus deformity of the great toe. We have resected the proximal—sometimes even part of the middle—phalanx and syndactylized the toe with its neighbor on either side. During surgery the toe is defatted. The operation is carried out in two steps, first on one side of the toe and several months later on the other. In four cases we explored the medial plantar nerve and found it normal. *Divergent second and third toes* are treated by partial proximal phalangectomy and surgical syndactylia (Fig. 15–48).

Microdactylic toes are usually accompanied by stunted metatarsal bones: they require no treatment. *Congenital webbing* of the toes should be regarded as a salutary anomaly. Because there is no fold, troublesome interdigital infections cannot obtain a foothold and flourish. Webbed toes are not known to become hammered or clawed and they are seldom accompanied by metatarsalgia.

At birth, the third toe of each foot is sometimes seen to bend plantarward; it begins to curl under the second digit and twist in such a way as to turn its terminal pulp toward the midsagittal plane. Trethowan (1925) classified this deformity as a *congenital form* of hammertoe. He considered it amenable to conservative treatment, passive movements beginning in infancy. Sweetman (1958) coined the term *congenital curly toe.* He regarded "the usual method of treatment with over-and-under strapping . . . without effect and unnecessary."

To date we have encountered six cases of bilateral curling third toes. We do not share Trethowan's optimism concerning the amenability of this deformity to passive massage and manipulation. We agree with Sweetman that the *over-and-under* strapping is useless, but disagree with him when he implies that no treatment is necessary. Almost all our patients had discomfort on wearing prefabricated shoes. One boy, age 20, had severe pain under the second metatarsal head because the underslung third toe would not permit its medial neighbor to touch the proffered surface. In children, we have been syndactylizing the curling third toe with its neighbor on the medial side. In adults, we combine partial proximal phalangectomy with surgical syndactylia of the toes.

Interdigital clavus between the fourth and fifth toes is not an uncommon accompaniment of hallux valgus. Manwaring (1930) ascribed soft corns to the "pressure by an enlarged joint." He recommended resection of the prominent lateral base of the proximal phalanx of the fourth toe. He considered the removal of the corn itself unnecessary and thought it would "disappear in time if freed sufficiently from pressure." We resect the corn and the surrounding avascular skin, and excise the basal half of the proximal phalanx of the fourth toe. If the small toe is de-

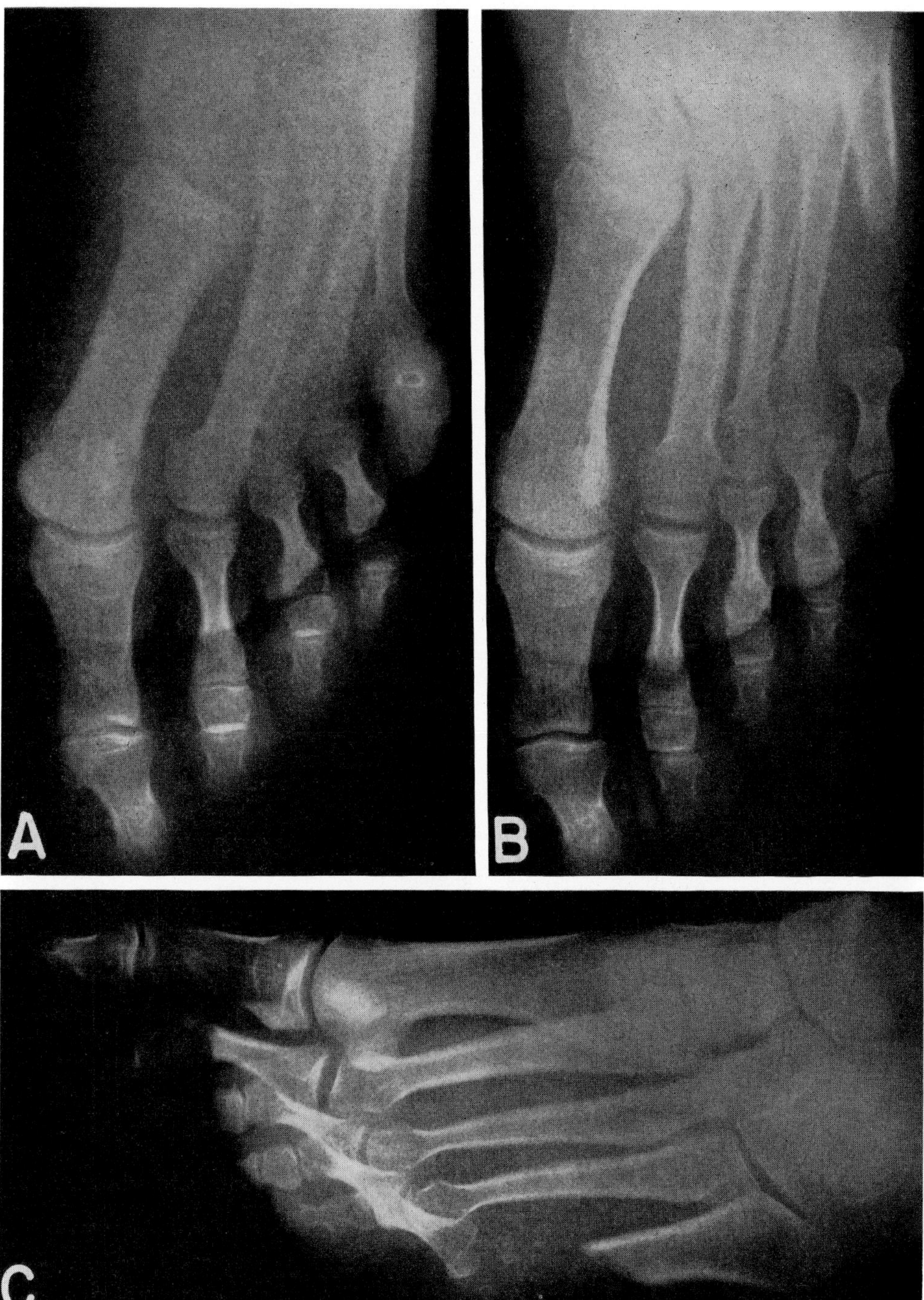

Figure 15–47. The same case as in Figure 15–46. Preoperative dorsoplantar roentgenogram of left forefoot (*A*). Dorsoplantar (*B*) and oblique (*C*) views of the same, showing the amount of bone resected and the beveled off end of the remaining segment of the fifth metatarsal bone. Patient is satisfied.

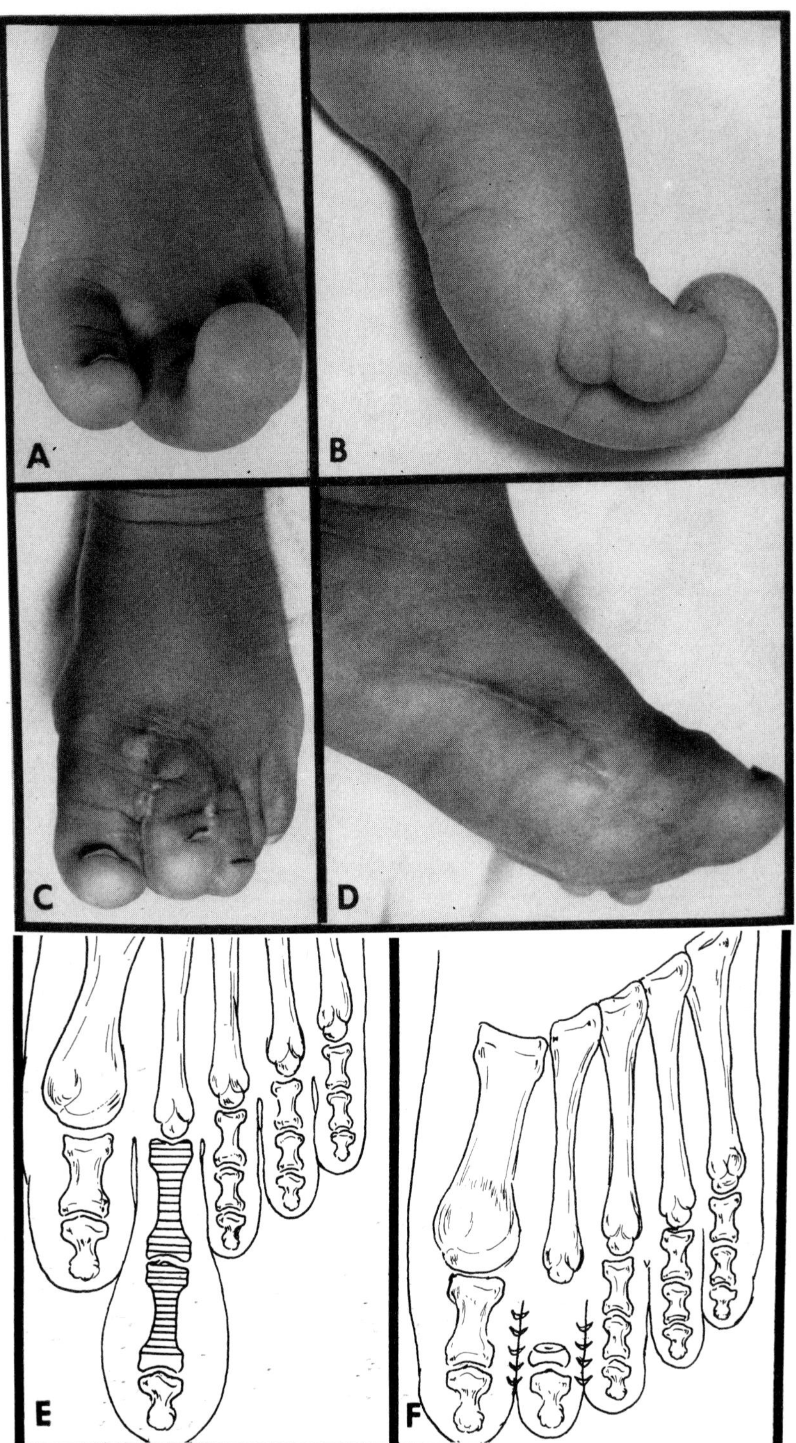

Figure 15–48. Female child with unilateral congenital gigantism of the left second toe. During the first sitting the medial plantar nerve was explored and found normal, and the proximal phalanx of the second toe was excised. The toe was defatted from its medial aspect and anastomosed with the hallux. At the second sitting, three month later, the middle phalanx of the second toe was excised almost in its entirety, and the toe was defatted again from its lateral aspect and syndactylized with the third digit. Preoperative frontal view photograph (*A*). Preoperative photograph taken from the medial side (*B*). Postoperative dorsal view photograph (*C*). Postoperative medial view photograph (*D*). Interpretative diagrams to show the amount of bone resected and the surgical syndactylia of the second toe to its neighbors on either side (*E* and *F*). The child can wear the same size of shoe on the left foot as on the right.

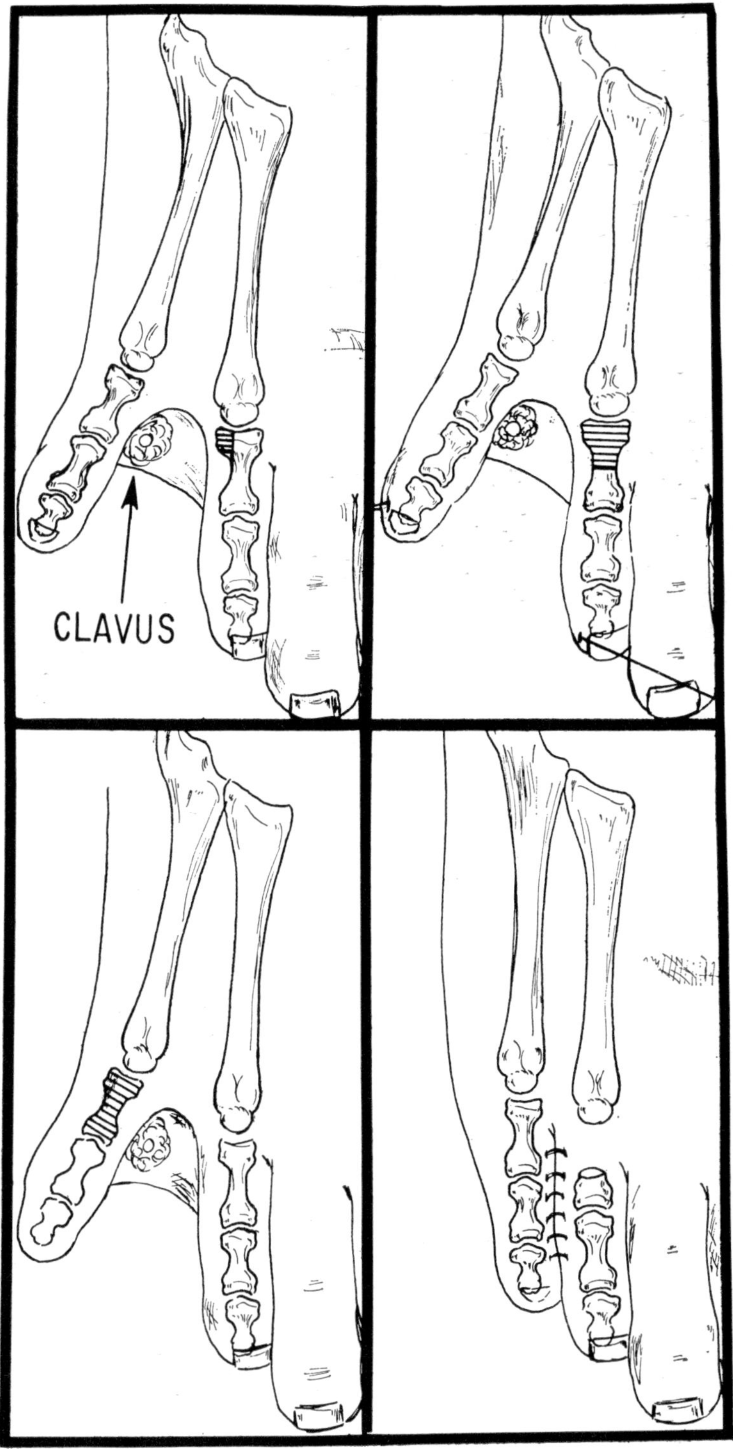

Figure 15–49. Diagrams demonstrating the bone resection and surgical syndactylia of the fourth and fifth toes for interdigital soft corn. Shaded areas indicate the amount of bone resected from the proximal phalanges of either the fourth or the fifth toes. The interdigital clavus is excised prior to bone resection and surgical syndactylia.

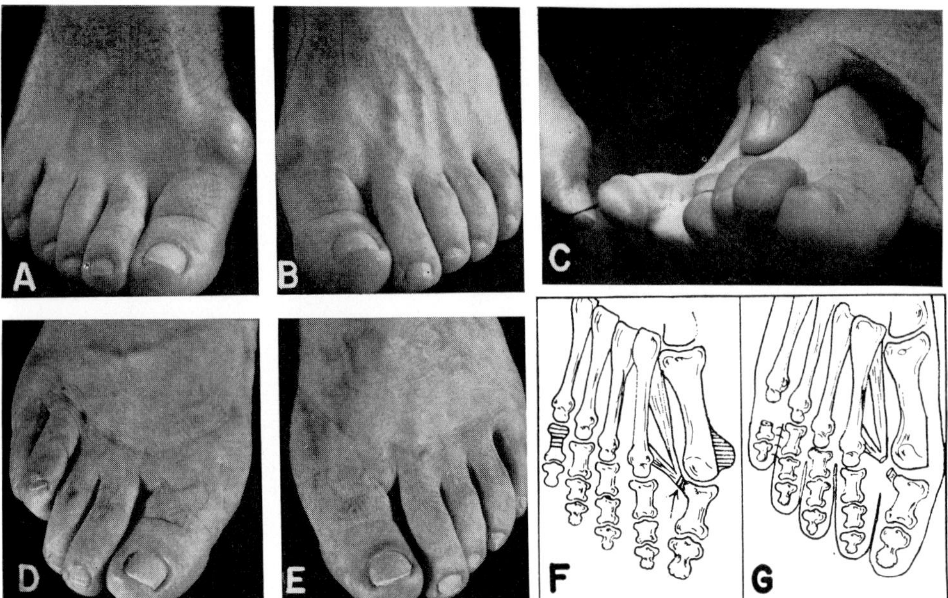

Figure 15–50. Woman with bilateral hallux valgus complicated with interdigital clavus between the right fourth and fifth toes. Surgery performed was the modified Silver operation to correct the bilateral hallux valgus. The soft corn was excised, the proximal half of the first phalanx of the fifth toe was resected, and the fourth and fifth toes were connected by surgical syndactylia. Preoperative photographs (*A* and *B*). Right foot showing interdigital clavus between fourth and fifth toes (*C*). Post-recovery photographs (*D* and *E*). Interpretative diagrams (*F* and *G*).

formed and bears a painful dorsolateral corn, we enucleate its basal phalanx instead. In either instance the fourth and fifth toes are syndactylized together (Figs. 15–49 and 15–50).

REFERENCES

Adams, W.: On the successful treatment of "hammer toe" by the subcutaneous division of the lateral ligaments. Brit. Med. J. *1*:645, 1888.

Anderson, W.: Hammer-toe and hallux flexus. Brit. Med. J. *1*:1129, 1887.

Anderson, W.: *The Deformities of Fingers and Toes.* London, J. & A. Churchill, 1897, p. 120.

Barwell, R.: Pes planus and pes cavus: an anatomical and clinical study. Edinburgh Med. J. *3*:113–124, 1898.

Bigg, H. H.: *Orthopraxy: The Mechanical Treatment of Deformities, Debilities, and Defficiencies of the Human Frame.* London, J. Churchill & Sons, 1865, pp. 565–575.

Blum, A.: De l'orteil en marteau. Bull. Mém. Soc. Chir. *9*:738–745, 1883.

Borg, I.: Operation for hammer toe. Acta Chir. Scand. *100*:619–625, 1950.

Boyer, B.: *A Treatise on Surgical Diseases, and the Operations Suited to Them* (translated from the French by Alexander H. Stevens). New York, T. & J. Swords, 1816, Vol. II, pp. 383–385.

Bragard, K.: Die Beseitigung der Hammerzehe durch juxtakapitale Resektion aus der Grundphalanx. Zeit. Orthop. Chir. *47*:283–286, 1926.

Brown, J. E.: Functional and cosmetic correction of metatarsus latus (splay foot). Clin. Orthopaed. *14*:166–170, 1959.

Davies, H.: Metatarsus quintus valgus. Brit. Med. J. *1*:664–665, 1949.

Decoppet, R. W.: Hammerzehen und vermeidbare Amputationen. Schweiz. Med. Wchnschr. *77*: 443–449, 1947.

Dickson, F. D., and Diveley, R. L.: Operation for correction of mild claw-foot, the result of infantile paralysis. J.A.M.A. *87*:1275–1277, 1926.

Duchenne, G. B.: *Physiology of Motion* (translated by E. B. Kaplan). Philadelphia, J. B. Lippincott Co., 1949, pp. 370–439. The original French edition appeared in 1867.

Ducroquet, C.: Le pied creux équin. Press. Méd. *59*:566–569, 1910.

DuVries, H. L.: *Surgery of the Foot.* St. Louis, C. V. Mosby Co., 1959, pp. 347–356.

Dwyer, F. C.: A new approach to the treatment of pes cavus. Sixième Congrès de Chirurgie Orthopédique, Berne, 30 août-3 septembre, 1954. *Société Internationale de Chirurgie Orthopédique et de Traumatologie.* Brussels, Lielens, 1955, p. 551.

Dwyer, F. C.: Osteotomy of the calcaneum for pes cavus. J. Bone Joint Surg. *41*:80–86, 1959.

Ely, L. W.: Hammer toe. Surg. Clin. N. Amer. *6*: 433–435, 1926.

Farkas, A.: Operative treatment of hollow foot. J. Bone Joint Surg. *17*:370–372, 1935.

Fisher, F. R.: Orthopaedic surgery: the treatment of deformities. In *International Encyclopaedia of Surgery* (J. Ashhurst, Jr., ed.). New York, W. Wood & Co., 1888, Vol. III, pp. 657–699.

Foley, T. M.: Pes cavus, due to paralysis of the extensor muscles, dorsal flexors of the feet. South. Med. J. *17*:798–800, 1924.

Forbes, A. M.: An operation for the relief of anterior metatarsalgia including Morton's disease. Am. J. Orthop. Surg. *8*:507–510, 1910.

Forbes, A. M.: Clawfoot, and how to relieve it. Surg. Gyn. Obst. *16*:81–83, 1913.

Forrester-Brown, M. F.: Tendon transplantation for the clawing of the great toe. J. Bone Joint Surg. *20*:57–60, 1938.

Garceau, G. J., and Brahms, M. A.: A preliminary study of selective plantar-muscle denervation for pes cavus. J. Bone Joint Surg. *38*:553–560, 1956.

Glassman, F., Wallin, L., and Sideman, S.: Phalangectomy for toe deformities. Surg. Clin. N. Amer. *29*:275–280, 1949.

Gocht, H., and Debrunner, H.: *Orthopaedische Therapie*. Leipzig, F. C. W. Vogel, 1925, pp. 238–247.

Goff, C. W.: The pes cavus of congenital syphilis. J.A.M.A. *86*:392–395, 1926.

Goodwin, F. C., and Swisher, F. M.: The treatment of congenital hyperextension of the great toe. J. Bone Joint Surg. *25*:193–195, 1943.

Gross, S. D.: Diseases and injuries of extremities. In *A System of Surgery*. Philadelphia, Blanchard and Lea, 1864, Vol. II, pp. 960–977.

Hackenbroch, M.: Der Hohlfuss. Ergebn. Chir. Orthop. *17*:457–515, 1924.

Heyman, C. H.: The operative treatment of clawfoot. J. Bone Joint Surg. *14*:335–338, 1932.

Hibbs, R. A.: An operation for "claw foot." J.A.M.A., *73*:1583–1585, 1919.

Higgs, S. L.: "Hammer-toe". Med. Press *131*:473–474, 1931.

Hoffmann, P.: An operation for severe grades of contracted or clawed toes. Am. J. Orthop. Surg. *9*:441–449, 1911.

Hohmann, G.: *Fuss und Bein*. Muenchen, J. F. Bergmann, 1951, pp. 145–192.

Jones, A. R.: Discussion on the treatment of pes cavus. Proc. Roy. Soc. Med. (Section of Orthopaedics) *20*:1118–1132, 1927.

Jones, R.: *Notes on Military Orthopaedics*. New York, P. B. Hoebber, 1917, pp. 38–57.

Kelikian, H., Clayton, L., and Loseff, H.: Surgical syndactylia of the toes. Clin. Orthop. *19*:208–231, 1961.

Kellock, T. H.: A modification of Phelps's operation for the relief of talipes equino-varus. Lancet *1*:805–806, 1895.

Kreuz, L.: Die Hammerzehen und ihre Operation nach Gocht. Arch. Orthop. Unfall-Chir. *21*: 459–472, 1923.

Kuhns, J. G.: The care of the feet in chronic arthritis. J.A.M.A. *109*:1108–1111, 1937.

Laforest: *L'Art de Soigner les Pieds*. 3rd Ed., Paris, Lebigre, 1782, pp. 87–95.

Lambrinudi, C.: An operation for claw-toes. Proc. Roy. Soc. Med. *21*:239, 1927.

Lambrinudi, C.: New operation on drop-foot. Brit. J. Surg. *15*:193–200, 1927.

Lambrinudi, C.: Use and abuse of toes. Post-Grad. Med. J. *8*:459–464, 1932.

Lambrinudi, C.: Deformities of the toes. Clin. J. Surg. *64*:57–61, 1935.

Lambrinudi, C.: Functional aspect: action of foot muscles. Lancet *2*:1480–1482, 1938.

Lambrinudi, C.: Metartarsus primus elevatus. Proc. Roy. Soc. Med. *31*:1273, 1938.

Lambrinudi, C.: Discussion on painful feet. Proc. Roy. Soc. Med. *36*:47–51, 1942.

Lambrinudi, C., and Stamm, T. T.: A report on the work in the orthopaedic department of Guy's Hospital. Guy's Hosp. Rep. *89*:184–225, 1939.

Lantzounis, L. A.: Congenital subluxation of the fifth toe and its correction by a periosteocapsuloplasty and tendon transplantation. J. Bone Joint Surg. *22*:147–150, 1940.

Lapidus, P. W.: Operation for correction of hammer-toe. J. Bone Joint Surg. *21*:977–982, 1939.

Lapidus, P. W.: Transplantation of extensor tendon for correction of overlapping fifth toe. J. Bone Joint Surg. *24*:555–559, 1942.

LeCocq, E. A.: Subtotal phalangectomy for relief of painful clavus. Northwest Med. *48*:398–399, 1949.

Lenggenhager, K.: Eine neue Operationsmethode zur Behandlung des Hallux valgus. Chirurg *7*:689–692, 1935.

Little, E. M.: Phelps's operation for club-foot. Brit. Med. J. (Section of Surgery) 977–981, October 17, 1903.

McElvenny, R. T., and Caldwell, G. D.: A new operation for correction of cavus foot; fusion of first metatarsocuneiformnavicular joints. Clin. Orthop. *11*:85–92, 1958.

McFadyean, K.: Prevention of hammer-toe bursitis. Lancet *1*:474, 1942.

McFarland, B.: Congenital deformities of the spine and limbs. In *Modern Trends in Orthopedic Surgery*, Sir Harry Platt, editor. New York, P. B. Hoeber, Inc., 1950, pp. 107–137.

McKeever, D. C.: Excision of the fifth metatarsal head. Clin. Orthop. *13*:321–322, 1959.

Manwaring, J. G. R.: Corns, hammer-toes and bunions. J. Michigan State Med. Soc. *29*:497–499, 1930.

Mellet, F. L. E.: *Manuel Pratique d'Orthopédie*. Paris, De Just Rouvier et E. Lebouvier, 1835, p. 488–519.

Merrill, W. J.: Conservative operative treatment of hammer toe. Am. J. Orthop. Surg. (Clinical Department) *10*:262–263, 1912.

Michele, A. A., and Krueger, F. J.: Operative correction for hammer toe. Mil. Surg. *103*:52–53, 1948.

Milgram, J. E.: Office measures for relief of the painful foot. J. Bone Joint Surg. *46*:1095–1116, 1964.

Mills, G. P.: The etiology and treatment of claw foot. J. Bone Joint Surg. *6:*142–149, 1924.

Nissen, K.: Excision of the head of a metatarsal bone—Morton's metatarsalgia: resection of a plantar digital nerve. Operat. Surg. *5:*317–323, 1957.

O'Donoghue, D. H., and Stauffer, R.: An improved operative method for obtaining bony fusion of the great toe. Surg. Gyn. Obst. *76:*498–500, 1943.

O'Neill, J.: An arthroplastic operation for hammertoe. J.A.M.A. *57:*1207, 1911.

Perkins, G.: *Orthopaedics.* London, Athlone Press, 1961, pp. 636–664.

Petri, C.: Zur Behandlung von Vorfussdeformitaeten. Ztschr. Orthop. Grenzgb. *70:*343–349, 1940.

Phelps, A. M.: The treatment of double talipes equino varus by open incision and fixed extension. Trans. Med. Soc. New York. Pp. 269–276, 1881.

Phelps, A. M.: A new method of curing inveterate soft corns between the toes. Trans. Am. Osthop. Assoc. *6:*237–238, 1894.

Post, A. C.: Hallux valgus, with displacement of the smaller toes. Med. Rec. New York *22:*120–121, 1882.

Ramstedt, C.: Vorschlag zur Behandlung gewisser Zehendeformitaeten mittels kuenstlicher Syndaktylie. Chirurg *17–18:*63–65, 1947.

Redard, P.: Du traitement du pied creux. Gaz. Méd. *3:*261–263, 1896; *3:*289–290, 1896.

Rosenzweig, A.: Die operative Behandlung des Hohlfusses. Zbl. Chir. *61:*2037–2041, 1934.

Rugh, J. T.: The plantar fascia: a study of its anatomy and of its pathology in talipes cavus; a new operation for its correction. Am. J. Surg. *2:*307–314, 1927.

Scherb, R.: Die transossaere Extensorenfixation bei Klauenhohlfuss. Klin. Wchnschr. *3:*787, 1924.

Schlaepfer: Die Hammerzehe. Deut. Zschr. Chir. *147:*394–413, 1918.

Schnepp, K. H.: Hammer-toe and claw foot. Am. J. Surg. *36:*351–359, 1937.

Scrase, W. H.: The treatment of dorsal adduction deformities of the fifth toe. J. Bone Joint Surg. *36:*146, 1954.

Selig, S.: Hammer-toe: a new procedure for its correction. Surg. Gyn. Obst. *72:*101–105, 1941.

Shattock, S. G.: Hammer toes. Tr. Path. Soc. London *38:*449, 1886.

Sherman, H. M.: The operative treatment of pes cavus. Am. J. Orthop. Surg. *2:*374–380, 1905.

Soule, R. E.: Operation for the cure of hammer toe. New York Med. J. pp. 649–650, March 26, 1910.

Spitzy, H.: Operative correction of claw-foot. Surg. Gyn. Obst. *45:*813–815, 1927.

Stamm, T. T.: In Memoriam of Constantine Lambrinudi. Guy's Hosp. Rep. *92:*45–49, 1943.

Stamm, T. T.: Foot—Surgery of. In *British Surgical Practice.* London, Butterworth & Co.; St. Louis, C. V. Mosby Co., 1948, Vol. IV, pp. 160–163.

Steindler, A.: Operative treatment of pes cavus; stripping of the os calcis. Surg. Gyn. Obst. *24:* 612–615, 1917.

Steindler, A.: Stripping of os calcis. J. Orthop. Surg. *2:*8–12, 1920.

Steindler, A.: The treatment of pes cavus (hollow claw foot). Arch. Surg. *2:*325–337, 1921.

Stephens, R.: Dorsal wedge operation for metatarsal equinus. J. Bone Joint Surg. *5:*485–489, 1923.

Stiles, H. J., and Forrester-Brown, M. F.: *Treatment of Injuries of the Spinal Peripheral Nerves.* London, F. Frowals, Hodder & Stoughton, 1922, pp. 166–171.

Straub, L. R.: Affections of the feet. In *The Specialties in General Practice* (R. L. Cecil, ed.). Philadelphia, W. B. Saunders Co., 1951, pp. 125–134.

Stuart, F. W.: Claw foot—its treatment. J. Bone Joint Surg. *6:*360–367, 1924.

Sweetnam, R.: Congenital curly toes—an investigation into the value of treatment. Lancet *2:*398–400, 1958.

Tamplin, R. W.: *Lectures on the Nature of Deformities, Delivered at the Royal Orthopaedic Hospital, Bloomsbury Square.* London, Longmans, Brown, Green, and Longmans, 1846, pp. 266–267.

Taylor, R. G.: An operative procedure for the treatment of hammer-toe and claw-toe. J. Bone Joint Surg. *22:*608–609, 1940.

Taylor, R. G.: The treatment of claw toes by multiple transfers of flexor into extensor tendons. J. Bone Joint Surg. *33:*539–542, 1951

Terrier: Orteils en marteau avec durillons et bourses séreuses sous-jacentes enflammées. Résection des deux côtés, et dans la même séance, de l'articulation phalango-phalangienne. Bull. Mém. Soc. Chir. *14:*624–626, 1888.

Tierny, A.: Traitement de l'orteil en marteau. Rev. Orthop. *33:*445–452, 1926.

Todd, A. H.: The treatment of pes cavus. Proc. Royal Soc. Med. (Section of Orthopaedics) *28:*117–128, 1934.

Trethowan, W. H.: Pes Cavus. In *A System of Surgery,* C. C. Choyce, editor. New York, P. B. Hoeber, 1923, pp. 1043–1046.

Trethowan, W. H.: The treatment of hammer-toe. Lancet *1:*1257; 1:1312, 1925.

Wallet: Structural redressing of the forefoot by multiple arthroplasties. Rev. Chir. Plastiq. *7:* 122–125, 1937.

Willens, C.: The technique of tarsectomy for talipes. Brit. Med. J. *2:*984–986, 1908.

Wilson, J. N.: V-Y correction for varus deformity of the fifth toe. Brit. J. Surg. *41:*133–135, 1953.

Young, C. S.: An operation for the correction of hammer-toe and claw-toe. J. Bone Joint Surg. *20:*715–719, 1938.

Young, J. K.: *A Manual and Atlas of Orthopedic Surgery.* Philadelphia, P. Blakiston's Son & Co., 1906, pp. 828–829.

Chapter Sixteen

METATARSALGIA

The voluminous literature on pain across the ball of the forefoot and the barren polemics as to whether it is caused by bone imbalance, muscle dysfunction, vasospasm, or nerve irritation, reminds one of small boys flying kites. Each boy runs after his toy and winds up in the woods; he sees nothing in the entire forest except the single tree or rather the slender twig that caught his kite. Every author writing on metatarsalgia has pursued a favorite decoy. T. G. Morton's (1876) neuralgia is one; D. J. Morton's (1924–1952) atavistic first metatarsal is another. We could name half a dozen more. Each protagonist tends to overstress his point and ignore other factors.

Pain is a subjective symptom. It is intangible, invisible. As such it permits a diversity of interpretations. Samuel Gross (1872) used the term *pododynia* to describe an obscure pain in the foot. He thought sedentary occupations had something to do with it and singled out tailors as being particularly prone. With his flair for modulated phrases, Weir Mitchell, (1872, 1878) coined the term *pedal pain* and described a form of it as vasomotor neurosis. Curtis (1881) discussed "irradiated or reflected pains" in the foot occurring in connection with general and genitourinary diseases. Dana (1885) distinguished "reflex neuralgias" from "neuralgia due to some mechanical fault in the foot." Hughes (1887) spoke of "pain localized on the balls of three toes supplied by the internal plantar nerve," occurring in the wake of fevers and caisson disease. Mills (1888) considered "spinal sclerosis" as the cause of shooting, lancinating, or lightning-like pain in the foot. More recently a number of authors have related the metatarsalgia of cavus foot to adhesions around the spinal cord. Too often it is forgotten that the burning sensation in the forefoot may be in the nature of projected pain caused by lumbar disk disturbance.

The pain in the forepart of the foot may be nothing more than the local manifestation of a systemic disease. Forefoot pain is not an uncommon symptom of arteriosclerosis, thromboangiitis obliterans, acrocyanosis, erythromelalgia, or some other disease. Rheumatoid arthritis often involves the joints of the toes and so does gonorrhea and gout. It would take us too far afield to detail all the general or remote causes of forefoot pain. We remain content to

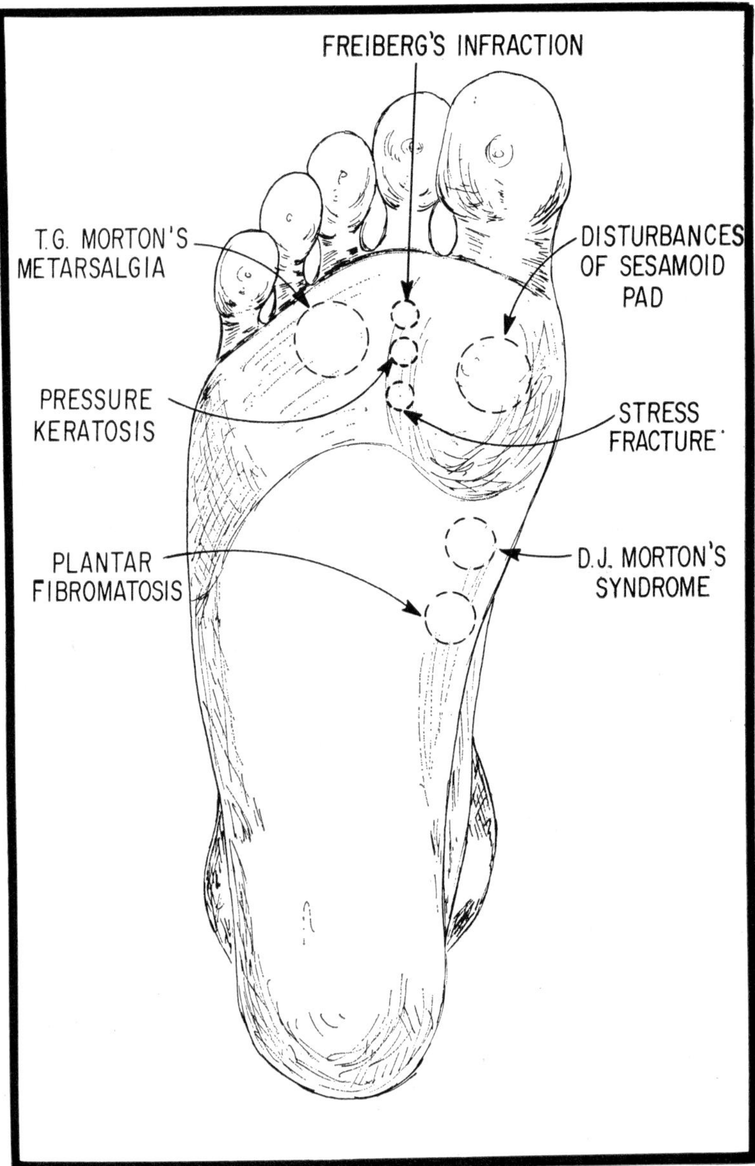

Figure 16–1. The location of the more common causes of metatarsalgia.

survey some of the more common—to be exact, more often discussed—regional disturbances that are held responsible for metatarsalgia, namely, derangements of the first plantar pad, plantar incarceration of the metatarsal heads and attendant pressure keratoses, verruca plantaris, T. G. Morton's metatarsalgia, D. J. Morton's syndrome, Freiberg's infraction, stress fractures of the metatarsal bones, tumors, scars, and ulcers (Fig. 16–1).

DERANGEMENTS OF THE FIRST PLANTAR PAD

In the forefoot there are five plantar pads, one for each metatarsophalangeal joint. Occasionally the second to fifth pads contain one or two sesamoid bones. These are not constant. The first pad is the only one that contains a pair of ossicles with constancy. Rarely, one of the pair may be missing. More commonly, either the medial or the lateral sesamoid is bi- or tripartite. This is explained by the fact that sesamoids may develop from several centers of ossification that fail to coalesce. The bony nuclei of pedal sesamoids become manifest around the age of nine in girls and a year later in boys. In both sexes ossification may be delayed until the age of eleven. Usually at twelve or thirteen ossification is complete (Figs. 16–2 and 16–3).

Because of their delayed ossification and their tendancy to become bipartite and undergo changes suggestive of chondromalacia, the sesamoids of the first plantar pad have been compared with the patella. Unlike the patella, pedal sesamoids are primarily designed to sustain weight. Accustomed to intermittent pressure and pounding, they can withstand considerable stress. Only rarely do these bones yield to excessive force and fracture; this they do after they have lost their hyaline coating and have become flat and brittle, as in later years of life.

The lateral sesamoid is frequently dislocated and becomes fragmented in its new and mechanically incongruous location. Fracture by sudden violence usually affects the medial sesamoid, which also is the bone that is often bipartite. A fractured sesamoid does not heal with exuberant callus, if at all. The broken fragments remain separated, and from studies of late roentgenograms one cannot positively state whether a fractured or bipartite bone is being dealt with. History of injury—as incurred by falling from a height or jumping—would be helpful, if authentic. The bipartite sesamoid is usually bilateral; study of roentgenograms of the opposite foot may lend a clue. In a fresh fracture of the sesamoid the shadows cast on x-ray films by the lines of separation of the fragments are jagged, serrated; in the bipartite sesamoid the shadows of junctional lines run parallel to one another and are smooth. Arthrography may be of some help. The fragments of the bipartite sesamoid are joined together with a band of fibrous or fibrocartilaginous tissue. Air injected into the first metatarsophalangeal joint will cast a shadow that is confined to the articular

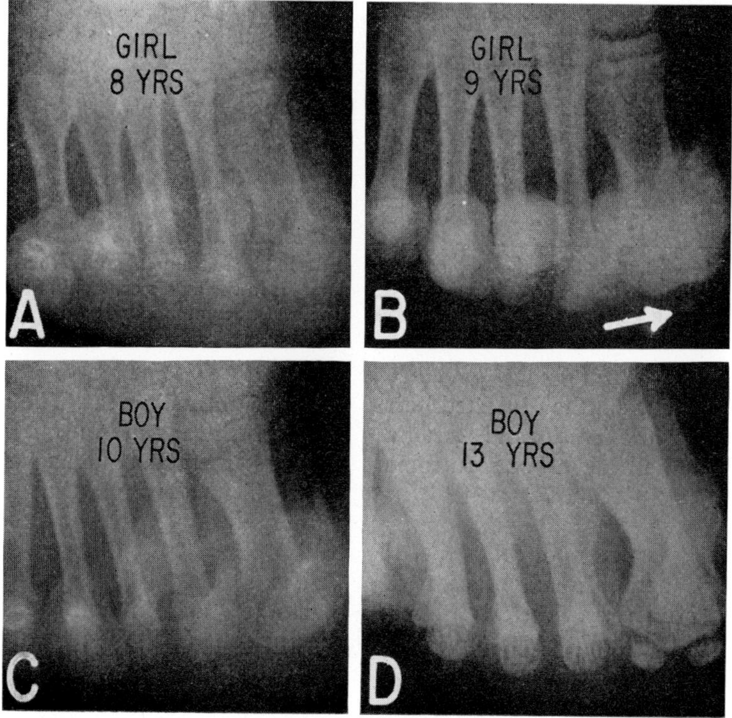

Figure 16–2. The appearance and maturation of the sesamoids of first plantar pad.

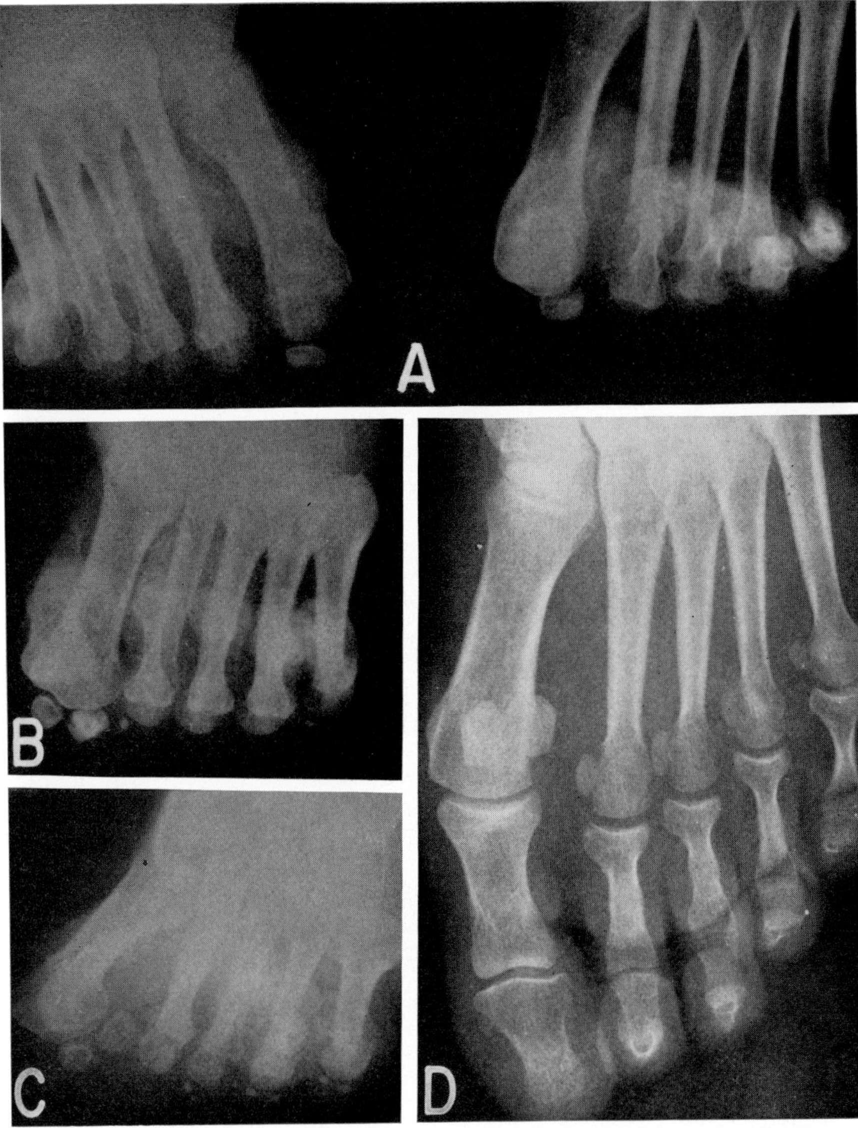

Figure 16–3. Numerical discrepancy of sesamoids. *A,* Single sesamoid under the first metatarsal head—the medial ossicle is missing on both sides. *B,* Sesamoids in the first, second, and fifth plantar pads. *C,* Sesamoids in first, third, fourth, and fifth plantar pads. *D,* Sesamoids under all five plantar pads.

cavity. In fracture, the injected air passes through the crack and casts a shadow below the broken bone. In some instances, differentiation between bipartite and a broken sesamoid is made only after surgical extirpation of the involved bone, roentgenographic examination of the pieces, or microscopic study of sections (Fig. 16–4).

As is true with other weight-bearing articular bones, the sesamoids of the first plantar pad are apt to manifest symptoms of untimely wear. The most important of these symptoms is pain under the first metatarsophalangeal joint. We have stated elsewhere that the sesamoid bones move with the great toe. In hallux valgus they are dislocated laterally, in hallux rigidus or flexus they have moved backward, and in hallux extensus they lie in front of the first metatarsal head. In their unaccustomed position—or when they have become fixed and immobile and hence functionally defunct—the sesamoids undergo arthritic changes. Bipartite sesamoids tend to degenerate prematurely (Fig. 16–5).

Metatarsalgia caused by degenerated or osteoarthritic sesamoids is usually confined to the ball of the great toe. Pain localized in this region is ascribed to what is called *sesamoiditis*. This is one of those nondescript terms that is made to mean more than it should. Pedal sesamoids are seldom involved in an inflammatory process; more often they wear out. When metatarsalgia can definitely be related to mushroomed or mechanically incongruous sesamoids, these bones may be removed surgically. One must rule out tenosynovitis of the flexor hallucis longus tendon and exaggerated plantar inclination of the first metatarsal bone, which also cause metatarsalgia around the ball of the big toe.

Another—more or less related—cause of metatarsalgia in this region is calcific deposits within the tendinous ring of the first plantar pad. When the great toe is extended, the segment of the flexor brevis tendon that connects the sesamoids to the proximal phalanx rubs against the head of the first metatarsal bone. Repeated friction against a hard surface in time induces degenerative changes in this portion of the tendon. One recalls the musculotendinous cuff of the shoulder, in particular the supraspinatus tendon, which also becomes chafed by friction against an articular surface and undergoes untimely degeneration. As in the case of the supraspinatus, calcific material accumulates within the frayed fibers of the flexor hallucis brevis tendon; it causes tension and pain. Injections and needling will occasionally relieve this pain. At times one may have to evacuate the calcific deposit surgically (Fig. 16–6).

PLANTAR INCARCERATION OF THE METATARSAL HEADS AND PRESSURE KERATOSES

By far the most common cause of

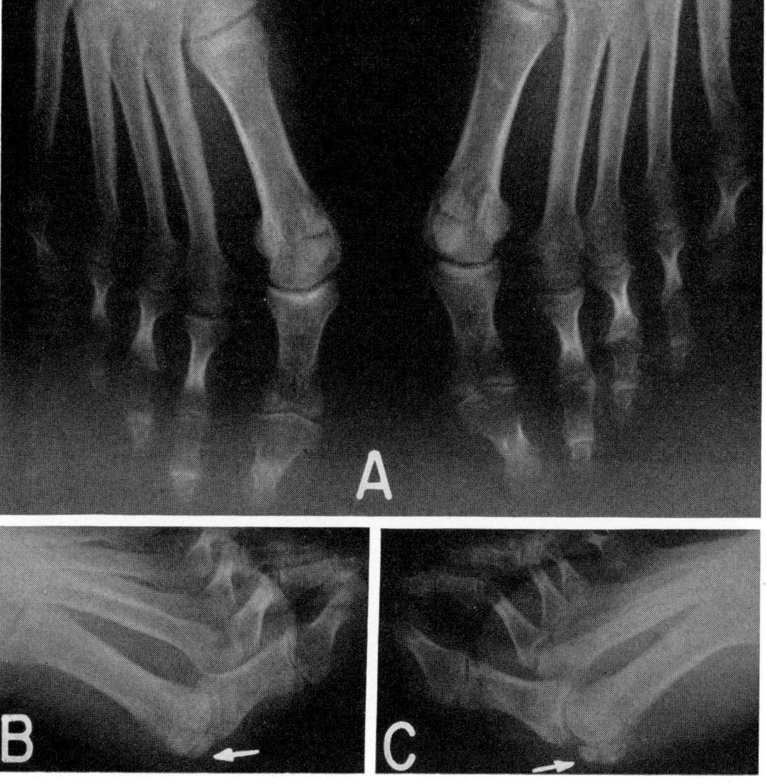

Figure 16–4. Bilateral bipartite medial sesamoids. *A*, Dorsoplantar view. *B* and *C*, Side views.

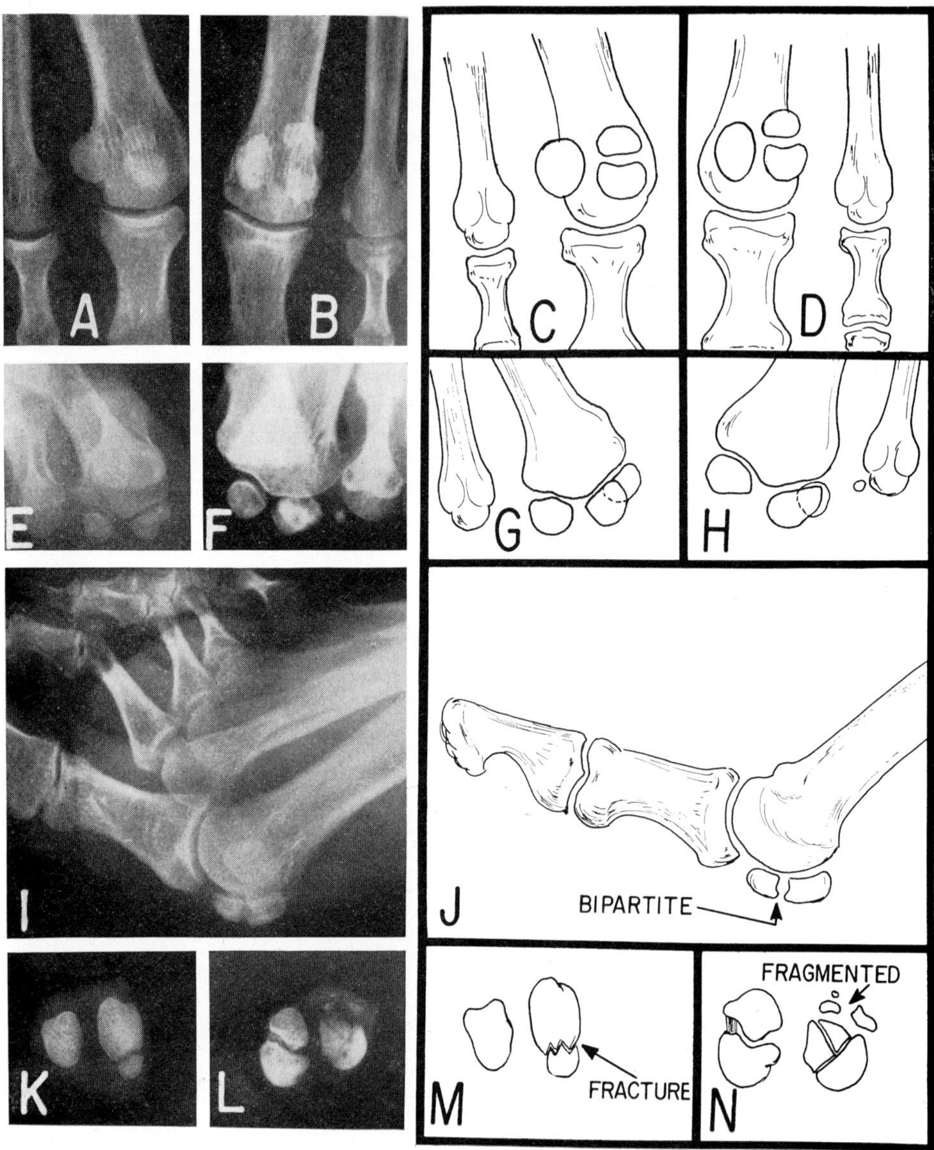

Figure 16–5. Bipartite, fractured or fragmented sesamoids. *A,* Bipartite medial sesamoid. *B,* Bipartite lateral sesamoid. *C,* Interpretative diagram of *A*. *D,* Interpretative diagram of *B*. *E,* Tangental view of *A*. *F,* Tangental view of *B*. *G* and *H,* Interpretative diagrams of *E* and *F*. *I,* Side view of bipartite medial sesamoid. *J,* Interpretative diagram of *I*. *K,* Fractured medial sesamoid. *L,* Bipartite medial sesamoid and fragmented lateral sesamoid. *M,* Interpretative diagram of *K*. *N,* Interpretative diagram of *L*.

metatarsalgia—in our estimation the most disabling deformity of the forefoot—is the fixed plantar prominence of the middle metatarsal heads. This is another manifestation of splaying of the forefoot; it is often associated with hallux valgus and hammered and clawed toes. At its inception the deformity is reversible. In time, it becomes rigid. The toes assume retracted positions; their joints stiffen, and painful keratoses form under the plantarly prominent metatarsal heads.

Historically, the symptom complex just described has been linked with the concept of a transverse arch across the span of the metatarsal heads. In an earlier chapter we discussed this matter briefly, reserving some of the pertinent details for the present section. It is not definitely known who first promulgated the idea of anterior transverse or anterior metatarsal arch. We note this arch mentioned in a book by C. H. Cleaveland (1862), dealing mainly with shoes and their construction. Peck (1871), too, spoke of the transverse metatarsal arch in his book, which also was devoted mostly to shoes. The concept presupposes that the middle three metatarsal heads do not touch the ground but sit on the dome of an arch for which the heads of the first and fifth metatarsals serve as side pillars.

The idea of an arch under the metatarsal heads seems to have been widespread. It was enthusiastically endorsed by almost all bootmakers, chiropodists, and surgeons. The anatomist, Henry Morris (1879), tried to stem the tide. "When the foot is firmly resting on the ground," Morris wrote, "the weight of the body is borne upon the extremities of all the metatarsal bones, and not simply upon those of the first and fifth, as has been sometimes stated." As all professional anatomists did, Morris recognized one transverse arch in the foot, which he said was "most marked across the cuneiform bones." Anatomists have made it clear that this arch gradually flattens as it approaches the forepart of the foot; it is nonexistent under the metatarsal heads. But there seems to have been no accord on this point between anatomists and clinicians.

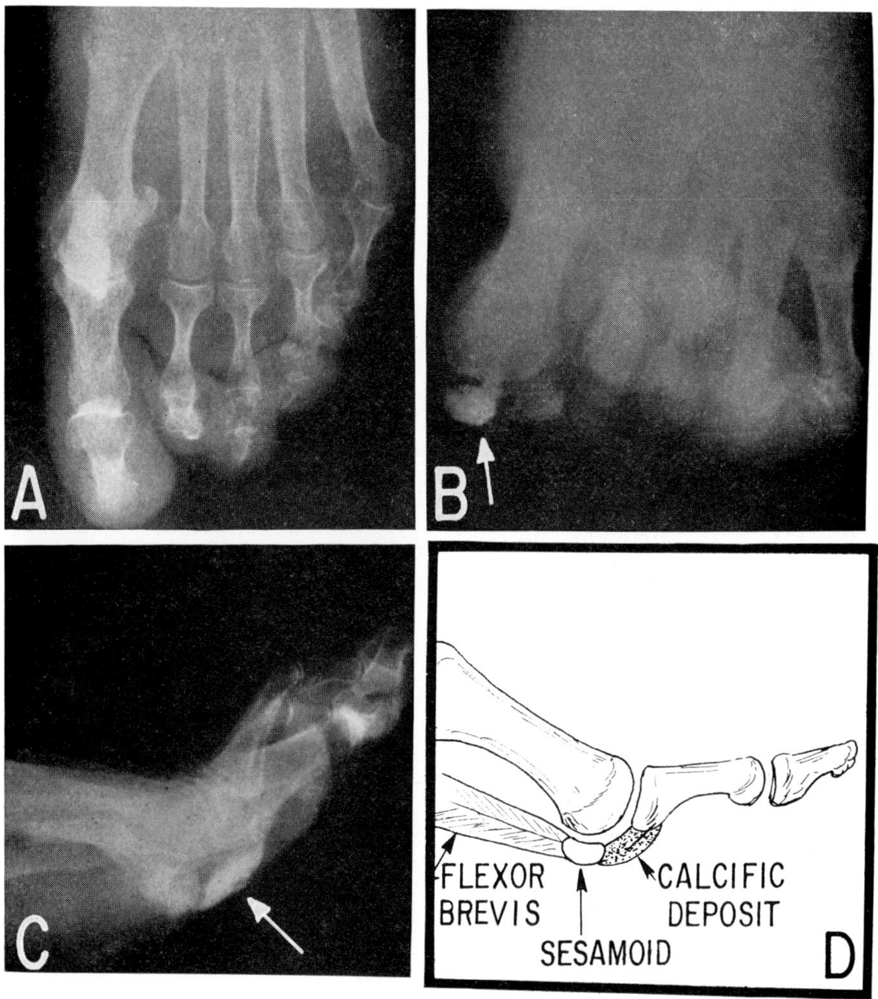

Figure 16–6. Calcific deposits at the junction of the first plantar pad and proximal phalanx of the great toe. *A,* Dorsoplantar view; *B,* tangental view; *C,* side view; *D,* interpretative diagram.

Auguste Pollosson (1889)—not Poullosson as T. S. K. Morton (1893) and Whitman (1898) spelled it—gave the name *anterior metatarsalgia* to the pain under the ball of the forefoot. "The cause of this affection," Pollosson wrote, "is evidently a certain laxity of the transverse metatarsal ligament, which permits a partial infraction of the arch formed by the heads of the five metatarsals." Pollosson's article was favorably reviewed by *The Lancet* (1889) and his views were endorsed by Roughton (1889). In one case he reported, Roughton found that "the transverse arch formed by the heads of the metatarsal bones had sunk, so that a distinct convexity replaced the concavity normally found in this situation."

Pollosson had used the adjective *anterior.* Goldthwait (1894) employed the same epithet to distinguish the alleged transverse arch under the metatarsal heads from the one farther back under the distal row of tarsal bones. Without mentioning Cleaveland, Pollosson and others, Goldthwait pontificated: "At the metatarso-phalangeal articulations there is an arch, called by the writer the anterior transverse arch. This, at times, becomes flattened and symptoms develop which are characteristic. The symptoms most commonly met are pain, referred to the anterior portion of the foot . . . and . . . painful callous in the centre of the ball of the foot. . . ." Coming from a veritable Boston Brahmin, this statement was met with uncritical endorsement. No less an authority than Whitman (1898) considered Goldthwait's explanation "more thorough and convincing . . . than had been done before." In his book, Whitman (1907) took pains to elucidate Goldthwait's already oversimplified platitudes.

Goldthwait's concept found echoes in other countries. In England, in the course of his lecture on hallux valgus, Sir Robert Jones (1924) spoke about "flattened arches." During the discussion that followed, Roth confessed being in the past year converted by Muirhead Little, who had pointed out that there was no anterior transverse arch. Venerable Bristow retorted saying Roth would retract in a year or two his remark about the transverse arch of the foot, the existence of which he had denied. Back in America, during a similar symposium following Freiberg's (1924) paper on hallux valgus, Porter stressed the importance of restoring the anterior transverse arch in the postoperative care of bunions. Henderson retorted: "All this talk about transverse arch is more or less nonsense. It does not make any difference what one does to it. It exists only in anatomical drawings." In closing, Freiberg said: "Dr. Porter errs in stating that he restores the transverse arch, because there is no such entity. The transverse arch is maintained wholly by muscle action. When the toes are flexed there is a transverse arch, and when they are extended it disappears."

The rebellion—if it can be called one—was weak. The orthodox views of Goldthwait and Whitman in America and of Jones and Bristow in England went on unchallenged until the fourth decade of the present century. In numerous articles and two books, D. J. Morton (1930–1952) categorically denied the existence of an arch under the metatarsal heads. He insisted that, through the intermediary of underlying soft tissues, the middle three metatarsal heads did contact the ground and sustained their share of the body weight. Morton considered the arched conformation of the metatarsal heads a physical impossibility and the persistence of the concept of an anterior metatarsal arch "faulty" and "unfortunate."

Elftman (1934) arrived at a similar conclusion. Cotton (1935) considered the "ascent" of the first metatarsal head rather than the "descent" of the central bones as the basic change and this view was shared by most German authors. Bruce and Walmsley (1938) and Russell Jones (1941) concurred with Morton. Speaking of the anatomical transverse arch of the foot, Grant (1958) wrote: "Since the heads of all metatarsals make contact with the ground, it is evident that they do not contribute to this arch." Wood Jones (1949) reiterated what Henry Morris had said three quarters of a century earlier—that the true anatomical transverse arch of the foot "reaches the maximum beneath the cuneiforms and the anterior extremity of the cuboid. The arched form is still present at the bases of the metatarsals, but it disappears altogether at the heads of these bones, which are all on the same level when the foot is supporting the body weight."

As yet there appears to be no complete accord between clinicians and anatomists. Most clinicians still cling to the concept of anterior transverse or anterior metatarsal arch. They seem reluctant to part with the idea. Lewin (1941) —a former assistant of Porter's—regarded the structure formed by the metatarsal heads as a "true arch." Dickson and Diveley (1944) wrote: *"The transverse or metatarsal arch,* as is commonly accepted, is formed by the heads of five metatarsals. . . . Notwithstanding the doubt as to the presence of a metatarsal arch which has been expressed by a number of investigators, the concept that such a metatarsal arch does exist is widely held. Because of the general acceptance of such an arch and because so many functional ailments of the foot affect the metatarsal region, it seems best to retain for the present at least the theory of a metatarsal arch as part of the structures of the foot." DuVries (1959) wrote: *"The transverse metatarsal arch* is formed by the five metatarsal heads, the first and fifth form the inner and outer pillars. The transverse metatarsal ligament forms the bowstring of this arch."

When a normal forefoot—by this we mean one that has retained its resilience and is not marred by hallux valgus or hammered and clawed toes—when such a forefoot is lifted off the ground and viewed from the bottom, one may discern a shallow depression in the area under the necks of the middle metatarsal bones. This dimple is due to the relative abundance of soft tissues under the marginal bones and is accentuated when the toes are actively flexed. Obviously the foot does not function off the ground but when planted upon it, and it would be difficult to walk with flexed toes. If the patient is asked to stand on a transparent plate and the examiner inspects the foot from under the glass, he will at once see that the soft tissue prominences under the first and fifth metatarsals flatten out and the central dimple disappears. In fixed plantar incarceration of the central metatarsal heads, the dimple is absent even when no weight is borne on the forefoot. When such a foot is viewed from the plantar aspect, the area under the middle metatarsal heads presents a genuine convexity.

The central metatarsals—especially the second and third—are rigid; the marginal bones enjoy greater mobility. It would seem more rational to suppose that the "reversed transverse metatarsal arch" of orthopedists—or the "biplane forefoot imbalance" of podiatrists—is caused by the dorsal shift of the marginal capitalia, rather than be the plantar displacement of the central heads. In these cases the toes usually are hammered or clawed and the proximal phalanges hyperextended; the retraction of the toes accentuates the apparent plantar bulge of the central metatarsal heads.

Elsewhere we noted that plantar pads under the metatarsal heads are firmly attached to the proximal phalanges and move with them. In hammered and clawed toes the proximal phalanges have pulled the plantar pads—and with them the cushions of fat—forward from under the metatarsal heads. These bones now come to rest on the underlying skin, which reacts to the pressure from above and below by becoming keratotic. What really matters is whether the proximal phalanges can bend sufficiently plantarward and permit the plantar pads and cushions of fat to slip back under the metatarsal heads. The flexibility of the metatarsophalangeal joints and the pressing-down power of the toes provide the key to the treatment of metatarsalgia due to static disturbances of the forefoot.

Palliative measures. Numerous palliative measures have been advocated for the relief of metatarsalgia caused by the resilient or fixed plantar bulge of the central metatarsal heads—exercise, mas-

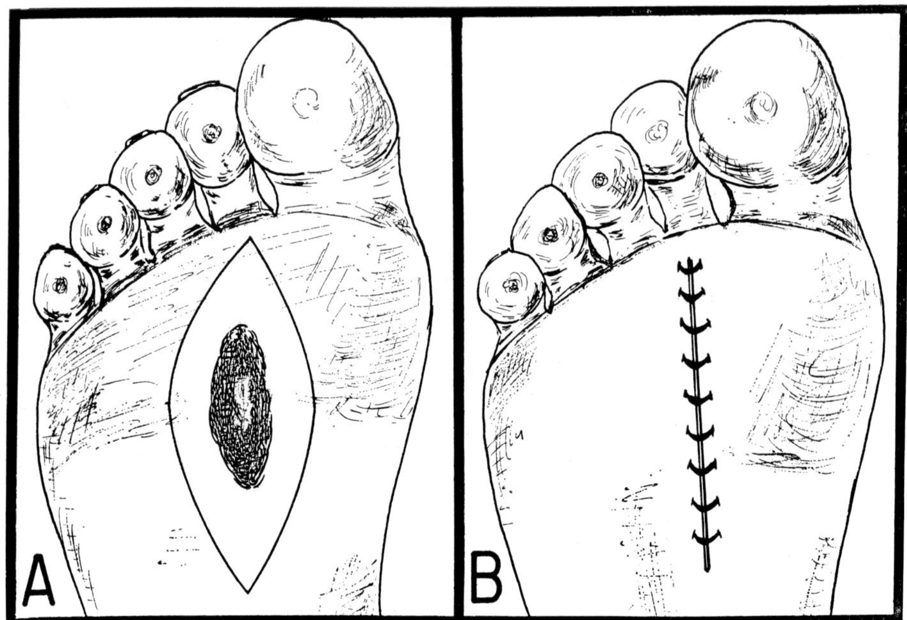

Figure 16–7. Diagrams illustrating excision of pressure ketatosis. *A*, Elliptical skin cuts; *B*, closure.

sage, manipulation, metatarsal pads, use of a transverse bar and wrenching followed by a cast, and so on. Podiatrists have concentrated their attention on the most obvious lesion—pressure keratoses, or as some prefer to call them, plantar calluses. Cornified skin is pared down and the area is protected with a pad or cushion. These measures obtain only temporary relief. Years ago Roux (1920) advised inserting a free graft of fat pad between the plantarly prominent metatarsal heads and the underlying callused skin. No one else appears to have practiced this method.

Excision of plantar keratoses. This procedure has been recommended by many surgeons. Blair and his associates (1937) saw "no reason for not eliminating the callous spot by excision." Excision of pressure keratosis is feasible in the young, who have pliable forefoot and yielding skin. The cornified area is resected with a pair of elliptical incisions, the wound is closed with interrupted wire sutures, a walking cast is worn for 3 weeks, stitches are removed, and the patient is advised to have a metatarsal pad put inside the shoe or transverse bar outside of it. In the aged with fixed incarceration of the metatarsal heads, recurrence of keratosis is inevitable unless the pressure by the overlying bone is eliminated (Fig. 16–7).

Condylectomy or resection of the plantar half of the offending metatarsal head. This procedure was recommended by DuVries (1953) for what he called *intractable verruca plantaris (plantar wart)*. Obviously DuVries had in mind pressure keratoses and not verruca plantaris or plantar wart, as indicated by the title of his article. He resected the projecting plantar condyles of the offending metatarsal head through a dorsal incision. Billig (1956) excised the condyles by either "a dorsal or ventral (sic) approach." Using the same unfortunate title, *intractable plantar wart,* Anderson (1957) supplemented excision of the plantar keratosis and condylectomy with resurfacing the soft tissue defect with a pedicle flap rotated from the nearby non-weight-bearing portion of the sole. Giannestras (1958) reported that in a personal communication, McElvenny had reviewed his results of "resection of the plantar half of the metatarsal heads" and had found such a great number of recurrences of pressure keratoses that he had discarded the procedure altogether (Fig. 16–8).

Osteotomy of the central metatarsals. This procedure was recommended by Meisenbach (1916). He spoke two types of "anterior, or transverse arch" causing symptoms—flexible and rigid. For the former he prescribed "proper plates, proper shoes and exercises." For "rigid, reversed arch"—with the "second, third and fourth metatarsal heads" lying "at a lower level than the first and the fifth" —he advised angulation osteotomy of each shaft in order to raise the head to a higher plane. Mau (1940) removed a trapezoid piece from the base of the metatarsal and tilted the distal fragment up. Borggreve (1949) performed a similar osteotomy at the distal end of the metatarsal. McKeever (1952) carried out subcapital osteotomy of the metatarsal and telescoped the spiked end of the shaft fragment into the capital piece. Giannestras (1954, 1958) said he had operated on a number of patients by this method and following surgery, stiffness in the metatarsophalangeal joint had developed. "Several years ago," Giannestras wrote, "the author resected the metatarsal head overlying plantar keratoses. Although there was relief from pain, in many patients a cock-up or a hammer toe deformity of the involved digit developed." Giannestras recommended shortening the metatarsal by what has come to be known as *step-cut osteotomy* (Figs. 16–9 to 16–11).

Excision of the offending metatarsal head. This procedure was recommended by George Davis (1917). Dickson (1948) extended this operation to include the entire metatarsal bone and the corresponding toe. Commenting on Dickson's "pie" operation, Robinson (1953) had this to say: "The operation is designed to eliminate the scarred ulcerated area on the sole by elliptical excision and longitudinal closure. It removes the underlying bony prominence of the metatarsal head by removing the entire metatarsal beneath the ulcer and the attached toe distal to the defect. The foot is collapsed and narrowed by sutures. . . . The principle of making long scars against the cleavage lines on the plantar skin is violated, and furthermore the arch is depressed so that new pressure points are produced." Anderson's (1957) objection to this operation was that it narrowed the foot. A more cogent criticism to Dickson's operation is that it deprives the great toe of its lateral buttress and paves the way for hallux valgus. This can be obviated by retention of the second toe and surgical syndactylia with the hallux (Figs. 16–12 and 16–13).

Dickson entitled his article "Surgical Treatment of Intractable Plantar Warts." In the discussion that followed Key said: "It seems to me that most of the lesions which Dr. Dickson showed were not plantar warts . . . were calluses which

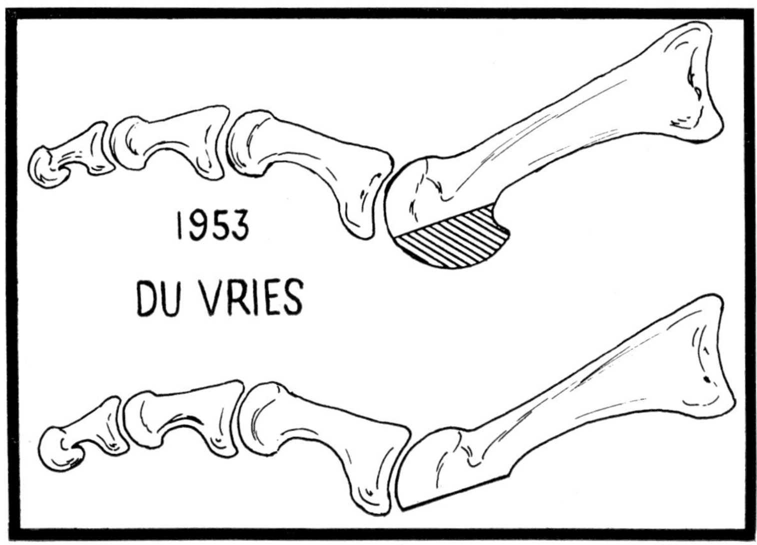

Figure 16–8. DuVries' condylectomy.

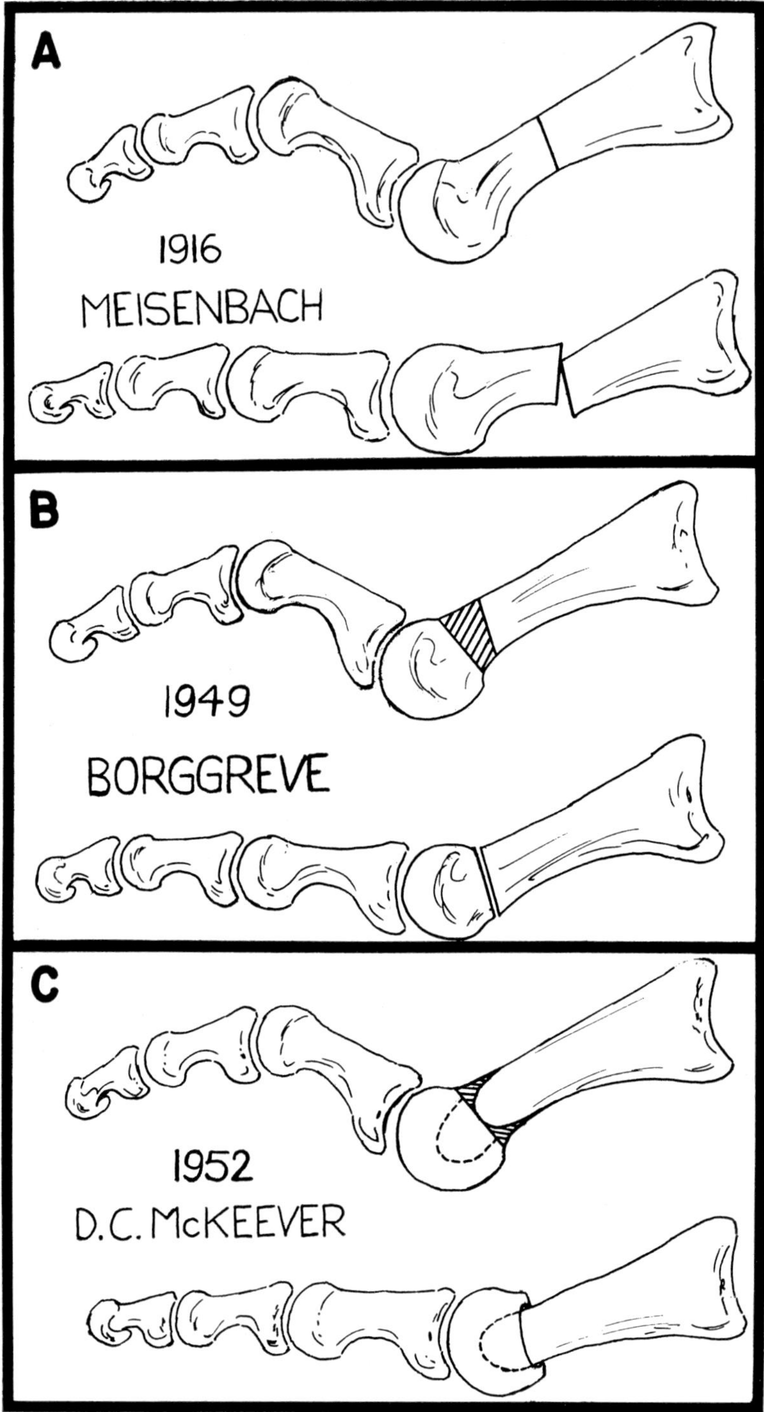

Figure 16–9. Osteotomy of the middle metatarsals. *A,* Angulation osteotomy of the shaft. *B,* Recession and angulation osteotomy of the distal extremity. *C,* Telescopic recession of the head.

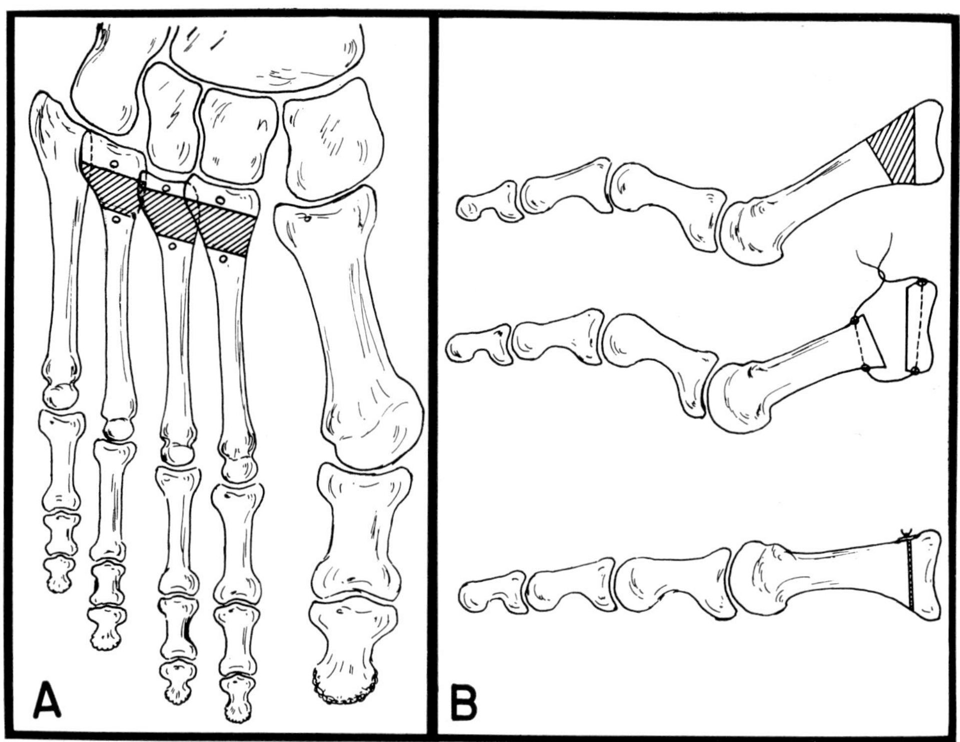

Figure 16–10. Recession and dorsal angulation of the distal fragment following osteotomy of the middle metatarsals at their proximal ends—Mau operation.

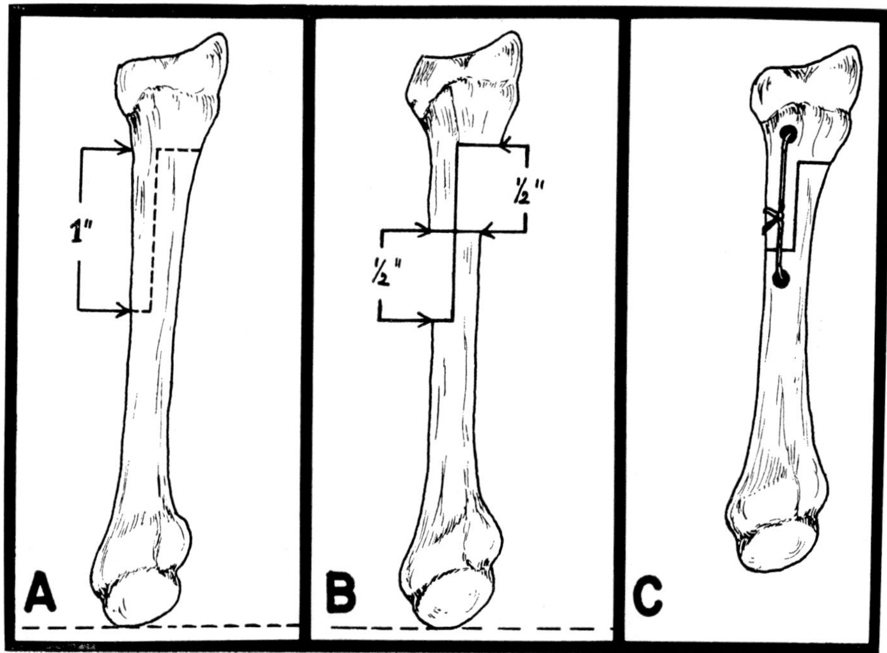

Figure 16–11. Giannestras' step-cut recession for pressure keratosis.

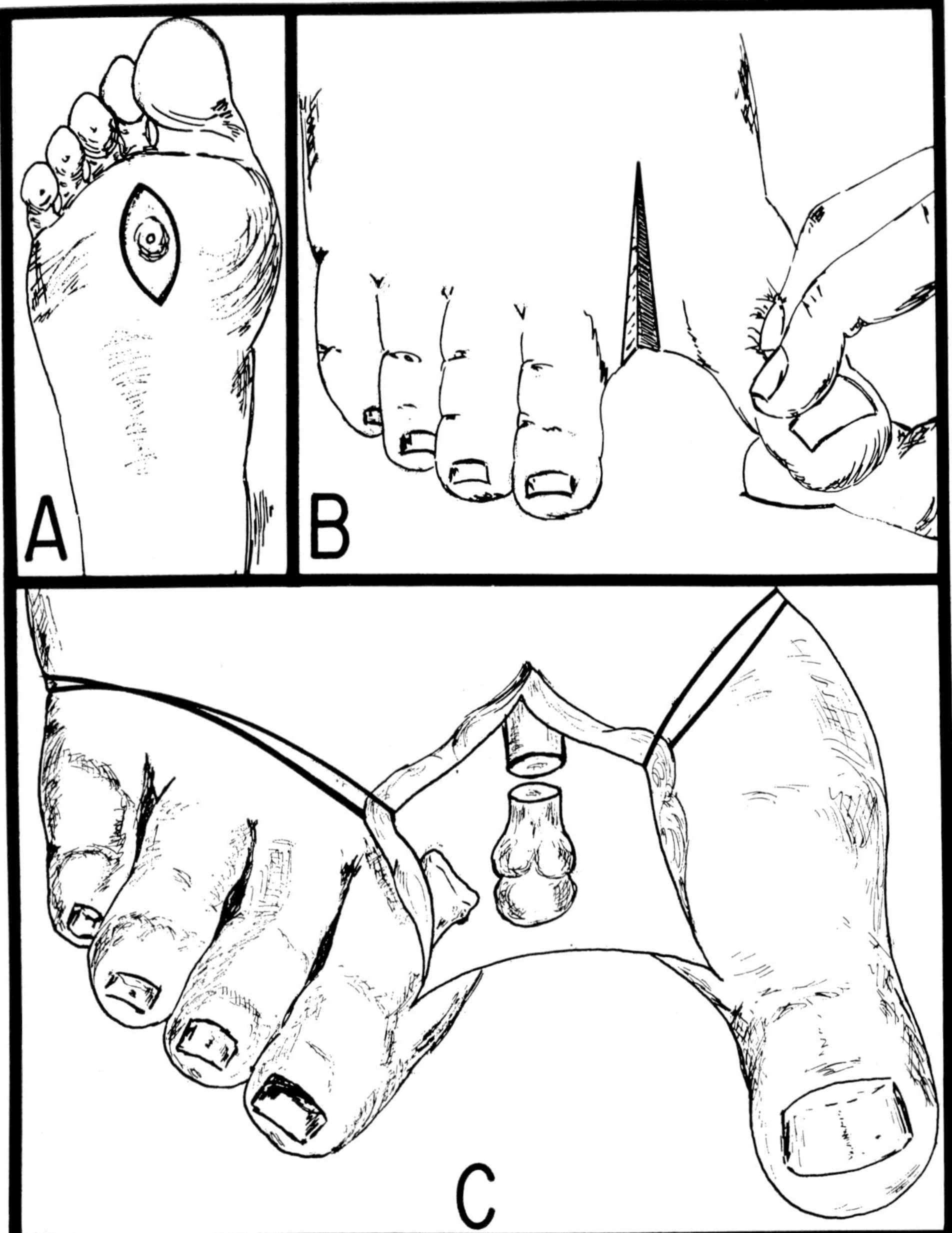

Figure 16–12. *A,* Davis' method of excision of pressure keratosis. *B,* Interdigital incision. *C,* Resection of distal extremity of second metatarsal.

I would correct by operating upon hammertoe or by removing the head of the metatarsal." Unaware of the operation described by Davis and taking their cue from Key, Rutledge and Green (1957) wrote: "We believe that removal of the metatarsal head and at least one third of the shaft is an adequate procedure for treatment of intractable corns in these areas"—meaning under the metatarsal heads. They conceded that the corresponding toe receded "one eighth to one fourth of an inch." They did not say how long they had observed the 30 patients thus operated. They merely said: "A five-year follow-up is planned." Kelikian and associates (1961) have noted more extensive recession of the toes and advised surgical syndactylia of adjacent digits to obviate this complication.

In connection with hallux valgus and hammered and clawed toes, we discussed some of the *surgical measures* utilized for mobilizing the metatarsophalangeal joints to enable the digits to contact the proffered surface. In metatarsalgia associated with hallux valgus without incarceration of the central heads, the preferred operation is osteotomy of the first metatarsal followed by lateral shift and plantar displacement of the capital fragment. In metatarsalgia accompanying hammertoes we combine partial proximal phalangectomy with surgical syndactylia of adjacent toes. In clawtoes and fixed incarceration of metatarsal heads we resect the segment of the offending metatarsal distal to the origin of the interossei and syndactylized the corresponding toe with its more sturdy neighbor (Figs. 16–14 to 16–16).

VERRUCA PLANTARIS

Pressure keratoses under plantarly bulging metatarsal heads have often been confused with papillomatous warts

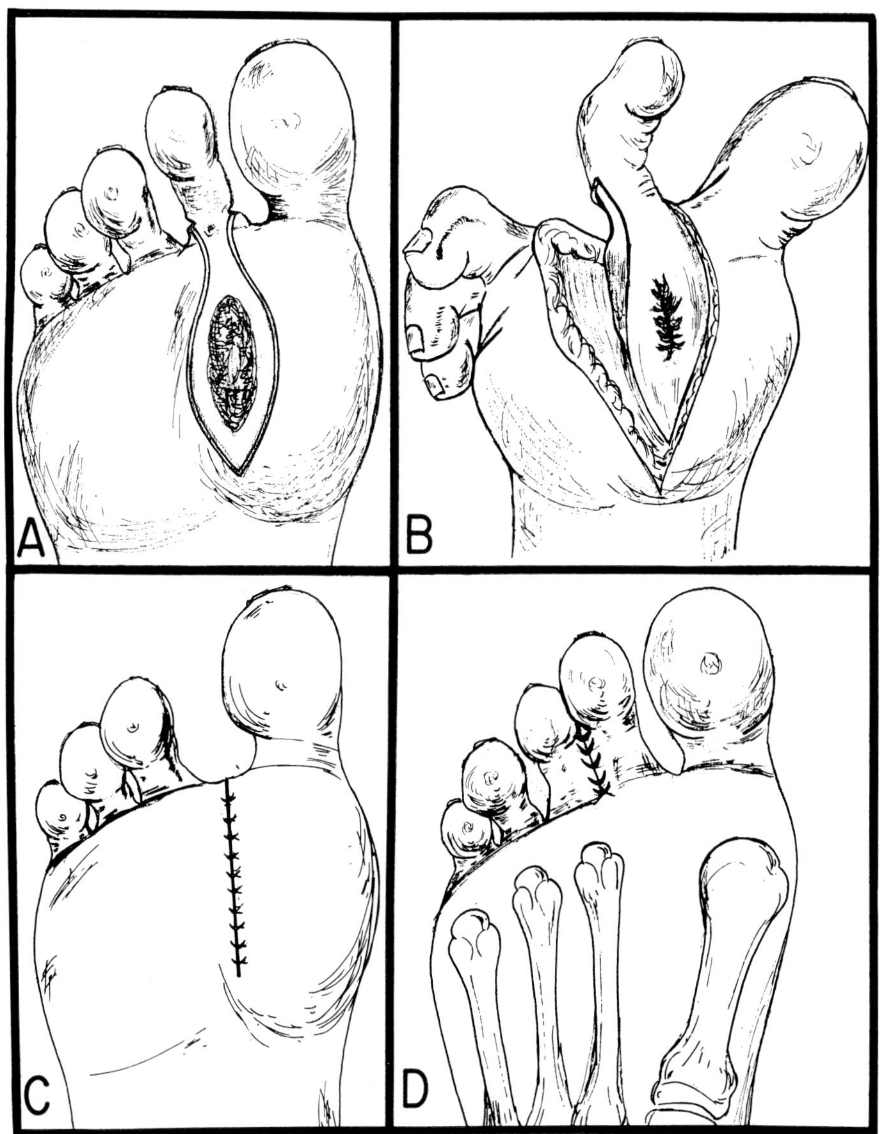

Figure 16–13. *A, B,* and *C,* Dickson's operation. *D,* Suggested modification.

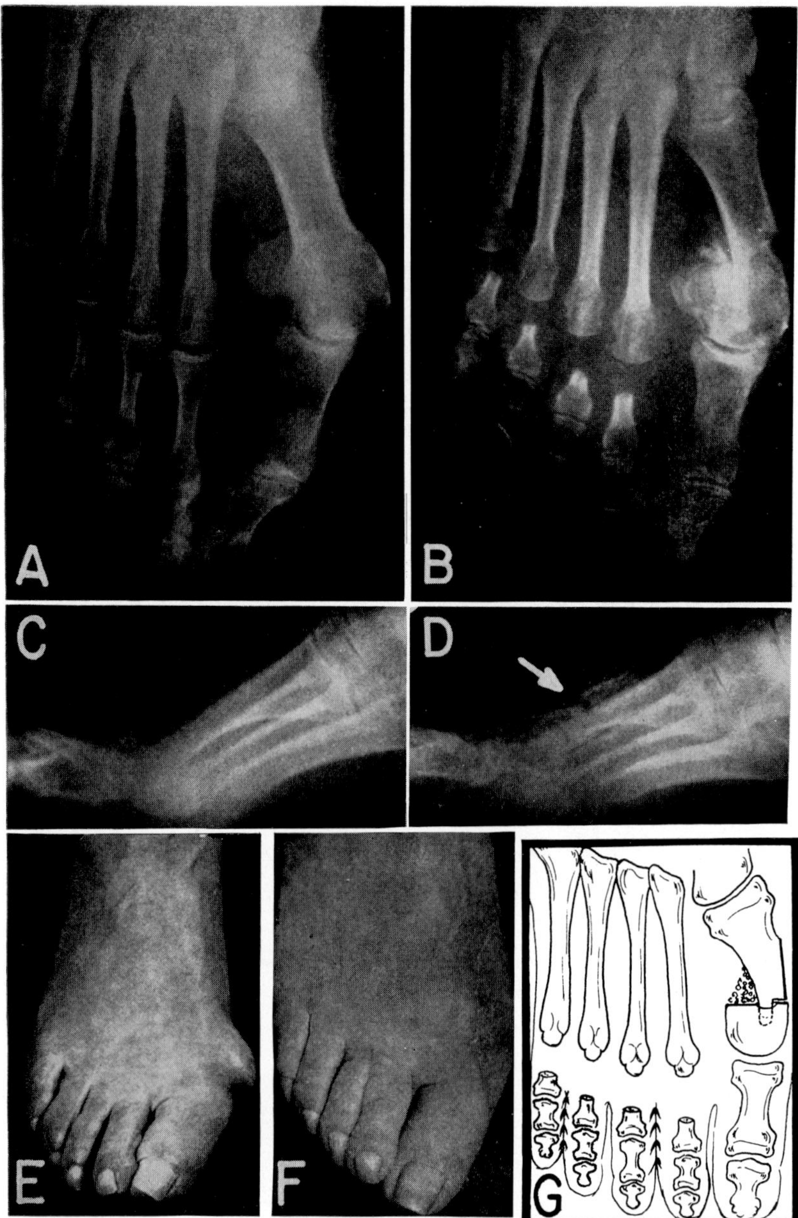

Figure 16–14. Woman, 51 years of age, with hallux valgus, hammertoes, and metatarsalgia, but no fixed incarceration of the middle metatarsal head. Surgery: distal osteotomy of the first metatarsal with lateral and plantar shift of the capital fragment; partial proximal phalangectomy of the lesser toes; surgical syndactylia of adjacent pair of digits. *A,* Dorsoplantar roentgenogram before surgery. Note the varus deformity of the first metatarsal. *B,* Same patient after recovery. *C,* Preoperative side view. *D,* Post-recovery side view. Note the plantar displacement of capital fragment. *E,* Preoperative photograph. *F,* Postoperative photograph. *G,* Interpretative diagram. Postoperative complaint: "bunion" pain. This was remedied by sagittal resection of the medial eminence. The patient works 8 hours a day and has no more complaints.

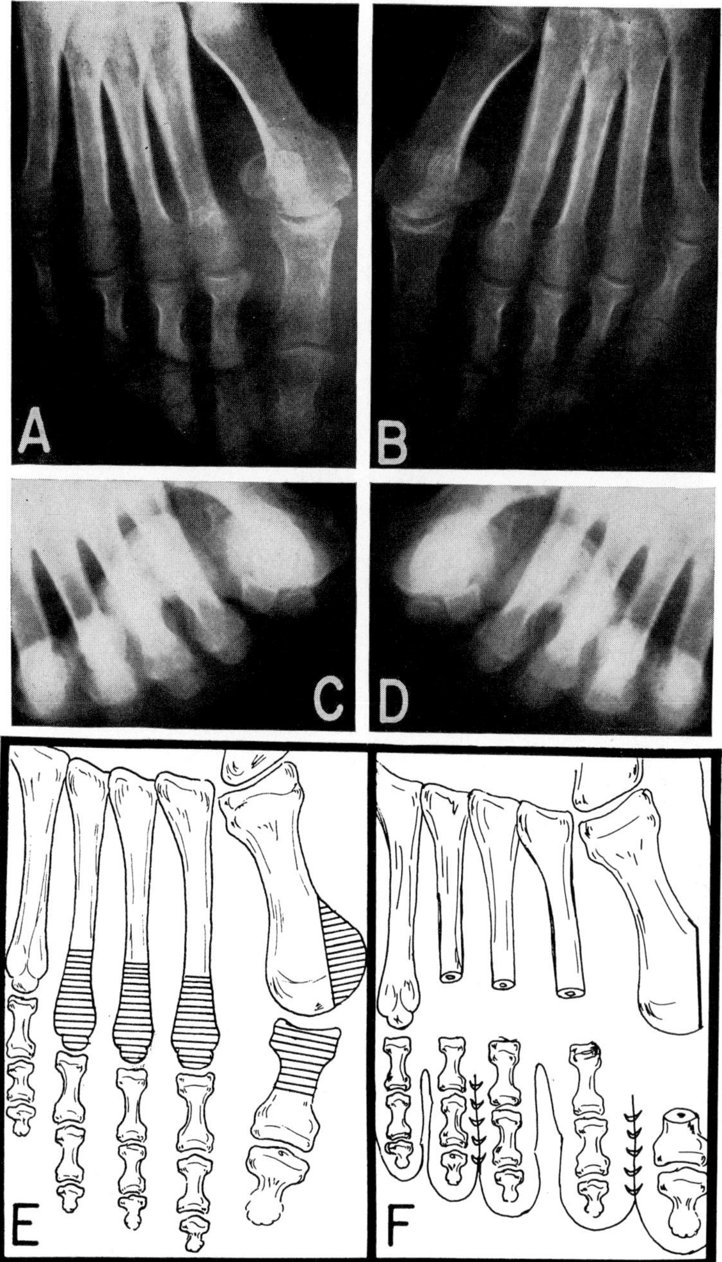

Figure 16–15. Woman, 44 years of age, with bilateral fixed plantar incarceration of the middle metatarsal heads, hallux valgus, and stiff first metatarsophalangeal joints. Complaint: pain over the first metatarsophalangeal joints—metatarsalgia. Surgery: Keller's resection on both sides, resection of distal thirds of the middle metatarsals, and surgical syndactylia of first with second and third with fourth toes. *A* and *B,* Preoperative dorsoplantar views of the forefeet. *C* and *D,* Tangential views. Note the advanced position of the middle metatarsal heads. *E* and *F,* Interpretative diagrams of the surgery on one foot. The other foot was similarly operated on.

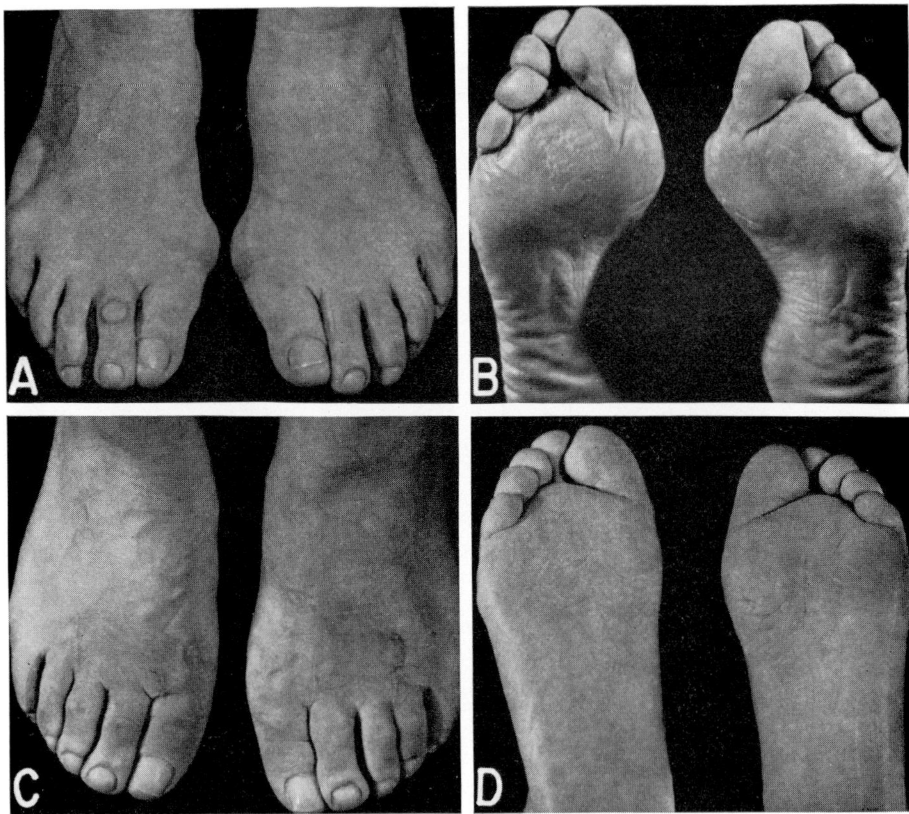

Figure 16–16. The same case as in Figure 16–15. *A,* Preoperative dorsal view of both feet. *B,* Plantar view. *C,* Postrecovery dorsal view. *D,* Postrecovery plantar view. The patient is satisfied.

of the skin below these bones. In the preceding section we mentioned several authors who, under the subject *Verruca Plantaris* or *Plantar Wart,* discussed treatments considered appropriate for callosities caused by excessive pressure. Conversely, pressure keratoses have been subjected to chemical escharification, electrocautery, or x-ray or radium therapy with disastrous consequences. The differentiation of these two lesions—plantar warts and pressure keratoses—from one another is paramount.

Differentiation of verruca plantaris from pressure keratosis. *Pressure keratoses* occur in older individuals with established forefoot deformities, the most obvious being hallux valgus and hammered and clawed toes. The pain appears after the patient is on his feet for some time, usually toward the end of the day. The cornification of the skin may be diffuse, involving the area under all five metatarsal heads. More often it is confined to the region under one or two metatarsal heads. In most instances the thickened skin does not contain a central core and the callus as a whole is not acutely tender to pressure. Plantar callosities containing cores are more painful. The core is pale, pearly white, and very hard. It can be distinguished from the surrounding, less cornified skin, but there is no distinct line of demarcation between the two. Tightly packed cornified cells of the central core blend into the less condensed cells of the periphery. The core is tender on direct, but not on lateral, pressure; it only bleeds when pared down deeply. Pressure keratoses do not disappear spontaneously; they persist as long as there is weight borne on them. They are radioresistant.

Verrucae plantaris occur more commonly in children and young adults with soft moist skin, pliable feet, and no retracted or malformed toes. These warts are most painful in the morning, when one starts to walk. The verruca may be single or solitary. Several of them may exist in clusters or may be disseminated all over the sole. Each wart contains a central core, which is demarcated from the surrounding skin by a definite ring of reactive dense dermis. The core is dark brown in color, often specked with black spots; it is pulpy and soft—softer than the surrounding zone of keratosis. The core is exquisitely tender, both on direct pressure and when an attempt is made to move it sideways. It bleeds even when shaved superficially. Some plantar warts tend to disappear spontaneously, and with a few exceptions, they are radiosensitive.

Verruca plantaris is akin to warts elsewhere on the body, but instead of burgeoning into a cauliflower shaped excrescence it has become flattened by the pressure. At weight-bearing points, under the metatarsal heads, the wart seldom projects beyond the surface of the skin. It appears to have been pushed in the opposite direction, buried behind a thin film of keratinized skin. When this superficial covering is shaved off, the reddish brown core at once comes into view. The core consists of dilated blood vessels and the punctate black spots represent the residues of repeated interstitial hemorrhages.

Etiology. The cause of verruca plantaris has been scrutinized by many. Wile and Kingery (1919) injected sterile filtrate of wart material intracutaneously and produced localized hyperkeratoses. They conceded that hyperkeratoses resembling verruca may be due to trauma or foreign bodies, but they did not consider these as inciting factors. They implied that trauma merely initiated a point of entrance for the infectious agent—most likely a filtrable virus. Whitfield (1932) advanced the theory of "small traumatic aneurysm" being brought about by bruises and other minor injuries. He did not think "single warts" had anything to do with infection. Sulkin and Harford (1943) reported "the presence of spherical virus-like particles in crystalline arrangements" in plantar warts. Strauss and associates (1951) centrifuged ground wart tissue and found "elementary bodies" in some warts. Lyell and Miles (1951) discovered "inclusion bodies" in several warts, not in all. Kile (1956) considered some strains of "virus wart" as being more communicable than others. He examined the inmates of an orphanage for children and of a seminary college for adults. According to him, warts "affected at least 20 per cent of residents in the seminary college and more than 25 per cent of the children in the orphanage." Kile thought "simple precautions" would help to prevent the spread of warts. It is generally agreed that multiple, disseminated warts are infectious as well as contagious. They are probably caused by some form of filtrable virus.

Prophylaxis. The prophylaxis against the spread of plantar warts was taken up by Lake (1952). "The infected patient," he wrote, "should not be allowed to walk barefooted anywhere where others are likely to follow; this applies particularly to dormitories and baths. All the patient's footwear must be kept separately, and on no account any interchange be allowed. Even the transference of a stocking from one foot to the other may lead to further infection. On the foot itself, the daily application of some suitable antiseptic is probably of value in the prevention of local spread. Ordinary spirit may be used, since it has the double advantage of being antiseptic and of drying and hardening the skin, so rendering it less liable to inoculation. Bath mats, and the like, which have been exposed to infection, should be treated with antiseptics, and reinfection guarded against. The use of thick paper and cardboard slippers, which can be easily destroyed after a day or two's use, is frequently advisable in households where the other precautions may be difficult to carry out."

Treatment. *Radiotherapy.* X-ray and radium have been recommended by many—Osborne and Putnam (1931), Degrais and Bellot (1931), Popp and Olds (1938), Marks and Franseen (1940), Pendergrass and Hodes (1941), Pipkin and associates (1949), and others. Reeves and Jackson (1956) regarded radiation therapy the treatment of choice for plantar warts, except in persons over 50 years of age "because of possible changes in skin nutrition."

In experienced hands radium or x-ray may perhaps be safely utilized in the treatment of verruca plantaris. Some warts are radioresistant. The patchy variety occurring in the area under metatarsal heads—described by Montgomery and Montgomery (1937) as "mosaic wart"—is an example. There have been numerous reports of radiodermatitis, actinonecrosis, and even sloughing of the metatarsal bones due to prolonged or repeated exposures. Shaw (1948) reported several tragic sequelae of improper radiation. "Plantar warts," McLaughlin (1948) wrote, "are both common and crippling; they are also essentially curable. Yet as a result of irrational treatment they are widely regarded as intractable and worthy of the radiotherapist's most ardent efforts; and also in turn often produce x-ray and radium burns of great severity, utterly disproportionate to such a simple condition."

Curettage and cautery. McLaughlin (1948) offered curettage and cautery as a safe alternative to radiotherapy. He pared down the hardened skin surrounding the central core and curetted the core. "The hyperkeratinized collar at the neck of the cavity is trimmed with scissors," McLaughlin wrote, "and the whole is converted into a 'saucer.' The base, which is tough, must then be scraped until smooth and repeatedly touched with a diathermy needle or electric cautery using a fine point (not too hot) with a light touch. This is the most essential step, which prevents recurrence and controls bleeding. . . ." Ducourtioux (1950) also favored *electrocautery*. Nissen (1957) described a method similar to McLaughlin's.

Chemical agents. Silver nitrate, phenol formalin, podophyllin, nitric acid, trinotrophenol, bichloracetic acid, trichloracetic acid, and others have been tried and are still used with varying success. Carpenter (1942) described a special apparatus for spraying carbon dioxide snow under pressure. This method has come to be known as *cryotherapy*. Carpenter (1943) advised paring the wart down with a knife or softening it by salicylic acid ointment. He then sprayed the wart with carbon dioxide snow for 2 to 5 seconds, depending on the size of lesion. Duthie and McCallum (1951) also pared down the wart and then applied elastoplast. In resistant cases they supplemented this with application of "podophyllin." An editorial in New England Medical Journal (1953) discussed Branson's (1953) method of treating "early" plantar warts. It consisted of injection of 1 per cent procaine under pressure. The bevel of the needle used for injection was made to reach stratum germinativum under the wart. A sufficient quantity of procaine was injected to cause blanching of the skin and elevate the wart. Procaine itself was said to act merely as an analgesic. The pressure of the liquid injected supposedly caused ischemic necrosis of the wart.

Psychotherapy. As a method of treating plantar warts, psychotherapy was discussed by Zwick (1932), Montgomery and Montgomery (1944), and many others. The subject was extensively reviewed by Allington (1952). We confess complete lack of experience with this method.

Surgical extirpation. The surgical extripation of persistent plantar warts is frowned on by many. The statement that the excision of plantar warts results in painful scars and recurrences is repeated in article after article, without citation of a single such case or the photograph of keloids, which are said to be common sequelae of incisions on the sole of the foot. Incisions utilized for resection of solitary plantar warts on the ball of the forefoot are usually elliptical, running more or less in a longitudinal direction. It is often stated that these long incisions cross the cleavage lines or flexion creases and that they violate canonized surgical principles and pave the way for painful keloids and contractures.

Once again we repeat: the hand and

the foot are two different organs and the sole of the foot is never used as a palm. In the palm there are at least two flexion creases disposed transversely. As demonstrated by Cox (1941) and reaffirmed by Wood Jones (1949), the cleavage lines of the sole run in the long axis of the foot with only slight convexity toward the fibular border. In infants there may be a suggestion of incomplete flexion creases across the ball of the forefoot; these disappear after

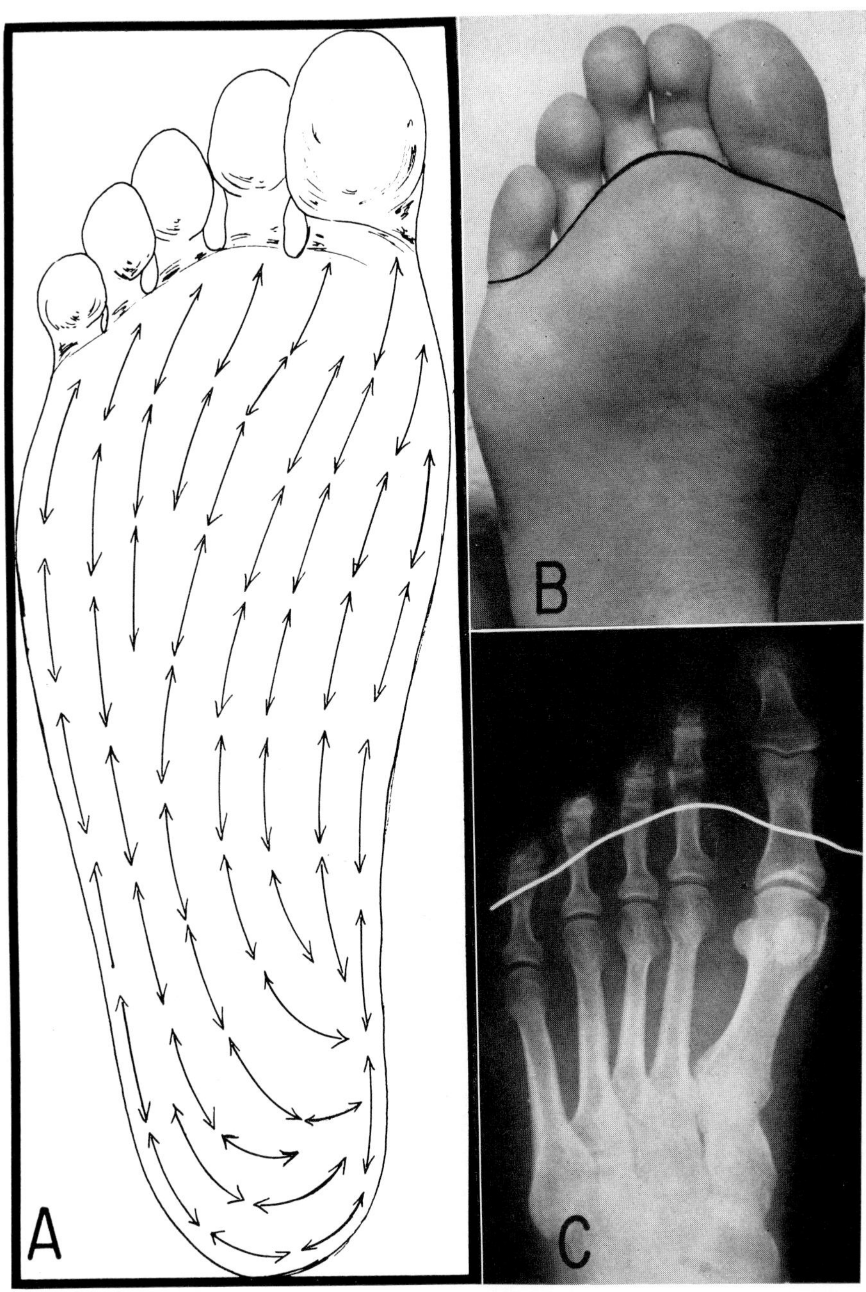

Figure 16–17. The cleavage lines and the flexion crease of the sole. *A*, Diagrams of longitudinally disposed cleavage lines of the sole. *B*, Position of the transversely disposed flexion crease. *C*, A metallic wire was taped into the flexion crease and a roentgenogram was taken. The crease lies at least an inch distal to the line of the metatarsophalangeal joints. Longitudinal incisions to resect pressure keratoses or plantar warts need not cross this crease; even if they do, contractures of the toes do not seem to develop.

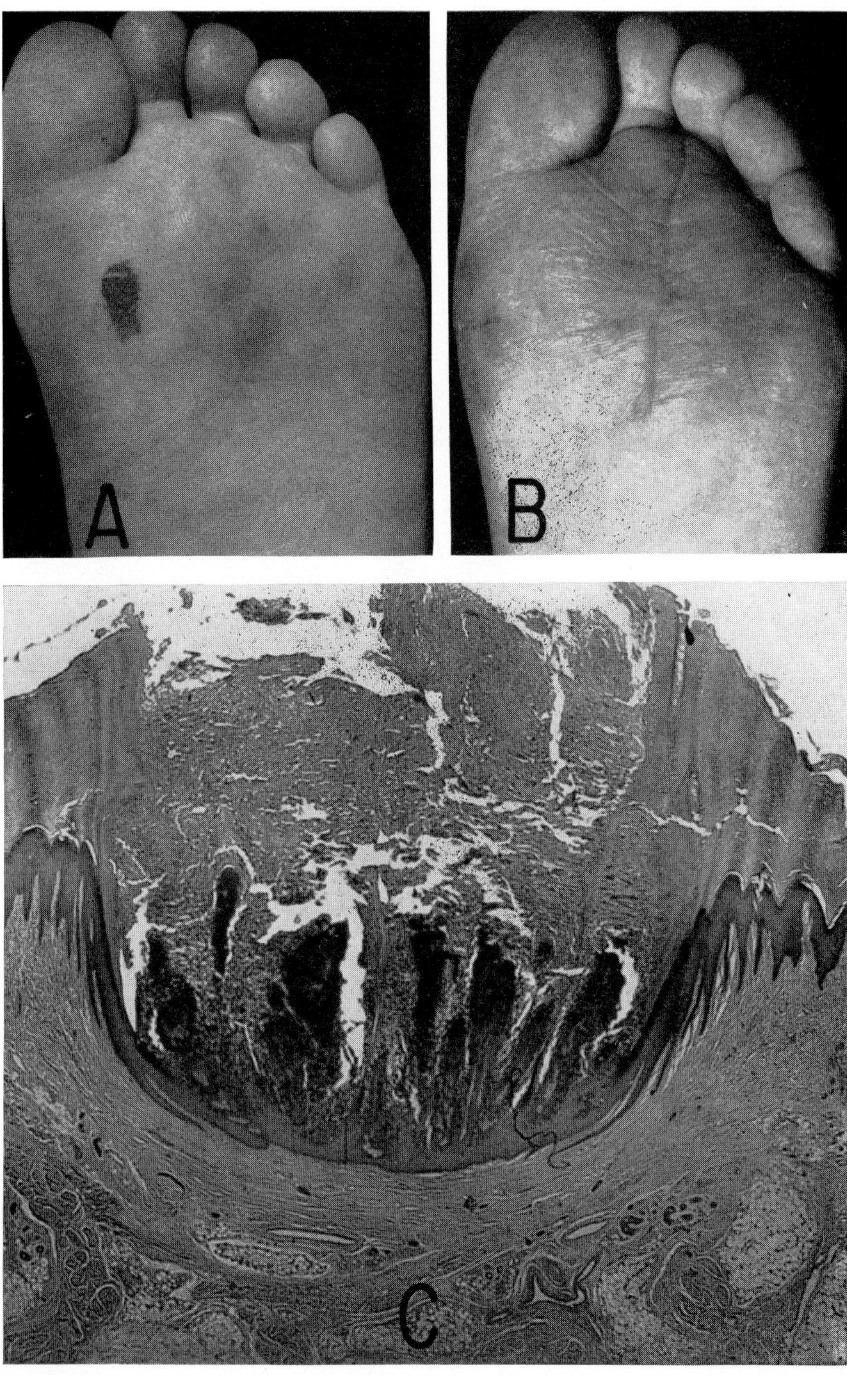

Figure 16–18. Girl, 7 years old, with painful, inflamed multiple verrucae. Treatment: antibiotics until inflammation subsided and resection of the warts by three separate longitudinally disposed pairs of elliptical cuts. *A,* Before surgery. *B,* After recovery. Note that only one scar shows. *C,* Photomicrograph of one of the warts (× 10). There has been no recurrence.

ambulation. Where the ball of the forefoot ends and the toes begin there is a deep transverse crease that is at least a whole inch distal to the line of the metatarsophalangeal joints. Longitudinally disposed elliptical incisions used for resection of painful persistent verrucae do not violate any surgical principle. Our next case may develop painful scar or keloid, but thus far we have not met with one. In fact a few months after surgery one hardly sees where the incision was made (Figs. 16–17 to 16–19).

T. G. MORTON'S METATARSALGIA

More than two decades before T. G. Morton's (1876) classic article appeared, Durlacher (1845) spoke of a "form of neuralgic affection" involving "the plantar nerve . . . between the third and fourth metatarsal bones." Morton related the "neuralgic paroxysms" to the region of the fourth metatarsophalangeal joint and suspected "a neuroma or some form of nerve hypertrophy" of digital

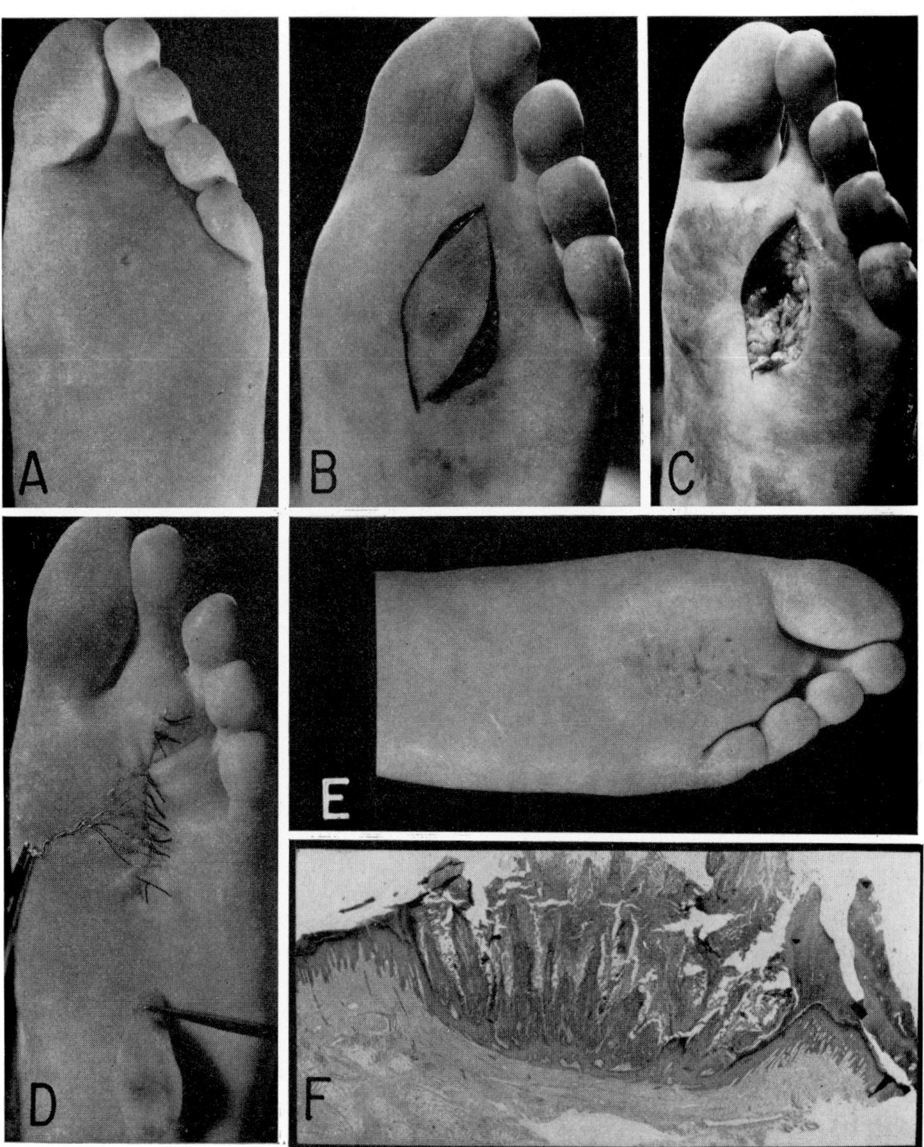

Figure 16–19. Girl, 12 years of age, with painful solitary verruca. *A,* Before surgery. *B, C,* and *D,* During surgery. *E,* Four weeks later. *F,* Photomicrograph (× 10). There has been no recurrence.

branches of the lateral plantar nerve. He supposed that the nerve was pinched by the flanking metatarsal bones, mainly by the fifth, which being short and mobile, was said to slip under the fourth following sudden twists of the foot.

In years to come what Morton called *painful affection of fourth metatarsophalangeal joint* was accepted as a definite clinical entity. It was variously named *luxation podalgia, Morton's toe, Morton's disease,* or *Morton's neuralgia.* At first it was thought that only the branches of the lateral plantar nerve were involved. Mason (1877) reported a case with pain around the second metatarsophalangeal joint and suspected involvement of the digital branch of the medial plantar nerve.

Pollosson (1889) introduced the term *anterior metatarsalgia* and suspected compression of the digital nerve by the plantar dislocation of one of the metatarsal bones, "probably the third." Woodruff (1890) advanced the view of dislocation at the metatarsophalangeal joint. Bradford (1891) endorsed Morton's original contention. An editorial in the New York Medical Journal—ascribed to Dana (1892)—sanctioned the symptom complex as a definite clinical entity. T. S. K. Morton (1893)—referred to by some as the younger Morton—gave the name *Morton's metatarsalgia.*

Evolution of the concept of plantar neuroma. Neither T. G. Morton, Mason, nor Pollosson explored the digital nerves they suspected of being the conveyors of paroxysmal pain. Mills (1888) suggested resecting or stretching "the external plantar nerve going to the fourth and fifth toes," but gave no indication that this suggestion had ever been carried out. It was perhaps on account of the domineering influence of the eastern group of orthopedic surgeons—of Boston, New York, and Philadelphia—that the findings of a relatively unknown midwesterner passed unnoticed. Hoadley (1893) of Chicago explored the digital nerve under the painful area, "found a small neuroma," resected it, and obtained "prompt and perfect cure."

Orthopedic surgeons of eastern hegemony—Gibney (1894), Goldthwait (1894), T. G. Morton (1897), Whitman (1898), and others—completely ignored Hoadley. Perhaps they did not even condescend to thumb the pages of that midwestern upstart, *The Chicago Medical Recorder,* in which Hoadley's article appeared. In England, Robert Jones (1897) echoed some of Hoadley's ideas but made no mention of his name. "In conversation with Mr. Tubby," Jones wrote, "he tells me that he has just operated on a case of advanced metatarsalgia and found the nerve swollen and congested." Hoadley's name appeared in the bibliography but not in the text of the article Jones and Tubby (1898) authored a year later.

The twentieth century dawned with several indifferent papers on this subject—one by Peckham (1901), another by Lovett (1903), a third by Stern (1904). None mentioned Hoadley. In the third edition of his book, Whitman (1907) repeated what he had said 9 years earlier. In the second edition of his *Deformities,* Tubby (1912) wrote: "As a rule, if the plantar digital nerves are examined, no change is visible in them, but in the course of operation of this condition the writer has twice seen the plantar digital nerves thickened and red; and once not red only but swollen, intensely congested, and dark, thus giving the evidence of persistent neuritis."

Tubby thus gave a clue as to the true cause of the paroxysmal pain. Maffei (1924) discussed Morton's metatarsalgia at some length, spoke about resecting the nerve, but said nothing about a tumor. Betts (1940) categorically stated: "Morton's metatarsalgia is a neuritis of the fourth digital nerve, with a pronounced neuroma in all cases." McElvenny (1943) wrote: "Morton's toe is a painful affliction of the foot which is often resistant to conservative treatment. It is caused by a tumor involving the most lateral branch of the medial plantar nerve. Careful palpation will usually reveal the tumor which lies high in the web between the third and the fourth toes. . . ." None of these authors mentioned Hoadley, who had pioneered the concept of nerve tumor as the cause of paroxysmal pain around the bases of third and fourth toes. Bickel and Dockerty (1947) mentioned Hoadley at long last, after 54 years of neglect.

Pathomechanics. In his original communication, T. G. Morton (1876) localized the paroxysmal pain around the vicinity of the fourth metatarsophalangeal joint. He explained this selective localization on the bases of comparative mobility of the two outermost metatarsal bones and the relative discrepancy of their lengths. He said that the fifth metatarsal was from three-eighths to one-half inch behind the fourth, which would place the fifth metatarsophalangeal joint closer to the heel than the fourth, and the base of the proximal phalanx of the small toe would be on a level with the neck of the fourth metatarsal bone. As compared to the three medial bones, Morton stated, the fourth metatarsal enjoyed greater mobility, the fifth still more than the fourth. According to him, lateral pressure brought the head of the fifth metatarsal and the base of the proximal phalanx of the small toe in contact with the neck of the fourth metatarsal. Morton even visualized the fifth metatarsal rolling "above and under" the fourth and pinching "the digital branches of the external plantar nerve." In his second paper on this subject, Morton (1897) interpolated several roentgenograms to reaffirm what he had said two decades earlier. He said he had no reason to change his views on this subject, expressed 20 years earlier.

Hoadley (1893) questioned the accuracy of Morton's contention that the digital nerve in the fourth intermetatarsal groove was pinched by the flanking metatarsal bones. He pointed out that the fourth and fifth metatarsal bones could not possibly "roll up and down . . . slide above or underneath," as claimed by Morton. These bones could not squeeze the nerve; the nerve lay below the transverse ligament, hence below the metatarsal heads and could not be pinched by these bones. Moreover, Hoadley argued, it was not the nerve in the fourth intermetatarsal groove but the one in the third—"the internal branch of the external plantar nerve" that was usually injured as it lay "just below where the foot makes the sharpest fold" (Figs. 16–20 and 16–21).

Jones (1897) made ample use of Hoadley's arguments. As had Hoadley, Jones pointed out that the plantar digital nerves lay below the deep transverse ligament and could not be pinched by the metatarsal bones. Jones and Tubby (1898) spoke of a communicating twig that passes beneath the fourth metatarsal bone and connects the neighboring branches of the medial and lateral plantar nerves. They thought this branch was the seat of neuralgic pain and advanced the view that it was compressed between the head of the fourth metatarsal bone and the ground.

Betts (1940) referred to both Jones and Tubby and appeared to agree with them. He himself explained "the mechanics that produce pain" on the basis of stretching and not compression of the digital nerve. "The fourth nerve," Betts wrote, "is formed by the external plantar, each coming around from opposite sides of the belly of the *flexor brevis* and crossing this obliquely before they unite. Two to three centimetres distally the nerve divides, to pass to the adjacent sides of the third and fourth toes. The nerve is thicker than the other digital nerves, owing to its double origin and early division requiring more fibrous sheath, and this thicker part lies immediately on the transverse ligament, which is a very firm structure. This anatomical difference from the other digital nerves explains why the fourth nerve is subject to this neuritis. When the foot is in action the *flexor brevis* contracts, fixing the origin of the nerve, while dorsiflexion of the toes in walking stretches it around the unyielding transverse ligament. The neuritis probably arises in the first place from minor trauma, the head of the fourth metatarsal taking most of the weight on the outer side and being the part of the tread most exposed to such injuries. Once the nerve is swollen from neuritis a vicious circle is set up. . . ."

Betts called this swollen nerve "neu-

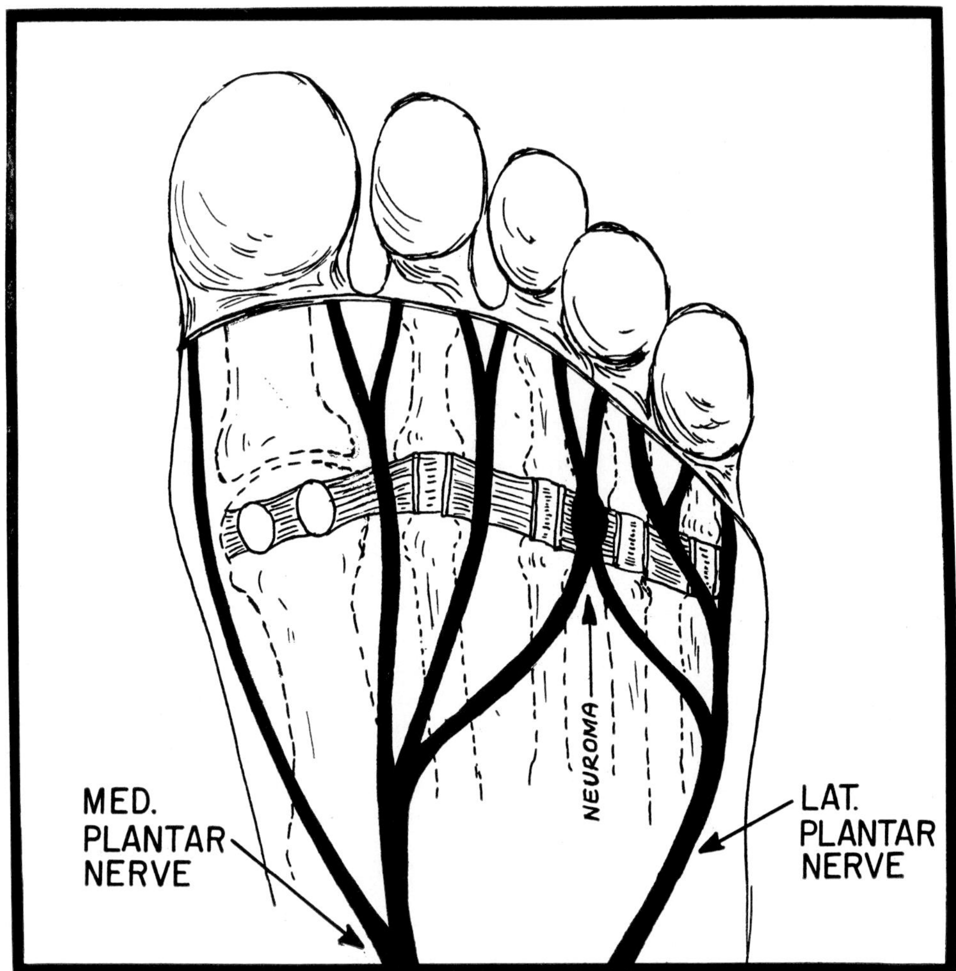

Figure 16–20. Diagram illustrating that both medial and lateral plantar nerves contribute to the formation of the fourth digital nerve, which usually bears the neuroma.

roma." He made no commitment as to the true nature of the tumors except to say that microscopic section revealed a great increase in the fibrous tissue element of the nerve. McElvenny (1943) was equivocal. He wrote: "A number of pathologists have studied sections from these tumors. Agreement amongst these men has not been forthcoming. Some of these tumors are thought to be neurofibroma and others resemble glomus tumore. . . ." Baker and Kuhn (1944) advanced the concept of "degenerative fibrosis of the nerve with neuromatous proliferation resulting from, or irritated by, repeated trauma." King (1946) considered chronic trauma as the cause and drew an analogy with Koloid; he suggested the term "sclerosing neuroma." Bickel and Dockerty (1947) recorded the following findings: edema, demyelinization and cystic vacuolization of the nerve, and endarteritis of the vessels. Winkler and associates (1948) arrived at a similar conclusion. "We do not," they wrote, "find changes which could be interpreted as evidence of active proliferation of either nerve or connective tissues. The deposition of hyaline and collagenous material in itself accounts for the enlargment . . . the process is essentially degenerative in nature, trauma being its most probable cause."

Nissen (1948) said that in every case of Morton's metatarsalgia on which he operated, he found "a fibrous swelling of the nerve. . . . The primary lesion," Nissen added, "is one of local vascular degeneration leading to a variety of changes in and around the cutaneous nerve. . . ." At a later date Nissen (1951) wrote: "The pain coming after perhaps half a mile of walking and persisting as a severe ache for a number of minutes after rest bears the stamp of ischaemia. . . ." Histologically, he thought the nerve lesion was "ischemic." Ringertz and Unander-Scharin (1950) did not think "the theory expounded by Nissen, that Morton's disease depends on primary endarteritis and secondary fibrosis as a consequence of circulatory disturbances" gave "full explanation." Mulder (1951) found the neuroma to be adherent to the intermetatarsal bursa and suggested prolapse of the plantar digital nerve into the bursa as the basic disturbance. Venturi (1960) reviewed the subject at some length and said very little that had not been said before.

These controversies have merely augmented the confusion. Notwithstanding numerous articles on the subject with photomicrographic illustrations of sections of the nerve resected, one cannot say it has as yet been definitely estab-

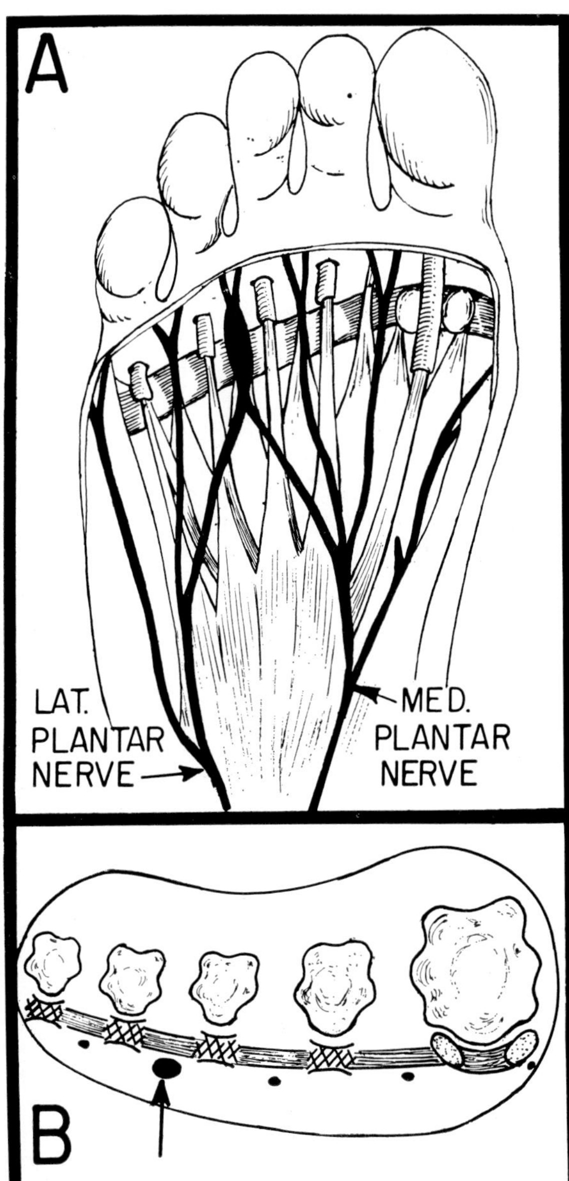

Figure 16–21. Diagrams illustrating that the neuroma lies on the plantar aspect of the deep transverse ligament, hence, below the level of the metatarsal heads and cannot be pinched by the flanking bones.

lished that the swollen interdigital nerve so often seen in the course of surgical exploration is in the nature of neoplastic growth. Many consider the thickening of the nerve as a response on the part of fibrous tissue elements to mechanical irritation.

Clinical features. Morton (1876) characterized the pain around the fourth metatarsophalangeal joint as being paroxysmal. He reported 12 cases and said he had 3 more patients under his care. Thirteen of 15 were females; 8 related their discomfort to direct injury of the fourth toe; 3 or 4 spoke of shoe pressure; the remainder could not give any cause. "All of the patients," Morton wrote, "were surrounded not only by the comforts, but in most instances were accustomed to the luxuries of life." Pollosson's (1889) patient was a medical man. He had no pain when the foot was at rest and unshoed. The pain came on suddenly in attacks upon wearing shoes and taking long walks. It was more likely to occur when going downhill than when going uphill. Pollosson explained this stating that in the former instance greater load was thrown on the forepart of the foot. Grün (1889), himself a surgeon, described his own metatarsalgia as being "cramping . . . causing the unhappy patient to remove his boots without regard to place or circumstances, often most inconvenient. On first removal of the boot," he said, "the pain is intensified, and has been so great as to almost cause fainting, necessitating at least a quarter of an hour's rest, after which it will gradually wear off." Guthrie (1892), another sufferer and also a medical man, described his pain as a sense of something having given away at the site of the affected joint. The pain, he said, was relieved by removing the shoe and gently pressing the displaced bones into proper position. According to him, "the reduction" was always accompanied by a sharp twinge of pain, followed by instantaneous relief. Guthrie then spoke of a patient whose pain was under the third metatarsal head; he could relieve it by taking his shoes off and flexing his toes while pressing gently with his finger on the site of discomfort. The patients reported by Robert Jones (1897) variously described their pains as "sickening, like treading on something hot," "as if walking on hot marble," "excruciating martyrdom," burning, and so on. Some obtained relief by the removing of their shoes and squeezing the forefoot or flexing the toes.

Most of the earlier authors did not make a clear distinction between T. G. Morton's metatarsalgia and other forms. Morton's metatarsalgia is confined to the region between the third and the fourth toes, rarely between the more medial digits. The pain is paroxysmal; it comes in spells. It is described as being knifelike, stabbing, or burning. It comes when walking in shoes and radiates to the tips of one or both adjacent toes and sometimes up toward the leg. Pressure in the web between the involved toes, or slightly proximal, may elicit pain. Occasionally, tumor mass is palpated; rarely the sensation along the contiguous surfaces of the third and fourth toes is dulled or diminished. The foot appears normal. The condition affects women more often than men. Metatarsal pad and injection of hydrocortisone may temporarily alleviate the pain but it soon recurs.

Treatment. "In chronic cases," T. G. Morton (1876) wrote, "complete excision of the irritable metatarsophalangeal joint with the surrounding soft parts will be likely to prove permanently successful." Hoadley (1893), we noted, resected the neuroma. Gibney (1894) manipulated the foot, grasping the metatarsal bones at their base and exerting enough pressure to cause separation of the distal ends. He prescribed shoes with Spanish last. Robert Jones (1897) recommended thick-soled boots provided with a transverse bar half an inch behind the metatarsal heads. He considered the following operations efficient: excision of the metatarsal head, excision of the joint, and amputation of the metatarsal head and the toe. "Short of these radical measures," he wrote, "we may employ any or all the following measures: (1) Actual cautery. (2) Heated needle into painful site to destroy the nerve. (3) Hypodermic injections of carbolic acid. (4) Part exsection of digital plantar nerve."

Now almost three-quarters of a century after he described it, Hoadley's neurectomy is considered the operation of choice for Morton's metatarsalgia. Hoadley approached the nerve through a plantar longitudinal incision. This approach has also been utilized by Betts (1940), Nissen (1948–1957) and many others. McElvenny (1943) advocated a dorsal web-bisecting incision. McKeever (1952) referred to Betts as having depicted in his article a transverse incision on the sole. "By instinct and training," McKeever commented, "the author has an aversion to making an unnecessary incision in the plantar surface of the foot. The beauty of the anatomical demonstration possible through such an incision, extolled as one of its advantages

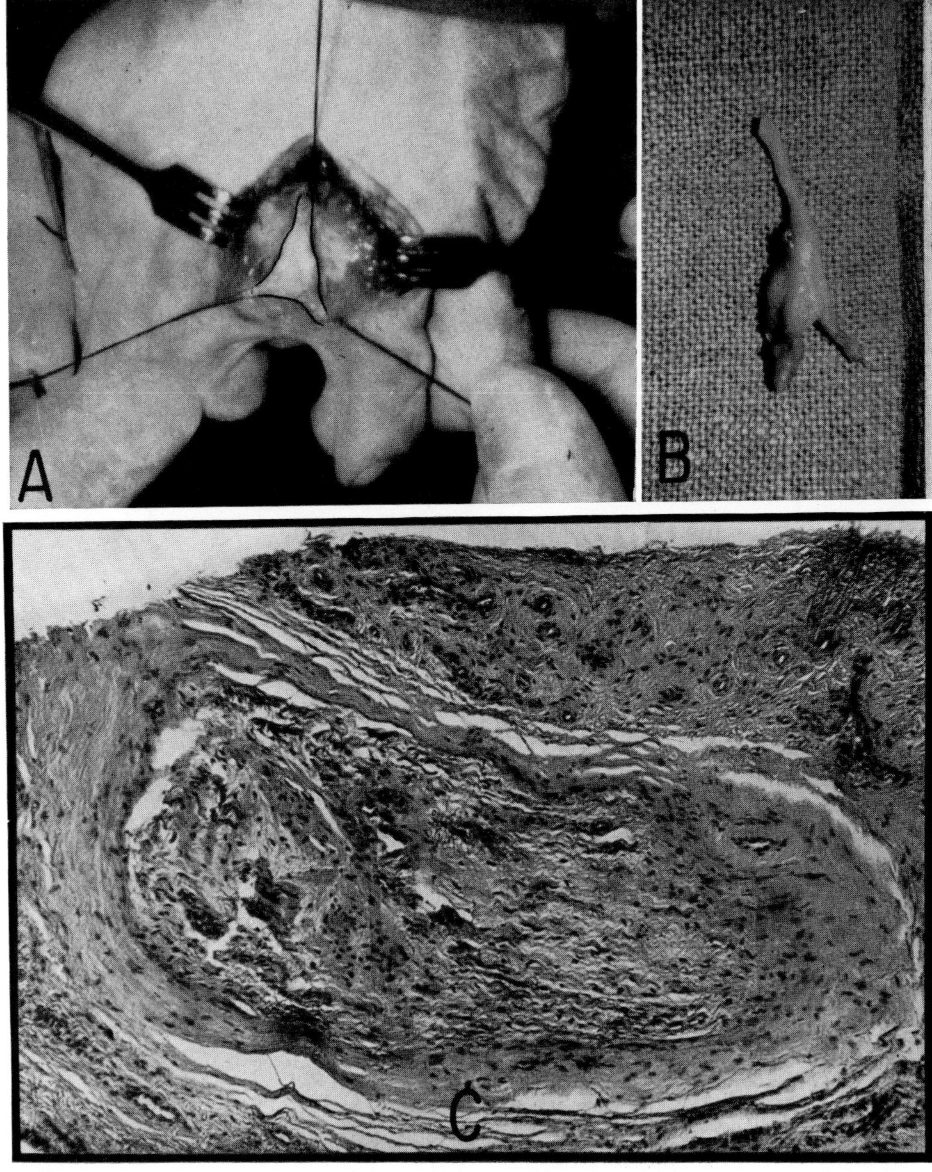

Figure 16–22. Woman, 67 years of age, with paroxysmal metatarsalgia between the bases of third and fourth toes. Duration: 4 months. *A,* Delivery of the neuroma through a dorsal approach. *B,* Resected neuroma. *C,* Photomicrograph (× 75). Complete relief resulted.

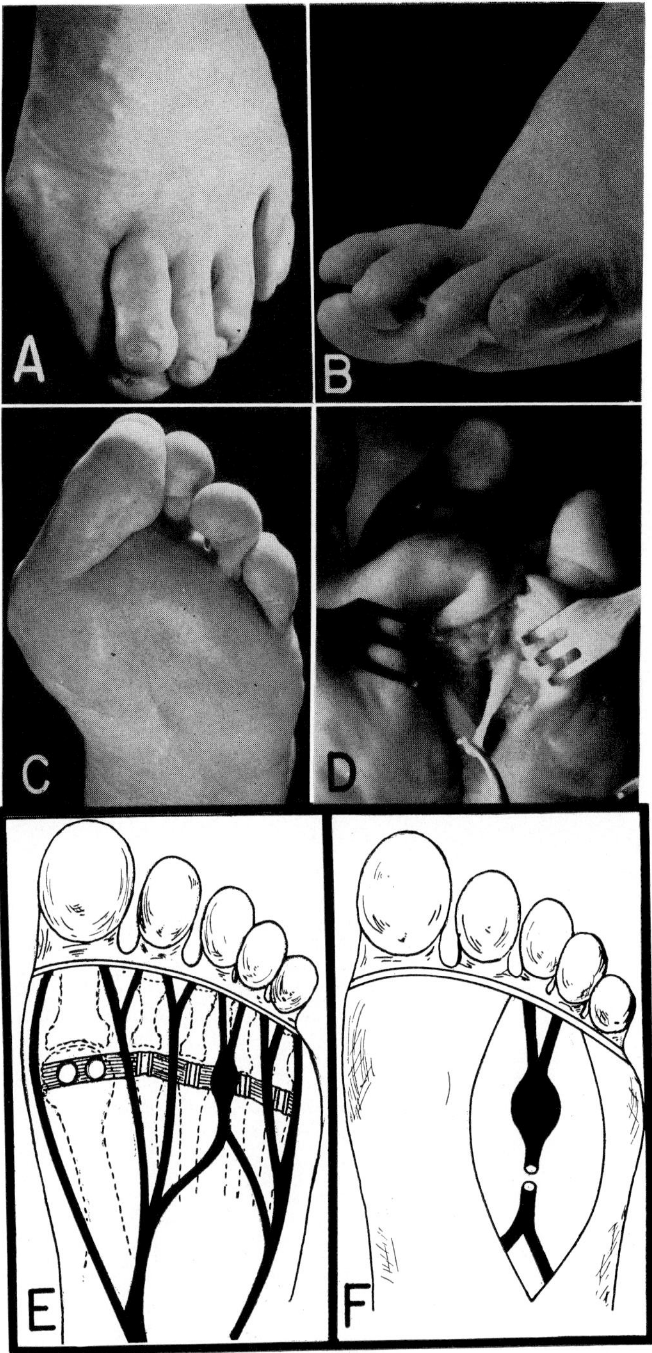

Figure 16–23. Woman, 58 years of age, with hallux valgus, overriding second toe, plantarly bulging middle metatarsal heads, diffuse metatarsalgia, and numbness of third and fourth toes. In view of uncertain diagnosis, the area was approached through the plantar incision. *A, B,* and *C,* Various views of the forefoot. *D,* During surgery. *E* and *F,* Interpretative diagrams. In *E* the nerve is shown as sectioned only. It was dissected out. The digital deformities were simultaneously corrected. Metatarsalgia was relieved.

hardly justifies it. Such anatomical demonstrations had better be made on cadavers."

McKeever resected the nerve through a small "not . . . more than one inch in length" dorsal incision between the bases of the third and fourth toes. "Blunt dissection between the metatarsal heads can be made easily with a hemostat," McKeever continued. "The metatarsal heads can then be separated with two rake retractors and pressure on the sole of the foot will present the neuroma, or neuromata, in the space between the metatarsal heads where it can be grasped with a hemostat, cut loose at both ends, and removed. . . . The entire procedure, including closure, takes less than five minutes."

Admire as we do McKeever's ability to finish the operation "in less than five minutes," it must be admitted that watching the time while one operates, favoring small skin cuts, and instinctive aversions toward other incisions are not commendable surgical traits. McKeever must have misread the article by Betts, whom he blamed as having used a

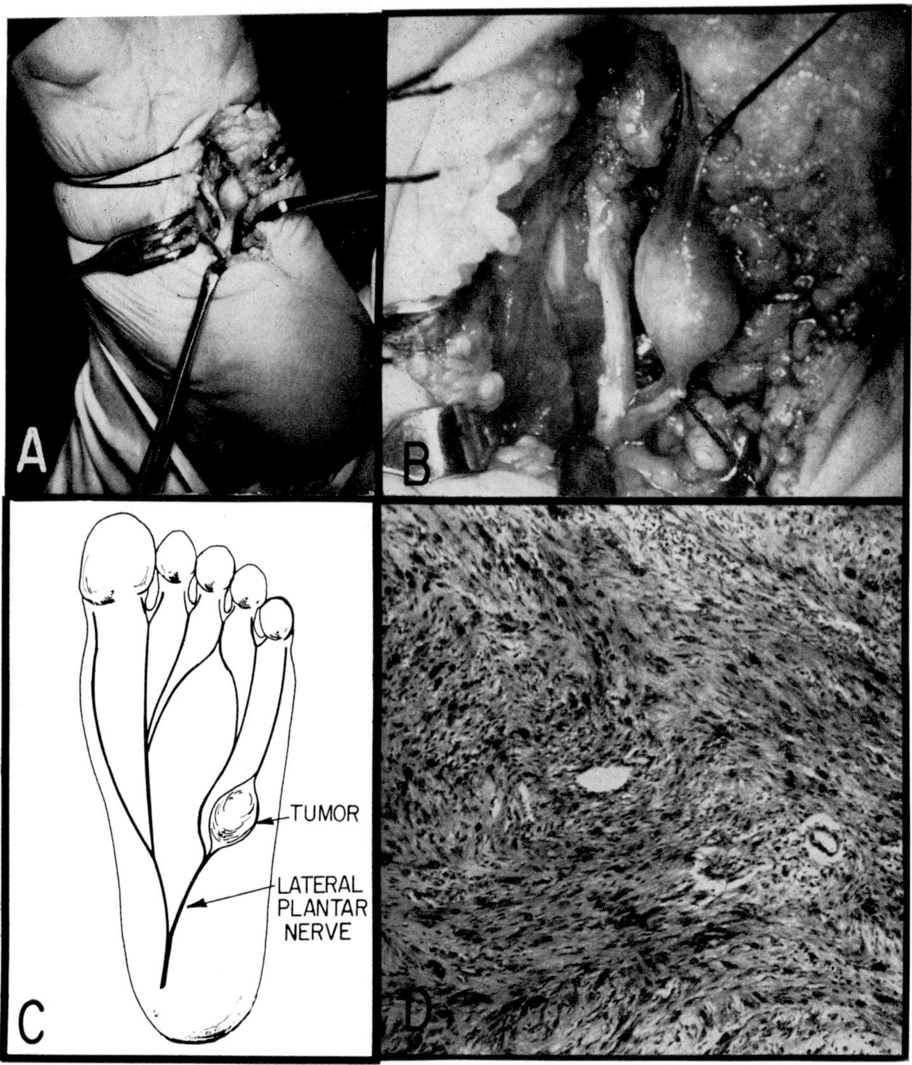

Figure 16–24. Woman, 38 years of age, with paroxysmal metatarsalgia on the lateral aspect of the sole radiating to the fifth toe. In view of the unusual location of pain, a plantar approach was chosen. A large neuroma was found on the outermost branch of the lateral plantar nerve. It was resected. *A,* Photograph after exposure of neuroma; *B,* the same, enlarged. *C,* Interpretative diagram. *D,* Photomicrograph (× 130). Complete relief of pain resulted.

transverse incision across the ball of the forefoot. Betts spoke of the objection by Robert Jones against placing "the scar on the tread of the foot." In practice Betts (1940) wrote, "Jones's (sic) objection has proved to be without foundation. A longitudinal incision between the heads of the third and fourth metatarsals heals well, and the scar almost disappears in a few months . . . in performing neurectomy I remove about an inch of the nerve, cutting it back proximally as far as possible to prevent any chance of painful neuroma under the head."

McKeever might have had Nissen, and not Betts, in mind when he castigated the transverse plantar incision "described and illustrated in a recent article." In this first paper on the subject, Nissen (1948) wrote: "An Esmarch bandage is fixed round the thigh and the patient is turned into the prone position with the ankle resting over a sandbag at the end of the table. The third and fourth metatarsophalangeal joints are palpated, and an incision two inches or more in length is made between them, down to the web." In the footnote Nissen added: "A transverse incision in the tread has some advantages, especially when a neighboring cleft may have to be explored." Ordinarily Nissen favored a longitudinal plantar cut. This incision is well described and illustrated in a later communication by Nissen (1957). It gives an excellent view of the field. "The source of the pain," Nissen commented, "may prove to be a cyst, not a neuroma."

There is something to be said in favor of both dorsal and plantar incisions. The former is not attended with as long a period of postoperative disability, but one occasionally has to cut the deep transverse metatarsal ligament to deliver the neuroma. Too often not enough of the main trunk can be seen and cut to prevent the proximal stump from becoming involved in the surgical scar or from forming another neuroma under the area where weight is borne. We have operated on two such patients with recurrent metatarsalgia. In both, the nerve was bound down in adhesions. When certain of the diagnosis, we utilize dorsal incision. When something else is suspected or two nerves are to be exploited, we use a longitudinal plantar cut (Figs. 16–22 to 16–24).

D. J. MORTON'S SYNDROME

T. G. Morton ascribed the pain in the forefoot to the comparative shortness and mobility of the fifth metatarsal bone. Years later his namesake, D. J. Morton, drew attention to the brevity and hypermobility of the first metatarsals and considered them as causes of forefoot pain. Henry Kemp Randell (1831) had long ago written: "The meta-tarsal bone of the *great toe* is the thickest, shortest, and strongest of the whole." Ninety-nine years later, in the course of the discussion following one of D. J. Morton's (1930) papers, Mather Cleveland said: "The first metatarsal is always described as the shortest and the thickest of the metatarsals. I should like to ask Dr. Morton when he considers a first metatarsal abnormally short."

Dudley Morton (1924–1952) made it clear that he identified shortness by the distance the most advanced point of the second metatarsal extended beyond the first. With his known preoccupation with the evolution of the human foot, it was inevitable—in a way predictable—that he should choose such an epithet as *atavicus* for the comparatively short first metatarsal, which he considered the cause of forefoot pain. Subsequently, D. J. Morton added two other structural factors contributing to metatarsalgia: hypermobile first metatarsal segment and posteriorly located sesamoids. Morton ascribed the laxity of the first metatarsal segment to the unusually free motion in the joint between the medial and middle cuneiforms. He argued that the two sesamoids served as bearing points for the first metatarsal and augmented its potential length. When these two ossicles lay under the neck rather than the head, the effect upon the distribution of weight in the foot was that of a short first metatarsal.

According to Dudley Morton, short

first metatarsal, hypermobile first segment, and retroplaced sesamoids upset the balance of weight distribution in the foot. The lateral metatarsal bones were subjected to more than their share of stress. The second metatarsal responded to excessive load by gaining in girth; the skin under its head formed a painful callus. The basal joint of the second metatarsal became painful. Morton explained this pain by the proximity of the medial plantar nerve and its irritation.

From Morton's many communications we cull the following as manifest effects of his syndrome: (1) pain and keratosis under the second and sometimes the third metatarsal heads; (2) tenderness around the base of the second metatarsal; (3) pain projected into the toes because of irritation of the medial plantar nerve, the discomfort being diffuse but occasionally simulating the paroxysmal neuralgia of T. G. Morton; (4) roentgenographic evidence of posteriorly located sesamoids, thickened second metatarsal shaft, and wide joint space between middle and medial cuneiforms; and finally (5) evidence of concentrated pressure under the second metatarsal head in kinetographic prints (Fig. 16–25).

D. J. Morton's contention that the syndrome he described should be recognized as a definite clinical entity has been questioned. After their survey of soldiers' feet in the Canadian Army, Harris and Beath (1949) arrived at the conclusion that "shortness of the first metatarsal is not a cause of any disability," that "the hypermobility of the first metatarsal segment could not be identified as a clinical entity," and that "posterior displacement of the sesamoids of the hallux gave no evidence that it is a cause of disability."

By way of countercriticism, Morton (1952) pointed out that the survery conducted by Harris and Beath had been carried out on comparatively young soldiers. In his book published in 1935, Morton said he had stated that shortness of the first metatarsal rarely produced symptoms in the very young, especially in men. "Consequently," Morton wrote, "their results in showing the usual lack of disabling symptoms in young military groups is in accord with, and confirms, my findings as previously published. In view of the critical position assumed by the authors," Morton continued, "their failing to mention *corroborating* nature of the survey can be explained by one of the following reasons: Unfamiliarity with the contents of the book, an unintentional oversight or less gracious desire to strengthen their arguments by false and misleading implication."

A more valid criticism of Morton's views was leveled by Wood Jones (1943). Wood Jones had run across an article by Flavell (1943), who had quoted Bruce (1937) to the effect that in a normal foot the head of the first metatarsal was "on the same transverse plane or even a little distal than the second." In his turn Flavell had reiterated some of D. J. Morton's views concerning the evolution of the human foot and had flaunted such exalted phrases as "metatarsus atavicus" and "humanoid line."

Not without ire, Wood Jones (1943) commented: ". . . Flavell follows Mr. John Bruce, who follows Dudley J. Morton . . . in blaming a short first metatarsal for many forefoot disabilities. They blame this bone because one and all assume that 'the head of the first metatarsal' is 'on the same transverse plane, or even a little more distal, than that of the second.' It cannot be insisted too strongly that in the normal human foot the head of the first metatarsal is always behind that of the second and usually behind that of the third. It is true that the normal human metatarsal formula is what Morton in his book mistakenly regards as a deformity of 'fourth degree shortening' of the first metatarsal, but that does not justify orthopedic surgeons failing to recognize the normal when they see it. . . . The apparent profundity of such expressions as Morton's 'humanoid line' and Morton's 'metatarsus atavicus,' when founded on a failure to recognize a very commonplace condition of human osteology, fails to be impressive. Far from the first meta-

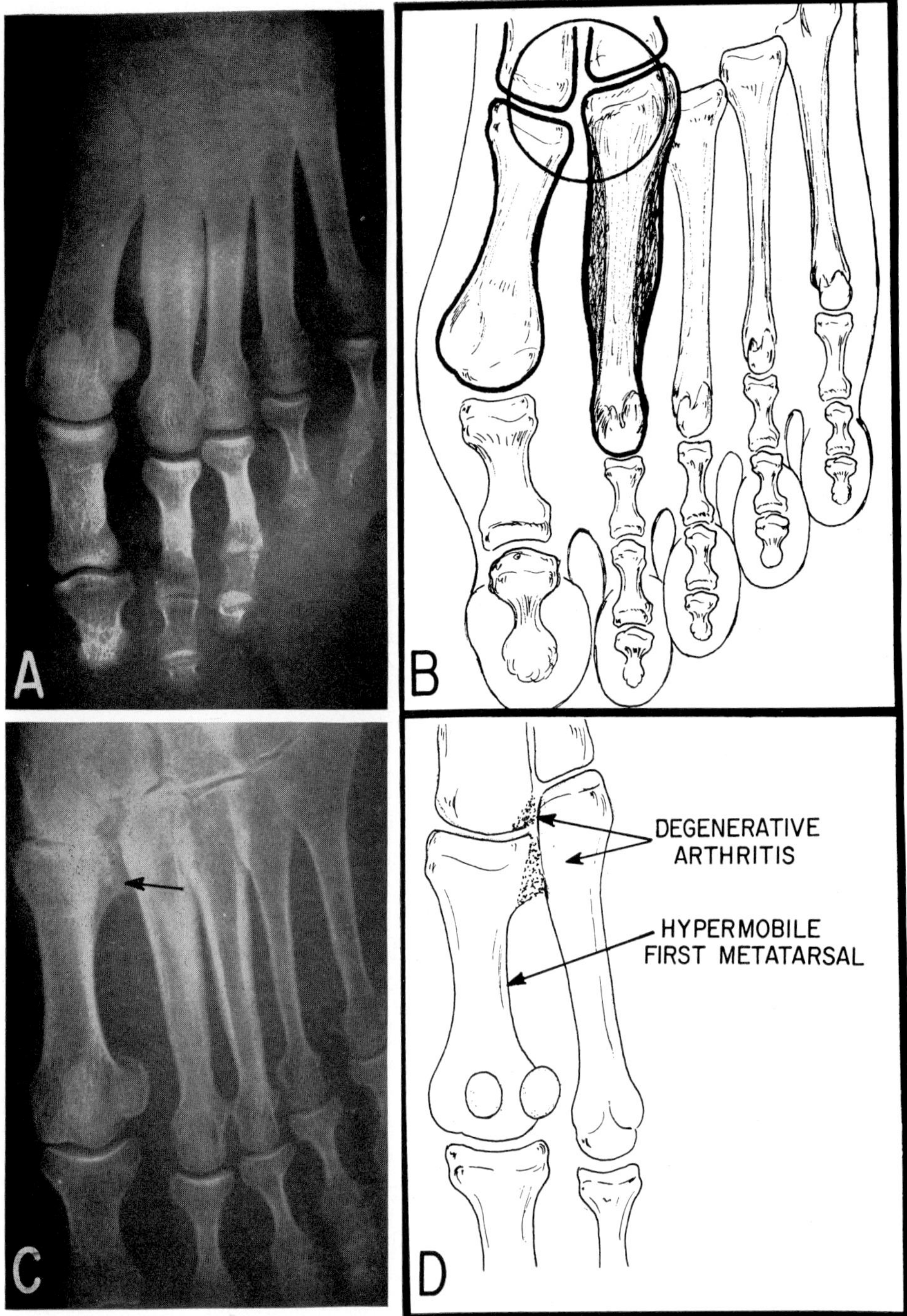

Figure 16–25. Some of the manifestations of D. J. Morton's syndrome. *A,* Roentgenograph showing the "short" first metatarsal with thin medial and thick lateral cortex and thickening of shaft of the second metatarsal. *B,* Interpretative diagram with a circle around where Morton said tenderness was located. *C,* Roentgenograph showing the late effect of hypermobile first metatarsal. *D,* Interpretative diagram.

tarsal bone equalling in length the longest metatarsal segment, it is *always the shortest* member of the series."

In his book *The Human Foot,* Morton (1935) had written: "One of the requirements for ideal foot function is an equidistance of the head of the first and second metatarsal bones from the heel." Wood Jones (1949) wrote: "It is difficult to know why the human foot should be selected as an organ that is assumed to have an ideal or perfect form differing from that which the anatomist finds to be normal in the vast majority of mankind. If we substitute "normal" for "ideal" in the above sentence, we must conclude that the bulk of humanity is condemned by the normal disposition of bones of the foot to show some departure from normal functioning of the foot. The only alternative is to assume that there is such a thing as ideal foot function and that this function could presumably be carried out by the ideal but not by the normal foot" (Fig. 16–26).

D. J. Morton gave no indication of having read the above criticism. One, however, senses a condescending note in

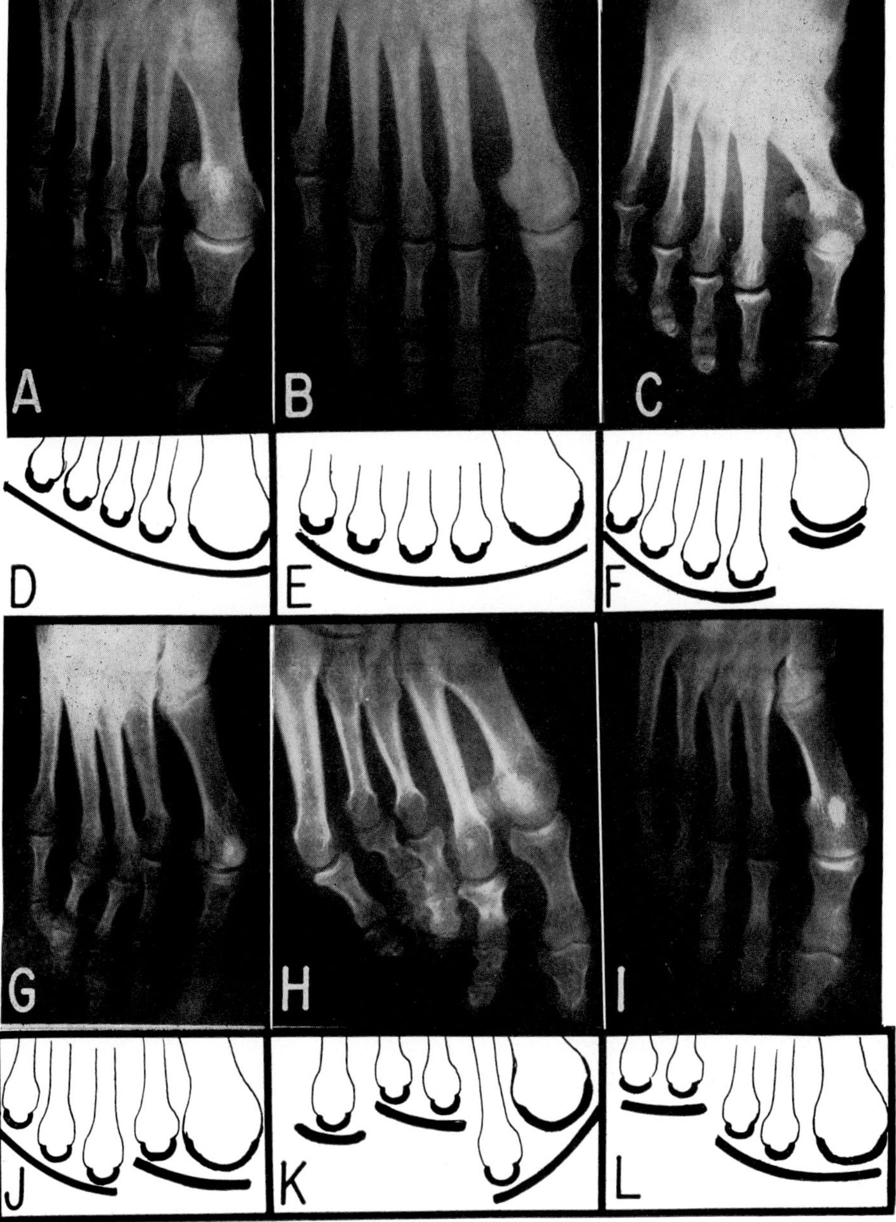

Figure 16–26. Asymptomatic variations of "the metatarsal formula." *A* and *D,* First metatarsal head slightly ahead of the second. *B* and *E,* Considered normal. *C* and *F,* Short first metatarsal. *G* and *J,* Short second metatarsal. *H* and *K,* Short third and fourth metatarsals. *I* and *L,* Short fourth and fifth metatarsals.

his later writings—and some confusion. "Of the two structural factors identified," Morton (1952) wrote, referring to the brevity and hypermobility of the first metatarsal, "a short first metatarsal invites primary consideration because it can readily be described as a definite morphological feature. . . . A spasmodic pain which characterizes the condition known as Morton's Metatarsalgia appears to have frequent origin from this source. Its cause has always been obscure. The typical location of the pain in the fourth, third, or second toes (in order of frequency) conforms with the distribution of the medial plantar nerve. This nerve lies in close proximity to the basal joints of Metatarsal II, which are subject to overloading strain. The consistent response of this condition to conservative treatment by improved weight distribution and general care, indicates its traumatic and chronic inflammatory nature. This spasmodic type of metatarsalgia may occur in either male or female feet; also it can quite frequently be identified in connection with disordered weight distribution caused by hypermobile first metatarsal segment." Morton did not mention neurectomy and gave the date of T. G. Morton's classic publication as 1875, which is not exactly correct.

Reading D. J. Morton's numerous articles and two books, one gets the impression that he definitely lacked surgical—not to say clinical—experience. His contribution must be assessed on the basis of his study of weight distribution in the forefoot and his justifiable crusade against the concept of the anterior transverse or anterior metatarsal arch. He also deserves credit for having stressed the importance of hypermobile first metatarsal segment. It is now generally agreed that metatarsus primus varus is conducive to hallux valgus and associated metatarsalgia. Oblique setting of the innermost cuneometatarsal joint as the basis of metatarsus primus varus has been sufficiently emphasized. But hypermobility of this joint as a cause of metatarsus primus varus and hence hallux valgus has not been sufficiently stressed by clinicians. The so-called "overbone," often shaved from the dorsal aspect of the medial cuneiform bone, is nothing more than proliferative response to articular erosion inside the joint caused by hypermobile first metatarsal. In time the resected "overbone" and the pain in the cuneometatarsal junction will recur. A more rational procedure is to stabilize this joint by arthrodesis. We also fuse the medial with the middle cuneiform and the first metatarsal with the second.

FREIBERG'S INFRACTION

Another form of metatarsalgia was described by Freiberg (1914). The pain was confined to the area under the second metatarsal head and it was not paroxysmal. Freiberg said these features differentiated the condition he spoke about from Morton's metatarsalgia, which was related to the fourth metatarsophalangeal joint and appeared in acute attacks. Freiberg also distinguished the pain he described from metatarsalgia due to *static incompetence of the foot* in that unlike metatarsalgia it was neither diffuse nor bilateral. On the x-ray films of the feet of six women with the type of metatarsalgia that Freiberg reported, the second metatarsal head showed a "crushed in" appearance. The shadow cast by the articular cortex of the head was not curved but flat, and there was some evidence of osteocartilaginous loose bodies.

The name and the question of priority of description. Freiberg (1914) named the condition he described as *infraction* of the second metatarsal head. Skillern (1915) called it *eggshell fracture.* In the continental literature the condition is called Koehler's No. 2 disease to distinguish it from Koehler's No. 1 disease of the tarsal navicular. Panner (1921–1922) studied this condition in some detail and many authors have connected his name with it. Lewin (1923) scrutinized the following titles: *metatarsal epiphysitis, metatarsal "Flathead"* and *osteochondritis deformans metatarsojuvenalis.* He finally concocted the ensuing: *juvenile metatarsophalangeal* *osteochondritis.* Bragard (1924) invented the term *malakopathy,* which Moutier (1925) considered an objectionable neologism. Moutier chose *metatarsal epiphysitis.* Mouchet (1929) also preferred the last term. Doub (1945) considered this disease under the general heading of *aseptic necrosis* and there are those who use the adjective *avascular* instead.

A recurrent controversy has been waged as to who—Freiberg or Koehler—described this condition first and therefore deserves to have his name attached to it. Lewin (1923), Moutier (1925), Mouchet (1929), and many others have presented documentary evidence to prove Freiberg's priority. Mouchet minced no words: ". . . it is not just," he protested, "to attribute the paternity of this disease to Koehler since it was first described by A. H. Freiberg . . . in 1914, six years before Koehler." Freiberg (1926) himself wrote: "The matters of priority of publication and of the attachment of an eponymic title to the condition seem to me of little importance."

Koehler did not seem to have felt the same way. "The second metatarsophalangeal joint," Koehler (1923) wrote, "is subject to a peculiar disease, to which I called attention in 1915 in the second edition of my book. . . . I described my cases more minutely in 1920. . . . Meanwhile a number of contributions have appeared. . . ." Koehler avoided any reference to Freiberg, whose name was mentioned by the editors of the *American Journal of Radiology and Radium Therapy,* in which Koehler's article appeared. Those who edited and translated the posthumous edition of his book into English appeared determined to perpetuate the myth of his priority. In the tenth edition of Koehler's (1956) book we read: "The affection of the metatarsal head which Koehler first described in the second edition of this book and described in great detail . . . in 1920. . . . For demonstration of Koehler's disease involving the second metatarsal, we reproduce Koehler's original roentgenograms as having historic value. . . ."

The last remark was undoubtedly aimed at those who may have nursed misgivings about Koehler's priority. The editors of the book committed a tactical error in mentioning Freiberg. "In English literature," they wrote, "the affection is also known as Freiberg's disease" (p. 208). In the reference after this number, 1914 was given as the date of publication of Freiberg's article. The apparent discrepancy between the text and the bibliography thus betrayed their unwilling admission of Freiberg's priority: 1914 comes before 1915, when Koehler vaguely referred to this condition. In 1914, Freiberg gave as comprehensive a description of this condition as has appeared since.

The seat and the nature of structural change. Another controversy pertains to the question of whether the disease primarily involves the head or the adjacent shaft of the metatarsal bone. According to Panner (1921–1922), Koehler thought that the diaphysial thickening was primary and the changes in the head were secondary. Panner placed the primary seat of the disease within the head or the epiphysis; he considered this condition analogous to Perthes' disease of the hip, Koehler's of tarsal navicular, Osgood-Schlatter's of the tibial tubercle, and Scheuermann's of the spine. "The diaphysis is never changed at the beginning of the disease," Panner wrote. He regarded periosteal stratification of the shaft as of late occurrence. Braddock (1959) also considered the thickening of the metatarsal shaft a later development; he ascribed it to the stress resulting from loss of motion of the involved metatarsophalangeal joint.

It is now generally agreed that Freiberg's infraction is a disease of the growing epiphysis, affecting most commonly—though not exclusively—the growth center of the second metatarsal bone. Campbell (1917) recorded involvement of the first metatarsal head, which of course is not an epiphysis. Moutier (1925) spoke of the other metatarsals being similarly affected as the second is. Koehler (1923) noted the occurrence of a bilateral lesion. Wagner (1930) reported "isolated aseptic necrosis of the ephiphysis of the first metatarsal bone." Burman (1933) wrote an article entitled "Epiphysitis of the Proximal or Pseudometatarsal Epiphyses of the foot" (Fig. 16–27).

Causal relations. Because the six cases Freiberg (1914) originally reported and three that he himself added had all been females, Willis Campbell (1917) categorically stated, "No case had been observed in males," the implication being that this disease affected women exclusively. It was not long after when Painter (1921) reported two cases occurring in males and the subject of Freiberg's (1926) second paper was a boy, aged 13. Numerous cases occurring in men have since been reported, though the condition is still considered prevalent in women. Smillie (1955) reviewed 41 cases—31 females and 10 males.

One often sees patients who place the inception of their discomfort at a period well past the time of epiphysial closure. Skillern's (1915) patient was a woman around 40 years old who reported having recently "stubbed" the second toe of her right foot against the floor. There was definite swelling over the head of the second metatarsal bone, and examination revealed "wincing" tenderness. The lateral view "skiagram" clearly showed "an oblique indentation" that resembled "that of the proverbial egg of Columbus. . . ." Skillern called the condition "eggshell" fracture of the second metatarsal bone, leaving no doubt as to its cause and acute inception. One of Painter's (1921) cases was a woman 60 years of age who had been free of discomfort until she injured her second toe 4 years previously—at 56 years of age. Van Demark and McCarthy (1946) reported a case of what they preferred to call Panner's disease, which presumably had its start in adulthood. They wrote: "The occurrence of aseptic necrosis in the adult metatarsal head is less frequent than in the juvenile case, and it is not so generally recognized. Gaitskell reported one case in which roentgenographic changes first occurred in adult life; the same is true in the present case."

Another question revolves about the causal connection of trauma to this disease. The first patient Freiberg reported had "stubbed" her toe while playing tennis. The second and the third patients also admitted having received "the injury" in the course of a tennis game. Two patients out of six could recall no injury; in two women Freiberg found "evidence of static incompetence of the feet," but he had "no reason to believe this stood in any particular relationship to the condition. "Under normal circumstances," Freiberg wrote, "the second metatarsal bone is slightly longer than the first. In the presence of a diminished power of toe flexion and especially of the great toe, it is apparent that the forcible impact of the ball of the foot against the ground not sufficiently guarded by the flexor power of the toes will cause the distal end of the second metatarsal to bear the brunt of the blow."

Skillern's (1915) patient "stubbed the second toe of her right foot against the floor." One of Campbell's (1917) cases also "stubbed" her foot, and the other injured it while playing basketball. Painter's (1921) second case—a boy of thirteen—"stumbled while running bases and had sudden sharp pain at the base of the second toe." Another—a woman of 60 years—"has been conscious of more or less discomfort, amounting at times to pain ever since she stubbed this toe three or four years ago." In these earlier reports one is struck by the recurrence of the word "stubbed," which Freiberg first used. One wonders if, in the course of questioning the patients, the word was not inculcated into them. It is also possible that the men who followed Freiberg in describing what at the time was a novel disease emulated his style. Kappis (1923) thought violent trauma was a cause. Schroeder (1923) considered intermittent injury over a period as an etiologic factor. Koehler (1923) did not think acute trauma was a cause but conceded that barely perceptible, frequently repeated strains and mechanical insults may have a cumulative effect in bringing about the osteochondritis.

Freiberg (1926) entitled his second article "The So-called Infraction of the Second Metatarsal Bone." The implication was clear; he was not as sure of the traumatic origin of this disease as before,

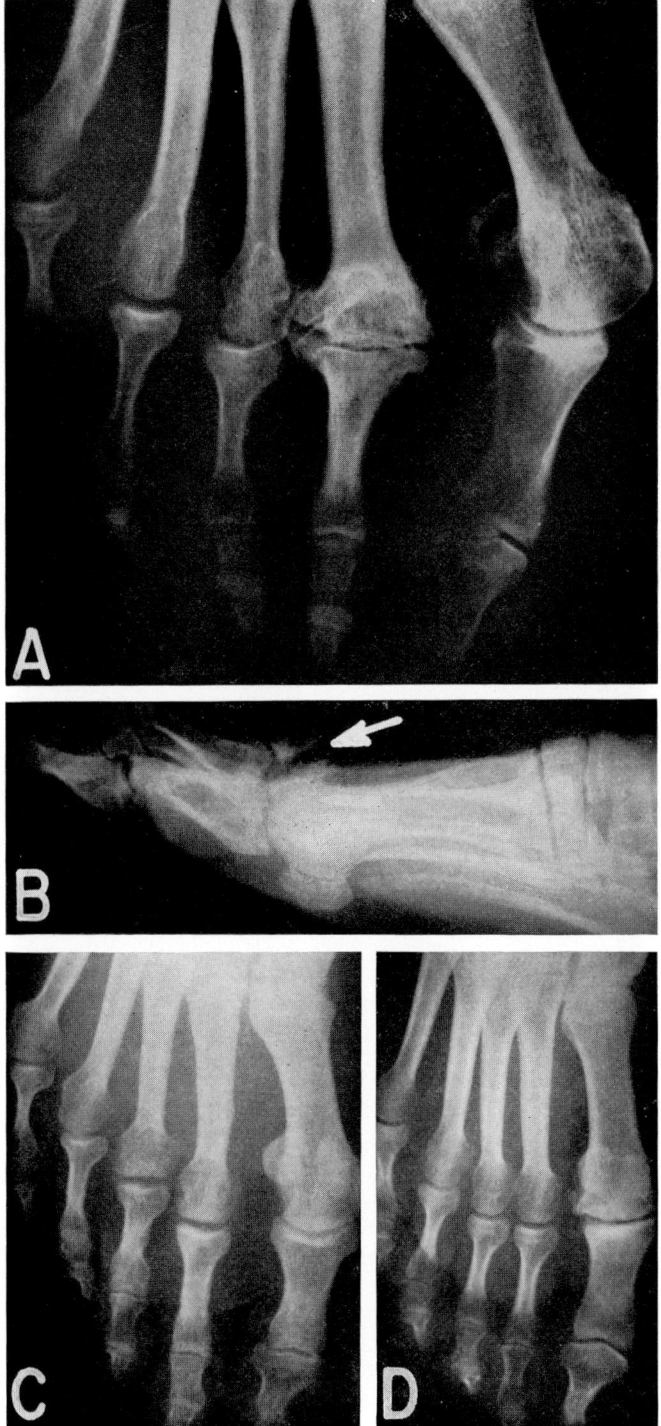

Figure 16–27. Localization of Freiberg's infraction. *A,* The most common location. *B,* Lateral view Note the detached piece of bone (arrow). *C,* Flat second and third metatarsal heads. *D,* Flat and arthritic first metatarsal head, which is not considered true Freiberg's infraction because it does not involve an epiphysis.

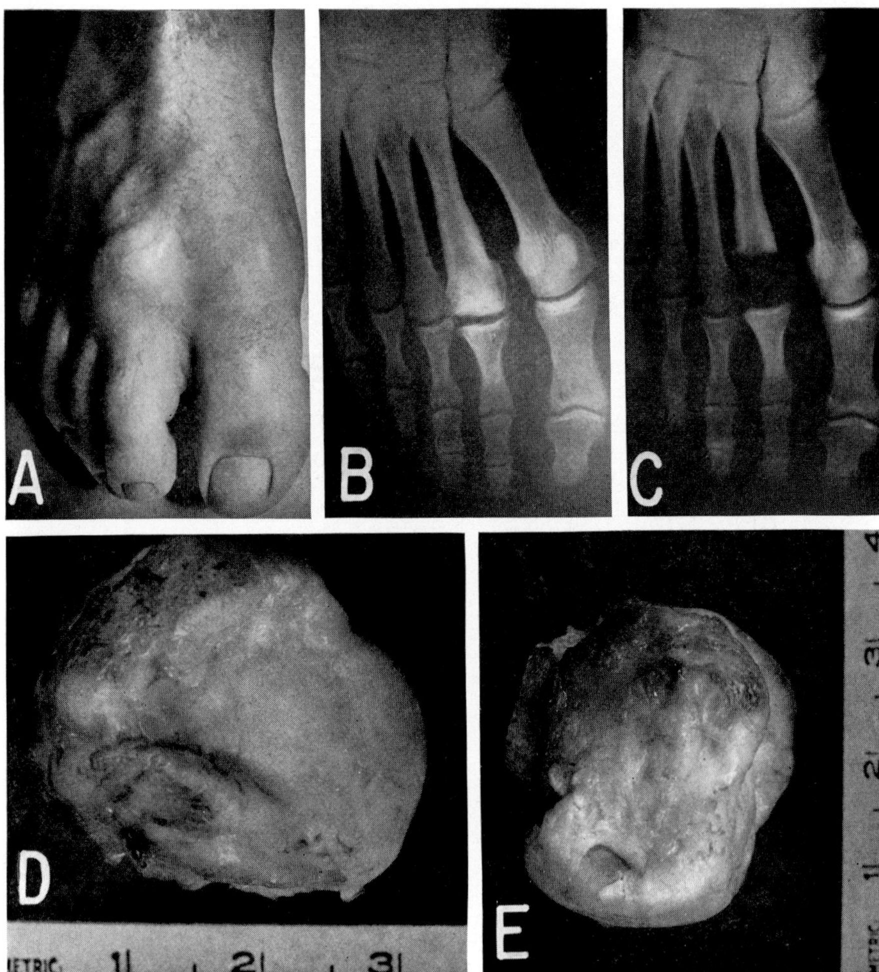

Figure 16–28. Man, about 23, soldier, swelling and pain in the forefoot. Duration: 2 years; diagnosis: Freiberg's infraction of the second metatarsal bone. Surgery: resection of the distal third of the second metatarsal and surgical syndactylia of the second and third toes. *A,* Dorsal view before surgery. *B,* Preoperative roentgenogram. Note the thickened shaft proximal to the flattened head. *C,* Roentgenogram after recovery. *D,* Resected head, seen from the front. *E,* Resected head seen from the side. Pain and swelling were relieved.

even though the patient he discussed "ascribed the condition to an injury sustained at play" about 9 months earlier. On the x-ray film, besides flattening of the metatarsal head, Freiberg now discerned definite evidences of the type of diaphysial thickening. "The interpretation of these changes in the second metatarsal, occurring within a period of eight months," Freiberg wrote, "is a difficult matter without more evidence than is at command. . . . I am ready to acknowledge that simple trauma is not a satisfying explanation of the clinical and roentgenographic phenomena. . . ."

Zeitlin (1935) linked Freiberg's infraction with stress fracture of the metatarsal bone, which he respectively called Koehler's No. 2 disease and Deutschlaender's disease. For a common etiologic factor he evoked Dudley J. Morton's syndrome and thought that the overloading of structurally inadequate feet played a very important role in both these conditions. "The difference in localization of the two conditions," Zeitlin wrote, "may be explained to a certain extent by the age of the patient. An alteration in the head is due to the fact that it develops earlier than in a diaphysis. . . . In young subjects it is the head of the metatarsal (Koehler's disease) which is most involved, while at a more advanced age the involvement is in the diaphysis (Deutschlaender's disease). The two processes are accompanied by thickening of the diaphysis."

Speaking of Freiberg's infraction Smillie (1955) is reported as having maintained that the condition "occurred in structurally weak feet with short, varus or hypermobile first metatarsals . . .

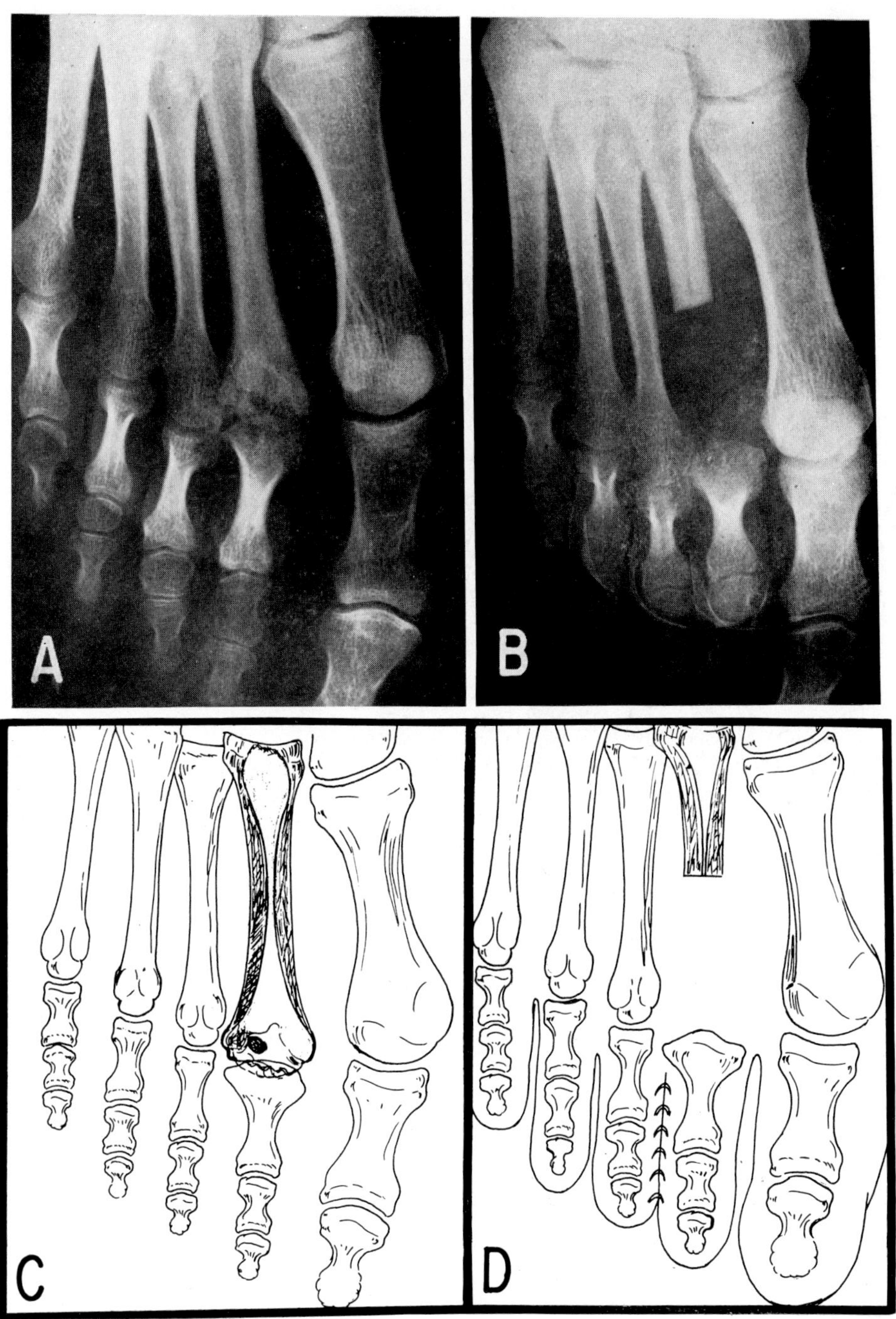

Figure 16–29. Man, 24 years of age, civilian, with pain and swelling at the bottom of the second toe. Duration of symptoms: 6 months; diagnosis: Freiberg's infraction of the second metatarsal. Surgery: resection of distal two-thirds of the second metatarsal and surgical syndactylia of second and third toes. *A* and *B*, Pre- and postoperative roentgenograms. *C* and *D*, Interpretative diagrams. Relief of pain and swelling resulted.

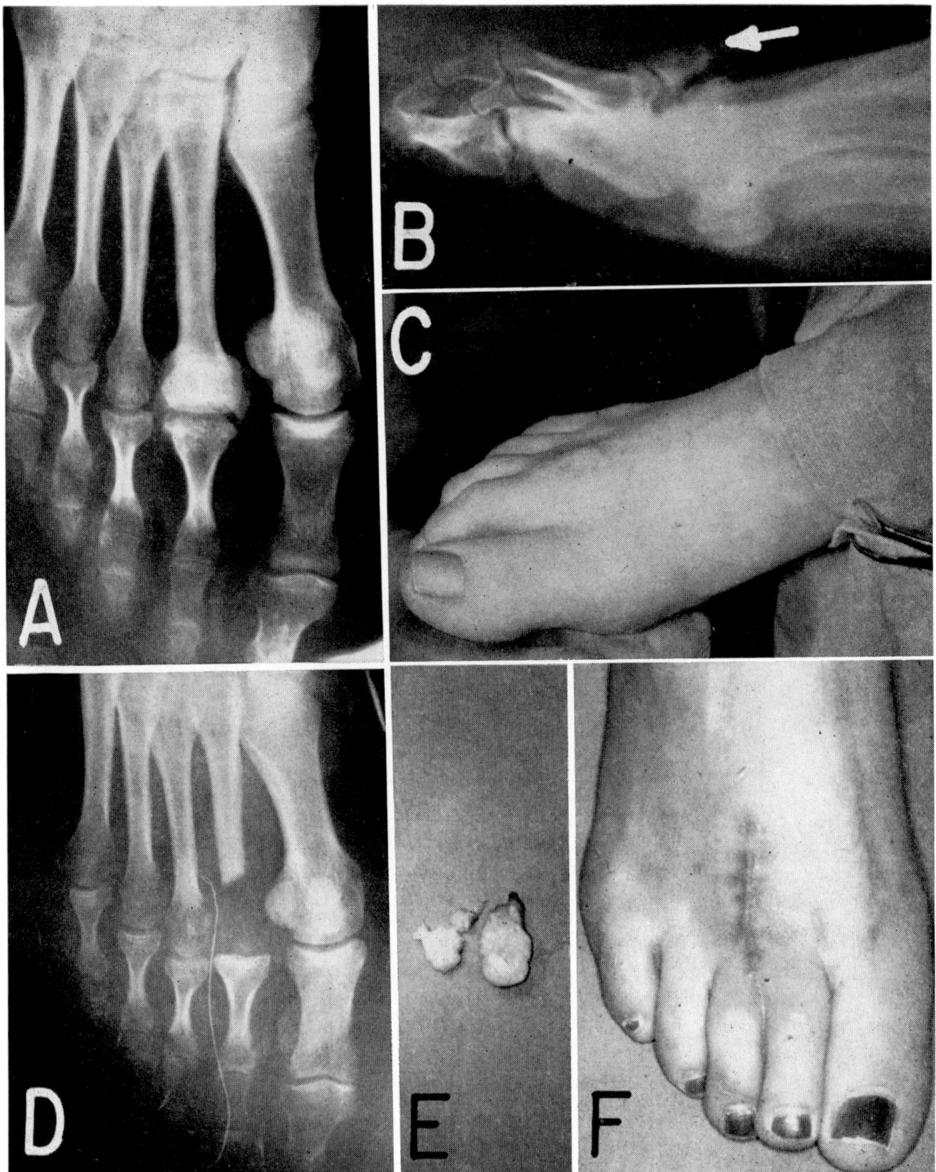

Figure 16–30. Woman, 21 years of age, with swelling at the base of the second toe and pain under the ball of the forefoot. Diagnosis: Freiberg's infraction of the second metatarsal bone. Surgery: resection of the distal third of second metatarsal and surgical syndactylia of the second and third toes. *A,* Dorsoplantar view roentgenogram before surgery. *B,* Preoperative side view roentgenogram. Note the detached osteophyte. *C,* Preoperative side view. *D,* Postoperative dorsoplantar view roentgenogram. *E,* Loose bodies seen in *B*. *F,* Postrecovery dorsal view. Swelling and metatarsalgia vanished.

and therefore, had the same etiology as march fracture." According to Braddock (1959), Smillie "favored the traumatic view, postulating stress rather than single injury." Braddock experimentally "attempted to assess the strength of the second metatarsal and proximal phalanx at varying ages" by subjecting these bones to pressure. As a result of his investigation, he concluded that the second metatarsal epiphysis was vulnerable and that Freiberg's infraction . . . was a fracture, somewhat modified by its proximity to the epiphyseal plate and articular cartilage."

Basic pathology. Not much is written about the primary disturbance that leads to the crumbling and collapse of the metatarsal head. Axhausen (1922) examined some specimens and found focal necrosis in the head and at times fibrous dysplasia of the bone marrow. He suggested embolic obstruction of the epiphysial end arteries by mildly virulent bacteria as the cause of necrosis. It is now known that infection has nothing to do with this condition but the concept of arterial insufficiency has been retained. The lesion is considered akin to aseptic or avascular necrosis of other bones.

The management. It is generally agreed that in adolescents the treatment of this condition should be conservative: immobilization with the aid of a walking cast during the acutely painful phase to be followed by a low-heeled shoe provided with a metatarsal pad or transverse bar. When there were loose bodies, Freiberg (1914) resorted to arthrotomy and removed the "corpora libra." Campbell (1917) resected the metatarsal head; Painter (1921) curetted it. In advanced cases with mushrooming of the metatarsal head and arthritic spurs on the opposed articular end of the proximal phalanx, Brandes and Ruschenburg (1939) advised remodeling both bones. DuVries (1959) excised "all the excess bone" and rounded "the head with a rasp." We find it more expeditious to simply resect the head with a portion of the adjacent shaft; the corresponding toe is surgically syndactlyized with its sturdy neighbor (Figs. 16–28 to 16–31).

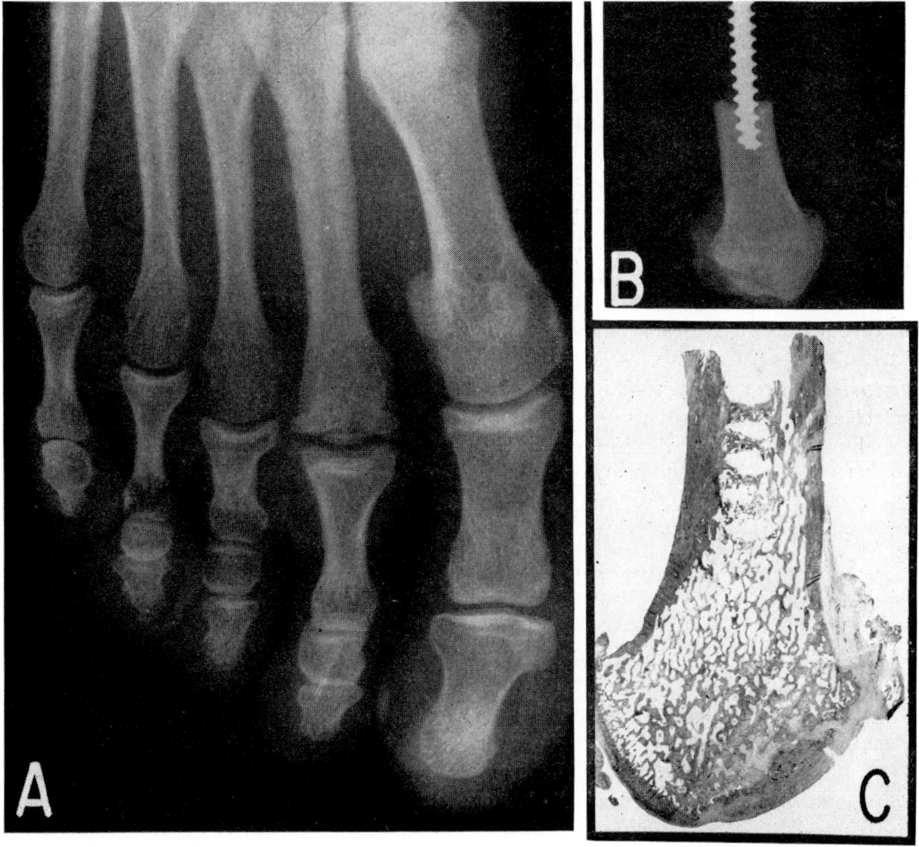

Figure 16–31. Woman, 18 years of age, with pain under the second metatarsal head. Surgery: resection of distal third of the metatarsal and surgical syndactylia of second and third toes. *A,* Preoperative roentgenogram. *B,* Roentgenogram of resected specimen. *C,* Sagittal section (× 21) of the resected bone showing focal necrosis under the articular surface of the second metatarsal head. The patient was relieved of metatarsalgia.

STRESS FRACTURE OF THE METATARSALS

Fractures of the bones of forefoot that can definitely be related to sudden violent injuries fall outside the domain of this study. Fracture of the metatarsal bones that passes unnoticed, until insidiously developing pain of the forefoot invites attention, cannot be left out of any discussion dealing with various causes of metatarsalgia. Meyerding and Pollock (1938) have rightly suggested that this last type of fracture should be considered as a possible diagnosis in every case of painful feet in which a complaint is made following unaccustomed and excessive exercise.

Synonyms. Metatarsalgia that appears after strenuous walks and is accompanied by fracture of one of the metatarsal bones has acquired numerous synonyms: Fussgeschwulst, Marchgeswulst, inderekten Metatarsalfraktur, Mittelfussgeswulst, morbus Deutschlaender and Marschfraktur—in German literature; pied forcé, pied de marche, l'enflure du pied, pied surchargé and fracture de recrue—in French; march foot, marching foot, marching fracture, crack fractures, insufficiency fracture, pseudofracture, march fracture and stress fracture—in English.

Historical perspective. The history of march or stress fractures of metatarsal bones has been well documented by Straus (1932), Dodd (1933), Speed and Blake (1933), Maseritz (1936), Edward (1936), and Meyerding and Pollock (1938). All that needs to be said here is that Breithaupt (1855) reported a number of cases of persistent pain and puffiness of the feet in soldiers following long hikes. He conjectured inflammation of the tendon sheath. Similar cases were reported: Weisbach (1877), Pauzat (1887), Poulet (1888), Martin (1891), and Busquet (1897). In the absence of roentgenography, they surmised sundry lesions: ligamentous injury, periostitis, rheumatism, synovitis, arthritis, and others. With the aid of roentgenograms, Stechow (1897) was able to demonstrate fracture of the metatarsal bones in the cases he studied. Schulte (1897), Thiele (1899), Boisson and Chapotot (1899), Loison (1900), Meiser (1901), Momburg (1904), Blecher (1902), and Kirchner (1905) confirmed Stechow's findings. Kirchner stated that this type of fracture also occurred in civilians. These earlier reports were either in German or French.

The first account of this condition to appear in English was an editorial in the New York Medical Journal (1899). It was a review of what German and French authors had said. Pirie (1917) was perhaps the first to report several cases in English. Trethowan (1921) wrote: "An interesting fracture is that of the middle shaft of the second and third metatarsal bones which may be due to trivial accident to the foot in ordinary walking, as for example, in soldiers on the march. No displacement occurs, and the patient may be unaware of its existence; a little pain and tenderness, and puffiness on the dorsum of the foot are all the symptoms, and an unsuspected fracture is revealed by the routine skiagraphic examination." Goldman (1928) credited this quotation to Sir Robert Jones. Dodd (1933), and Sloane and Sloane (1936) also ascribed this reference to Sir Robert Jones, who merely edited the volume in which Trethowan's comment appeared. Fame has a curious way of appropriating what belongs to others. Sir Robert Jones has been credited with many ideas first formulated by less famous men.

Etiology. The predisposing factors in stress fracture have become the subject of controversy. Pauzat (1887) considered the dorsal fold of the soldier's shoe a cause of what he thought to be inflammatory periostitis. Deutschlaender (1921) suggested hematogenous infection causing pariostitis. Jansen (1926) ascribed the lesion to the overfatigue of a preexisting weak foot. According to him excessive stress caused spasm of the interossei, which pulled the periosteum of the metatarsal shaft; subperiosteal hematoma formed and this in turn caused the bone to become brittle and break. Speed and Blake (1933) regarded pre-existing deformity as a factor. All their patients gave "history of foot ailments, the usual being bunions, calluses under metatarsal heads, and rigidity of tarsal and tarsometatarsal joints." Dodd (1933) evoked D. J. Morton's syndrome and considered march fracture "probably autotraumatic complication of subacute flat-foot in an architecturally weak foot rather than a separate entity." This view was also favored by Zeitlin and Odessky (1934), Zeitlin (1935), Bruce (1937), Meyerding and Pollock (1938), Flavell (1943), and many others. It is supposed that a short or hypermobile first metatarsal fails to sustain its share of stress and its weaker neighbor—the second metatarsal—bears the brunt of the overload. Bernstein and Stone (1944) found "no usual or unusual deformities of the foot"; the condition occurred in "soldiers irrespective of age, height, weight and general body build." They also reported march fracture in Negro soldiers but these were comparatively few. Bernstein and Stone felt that march fracture was due to "bone stress, following complete fatigue and exhaustion of supporting structures of the foot, which include the muscles, ligaments, and fascia."

Meyerding and Pollock (1938) reported stress fracture of the lateral metatarsals following decapitation of the first metatarsal for hallux valgus. Cleveland and Winant (1950) recorded the same complication after Keller's resection. We have had a similar experience with one of our cases of Keller's resection. We have also seen stress fracture of the metatarsal following triple arthrodesis for pes planus, and in connection with an unstable ankle due to Charcot's arthropathy (Fig. 16–32).

Undoubtedly a structurally weak or physiologically inadequate foot is more prone to fracture. An argument against tying stress fractures to Dudley Morton's syndrome is that in the latter the second metatarsal is said to have become "hypertrophied" and is not likely to fracture easily.

Localization. Almost all authors writing on this subject concede that the second metatarsal bone is involved most commonly; then come the third and less frequently the fourth metatarsals. Kirschner (1905) reported a spontaneous fracture of the fifth metatarsal—one case from 82. Nion (1903) recorded the involvement of the first metatarsal once in 575 stress fractures. Recurrent, bilateral, multiple and associated stress fractures have been recorded by many authors. Monteith (1934) reported an old healed fracture of the second metatarsal and a recent one of the third. Maseritz (1936) spoke of a case in which march fracture of the second metatarsal head and fracture of the fifth metatarsal base were associated with fragmentation of the medial cuneiform bone. In an as yet unpublished paper Kingsley (1964) detailed his experience with 750 march fractures. He came across three cases of multiple fractures involving both feet. The first patient had 7 fractures—4 on the right side and 3 on the left. The second patient had a total of 5 fractures—2 on the right side and 3 on the left. The third patient also had five fractures—two on the right side and 3 on the left. Of the total 17 fractures, the first metatarsal was involved twice; the second and third, each 4 times; the fourth, 5 times; and the fifth, twice. There were 9 complete and 8 incomplete fractures in this series. The base of the metatarsal was involved twice; the midshaft, twice, the distal shaft, 11 times; and the neck twice. In his second communication Kingsley (1964) reported multiple fractures in a single metatarsal.

Diagnosis. It seems incredible to us now that stress fracture of the metatarsal shaft could be mistaken for osteogenic sarcoma. Only three decades ago, within a year of each other, two such cases were reported—one by Straus (1932) and another by Dodd (1933). Both patients were civilian women; one was 36 and the other 51 years of age. The first woman was a cafeteria attendant; the second, an amateur golf player. Each complained of slowly developing pain and swelling of the foot and gave no history of sudden injury. The affected foot was edematous on the dorsum and tender over the second metatarsal. Fracture was not detected on x-ray films—in fact, not until biopsy material was

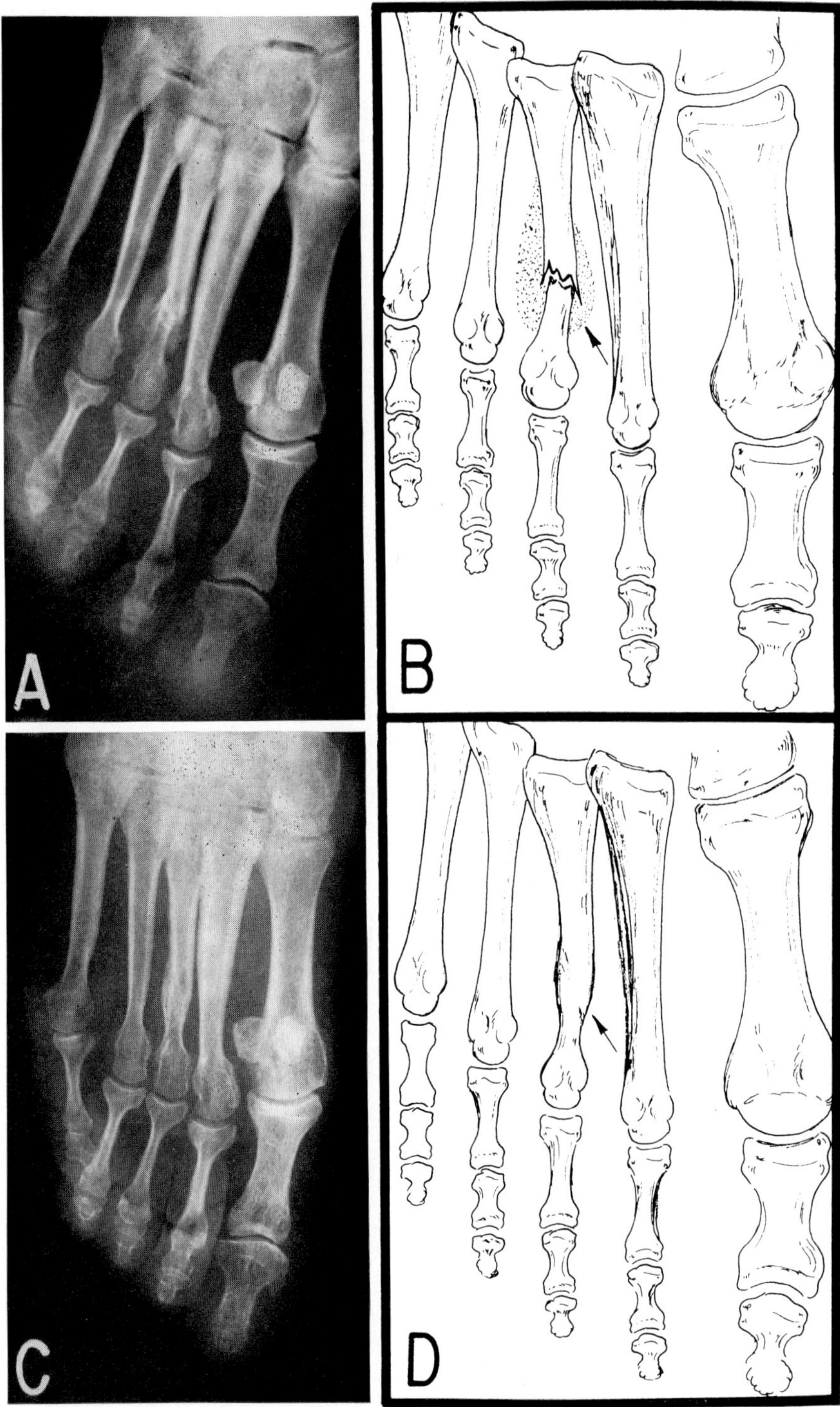

Figure 16–32. Woman, 44 years of age, with stress fracture of the third metatarsal following triple arthrodesis. This occurred 2 months after the cast was removed. *A*, Early callus around the fracture. *B*, Interpretative diagram of *A*. *C*, Shrinkage of the callus after 6 weeks' immobilization in a cast. *D*, Interpretative diagram of *C*.

obtained, in one case by resection of the affected metatarsal bone and in the other by amputation of the forefoot.

The case reported by Straus "had been previously seen by very good surgeons and roentgenologists who had said she was suffering from a sarcoma and had been sent to the hospital to have an amputation of the leg . . . The metatarsal was excised as a means of verifying the diagnosis. . . . Examination of the specimen . . . showed a bulbous enlargement 1.6 centimeters long by 1.7 centimeters wide at the junction of the distal and middle thirds of the shaft. . . . Microscopic sections through the new bone growth showed it to be well developed and partially calcified osteoid tissue. . . . The lesion was diagnosed as a fracture of the shaft of the bone due to lack of immobilization of the fragments."

Dodd's case was independently examined by two roentgenologists. One wrote: "The distal end of the shaft of the second metatarsal shows periosteal reaction perpendicular to the shaft; there is some localized rarefaction. The appearances lend suspicion to a new growth (sarcoma)." The second roentgenologist gave the following report: "My opinion is that she had an old ununited fracture and is now developing a periosteal sarcoma over the old callus which obscures the ordinary diagnostic appearances of new growth. I must admit that there is only a shred of evidence for this." A month later another radiograph was taken and the first radiologist "repeated his opinion of a probable new growth." The patient was subjected to a Lisfranc type of amputation. The specimen revealed a "considerably thickened metatarsal" consisting "of dense greyish-pink bone throughout, with evidence of a slight irregular crack in the shaft but none of localized growth. . . ."

Speed and Blake (1933) conceded that the circumscribed spindle shaped callus surrounding the metatarsal shaft may simulate sarcoma. Meyerding and Pollock (1938) spoke of "a case in which the patient's own physician reasonably enough had made the diagnosis of sarcoma and had advised immediate amputation." We are told that "the question of march fracture arose but the other features were so much in favor of the more serious condition that a preliminary biopsy was decided on and . . . the simpler condition was proved . . . on microscopic examination of tissue." Meyerding and Pollock felt "biopsy should be carried out when any doubt exists as to the true nature of the condition." Sirbu and Palmer (1942) made "the tentative diagnosis . . . of Ewing's sarcoma, based on the periosteal reaction, the 'onion-peel' appearance of the new bone and absence of fracture." Bed rest and elevation were soon followed with recession of swelling and tenderness and finally with complete disappearance of symptoms and consolidation of the callus.

Watson-Jones (1941) wrote: "If sarcoma of the metatarsals was not so rare as to be almost unknown, the periosteal elevation and ossification, and the absence of a history of injury might be confusing." In a later edition of his book Watson-Jones (1957) stated that ". . . nearly five hundred march fractures of the second metatarsal were recorded in one year alone in one country, and sarcoma of this bone has not been reported in thousands of years in any country. . . . " Someone should have reminded Watson-Jones that not long before the appearance of the first edition of his book, at least in one country and within a few years of each other, there were several reports of sarcomas involving the metatarsal bones, including the second. Coley and Higinbotham (1939) of New York included in their tabulation three such cases. Meyerding (1944) of Rochester, Minnesota, resected the second metatarsal in another case, and no less an authority than Broders diagnosed the sections as representing a "periosteal osteogenic sarcoma." Meyerding in his report included two photomicrographs. "I believe," he wrote, "that this is a case of multiple metatarsal (march) fractures of the right foot in which the tissue of the primary lesion of the second metatarsal bone had undergone malignant change."

In both editions of his book Watson-Jones (1941–1957) considered it far more

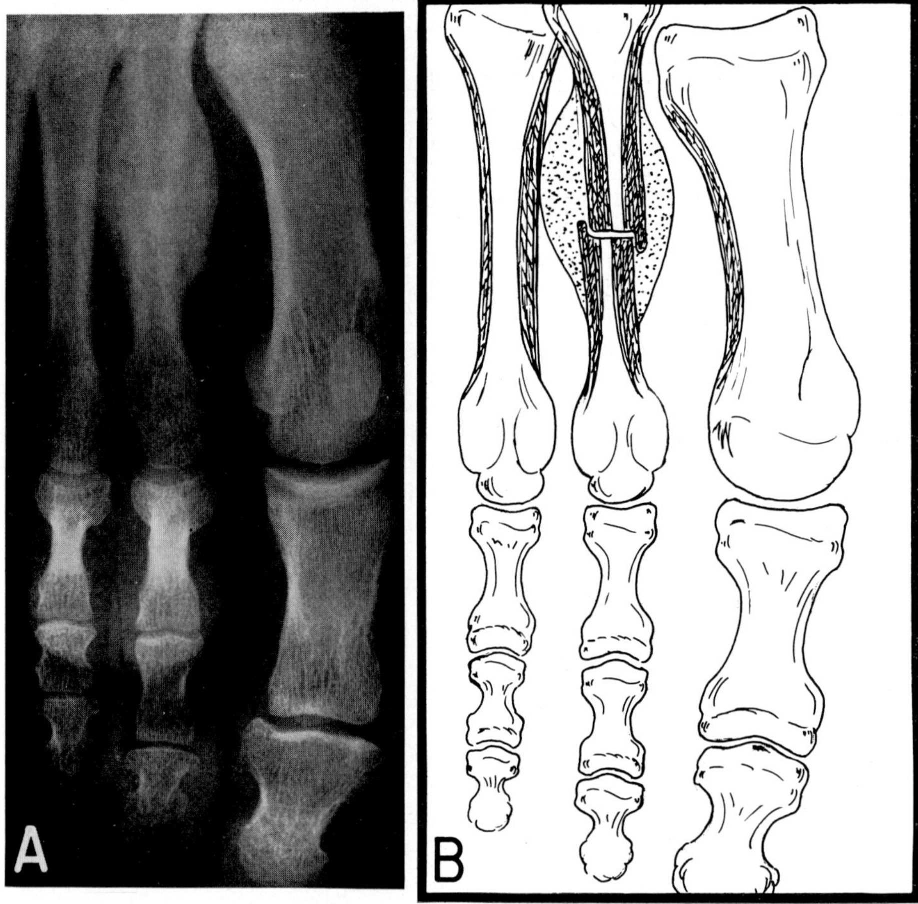

Figure 16–33. Man, 24 years of age, soldier, with pain and swelling of the forefoot after long marches. *A,* Roentgenogram showing the spindle-shaped callus around the fracture line. *B,* Interpretative diagram. He was treated with a cast and metatarsalgia was relieved.

difficult to differentiate stress fracture from "Panner's disease of the second metatarsal—an allied disorder in which there is periosteal thickening of the shaft of the second and sometimes third metatarsals. In this condition," he continued, "there is impairment of the blood supply of the bone and usually avascular necrosis of the metatarsal head causing rigidity of the joint." As we have noted, Panner's disease is another name for Freiberg's infraction with reactive thickening of the shaft behind the metatarsal head. Confusion of Freiberg's infraction with march fracture is not fraught with as serious consequences as mistaking march fracture for sarcoma. In the event of the remotest suspicion about the existence of malignant disease, the following therapeutic test may be put to use: rest and elevation or immobilization that will cause the periosteal thickening in march fracture to diminish in size.

Stress fracture of the metatarsal bones is diagnosed by the insidious development of metatarsalgia with puffiness on the dorsal aspect of the forefoot. Roentgenograms during the first few weeks may not show the fracture line. Soft tissue exposures at this stage may reveal a circumscribed shadow cast by the subperiosteal hematoma. Repeated roentgenograms will in time show the fusiform callus and the line of fracture. It is frequently stated that the fragments in march fracture do not become displaced. This is not true. Oblique view roentgenograms will often reveal angulation of the bone and sometimes definite displacement of fragments (Figs. 16–33 and 16–34).

Treatment. There appears to be a

widespread disinclination to immobilize the limb with a short leg cast as a method of treating stress fracture of the metatarsal bones. Excessive periosteal callus often observed in these cases is due to inadequate immobilization and continued trauma. We have seen refracture through supposedly consolidated callus. Six weeks of immobilization in a short leg cast provided with a heel for walking is the treatment we prefer.

TUMORS OF THE FOREFOOT

With the exception of papillary warts and Morton's neuroma—both of which are classed as neoplasms by some authors—tumors of the forefoot as causes of metatarsalgia are seldom mentioned in the literature. It is even stated that tumors of the foot are comparatively rare. A more accurate statement would be to say that they are rarely reported. This

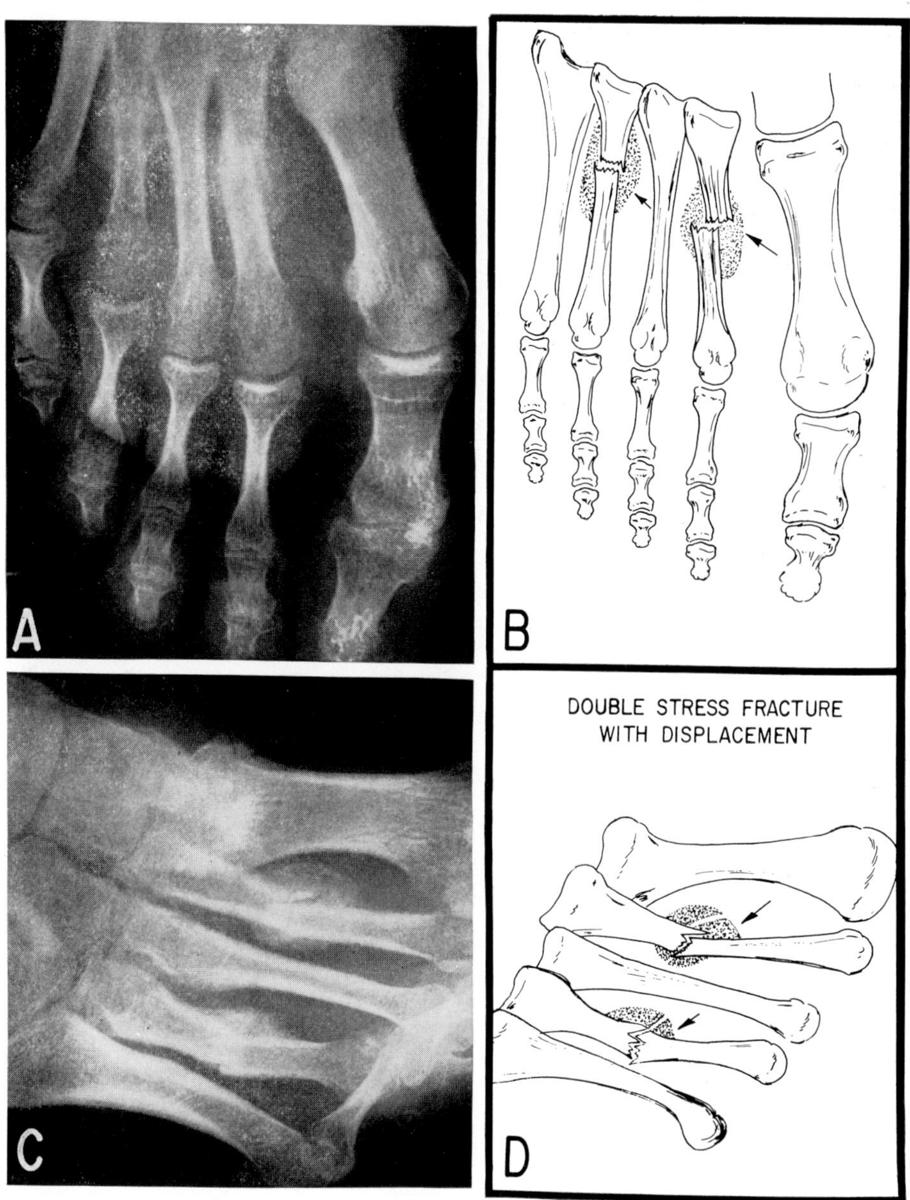

Figure 16–34. Male, 23 years of age, soldier, with pain and swelling of the forefoot after long hikes. Diagnosis: stress fracture of second and fourth metatarsal shafts with refracture through both calluses and displacement of fragments. *A*, Anteroposterior roentgenogram. *B*, Interpretative diagram of *A*. *C*, Oblique view roentgenogram. *D*, Interpretative diagram of *C*. Swelling and pain were relieved.

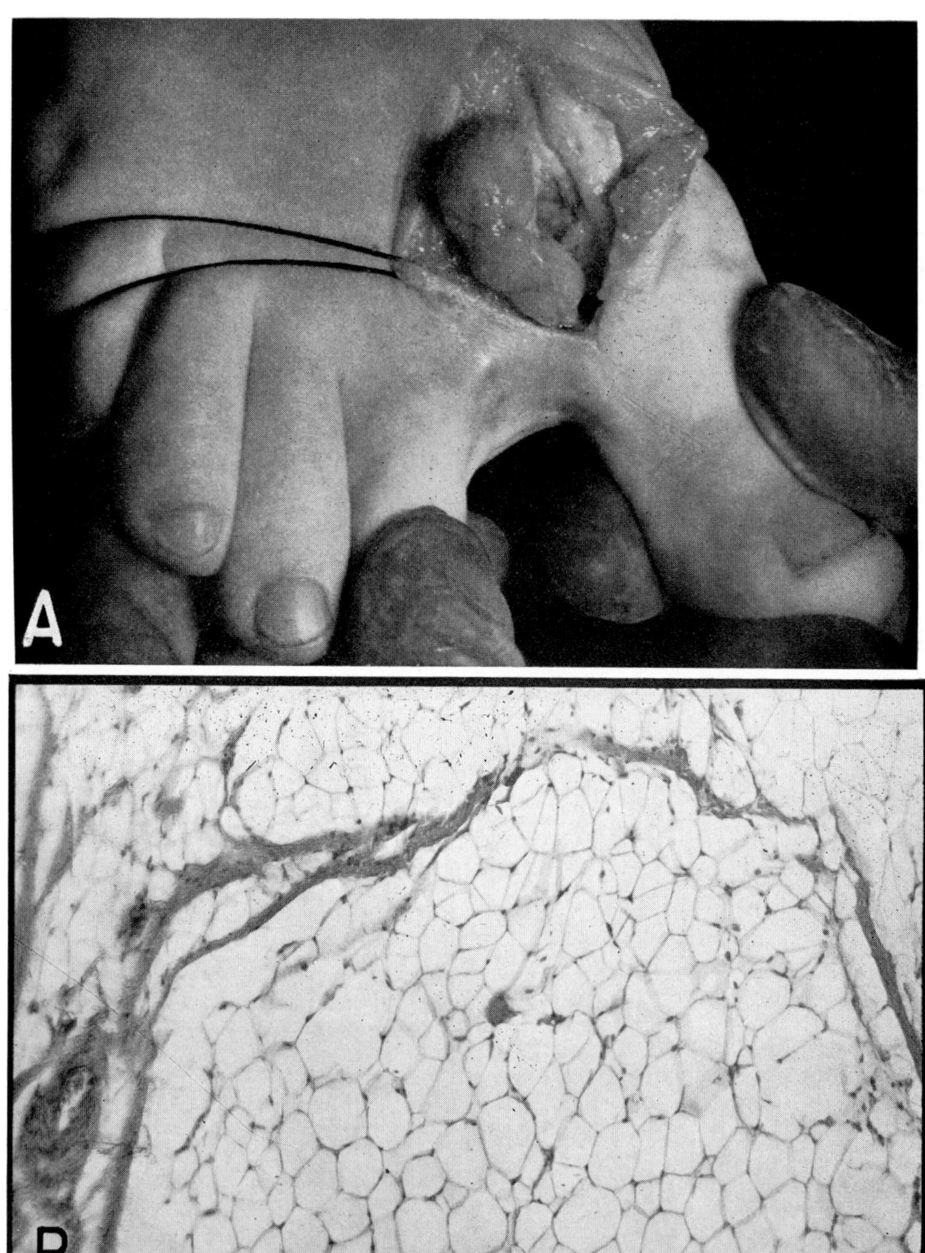

Figure 16–35. Woman, 33 years of age, with interdigital lipoma. *A,* Photograph after exposure. *B,* Photomicrograph (× 100).

is especially true of benign tumors, which hardly ever find their way into the literature (Figs. 16–35 to 16–42).

Too often tumors of the foot are coupled with those of the hand, and they invariably get overshadowed by discussions of the more glamorous member. In not a few articles, neoplasms of the foot are lumped with tumors of both extremities, and the discussion appears to fade out by the time the lowest segment of the lower extremity is reached. One also has to wade through many an article dealing with glomus tumor, hemangioma, carcinoma, or sarcoma in general to ferret out an occasional involvement of the foot, not to say the forefoot. When some of these authors finally mention the foot, they fail to specify exactly which part of it is involved. In the event of involvement of the forefoot, we are told almost nothing about the pain that most tumors cause.

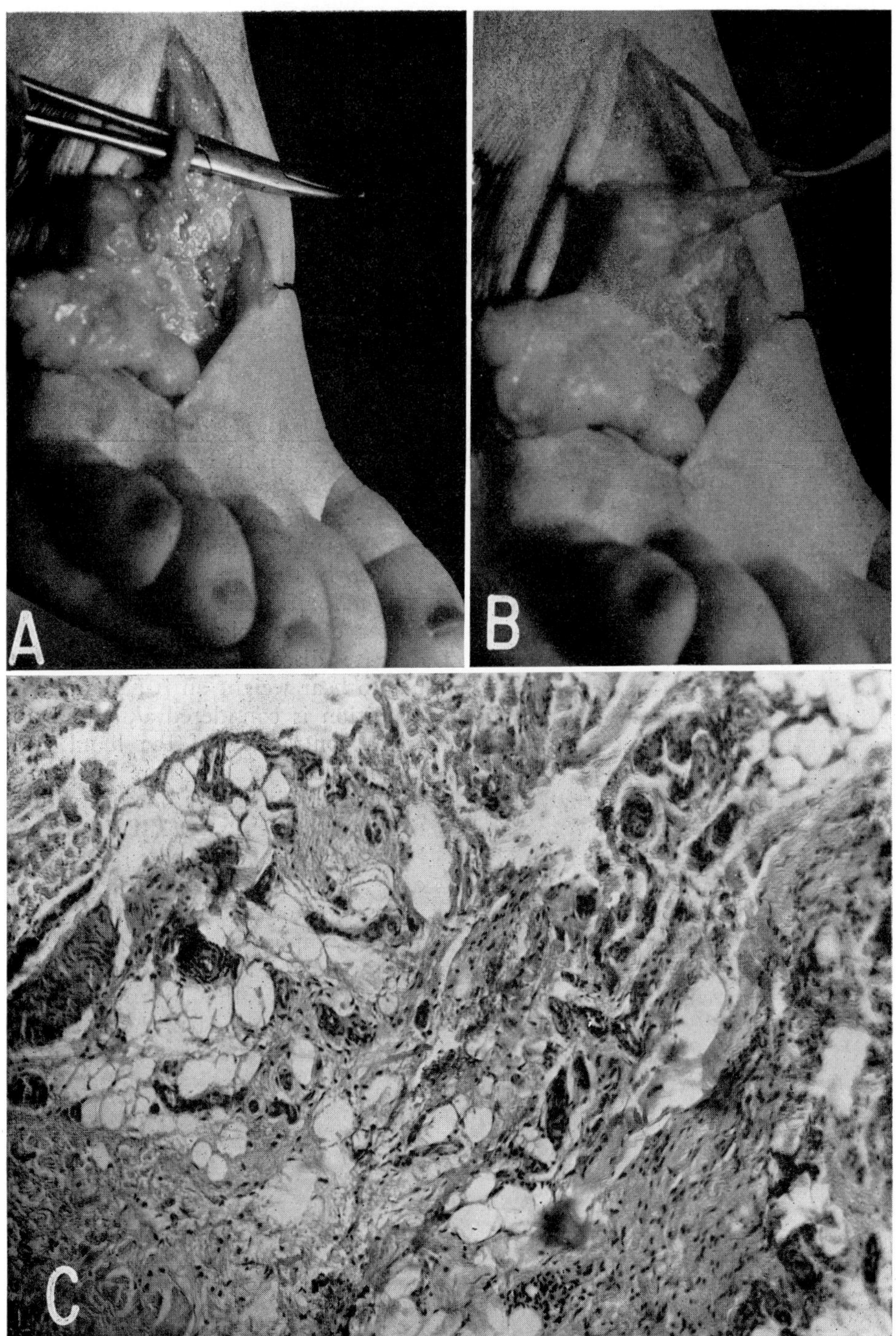

Figure 16–36. Dorsal digital nerve passing through a large tumor consisting of fibroadipose tissue with chronic inflammation. The woman was 42 years of age and obese. *A* and *B,* Photographs after surgical exposure. *C,* Photomicrograph (× 130).

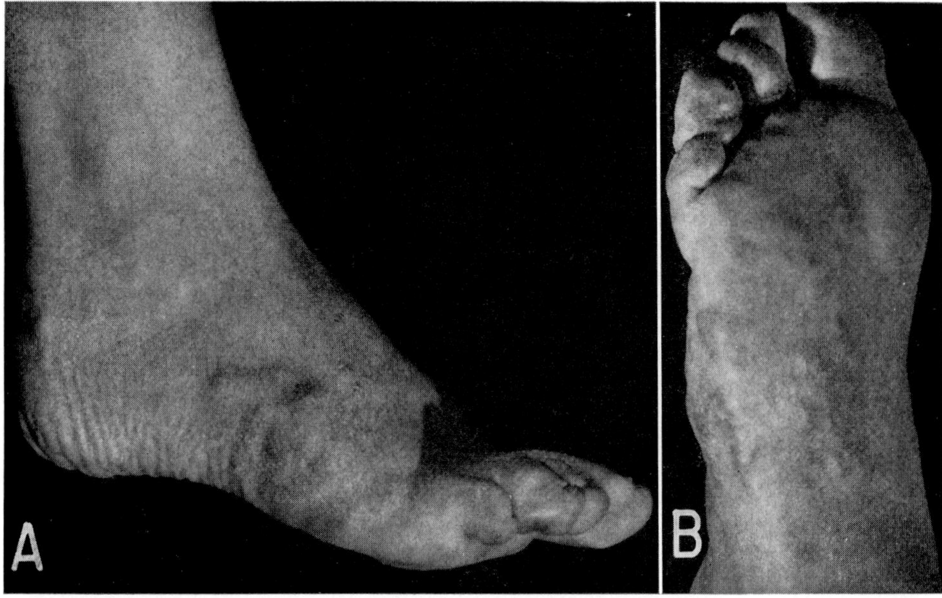

Figure 16–37. Congenital diffuse hemangioma, in a girl, 18 years of age.

Benign tumors. Kulchar (1944) stated that most benign tumors appearing on the skin and the subcutaneous tissue elsewhere are found in the foot. He mentioned the following: fibromas, lipomas, neuromas, myomas, koloids, the lesions of Recklinghausen's disease, molluscum contagiosum, various types of nevi, and sebaceous cysts. Aside from discomfort caused by pressure, Kulchar added that these benign tumors presented essentially the same problem of diagnosis and management as similar lesions elsewhere. Kulchar particularized the ensuing: foreign body granuloma, pyogenic granuloma, angioma, vascular nevi, angioneuromyoma or glomus tumor, synovial cysts, ganglioma, fibroma, xanthoma, and melanoma. Bergstrand (1937) reported two cases of "multiple glomic tumors" occurring in the foot, but they were confined to the region of the heel. From paucity of definite reports, glomus tumor of the forefoot must be regarded as being extremely rare. For some reason, in the section dealing with fibromas, Kulchar spoke of Recklinghausen's disease and "histocytoma cutis" and forgot to mention the more common fibromatosis of the plantar fascia, which most authors classify with benign tumors of the foot.

Plantar fibromatosis. This condition has deservedly received considerable attention in the literature. For one thing it is perhaps the most common benign tumor of the sole and is the cause of definite discomfort, since the sufferer has to bear weight on it and walk. The condition is considered akin to Dupuytren's contracture of the hand and is often called by the same eponym. At the end of his lecture on contracture of the fingers, Depuytren (1831) promised he would someday discuss the retraction of plantar fascia, which, he said, was more common and its effect on the toes no less important than that produced by the analogous affection of palmer aponeurosis on the fingers. Dupuytren (1839) later returned to this subject and reported a case of retracted second toe, which he said he had amputated in 1833. On a similar occasion, Dupuytren added, he would section the tendons and "the aponeurosis of the toe" instead of amputation.

Since Depuytren's time, often under different names, plantar fibromatosis has been discussed by numerous authors: Reeves (1881), Costilhes (1885), Madelung (1886), Souza-Leite (1886), Adams (1892), Davies–Colley (1894), Anderson (1897), Féré (1899), Ledderhose (1920),

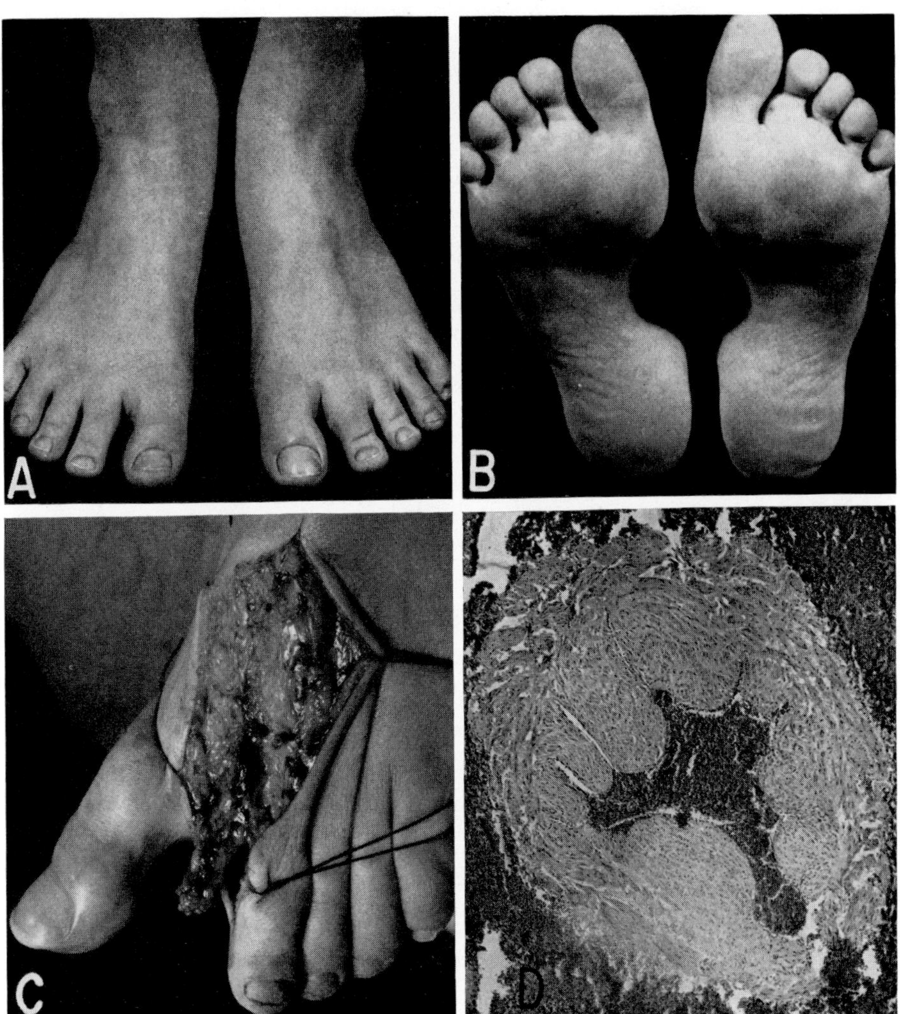

Figure 16–38. Congenital hemangioma, localized between the right first and second toes, extending plantarward, and causing metatarsalgia in a girl, 12 years of age. *A* and *B,* Before surgery. *C,* After exposure of tumor mass. *D,* Photomicrograph (× 50). Patient was relieved of pain, and there has been no recurrence.

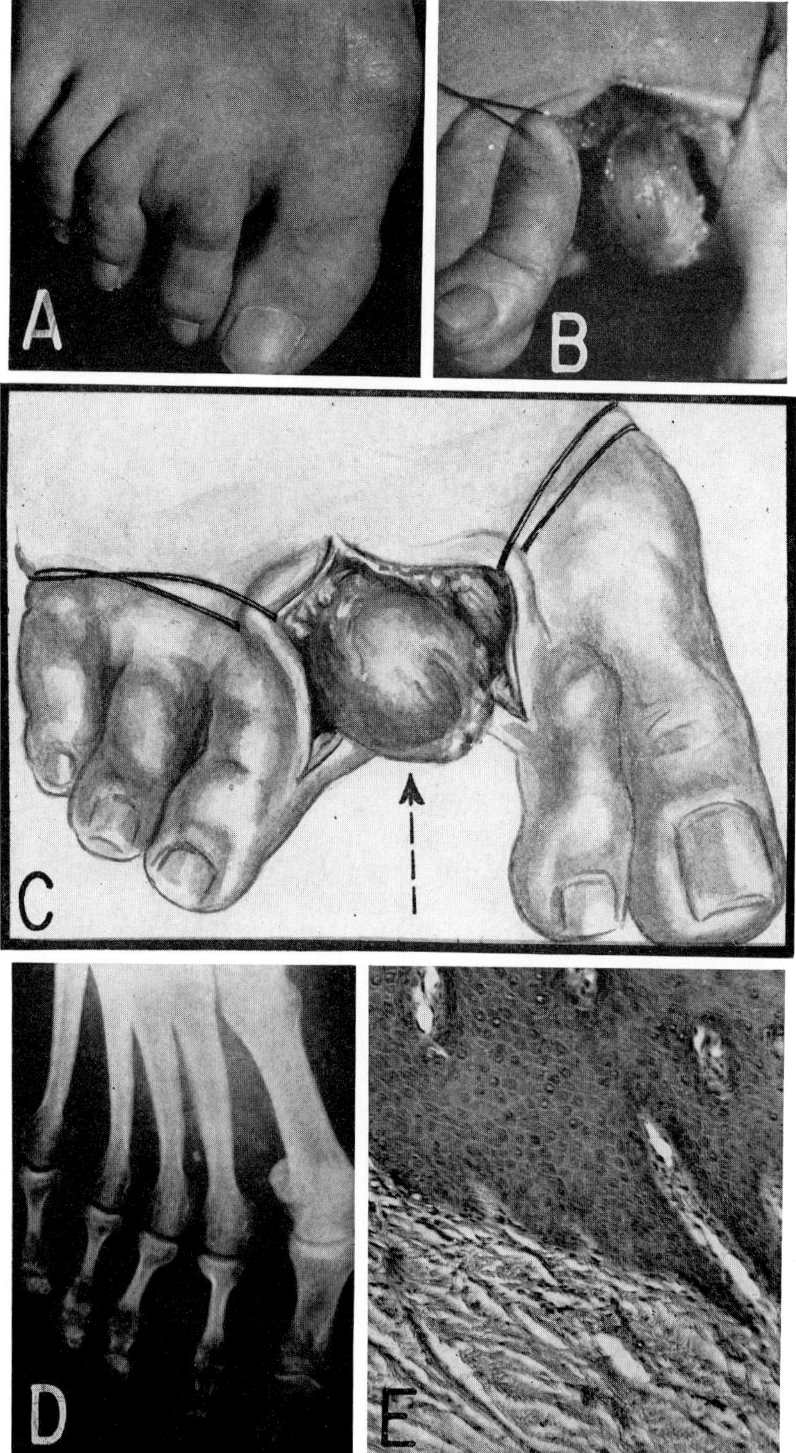

Figure 16–39. Interdigital epidermoid cyst in a woman, 40 years of age, with metatarsalgia and diverging second and third toes. *A,* Before surgery. *B,* After exposure of tumor. *C,* Diagram. *D,* Preoperative roentgenogram. Note the circular density between first and third metatarsal and the white spot between second and third metatarsals, suggestive of calcific deposit. *E,* Photomicrograph (× 130). Relieved of pain.

Specklin and Stoeber (1922), Cokkalis (1925–1926), Kinzel (1927), Auvray (1929), Kanavel and co-workers (1929), Rouillard and Schwob (1931), Fairbank (1932), Powers (1934), Greenberg (1939), Lund (1941), Hohmann (1941), Klossner (1944), Hammond and Dotter (1948), Skoog (1948), Meyerding and Shellito (1948), Pickren and associates (1951), Kapiloff and Prior (1952), Pedersen and Day (1954), Allen et al. (1955), Goetzee and Williams (1955), and perhaps a few others. Most of these authors concede that in some instances plantar fibromatosis coexists with the analogous lesion of the palmar fascia, and like Depuytren's contracture of the hand, it is often bilateral.

The main feature of plantar fibromatosis is the formation of modular tumors; contraction of the toes is rare or incidental. One wonders if the second toe Dupuytren (1839) amputated was not an ordinary hammertoe, which most often affects this digit. Concurrence of digital deformities and plantar fibromatosis have been reported by Ledderhose (1920), Powers (1934), Auvray (1934),

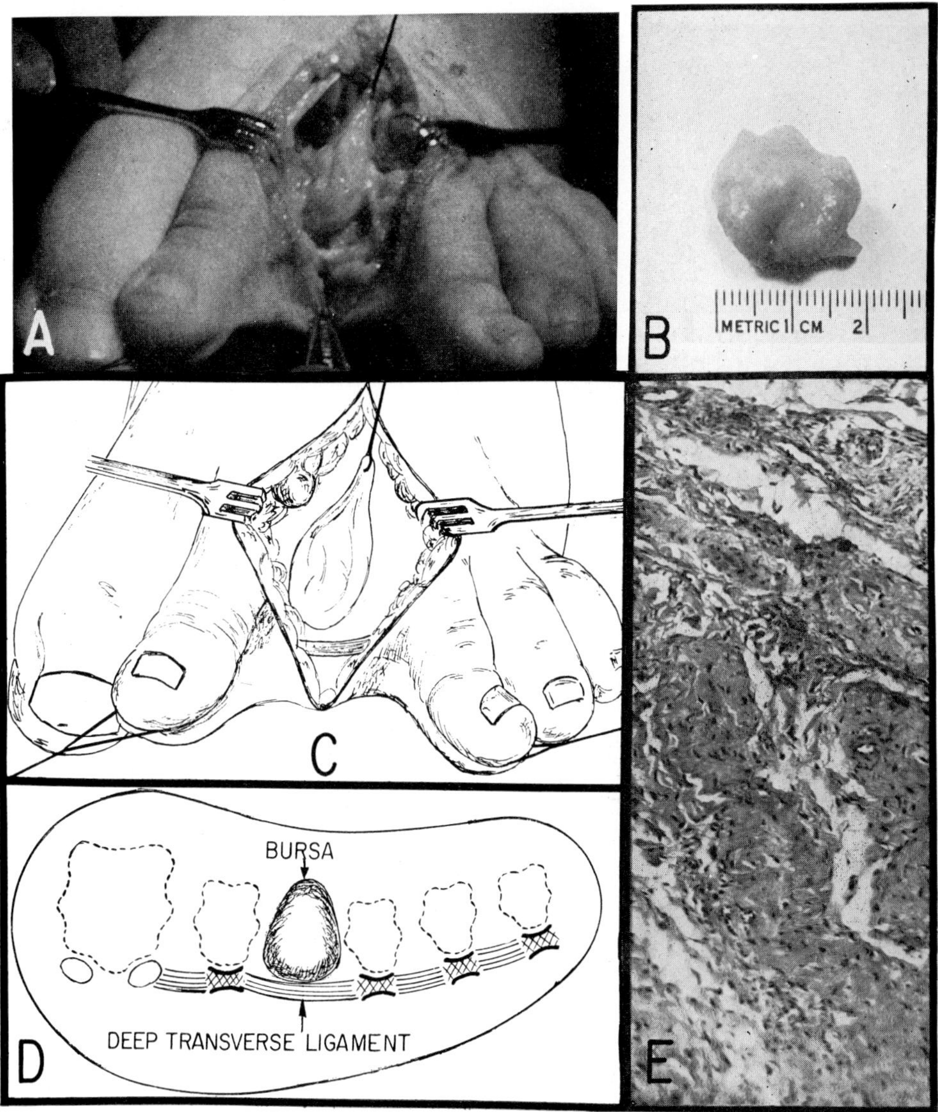

Figure 16–40. Intermetatarsal bursal tumefaction in a woman, 44 years of age, with pain between the bases of third and fourth toes. *A,* Surgically exposed tumor. *B,* Resected specimen. *C* and *D,* Interpretative diagrams. *E,* Photomicrograph (× 130). Discomfort was relieved after surgery.

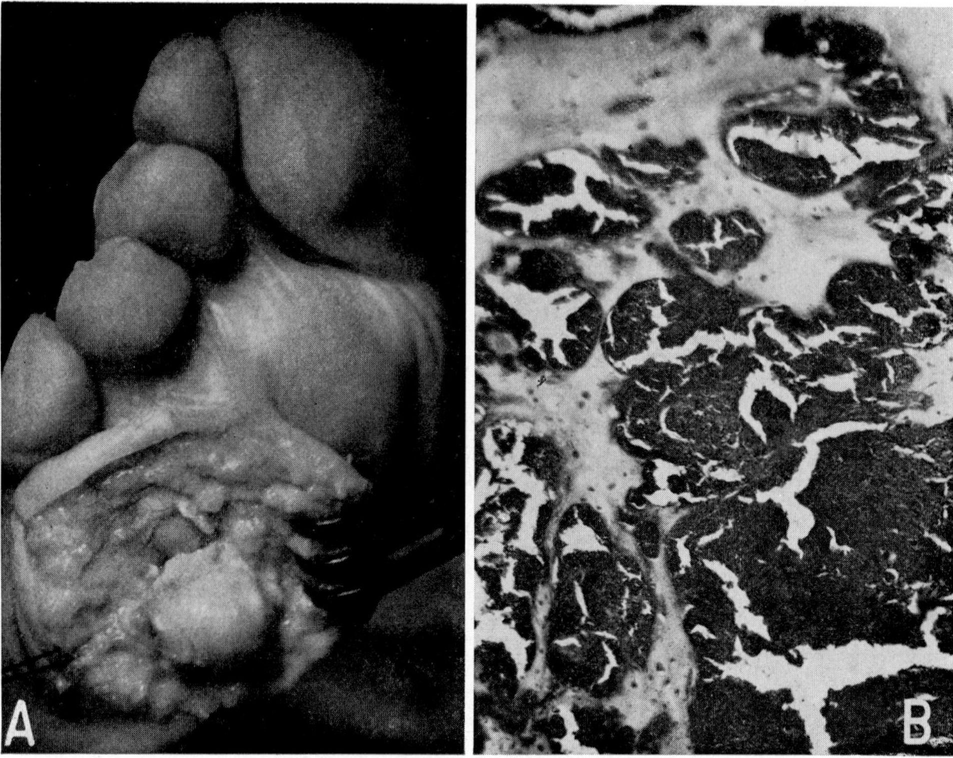

Figure 16–41. Plantar chondroma with calcification in a woman, 75 years of age, with a painful plantar mass of 9 years' duration. *A,* After exposure of the tumor. *B,* Photomicrograph (× 100). Patient was relieved of metatarsalgia after excision of tumor.

and Skoog (1948). It is to be remembered that deformities of the toes are very common, and plantar fibromatosis cannot be said to afford an immunity against them. "The scarcity of reports concerning an effect upon the toes," Pickren and associates (1951) wrote, "leads one to believe that it must be very uncommon."

The relative infrequency of digital deformities in plantar fibromatosis is explained on the basis of pressure from the ground or the shoe tending to hold the toes straight, thus counteracting the tendency of fascial bands to pull them into flexion. Fibrous extensions the plantar aponeurosis sends to the toes are at best rudimentary; they cannot be expected to form the tough cordlike structures seen so often in the hand between the palm and the involved finger. By way of analogy with Depuytren's contracture of the hand, it is presumed that the aponeurosis of the foot is contracted in plantar fibromatosis. If this were true, one would see a number of cavus feet in plantar fibromatosis. It may be that at the age when plantar fibromatosis occurs the skeletal framework of the foot is already established and cannot be changed by the contracted fascia. Unlike the analogous lesion of the hand, plantar fibromatosis is known to occur early in life, in growing children; congenital lesion has also been reported.

In Dupuytren's contracture of the hand, nodular thickenings of the fascia lie around the distal flexion crease of the palm, close to the metacarpophalangeal junction. The ulnar half of the aponeurosis is mainly involved, and in advanced cases the fourth and fifth fingers are drawn into the palm. In the foot the tibial sector of the fascia is thickened and the first and second toes are not known to curl plantarward and contact the sole. The nodular thickenings of the plantar fascia are located around the middle of the sole, at some distance from the line of metatarsophalangeal joints. The cases with nodular formation on both plantar and palmar aponeuroses do not seem to show the marked flexion deformity of the fingers that one sees in Depuytren's contracture of the hand without involvement of the feet. Plantar fibromatosis also appears to start at a comparatively younger age than uncomplicated Depuytren's contracture of the hand.

The palm possesses several flexion folds that are transversely disposed. These creases are intimately connected with the underlying fascia, which accounts for the puckering of the palmer skin in Dupuytren's contracture of the hand. From the deep surface of the palmar fascia several pairs of septal sheets pass in a dorsal direction on either side of the flexor tendons of the fingers and connect with the corresponding metatarsal bones. These tendons are often matted down by tough fibrous tissue. In the sole proper, there are no flexion folds, and a continuous sheet of fat intervenes between the cutis and the overlying aponeurosis. The skin of the sole is never puckered; the fleshy belly of flexor brevis sandwiches itself between

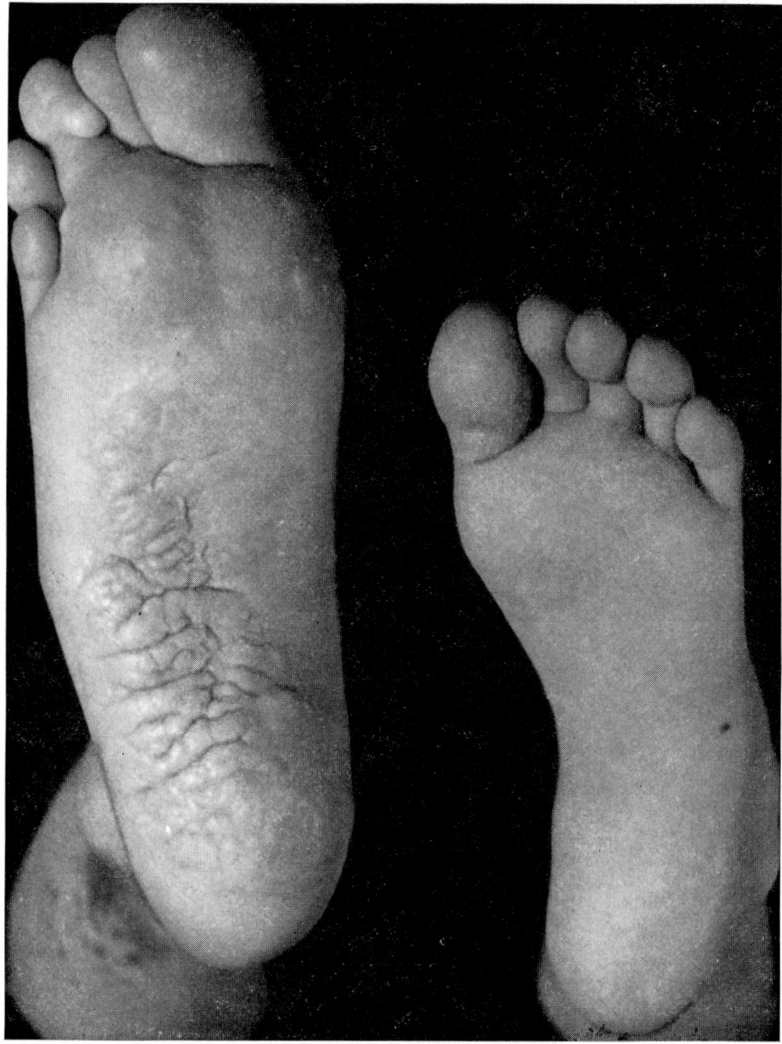

Figure 16–42. Osteocartilaginous tumors occurring in the hand and the foot of a young girl, 6 years of age, with unilateral gigantism. In the foot these tumors could be palpated under the third toe and second and third metatarsal heads. Note the corrugation of the plantar skin, which suggests von Rechlinghausen's neurofibromatosis. Tumors removed elsewhere in the body consisted of masses of bone covered with hyaline cartilage. They were interpreted as being benign. Compare the left with the right foot as to size.

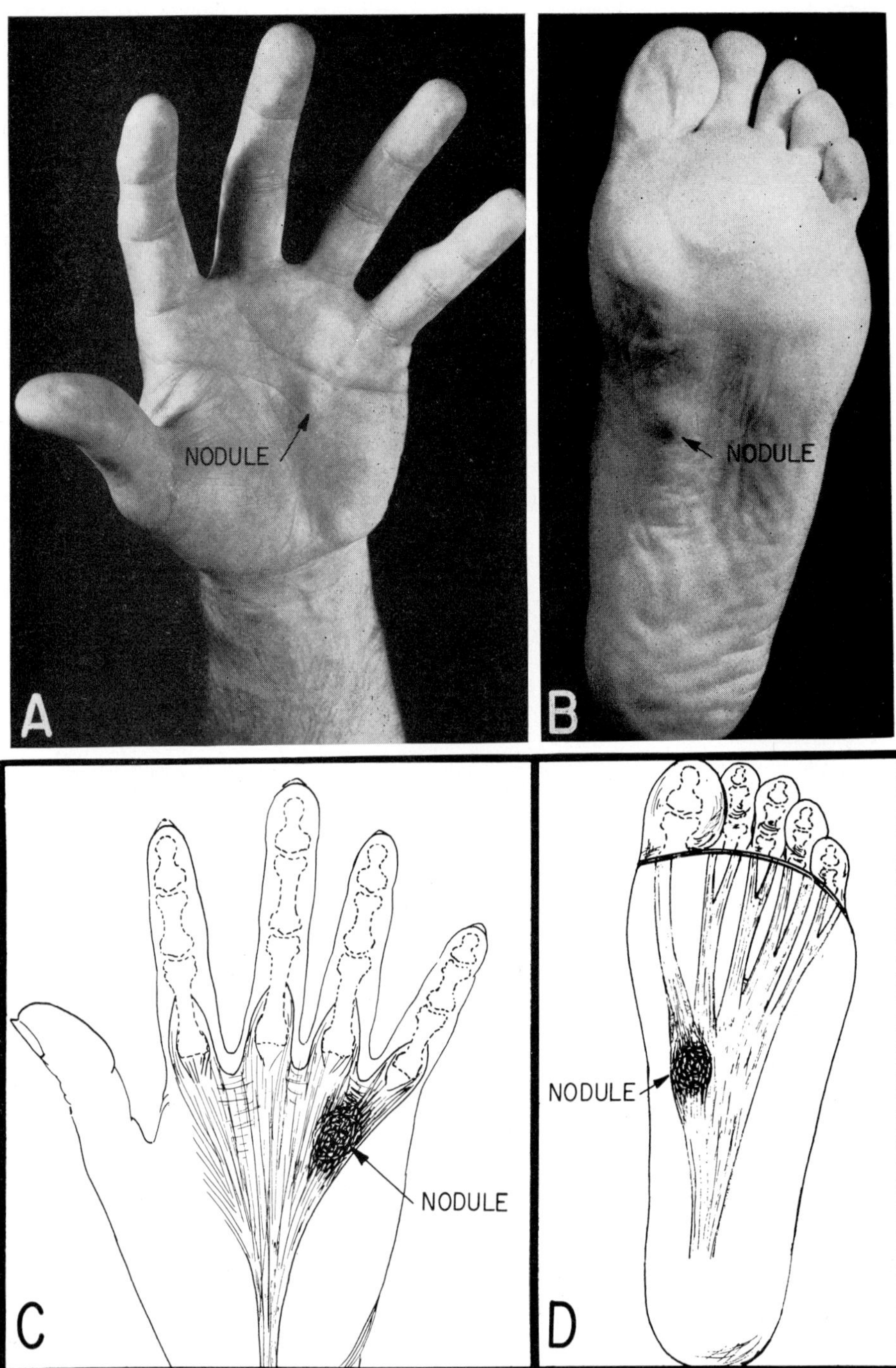

Figure 16–43. Localization of nodules in palmar (*A*) and plantar (*B*) aponeuroses of a woman who had both feet and one hand involved. *C* and *D,* Interpretative diagrams showing that in the hand the ulnar half of the aponeurosis is involved and in the foot the tibial portion is thickened. When Dupuytren's contracture of the hand occurs in the same patient with plantar fibromatosis, the fingers do not seem to be drawn into the palm.

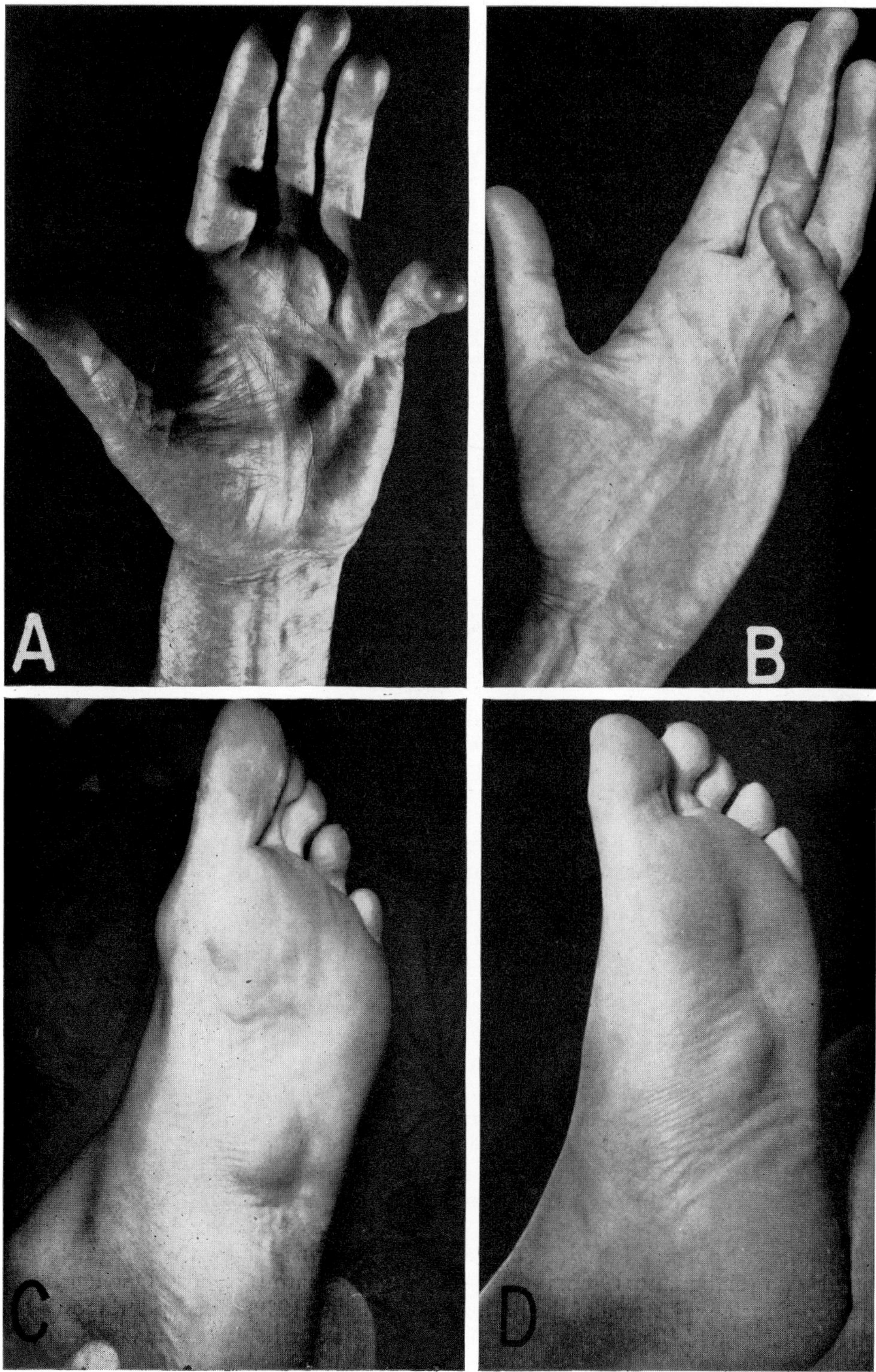

Figure 16–44. *A* and *B*, Dupuytren's contracture of the hand of a patient without concomitant plantar fibromatosis. *C* and *D*, the feet of two different patients with plantar fibromatosis. Note that the toes are not contracted.

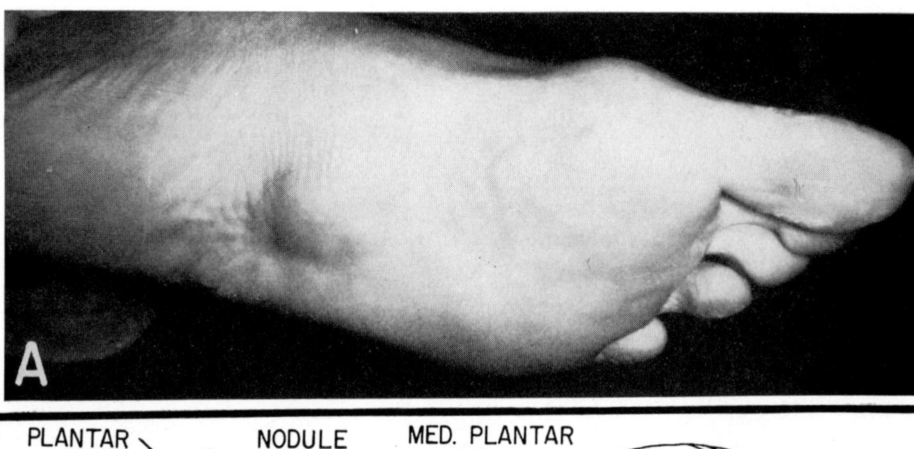

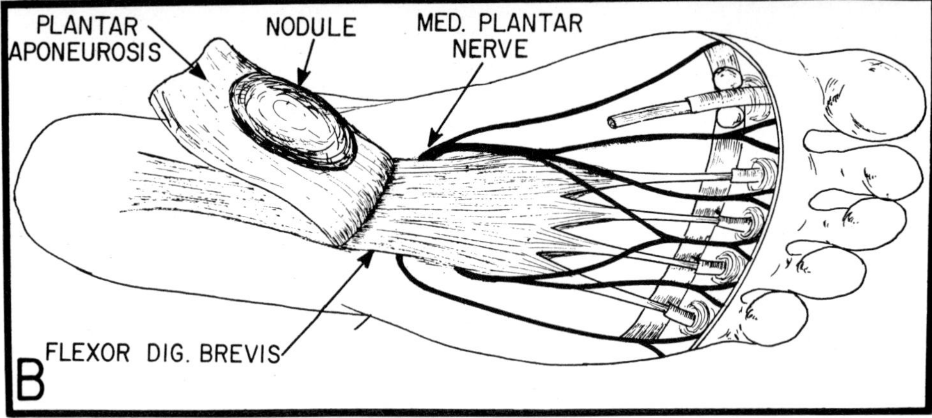

Figure 16–45. Photograph (*A*) and interpretative diagram (*B*) showing the nodule of the plantar aponeurosis in relation to the flexor digitorum muscle and the medial plantar nerve.

the aponeurosis and the long flexor tendons of the lesser toes. None of these tendons are matted down by fibrous tissue. Only one definite septal sheet emanates from the deep surface of the plantar aponeurosis and passes dorsally in the interval between the flexor digitorum brevis and abductor hallucis. It is to be remembered that the medial plantar nerve lies in this interspace; in plantar fibromatosis this nerve is sometimes involved in adhesions, which may account for the pain on weight-bearing and metatarsalgia referred to the forepart of the foot (Figs. 16–43 to 16–48).

Malignant tumors. Jaffé (1930) reported two malignant tumors of the forefoot—a melanoblastoma of the hallux and a squamous cell carcinoma of the small toe. Both were located in the nail bed. In the series surveyed by Schreiner and Wehr (1933), "nevus cell" carcinoma was the most common malignant tumor of the foot. Of 17 such cases only 2 originated in the forefoot—one under the nail of the hallux and the other at the tip of the fourth toe. These authors also reported a case of osteochondrosarcoma originating in the big toe. Coley and Pierson (1937) recorded 4 cases of synovioma of the foot proper; only 1 of these was said to definitely manifest itseft as a "painful swelling over the ball of the great toe." Charache (1939) reported 4 cases of squamous carcinoma of the foot but did not specify their location. Subungual melanoma was surveyed by Pack and Adair (1939). Thirty-four lesions involved the hallux and 3 the lesser digits. Under the general heading of angiomatous tumors, Oughterson and Tennant (1939) discussed Kaposi's multiple hemorrhagic sarcoma, which is also known to involve the forefoot. In their tabulation of bone tumors Coley and Higinbotham (1939) included 3 osteogenic sarcomas and 1 angiosarcoma of the metatarsal bones.

Collins (1940) reported a case of fibrosarcoma causing soreness over the midportion of the plantar surface of the right foot. Meyerding (1944) spoke of an osteogenic sarcoma of the second metatarsal causing swelling and tenderness "across the forepart of the dorsum of the right foot." Granville Bennett (1947) studied 37 specimens of "synoviomata"; in his tabulation he included 1 case involving the plantar aspect of the foot. Zarzecki (1949) surveyed 38 cases of fibrosarcoma of the extremities, 3 of which occurred in the foot. No mention was made of pain or metatarsalgia. Decker and Chamness (1951) reviewed 25 cases of melanocarcinoma of the plantar surface of the foot. Fahey and Bollinger (1953) reported a case of congenital sarcoma "attached at one point to the distal portion of the first metatarsal." Pascher and Sims (1954) wrote

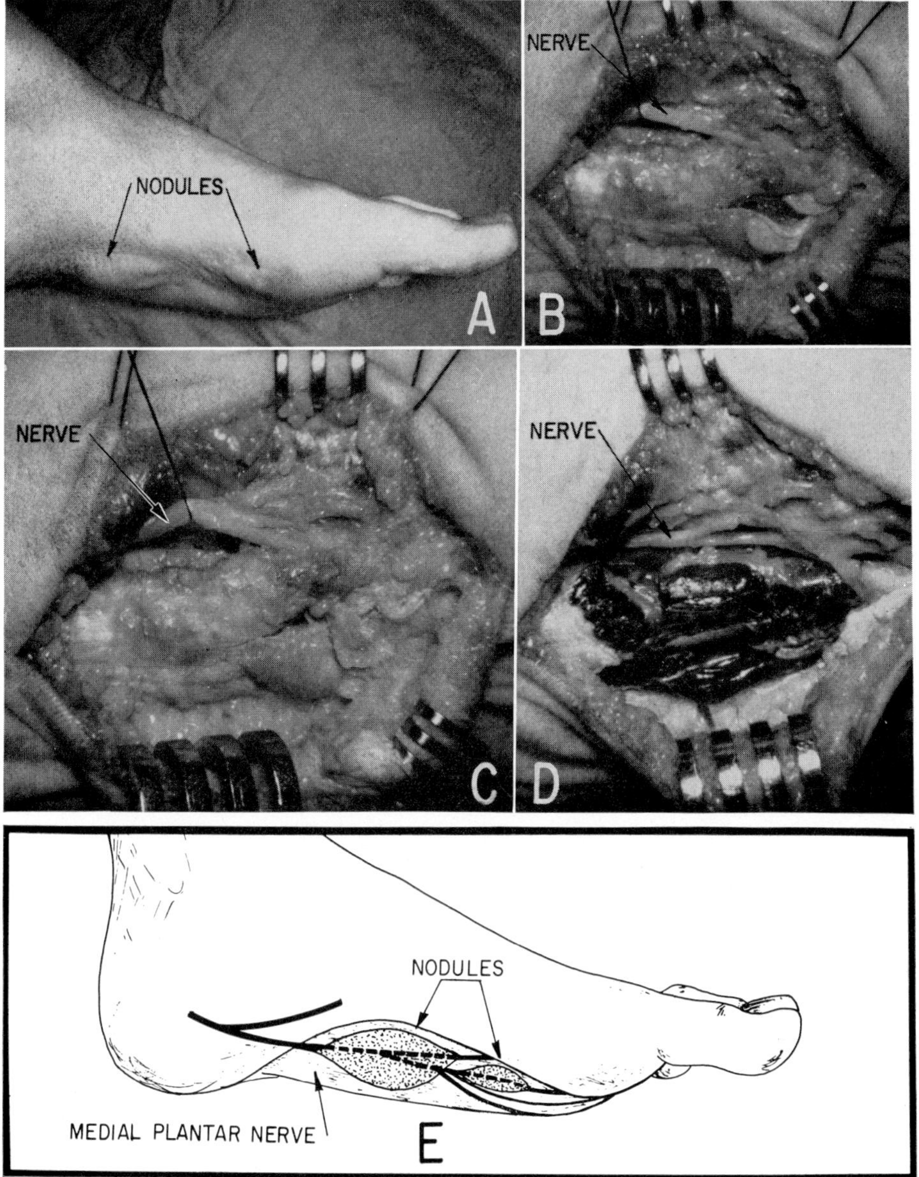

Figure 16–46. Multiple nodules of the plantar aponeurosis. *A,* Before surgery. *B,* After exposure of tumor and the medial plantar nerve. *C,* The nerve freed from the fibrous mass. *D,* The nodule-bearing plantar fascia resected. *E,* Interpretative diagram.

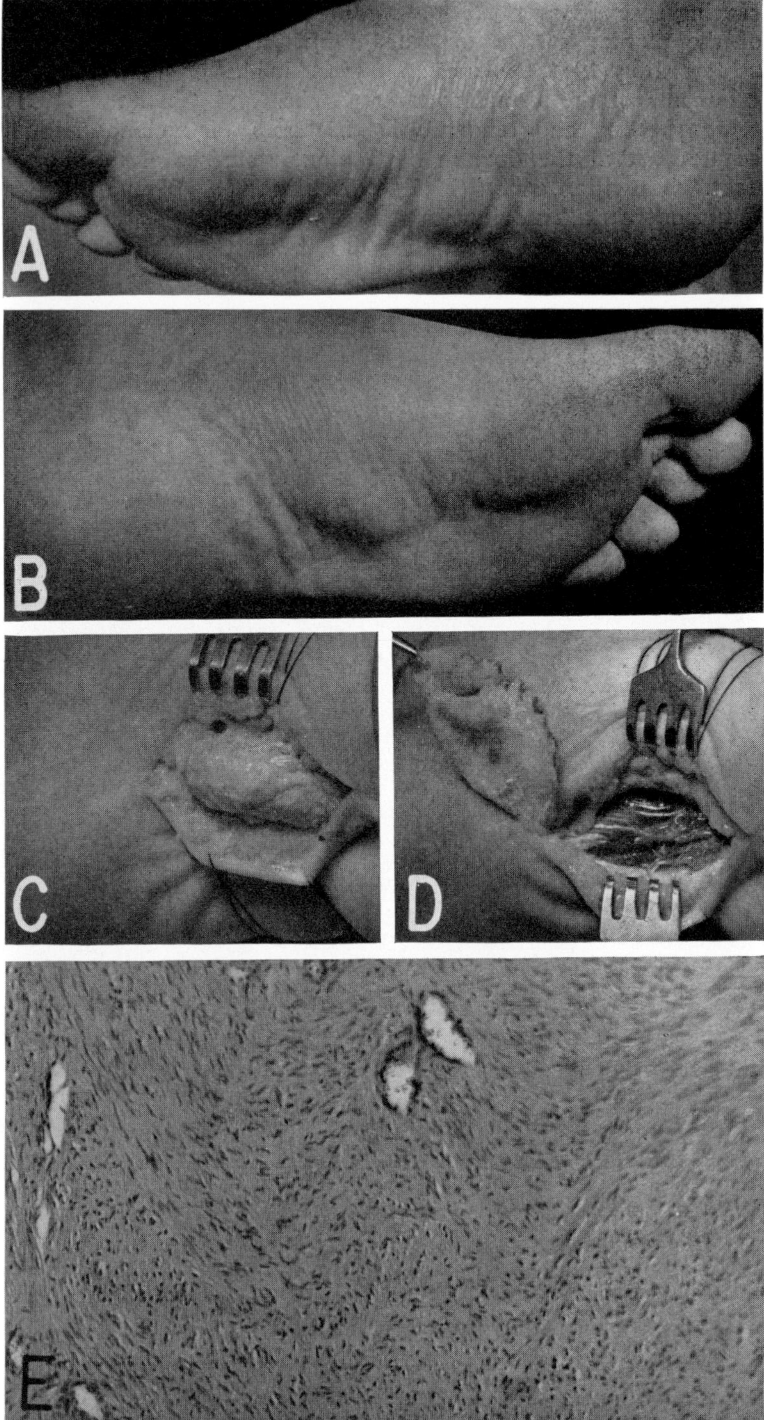

Figure 16–47. Bilateral plantar fibromatosis in a man, 37 years of age, with plantar pain on walking. *A* and *B,* Right and left feet. *C,* Surgically exposed tumor on the right side. *D,* Dissection of the tumor from the muscular belly of the short flexor of the toes. *E,* Photomicrograph (× 130). The patient had no recurrence; the pain was relieved.

about 2 cases of basal cell epithelioma of the sole of the foot. Allen and associates (1955) reported 9 cases of malignant soft tissue tumors of the sole of the foot—1 liposarcoma and 8 synoviomas. These authors were vague as to the exact location of the tumors. They merely stated whether a tumor occurred in the right or left sole. The closest they came to an exact localization was in the case

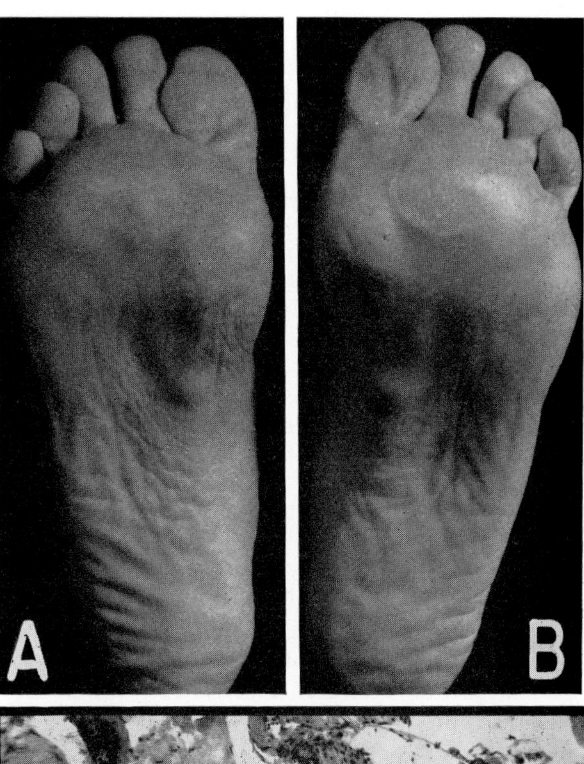

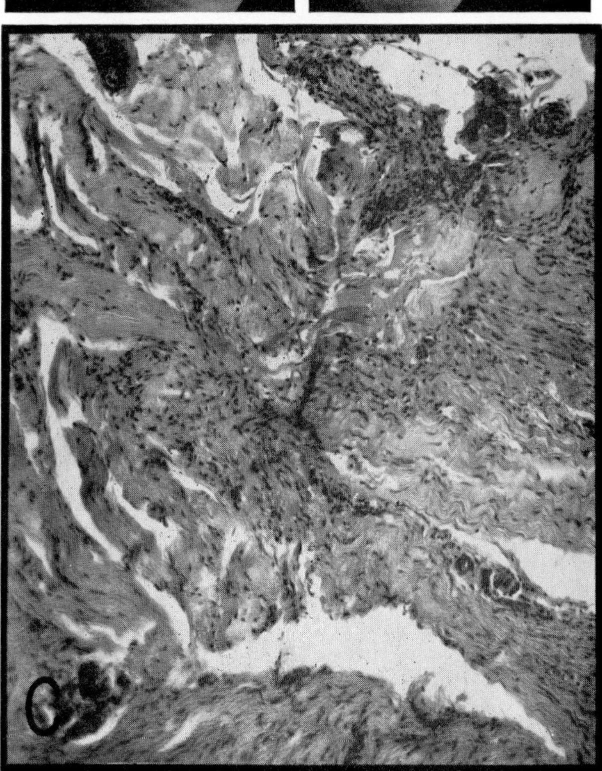

Figure 16–48. Bilateral plantar fibromatosis in a woman, 50 years of age, with plantar pain. *A* and *B*, Photograph of both feet. *C*, Photomicrograph (× 130). There has been no recurrence of the tumor. Mild pain has persisted on the right side.

of a synovioma that they said "occupied the entire mid-portion of the left sole."

Diagnostic clues. As a rule, malignant tumors are more painful than benign lesions. The glomus tumor constitutes an exception to this rule. It is excruciatingly painful, tender to touch or light pressure; it presents a smooth, slightly elevated surface and is purplish. Except for the glomus tumor, which as noted, must be extremely rare in the forefoot, severe pain in this area should arouse suspicions of a malignant lesion. This is especially true when the pain is felt at rest, without bearing weight on the foot, and if the pain becomes worse as time goes on. Coley and Higinbotham (1939) advised that persistent pain be regarded with deep suspicion, suggesting the possible existence of a primary bone tumor. Careful study of multiple view roentgenograms may aid in arriving at a fairly accurate diagnosis of tumors originating in the bones of the forefoot.

Pack (1939) wrote: "Perhaps no regions or organs in the body are so readily favored for early detection of tumors as are the hands and the feet. Constantly under inspection, always sensitive to pain, irritation, swelling, and impairment of function, it would seem that no tumor can grow for long without detection by the patient." Unfortunately this is only partly true. Unless they present themselves as visible and palpable masses, preoperative diagnosis of soft tissue tumors is mainly conjectural.

Roentgenograms taken by soft tissue technique will sometimes lend a clue as to the true nature of the tumor. Ordinary varicose veins do not occur in such active areas as the forefoot; on roentgenography shadow suggestive of phleboliths should arouse suspicion of hemangioma. Two lesions cast shadows denser than muscles and tendons but not as dense as those produced by bone—calcified tendonitis and extraskeletal chondromas. Fat is more radiolucent than muscle; a circumscribed soft tissue shadow of greater transparency than that cast by intrinsic muscles should suggest the presence of a lipoma. Almost all other soft tissue tumors of the foot are diagnosed after surgical exploration and biopsy.

Both Pack (1939) and Kulchar (1944) have stressed the multicentric tendency of tumors of the foot. When one tumor is found, another one should be searched for. Kulchar explained this multiplicity in the bases of the congenital origin of many tumors of the foot. One may look for other insignia of congenital anomalies—patchy pigmentation of the skin, or the so-called *café au lait* spots. Kulchar pointed out that the incidence of melanoma is comparatively rare among Negroes and the sole of the foot where pigmentation is least, is a common site. He advised that pigmented nevi of the foot be excised with a fair margin of the skin and subjected to microscopic examination because of the possibility of latent malignancy.

Plantar fibromatosis has been mistaken for fibrosarcoma. Meyerding and Shellito (1948) mentioned two such cases. "If the pathologist or the surgeon will bear in mind that the cellular microscopic appearance of Depuytren's contracture may show active fibroplasia and even mitoses," they said, "this error may be avoided." Pickren et al. (1951) spoke of two other patients who had undergone amputation of their feet—"one because of persistent recurrence of fibrous proliferation and the other because of erroneous diagnosis of fibrosarcoma." Allen and his group (1955) reported a case in which the patient had been subjected to amputation of the right foot for recurrence of nodular tumor of the plantar fascia. Six months later a similar nodule had appeared in the left sole. This was excised 2 years later and follow-up examination 14 years afterwards revealed no recurrence. Allen and associates considered diagnosis of plantar fibromatosis certain if the lesion is bilateral, if it is associated with involvement of a palmar aponeurosis or Peyronie's disease—fibromatosis of the corpus cavernosum of the penis. One should also search for knuckle pads. Allen and associates did not find any evidence that the thickened nodules of the plantar aponeurosis ever became malignant.

Melanoblastoma, squamous cell carcinoma, and synovioma are the most commonly reported malignant tumors of the forefoot. "Ulcerative lesions of the nail bed in elderly persons which do not show any tendency to heal," Jaffé (1930) wrote, "should be examined carefully for possible melanoblastoma or squamous cell carcinoma. In distinguishing melanoblastoma from benign granulomata and squamous cell carcinoma the demonstration of pigmented areas which may be very small is of great importance. In this location the carcinoma shows a dry and waxy surface." Mason (1939) went on record with the statement that "an irritation of . . . corns on the feet never produces carcinoma."

Coley and Pierson (1937) stated that diagnosis of synovioma was often exceedingly difficult. "When no palpable tumor exists," they wrote, "it may be impossible until operation has disclosed the condition. Where a definitely palpable tumor exists it must be differentiated from other soft tissue tumors, such as fibrosarcoma, myxosarcoma, neurogenic sarcoma, liposarcoma and xanthosarcoma of tendon sheath origin. The tumor is usually firm, well circumscribed. In none of the nine cases–

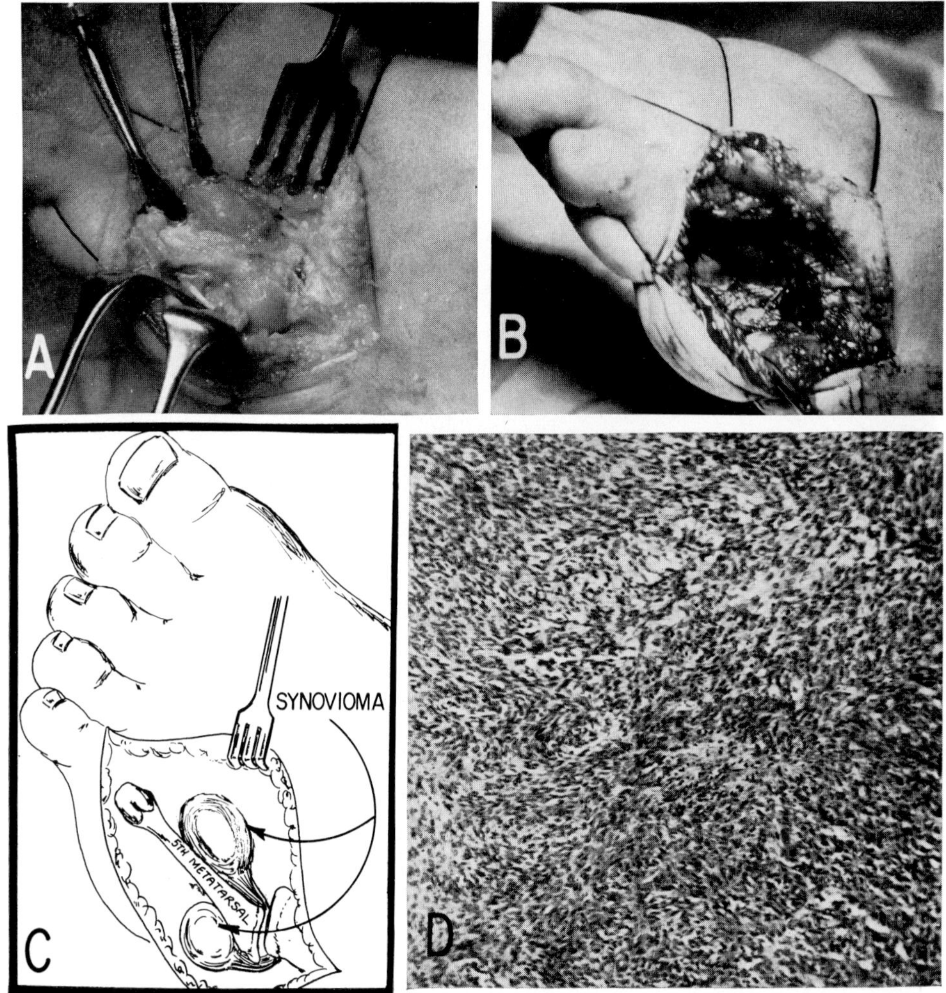

Figure 16–49. Synovioma of the forefoot in a woman, 25 years of age, with lateral metatarsalgia of several years' duration and recent appearance of swelling. Biopsy report: Synovioma. The foot was amputated through the leg. *A,* After tumor was exposed. *B,* Resection of the fifth metatarsal and surrounding tumor. *C,* Interpretative diagram. *D,* Photomicrograph (× 130). Death occurred within 2 years of pulmonary metastasis.

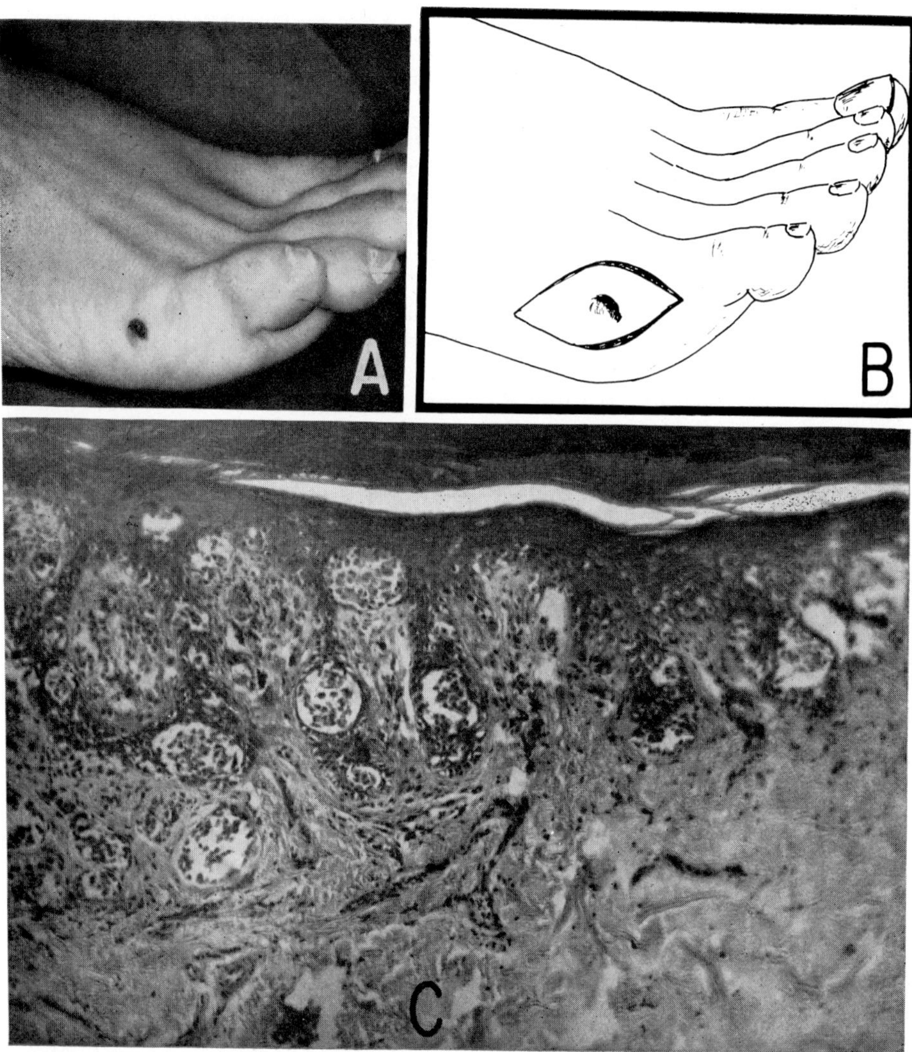

Figure 16–50. Malignant melanoma in white female, 49 years of age. Complaint: "mole" on the left foot, noticed first 20 years ago; 2 years ago it began to increase in size, and recently it appeared to have gotten darker. Surgery: wide excision. *A,* Before surgery. *B,* Interpretative diagram showing the area of excision. *C,* Photomicrograph (× 130). After 18 months there was no detectable evidence of recurrence or metastasis.

one of which was in the plantar surface of the foot—reported by Briggs (1942)—was diagnosis of synovioma made preoperatively.

The treatment. All pigmented nevi under the sole of the foot, between the toes, or around the area where the shoe rubs should be removed surgically with a wide strip of the surrounding skin. Other benign tumors are excised when they cause pain or interfere with wearing shoes. In excising fibromatous tumors of the plantar fascia, care must be taken to completely free the medial plantar nerve from adhesions. Melanoblastoma of the nail bed should be treated by amputation of the involved toe. When this tumor occurs on the dorsum of the forefoot and is not yet fixed, it may be excised with a generous portion of the surrounding skin and the underlying soft tissue. Indurated melanoblastoma, especially when it occurs on the sole, is treated by amputation through the leg. The same holds true with other malignant tumors of the forefoot.

Prognosis of the malignant tumors of

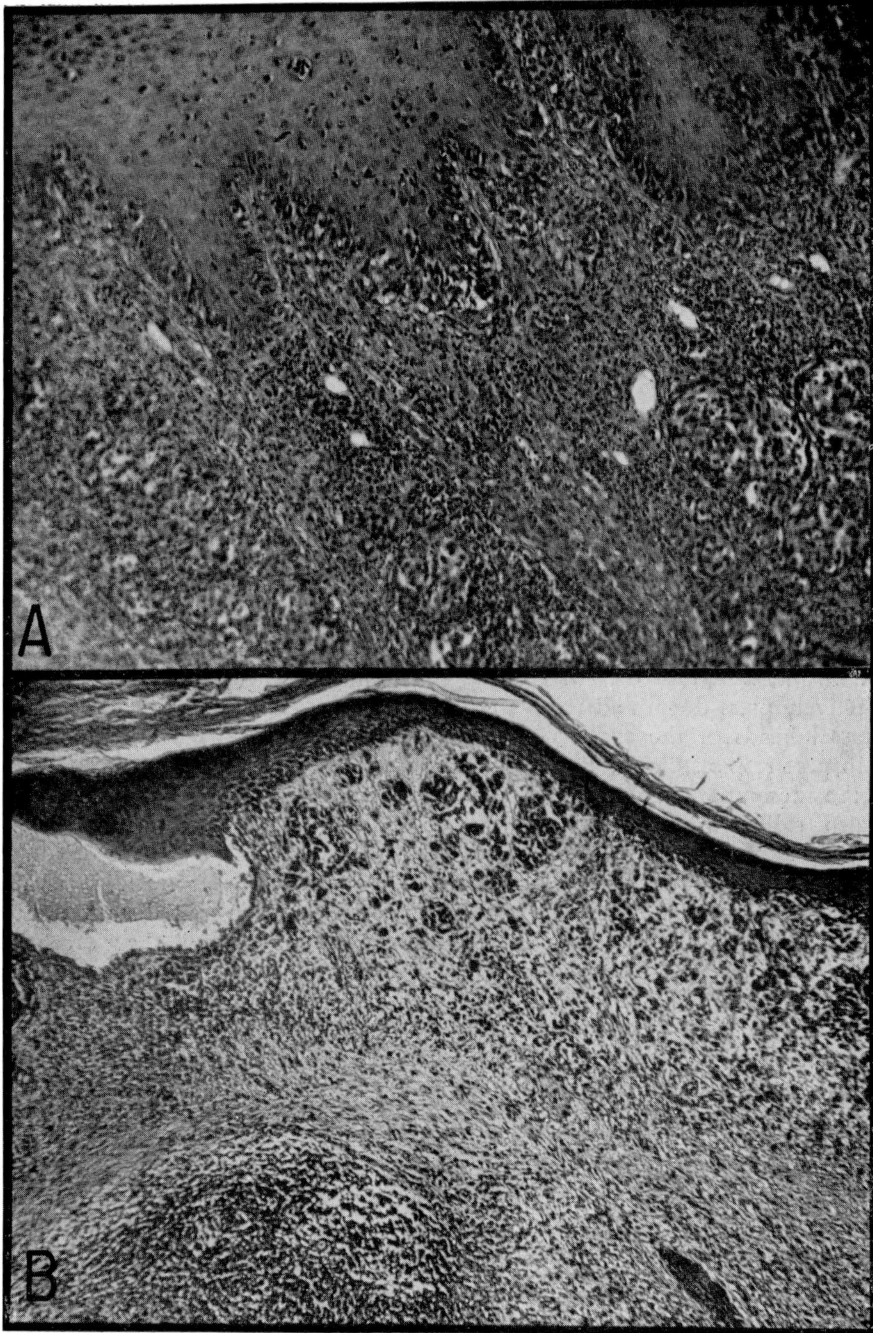

Figure 16–51. Malignant melanomas in two different patients. *A,* Photomicrograph (× 130) of the biopsy specimen from a white male, 49 years of age. He consulted a physician for what he thought was a painful corn on the ball of the foot; this was "cut." The surgical wound would not heal and metatarsalgia became unbearable. The foot was amputated through the midleg. He died of pulmonary metastasis exactly 3 years after the "corn was cut." *B,* Photomicrograph (× 60) of the biopsy specimen from a white female, 81 years of age. She developed a sore on the small toe 5 years previously. This would not heal and as time went on it grew larger. The toe was amputated through tarsometatarsal junction. Tissue examination was reported as malignant melanoma. After 9 months, there was no recurrence or sign of metastasis.

the foot is extremely poor even after amputation. Mason (1939) stressed the importance of examining the regional lymph nodes preoperatively. "When glandular enlargement is present," he wrote, "there is failure to obtain successful results in nearly 60 per cent, which if glands are not present this figure is reduced to 25 per cent (Figs. 16–49 to 16–51).

ULCERS AND SCARS

The most severe pain in the forefoot is caused by ulcers and scars that follow radionecrosis, chemical and mechanical injuries, or surgery. It is often erroneously stated that trophic ulcers due to spina bifida or diabetes are not painful. Elsewhere we pointed out that in these conditions there might be impairment of motor power with preservation of sensation. We said that toes that failed to effectively press down and relieve the metatarsal heads of the excessive stress were in part responsible for these ulcers and the accompanying metatarsalgia. We also called attention to another fallacious concept perpetuated by more than one author—that scars on the sole of the foot, especially when they are longitudinally disposed, are painful. In our experience the most disabling scars are the ones on the dorsum of the forefoot—scars that bind the extensor tendons, cause retraction of the toes, and prevent them from coming down and bearing effective pressure on the proffered surface.

Not many years ago it was a common practice to treat pressure keratoses, corns, kelloids, verruca fungus infections, and other skin diseases with x-ray or radium routinely. A single strong exposure or repeated exposures of the wart- or callus-bearing ball of the forefoot not only damaged the skin but also destroyed protective cushions of fat under the metatarsal heads. In some instances it even caused necrosis of these bones. Metatarsalgia accompanying radiodermatitis or actinonecrosis was unbearable. The patient was completely crippled and there was the ever present danger of malignant metaplasia. Fortunately these cases are becoming less common. But we still have to contend with ulcers and scars caused by mechanical, thermal, and chemical injuries, and there is always the hazard of skin slough incident to surgery.

Skin grafts. Haggart (1934) advocated the use of a cross-leg pedicle graft to cover sizable areas left after excision of plantar warts. Discussing mainly defects caused by excessive irradiation of plantar warts, Blair and associates (1937) advised excision of cornlike scars. Small defects were "closed by skin suture, perhaps with some drawing together or switching of the fat pad." For larger ulcers, they recommended a pedicle flap switched from the nearby non-weight-bearing surface of the sole. Ghormley and Lipscomb (1944) used "untubed" cross-leg pedicle grafts to repair deep defects of the foot caused both by trauma and actinodermatitis.

For repair of surface defects and replacement of scars of the foot, Brown and Cannon (1944) outlined the following methods: excision and resuture; free skin graft; direct local flaps; delayed cross-leg flaps; same-leg delayed flaps; distant "turn-over," "jump," or caterpillar flaps; and distant wrist-born flaps. "Tubed flaps," they wrote, "need special mention and application, *viz,* a large, long tube had often best be attached in a normal site close to the defect. Then when detached from the donor site, put in a second normal site close to the other end of the defect, so that a sort of suitcase handle of good tissue is lying close to the defect—getting its blood supply from two good sources."

Converse (1948) discussed various applications of "nontubulated" pedicle skin flaps. Braithwaite and Moore (1949) emphasized some of the technical details of cross-leg flaps and outlined their indications and contraindications. Pangman and Gurdin (1950) removed the bones from inside one of the toes and utilized its skin to cover the defect on the ball of the forefoot. Brown and Fryer (1951) also spoke of "filleted" toe flaps, among other grafts. Besides defects of the foot caused by actinonecrosis, they treated ulcers of the foot caused by freezing and atomic irradiation.

We have treated skin sloughs following surgery with Unna's paste boot, occasionally supplementing this with a walking cast. Trophic ulcers incident to spina bifida are treated by resection of the distal segments of metatarsal bones. In gangrene of the toes due to embolic accident, we resect sufficient bone to procure enough loose skin to cover the stump. An analogy may perhaps be drawn between the forefoot and a rock-ridden patch of ground: less rock, more

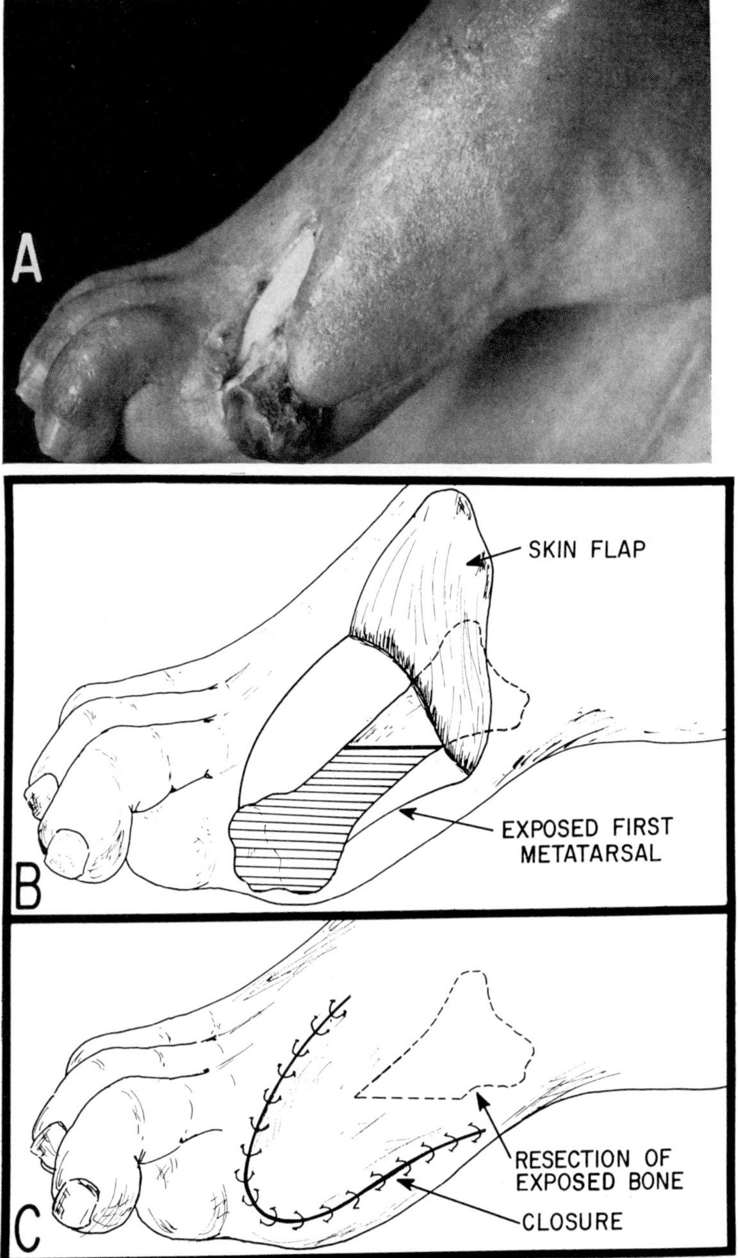

Figure 16–52. Defect left after embolic gangrene of the great toe in a woman, 33 years of age, suffering from mitral stenosis. She came from the Argentine presenting the picture shown in (*A*). The protruding distal half of the first metatarsal was resected, which permitted closure of the wound without tension. She returned to Argentina. *B* and *C,* Interpretative diagrams. Postrecovery photograph has not been available. According to her letters, the incision has remained closed.

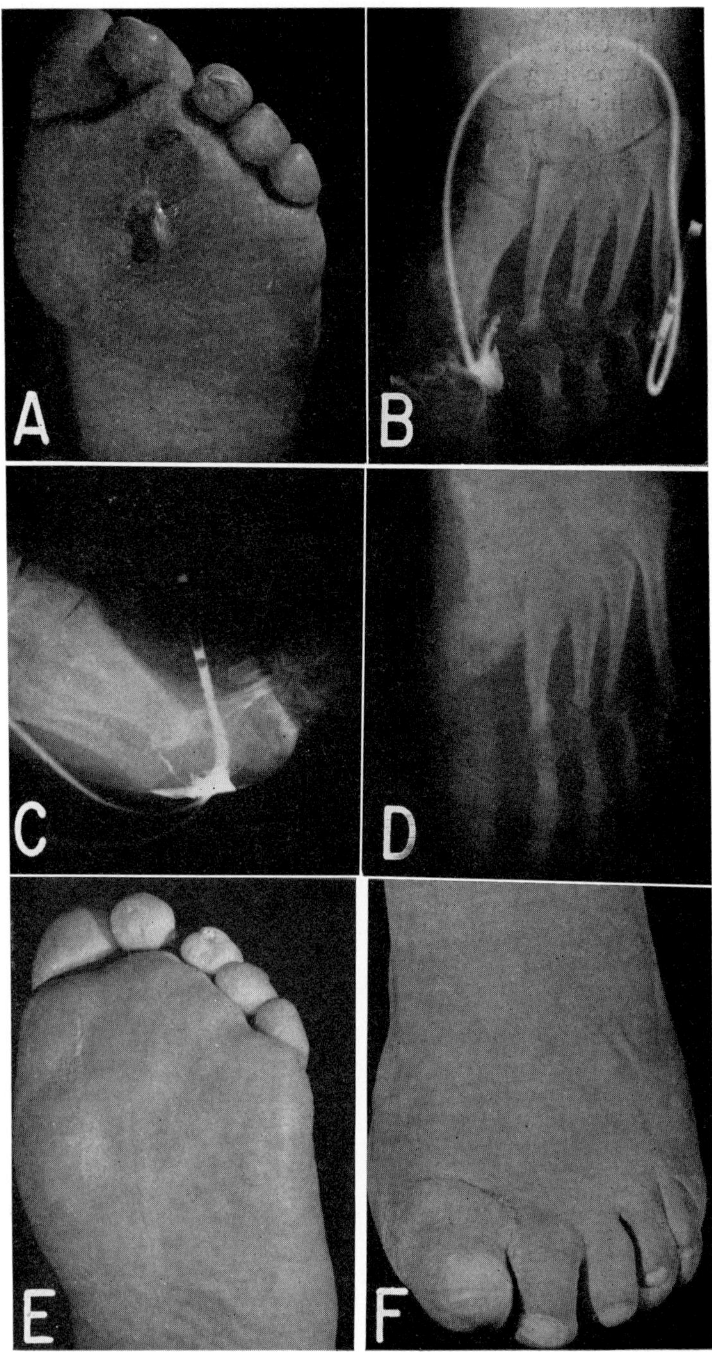

Figure 16–53. Pressure keratosis, plantar ulcer, and infected first metatarsophalangeal joint in a girl, 20 years of age, with spina bifida. *A,* Plantar ulcer. Iodized oil was injected through a catheter inserted into the sinus and roentgenograms (*B*) and (*C*) were taken. *D,* Roentgenogram after resection of the first metatarsophalangeal joint. *E,* Postrecovery plantar view. *F,* Dorsal view showing surgical syndactylia of first with second toe. After 6 years there has been no recurrence of ulcer or infection.

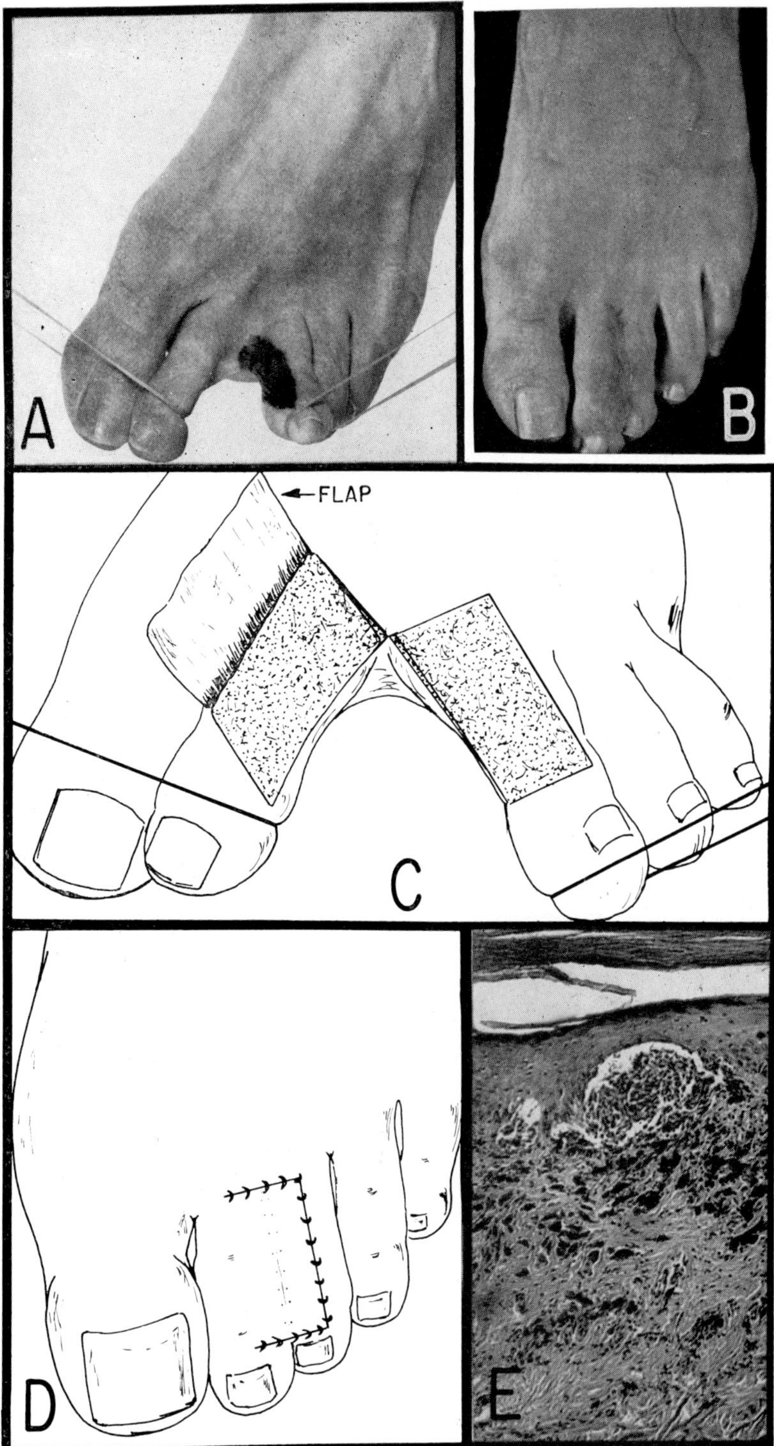

Figure 16–54. Closure of interdigital defect left by wide resection of pigmented nevus flap and surgical syndactylia of the toes in a man, about 50 years of age. No symptom. *A,* Before surgery. *B,* After syndactylia. *C* and *D,* Interpretative diagrams. *E,* Photomicrograph (× 75). There has been no recurrence.

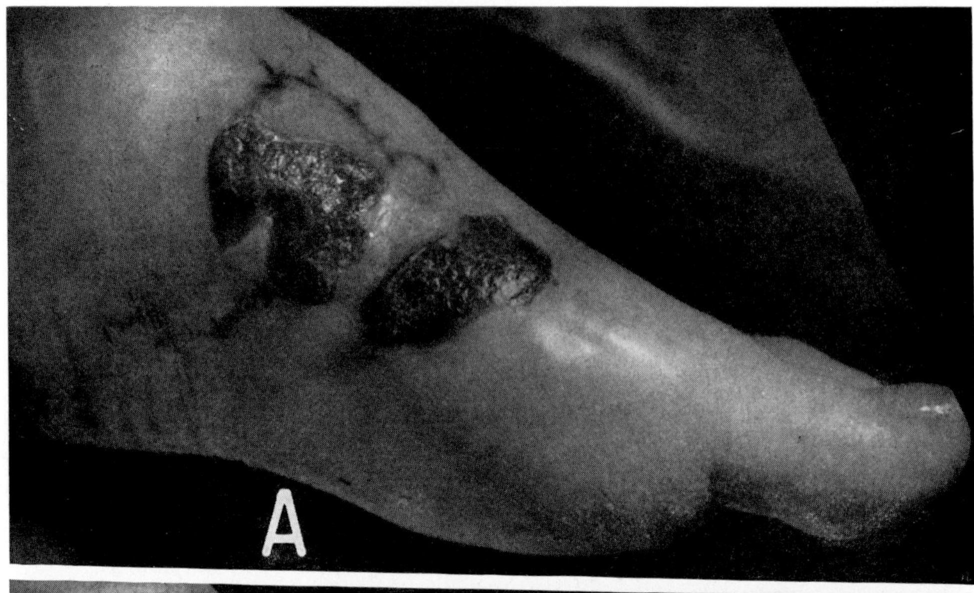

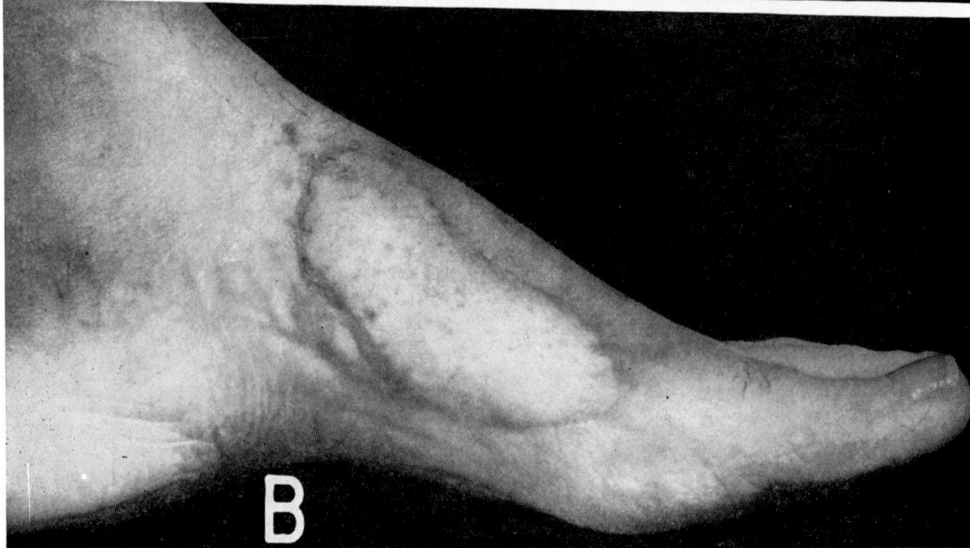

Figure 16–55. Skin defect closed by cross-leg flap in woman, 33 years of age. She gave the history of a mole resected elsewhere and treated with "skin graft." It did not take; the wound would not heal. The surgeon who had operated on her reported that he had removed a hemangioma. In view of failure of previous free graft, we decided to cover the area with a cross-leg flap. *A*, Before cross-leg flap. *B*, After recovery. The patient is satisfied.

soil; less bone, more soft tissue that can survive (Figs. 16–52 and 16–53).

We treat traumatic skin defects or ulcers that still possess a substratum of subcutaneous fat with a full thickness free graft. When the plantar cushion of fat is missing, the overlying metatarsal head is resected. In the event of a sizable defect on the interdigital aspect of one of the toes, we fashion a flap from the contiguous side of the neighboring digit and syndactylize the two members. Extensor tenotomy and dorsal capsulotomy may remedy the retraction of the toes by dorsal scars, and sometimes one also has to resect either the metatarsal heads or the basal portions of the proximal phalanges. Bone-bound, painful scars are replaced by cross-leg flaps. Extensive and deep ulcers on the dorsal or plantar aspect of the foot are treated by cross-leg flaps or tubes—using sometimes the so-called "caterpillar" or "waltzing" tube variety (Figs. 16–54 to 16–60).

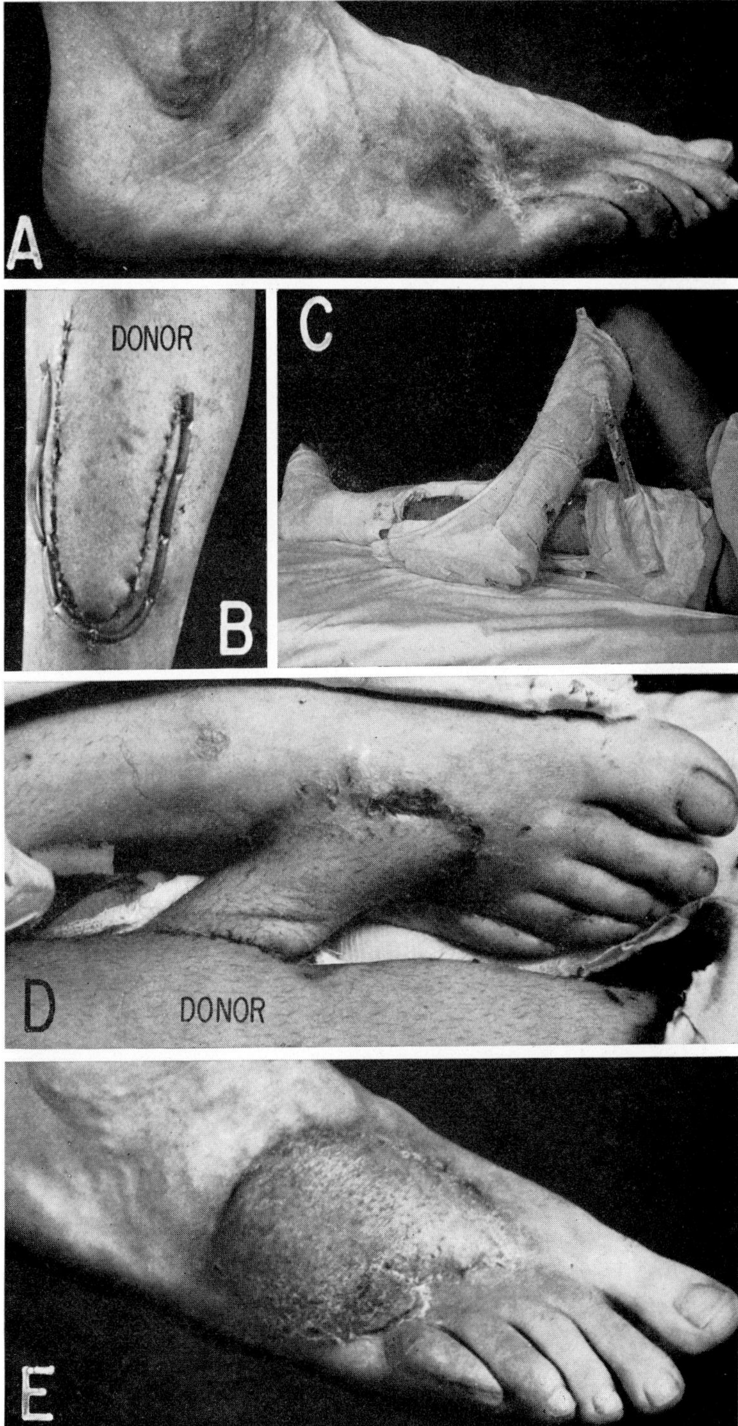

Figure 16–56. Replacement of painful dorsal scar adherent to bone in man, 27 years of age, with compound fracture of lateral metatarsals. *A,* Before cross-leg flap. *B,* delayed flap on the donor site. *C,* Plaster immobilization after anastomosis. *D,* Gradual weaning of the flap from the donor site. *E,* Postrecovery photograph.

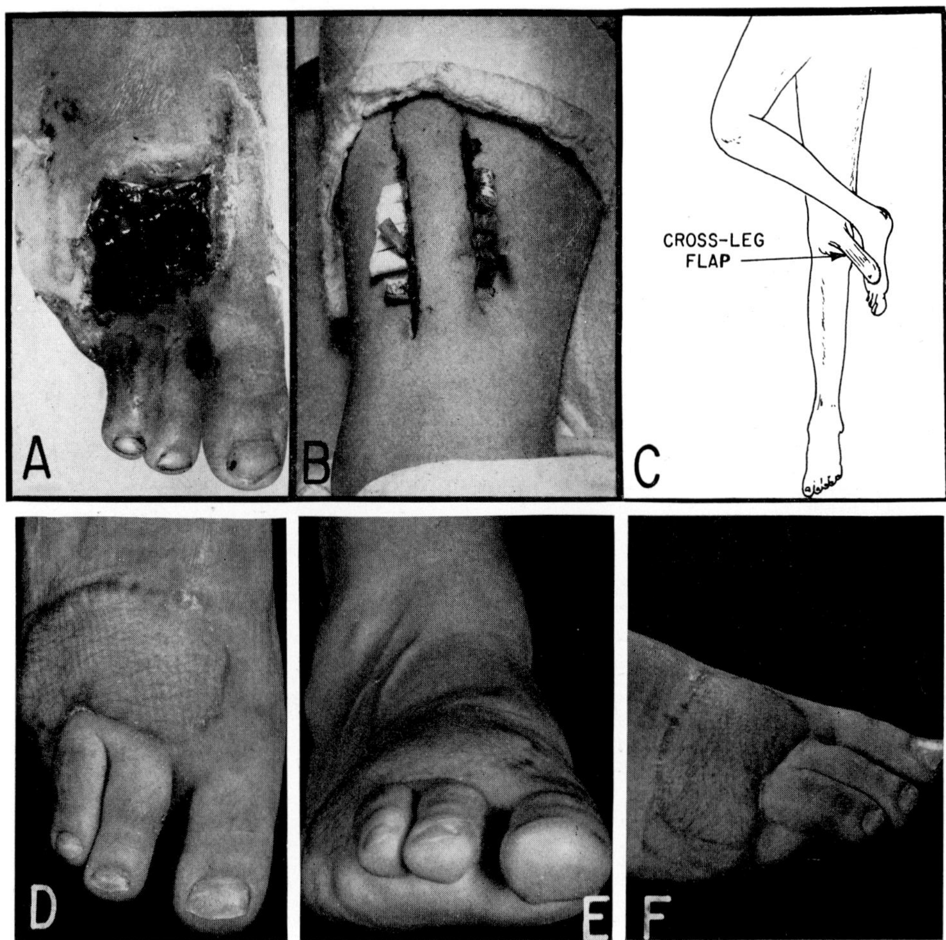

Figure 16–57. Large deep defect caused by lawnmower injury in a boy, 9 years of age. *A,* Before skin graft. *B,* Flap on the opposite thigh. *C,* Diagram of cross-leg anastomosis. *D, E,* and *F,* Postrecovery photographs.

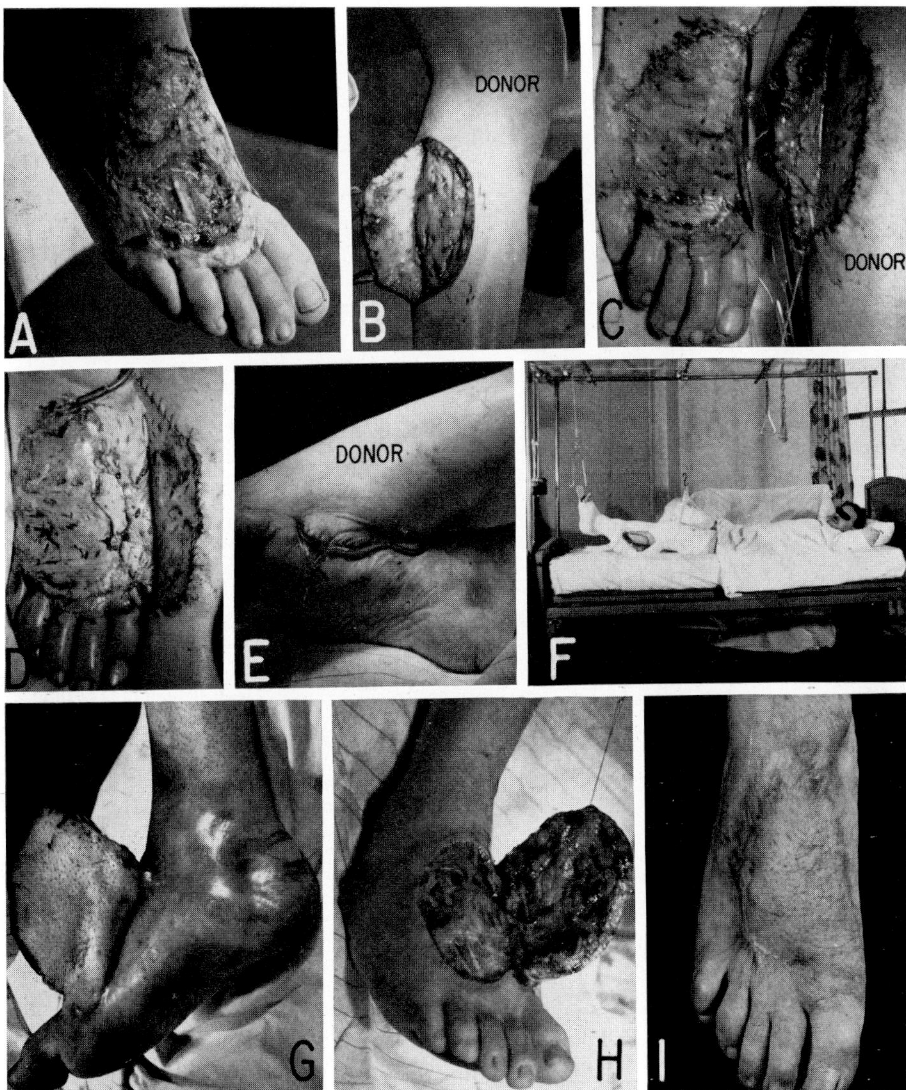

Figure 16–58. Large dorsal defect due to avulsion of skin. *A,* Before skin graft. Note the exposed extensor tendon. *B,* Elevation of flap on the opposite leg. *C,* The defects on the injured leg and the defect left by the elevation of flap have been surfaced with split thickness graft and anastomosis has begun. *D,* After suturing the flap to the injured foot. *E,* The same shown from the under aspect of the injured foot. *F,* Plaster immobilization and suspension with the aid of an overhead frame. *G,* Weaned graft. *H,* Same seen from the other side. Note that the temporary split graft has been dissected from both the injured foot and the flap. *I,* Postrecovery photograph.

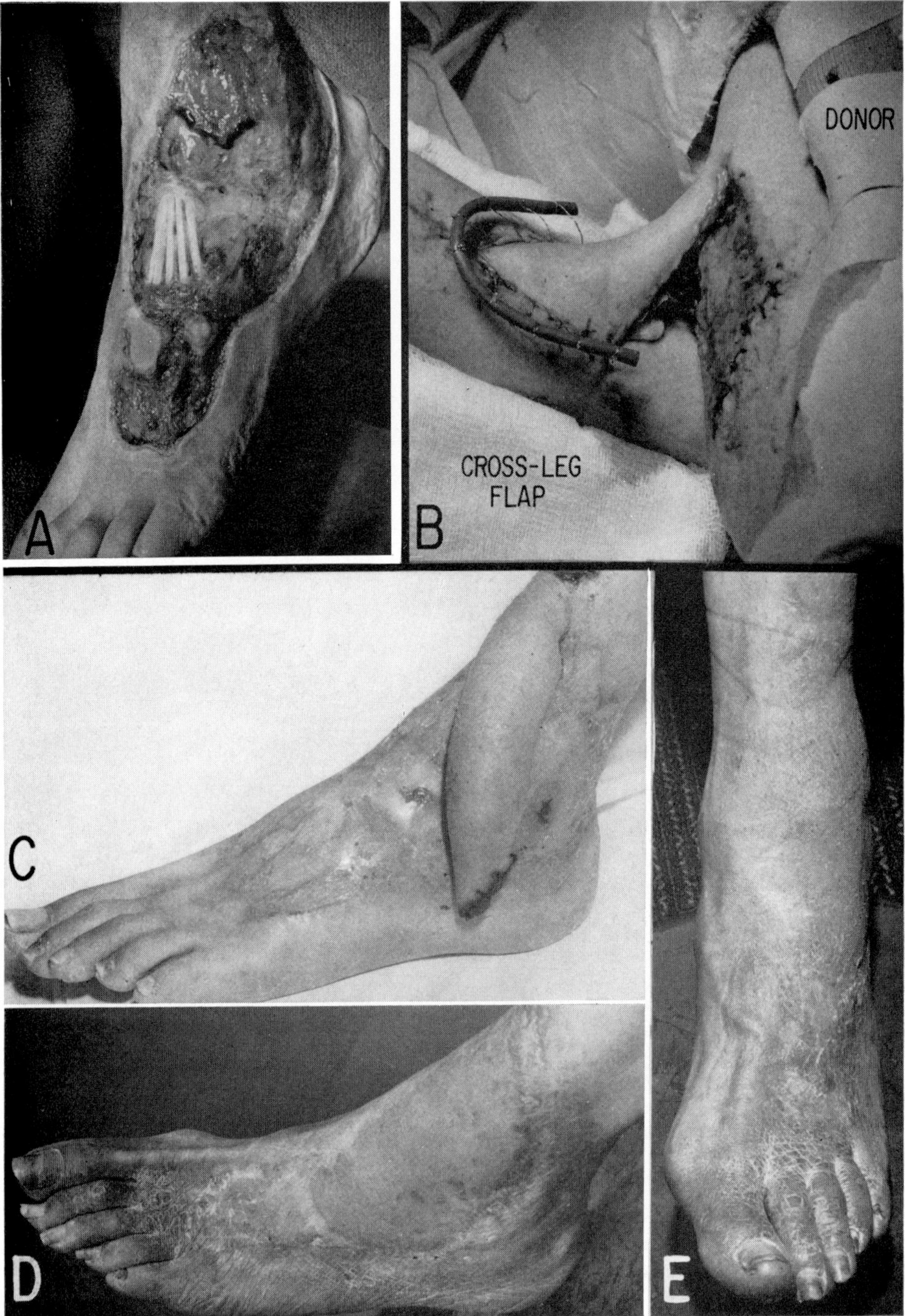

Figure 16–59. Skin slough caused by Levophed injection in the course of cardiac surgery in a man, 47 years of age. *A,* Before cross-leg flap. The defect was covered with split thickness graft as a temporary dressing. *B,* Anastomosis. *C,* The flap has been weaned. The previously applied split thickness graft was dissected from the underlying tendons and replaced by the fat-bearing flap. *D,* Several months after flattening the flap. *E,* Same after the flap has been defatted and coarse scars removed.

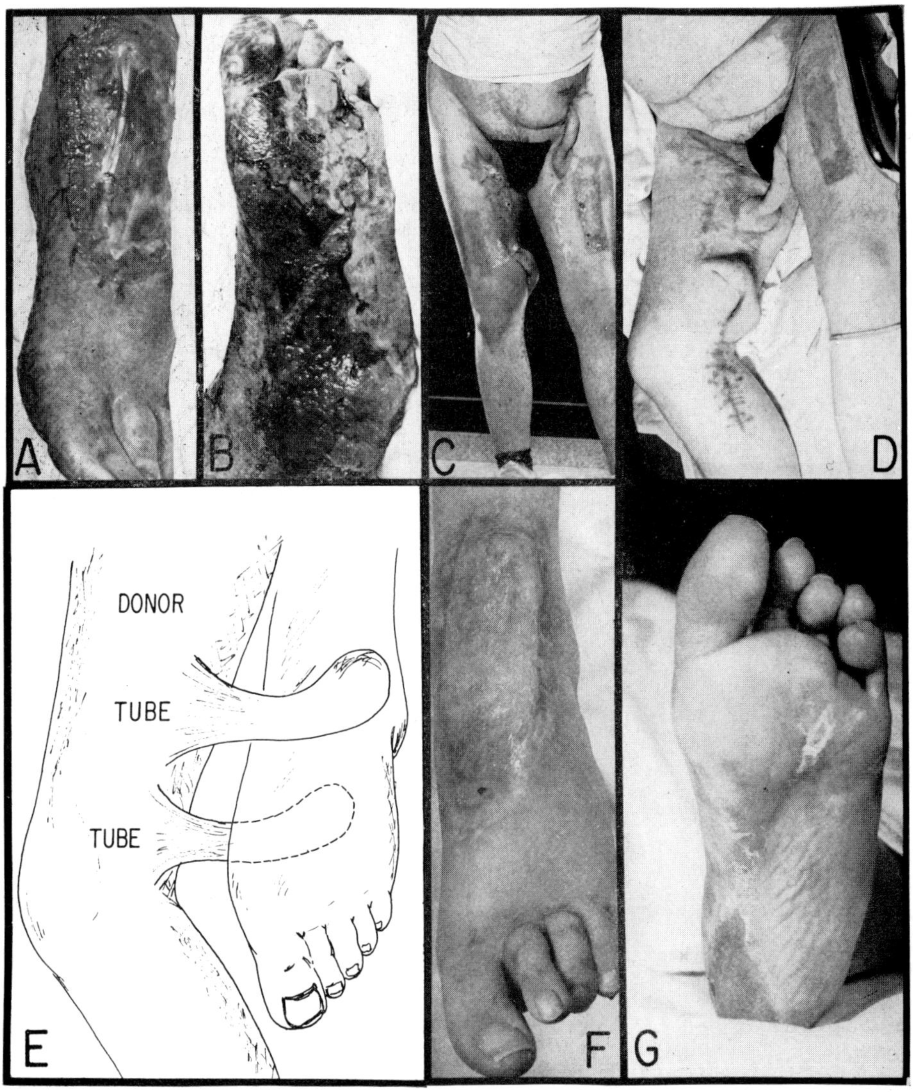

Figure 16–60. Large defects due to a rail injury on both the plantar and dorsal aspects of the left foot surfaced by waltzing tubes from the abdomen in a man, 28 years of age. *A,* Dorsal view. *B,* Plantar view. *C,* Two tubes had been "caterpillared" from the abdomen to the legs. *D,* Tube from the left thigh "jumped" to the right thigh. *E,* Diagram of anastomosis. One tube was connected to the dorsal and the other tube to the plantar aspect of the injured foot. *F* and *G,* Postrecovery photographs.

REFERENCES

Adams, W.: *On Contractions of the Fingers (Dupuytren's and Congenital Contractions), and on "Hammer-Toe."* London, J. & A. Churchill, 1892, pp. Introduction and 1–154.

Allen, R. A., Woolner, L. B., and Ghormley, R. K.: Soft tissue tumors of the sole—with special reference to plantar fibromatosis. J. Bone Joint Surg. *37:*14–26, 1955

Allington, H. V.: Review of the psychotherapy of warts. A.M.A. Arch. Derm. Syph. *66:*316–326, 1952.

Anderson, R.: The treatment of intractable plantar warts. Plast. Reconstr. Surg. *19:*384–388, 1957.

Anderson, W.: *The Deformities of Fingers and Toes.* London, J. & A. Churchill, 1897, pp. 86–149.

Auvray, M.: Double rétraction de l'aponévrose palmaire et de l'aponévrose plaintaire chez le même sujet. Bull. Mém. Soc. Chir. *55:*1026, 1929.

Auvray, M.: Volumineux fibrome du creux poplité. Bull. Mém. Soc. Chir. *60:*1236–1239, 1934.

Axhausen, G.: Die Koehlersche Erkrankung der Metatarsophalangealgelenke. Med. Klin. Wchnschr. *48:*318, 1922.

Baker, L. D., and Kuhn, H. H.: Morton's metatarsalgia; localized degenerative fibrosis with neuromatous proliferation of the fourth plantar nerve. South. M. J. *37:*123–127, 1944.

Bennett, G. A.: Malignant neoplasms originating in synovial tissues (synoviomata). J. Bone Joint Surg. *29:*259–291, 1947.

Bergstrand, H.: Multiple glomic tumors. Am. J. Cancer *29:*470–476, 1937.

Bernstein, A., and Stone, J. R.: March fracture—a report of three hundred and seven cases and a new method of treatment. J. Bone Joint Surg. *26:*743–750, 1944.

Betts, L. O.: Morton's metatarsalgia: neuritis of the fourth digital nerve. Med. J. Aust. *1:*514–515, 1940.

Bickel, W. H., and Dockerty, M. B.: Plantar neuromas, Morton's toe. Surg. Gynec. Obst. *84:* 111–116, 1947.

Billig, H. E.: Condylectomy for metatarsalgia: indications and results. J. Internat. Coll. Surgeons *25:*220–226, 1956.

Blair, V. P., Brown, J. B., and Byars, L. T.: Plantar warts, flaps and grafts. J.A.M.A. *108:*24–27, 1937.

Blecher: Fussgeschwulst, Knochenbruch und Knochenhautentzuendung. Deutsche mil-Ärtzl. Ztschr. *31:*321, 1902.

Boisson, A., and Chapotot, E.: Le pied forcé (étude sur la nature et la pathogénie des lésions de l'avant-pied provoquées par la marche chez les fantassins). Arch. Méd. Phar. Mil. *33:*81–103, 1899.

Borggreve, J.: Zur operativen Behandlung des kontrakten Spreizfusses. Zeitsch. Orthop. Grenzgb. *78:*581–582, 1949.

Braddock, G. T. F.: Experimental epiphysial injury and Freiberg's disease. J. Bone Joint Surg. *41:*154–159, 1959.

Bradford, E. H.: Metatarsal neuralgia, or "Morton's affection of the foot." Boston Med. Surg. J. *125:*52–55, 1891.

Bragard: Beitrag zur Malalopathie der metatarsalkopfchen Koehlersche Krankheit. Ztschr. Orthop. Chir. *46:*49–65, 1924.

Braithwaite, F., and Moore, F. T.: Skin grafting by cross-leg flaps. J. Bone Joint Surg. *31:*228–235, 1949.

Brandes, M., and Ruschenburg, E.: Eine operative Behandlung der (II.) Koehlerschen Krankheir am Koepfchen des Os metatarsale. Ztschr. Orthop. Grenzgb. *69:*353–361, 1939.

Branson, E. C., and Rhea, R. L., Jr.: Plantar warts: cure by injection. New Eng. J. Med. *248:*631–632, 1953.

Breithaupt: Zur Pathologie des menschlichen Fusses. Med. Ztg. *24:*169 and 175, 1855.

Briggs, C. D.: Malignant tumors of synovial origin. Ann. Surg. *115:*413–426, 1942.

Brown, J. B., and Cannon, B.: The repair of surface defects of the foot. Ann. Surg. *120:*417–430, 1944.

Brown, J. B., and Fryer, M. P.: Repair of surface defects of the foot—resurfacing the foot by plastic surgery for defects such as plantar warts and traumatic, thermal and radiation lesions. J.A.M.A. *146:*628–633, 1951.

Bruce, J.: Structural anomalies of the forefoot in relation to some metatarsal disturbances. Edinburgh M. J. *4:*530–547, 1937.

Bruce, J., and Walmsley, R.: Some observations on the arches of the foot and flat-foot. Lancet *2:* 656–659, 1938.

Burman, M. S.: Epiphysitis of the proximal or pseudometatarsal epiphyses of the foot. J. Bone Joint Surg. *25:*538–540, 1933.

Busquet, P.: De l'ostéo-périostite ossifiante des métatarsiens. Rev. Chir. *17:*1065–1099, 1897.

Campbell, W. C.: Infraction of the head of the second and third metatarsal bones: report of cases. Am. J. Orthop. Surg. *15:*721–724, 1917.

Carpenter, C. C.: A safe method of applying solidified carbon dioxide. J. Bone Joint Surg. *118:*296–297, 1942.

Carpenter, C. C.: Cryotherapy for common skin diseases. J. M. Soc. New Jersey *40:*354–357, 1943.

Charache, H.: Squamous cell carcinoma of the extremities. Surg. Gynec. Obst. *68:*1002–1006, 1939.

Cleaveland, C. H.: *Causes and Cure of Diseases of the Feet.* Cincinnati, Bradley & Webb, 1862, pp. 42–111.

Cleveland, M., and Winant, E. M.: An end-result of the Keller operation. J. Bone Joint Surg. *32:*163–175, 1950.

Cokkalis, P.: Dupuytrensche Kontraktur der Palmar- und Plantaraponeurose. Deutsche Ztschr. Chir. *194:*256–258, 1925–26.

Coley, B. L., and Higinbotham, N. L.: Tumors primary in the bones of the hands and feet. Surgery *5:*112–128, 1939.

Coley, B. L., and Pierson, J. C.: Synovioma—report of fifteen cases with review of literature. Surgery *1:*113–124, 1937.

Collins, N. C., and Anspach, W. E.: Fibrosarcoma of plantar tissues. Am. J. Cancer *39:*465–470, 1940.

Converse, J. M.: Plastic repair of the extremities by non-tubulated pedicle skin flaps. J. Bone Joint Surg. *30:*163–194, 1948.

Costilhes, J.: De la rétraction de l'aponévrose palmaire (maladie de Dupuytren). Thèse. Paris, 1885.

Cotton, F. J.: Foot statics and surgery. Tr. New England Soc. *18:*181–208, 1935.

Cox, H. T.: The cleavage lines of the skin. Brit. J. Surg. *29:*234–240, 1941.

Curtis, T. B.: Pododynia: its causes and significance. Boston Med. Surg. J. *104:*316–318, 1881.

Dana, C. L.: The acro-neuroses. Functional nervous affections of the extremities. Med. Rec. New York *28:*85–87, 1885.

Davies-Colley, N.: Fibroma of plantar fascia. Trans. Path. Soc. London *45:*150, 1894.

Davis, G. F.: Cure for hallux valgus: the interdigital incision. Surg. Clin. N. Amer. *1:*651–658, 1917.

Decker, A. M., and Chamness, J. T.: Melanocarcinoma of the plantar surface of the foot—a review of twenty-five cases. Surgery *29:*731–742, 1951.

Degrais, P., and Bellot, A.: La verrue plantaire—avantages de son traitement par le radium. Presse Méd. *99:*1840, 1931.

Deutschlaender, C.: Ueber entzuendliche Mittelfussgeschwuelste. Arch. Klin. Chir. *118:*530–549, 1921.

Dickson, J. A.: Surgical treatment of intractable plantar warts. J. Bone Joint Surg. *30:*757–760, 1948.

Dickson, F. D., and Diveley, R. L.: *Functional Disorders of the Foot.* Philadelphia, J. B. Lippincott Co., 1944, pp. 21–24.

Dodd, H.: Pied forcé or march foot. Brit. J. Surg. *21:*131–144, 1933.

Doub, H. P.: Aseptic necrosis of the epiphyses and short bones—roentgen studies. J.A.M.A. *127:* 311–321, 1945.

Ducourtioux, M.: La verrue plantaire et ses traitements. Presse Méd. *58:*1116, 1950.

Dupuytren, G.: De la r'traction des doigts par suite d'une affection de l'aponévrose palmaire. Description de la maladie. Opération chirurgicale qui convient dans le cas de la clinique chirurgicale de l'Hôtel-Dieu. Clinical lecture, 1831. This lecture appears in Medical Classics, *4:*127–141, 1939.

Dupuytren, G.: *Leçons Orales de Clinique Chirurgicale Faites a l'Hôtel—Dieu de Paris.* Paris, Baillière Co., 1839, Vol. IV, pp. 473–502.

Durlacher, L.: *A Treatise on Corns, Bunions, the Diseases of Nails and the General Management of the Feet.* London, Simkin, Marshall & Co., 1845, introduction and p. 52.

Duthie, D. A., and McCallum, D. I.: Treatment of plantar warts with elastoplast and podophyllin. Brit. M. J. *2:*216–218, 1951.

DuVries, H. L.: New approach to the treatment of intractable verruca plantaris (plantar wart). J.A.M.A. *152:*1202–1203, 1953.

DuVries, H. L.: *Surgery of the Foot.* St. Louis, C. V. Mosby Co., 1959, pp. 55 and 184–196.

Editorial: Treatment of plantar warts. New Eng. J. Med. *248:*659, 1953.

Editorial: Morton's painful affection of the foot. New York Med. J. *56:*410, 1892.

Editorial: Pied forcé in soldiers. New York Med. J. *63:*783–785, 1899.

Edward, J. F.: March foot. Am. J. Roentgenol. *36:*188–193, 1936.

Elftman, H.: A cinematic study of the distribution of pressure in the human foot. Anat. Rec. *59:*481–491, 1934.

Fahey, J. J., and Bollinger, J. A.: Congenital sarcoma of the foot; case report and review of literature. A.M.A. J. Dis. Child. *86:*23–27, 1953.

Fairbank, H. A. T.: Dupuytren's contraction of plantar fascia. Proc. Roy. Soc. Med. *26:*103, 1932.

Féré, C.: Note sur la rétraction de l'aponévrose plantaire. Rev. Chir. Paris *20:*272–277, 1899.

Flavell, G.: March fracture—a series of fifteen cases from the RAF. Lancet *2:*66–69, 1943.

Freiberg, A. H.: Infraction of the second metatarsal bone—a typical injury. Surg. Gynec. Obst. *19:*191–193, 1914.

Freiberg, A. H.: Again, the operation for hallux valgus. J.A.M.A. *83:*908–911, 1924.

Freiberg, A. H.: The so-called infraction of the second metatarsal bone. J. Bone Joint Surg. *8:*257–261, 1926.

Ghormley, R. K., and Lipscomb, P. R.: The use of untubed pedicle grafts in the repair of deep defects of the foot and ankle. J. Bone Joint Surg. *26:*483–488, 1944.

Giannestras, N. J.: Shortening of the metatarsal shaft for the correction of plantar keratosis. Clin. Orthopaed. *4:*225–231, 1954.

Giannestras, N. J.: Shortening of the metatarsal shaft in the treatment of plantar keratosis. J. Bone Joint Surg. *40:*61–71, 1958.

Gibney, V. P.: The non-operative treatment of metatarsalgia. J. Nerv. Ment. Dis. *19:*589–596, 1894.

Goetzee, A. E., and Williams, H. O.: Case of Dupuytren's contracture involving hand and foot in child. Brit. J. Surg. *42:*417–420, 1955.

Goldman, S. E.: March foot, with fracture of metatarsal bone—report of case. J. Bone Joint Surg. *10:*228–230, 1928.

Goldthwait, J. E.: The anterior transverse arch of the foot: its obliteration as a cause of metatarsalgia. Boston Med. Surg. J. *131:*233–234, 1894.

Grant, Boileau J. C.: *A Method of Anatomy.* Baltimore, Williams & Wilkins Co., 1958, p. 498.

Greenberg, L.: Dupuytren's contracture of palmar and plantar fasciae. J. Bone Joint Surg. *21:* 785–788, 1939.

Gross, S. D.: *A System of Surgery.* Philadelphia, Henry C. Lea, Vol. II, pp. 1054–1055, 1872.

Grün, E. F.: Metatarsalgia. Lancet *1:*707, 1889.

Guthrie, L. G.: On a form of painful toe. Lancet *1:*628, 1892.

Haggart, G. E.: The conservative and surgical treatment of plantar warts. Surg. Clin. N. Amer. *14:*1211–1218, 1934.

Hammond, G., and Dotter, W. E.: Quadrilateral Dupuytren's contracture. Guthrie Clinic Bull. *18:*34–38, 1948–1949.

Harris, R. I., and Beath, T.: The short first metatarsal—its incidence and clinical significance. J. Bone Joint Surg. *31:*553–565, 1949.

Hoadley, A. E.: Six cases of metatarsalgia. Chicago M. Rec. *5:*32–37, 1893.

Hohmann, G.: Dupuytrensche Kontraktur an beiden Haenden und beiden Fuessen. Eine Mitteilung. Ztschr. Orthop. *73:*45–47, 1944.

Hughes, C. H.: Quoted by Mills (1888).

Jaffé, R. H.: Malignant tumors of the nail bed. Surg. Gynec. Obst. *50:*847–850, 1930.

Jansen, M.: March foot. J. Bone Joint Surg. *8:* 262–271, 1926.

Jones, F. Wood: March fracture. Lancet *2:*116, 1943.

Jones, F. Wood: *Structure and Function as Seen in the Foot.* London, Baillière, Tindall & Cox, 1949, pp. 37–43, 46–49 and 246–265.

Jones, Robert: Plantar neuralgia. (Metatarsalgia—Morton's painful affection of the foot). Liverpool Med.-Chirur. J. *27:*1–46, 1897.

Jones, Robert: Discussion on the treatment of hallux valgus and rigidus. Brit. M. J. *2:*651–656, 1924.

Jones, R., and Tubby, A. H.: Metatarsalgia or Morton's disease. Ann. Surg. *28:*297–328, 1898.

Jones, R. L.: The human foot. An experimental study of its mechanics, and the role of its muscles and ligaments in the support of the arch. Am J. Anat. *68:*1–39, 1941.

Kanavel, A. B., Koch, S. L., and Mason, M. L.: Dupuytren's contraction; with a description of the palmar fascia, a review of the literature, and a report of twenty-nine surgically treated cases. Surg. Gynec. Obst. *48:*145–190, 1929.

Kapiloff, B., and Prior, J. T.: Fibromatosis in children. Plast. Reconstr. Surg. *10:*276–282, 1952.

Kappis, M.: Die Ursache der Koehler'schen Krankheit an den Koepfchen der Mittelfussknochen. Beitr. Klin. Chir. *129:*61–70, 1923.

Kelikian, H., Clayton, L., and Loseff, H.: Surgical syndactylia of the toes. Clin. Orthopaed. *19:*208–231, 1961.

Kile, R. L.: How communicable are warts? J.A.M.A. *162:*1222–1224, 1956.

King, L. S.: Pathology of Morton's metatarsalgia. Am. J. Clin. Path. *16:*124, 1946.

Kingsley, D. M.: March fractures of the metatarsals—multiple fractures involving five or more bones. 1964. Unpublished paper.

Kingsley, D. M.: Multiple march fractures of a single metatarsal bone. 1964. Unpublished paper.

Kinzel, H.: Dupuytrensche Kontraktur an Hand und Fuss. Inaugural-Dissertation, Breslau, 1927.

Kirchner, A.: Die Aetiologie der indirecten Metatarsalfracturen. Arch. Klin. Chir. *77:*241–267, 1905.

Klossner, A. R.: Dupuytrensche Kontraktur bei derselben Persongleichzeitig in beiden Haenden und im Linken Fuss. Acta Soc. Med. Fenn. Duodecim. *34:*1, 1944.

Koehler, A.: Typical disease of the second metatarsophalangeal joint. Amer. J. Roentgenol *10:*705–710 1923

Koehler, A.: *Borderlands of the Normal and Early Pathologic in Skeletal Roentgenology.* English translation, J. T. Case. New York, Grune & Stratton, 1956.

Kulchar, G. V.: Benign and malignant tumors of the foot. J.A.M.A. *124:*761–766, 1944.

Lake, N. C.: *The Foot.* London, Baillière, Tindall & Cox, 1952, p. 272.

Ledderhose, G.: Die Aetiologie der Fasciitis palmaris (Dupuytrensche Kontraktur). München. Med. Wchnschr. *67:*1254–1256, 1920.

Lewin, P.: Juvenile deforming metatarsophalangeal osteochondritis. J.A.M.A. *81:*189–192, 1923.

Lewin, P.: *The Foot and the Ankle.* Second edition. Philadelphia, Lea & Febiger,1941, p. 161.

Loison, E.: Les fractures du métatarse—par causes indirectes, ou à distance. Rev. d'Orthop. *1:* 342–360, 1900.

Lovett, R.: The occurrence of painful affections of the feet among trained nurses. Am. Med. *6:*15–20, 1903.

Lund, M.: Dupuytren's contracture and epilepsy. Acta Psychiat. Neurol. *16:*465–492, 1941.

Lyell, A., and Miles, J. A. R.: The Myrmecia—a study of inclusion bodies in warts. Brit. M. J. *1:*912–915, 1951.

McElvenny, R. T.: The etiology and surgical treatment of intractable pain about the fourth metatarsophalangeal joint. (Morton's toe). J. Bone Joint Surg. *25:*675–679, 1943.

McKeever, D. C.: Surgical approach for neuroma of plantar digital nerve (Morton's metatarsalgia). J. Bone Joint Surg. *34:*490, 1952.

McLaughlin, C. R.: Plantar warts—a plea for rational treatment. Lancet *1:*168–169, 1948.

Madelung, O. W.: Ueber eine der Dupuytren'schen Palmarkontraktur entsprechende Erkrangung der Planta. Cbl. Chir. *13:*758, 1886.

Maffei: Métatarsalgie ou maladie de Morton. Rev. d'Orthop. *11:*638–659, 1924.

Marks, J. H., and Franseen, C. C.: Radiation treatment of plantar warts. New Eng. J. Med. *223:*851–853, 1940.

Martin, A.: Inflammation periostito-arthritique du pied à la suite des marches. Arch. Med. Pharm. Mil. *28:*336–343, 1891.

Maseritz, I. H.: March foot associated with undescribed changes of the internal cuneiform and metatarsal bones. Arch. Surg. *32:*49–64, 1936.

Mason, E.: A case of neuralgia of the second metatarsophalangeal articulation—cured by resection of the joint. Am. J. Med. Sci. *74:*445–446, 1877.

Mason, M. L.: Carcinoma of the hands and feet. Surgery *5:*27–46, 1939.

Mau, C.: Eine Operation des kontrakten Spreizfusses. Zbl. Chir. *67:*667–670, 1940.

Meisenbach, R. O.: Painful anterior arch of the foot: an operation for its relief by means of raising the arch. Am. J. Orthop. Surg. *14:*206–211, 1916.

Meiser: Die Brueche der Mittelfussknochen als Ursache der Fuss—oder Marschgeswulst. Fortschr. Geb. Roentgenstr. *4:*105–112, 1901.

Meyerding, H. W.: Multiple metatarsal fractures associated with osteogenic sarcoma. J.A.M.A. *124:*228–230, 1944.

Meyerding, H. W., and Pollock, G. A.: March fracture. Surg., Gynec. Obst. *67:*234–248, 1938.

Meyerding, H. W., and Shellito, J. G.: Dupuytren's contracture of the foot. J. Internat. Coll. Surgeons *11:*595–603, 1948.

Mills, C. K.: Pain in the feet. J. Nerv. Ment. Dis. *13:*3–20, 1888.

Mitchell, W.: On certain painful affections of the feet. Philad. Med. Times *3:*81–82, 1872; *3:* 113–115, 1872.

Mitchell, W.: On a rare vaso-motor neurosis of the extremities, and on the maladies with which it may be confounded. Am. J. Med. Sci. *76:* 17–36, 1878.

Momburg, F.: Die Enstehungsursache der Fussgeschwulst. Deutsche Ztschr. Chir. *73:*425–437, 1904.

Monteith, W. B. R.: A case of march foot (pied forcé) with signs of old and recent injury. Brit. J. Surg. *21:*708, 1934.

Montgomery, A. H., and Montgomery, R. M.: Mosaic wart: an unusual type of plantar wart. New York J. Med. *37:*1978, 1937.

Montgomery, R. M., and Montgomery, A. H.:

Common hyperkeratotic lesions of the foot. J.A.M.A. *124*:756–761, 1944.

Morris, Henry H.: *Anatomy of the Joints of Man.* London, J. & A. Churchill, 1879, p. 401.

Morton, D. J.: Evolution of the longitudinal arch of the human foot. J. Bone Joint Surg. *22*:88–89 and conclusion, 1924.

Morton, D. J.: Metatarsus atavicus—the identification of a distinctive type of foot disorder. J. Bone Joint Surg. *9*:36, 1927.

Morton, D. J.: Hypermobility of the first metatarsal bone: the interlinking factor between metatarsalgia and longitudinal arch strains. J. Bone Joint Surg. *10*:196, 1928.

Morton, D. J.: Structural factors in static disorders of the foot. Am. J. Surg. *9*:315–328, 1930.

Morton, D. J.: *The Human Foot.* New York, Columbia University Press, 1935, pp. 179–195.

Morton, D. J.: Foot disorders in general practice. J.A.M.A. *109*:1112–1119, 1937.

Morton, D. J.: Functional disorders of the feet and their treatment. New York J. Med. *42*:2119–2123, 1942.

Morton, D. J.: Biomechanics of the human foot. Instructional Course Lectures American Academy of Orthopaedic Surgeons, Ann Arbor, pp. 92–104, 1944.

Morton, D. J.: *Human Locomotion and Body Form.* Baltimore, Williams & Wilkins Co., 1952, pp. 46–113.

Morton, T. G.: A peculiar and painful affection of the fourth metatarsophalangeal articulation. Am. J. Med. Sci. *71*:35–45, 1876.

Morton, T. G.: The application of the x-rays to the diagnosis of Morton's painful affection of the foot, or metatarsalgia. Internat. Med. Mag. *5*:322–324, 1897.

Morton, T. S. K.: Metatarsalgia (Morton's painful affection of the foot), with an account of six cases cured by operation. Ann. Surg. *17*:680–699, 1893.

Mouchet, A.: Metatarsal epiphysitis. J. Bone Joint Surg. *11*:87–93, 1929.

Moutier, G.: L'épiphysite métatarsienne. Rev. Orthop. *12*:235–253, 1925.

Mulder, J. D.: The causative mechanism in Morton's metatarsalgia. J. Bone Joint Surg. *33*: 94–95, 1951.

Nion: Mitteilungen aus der Roentgenabteilung—(ZurStatistik der Mittelfussknochenbrueche). Deutsche Mil.-Ärztl. Ztschr. *32*:200–201, 1903.

Nissen, K. I.: Plantar digital neuritis. Morton's metatarsalgia. J. Bone Joint Surg. *30*:84–94, 1948.

Nissen, K. I.: Correspondence (Morton's metatarsalgia). J. Bone Joint Surg. *33*:293–294, 1951.

Nissen, K. I.: Morton's metatarsalgia—resection of a plantar digital nerve. Operat. Surg. *5*:320–323, 1957.

Osborne, E. D., and Putnam, E. D.: The treatment of warts. Radiology *16*:340–345, 1931.

Oughterson, A. W., and Tennant, R.: Angiomatous tumors of the hands and feet. Surgery *5*:73–100, 1939.

Pack, G. T.: Symposium: Tumors of the hands and feet; Introduction. Surgery *5*:1–26, 1939.

Pack, G. T., and Adair, F. E.: Subungual melanoma—the differential diagnosis of tumors of the nail bed. Surgery *5*:47–72, 1939.

Painter, C. F.: Infraction of the second metatarsal head. Boston Med. Surg. J. *184*:533–537, 1921.

Pangman, W. J., and Gurdin, M.: The treatment of complicated plantar lesions. Plast. Reconstr. Surg. *5*:516–519, 1950.

Panner, H. J.: A peculiar characteristic metatarsal disease. Acta Radiol. *1*:319, 1921–1922.

Pascher, F., and Sims, C. F.: Basal cell epitheliomas of the sole; a report of two cases. A.M.A. Arch. Dermat. Syph., *69*:475–481, 1954.

Pauzat, J. E.: De la périostite ostéoplasique des métatarsiens à la suite des marches. Arch. Méd. Pharm. Mil. *10*:337–353, 1887.

Peck, J. L.: *Dress and Care of the Feet.* New York, S. R. Wells, 1871, pp. 54–86.

Peckham, F. E.: General remarks on painful affections of the feet. Trans. Am. Orthop. Assoc. *14*:201–210, 1901.

Pedersen, H. E., and Day, A. J.: Dupuytren's disease of foot. J.A.M.A. *154*:33–35, 1954.

Pendergrass, E. P., and Hodes, P. J.: Roentgen irradiation in the treatment of inflammations. Amer. J. Roentgenol. *45*:74–106, 1941.

Pickren, J. W., and Stevenson, T. W., Jr.: Fibromatosis of the plantar warts. Cancer *4*:846–856, 1951.

Pipkin, J. L., Lehmann, C. F., and Ressmann, A.: The treatment of plantar warts by single dose method of roentgen ray. South. M. J. *42*:193–202, 1949.

Pirie, A. H.: March fractures. Lancet *2*:45–46, 1917.

Pollosson, A.: De la métatarsalgie antérieure. La Province Méd. *6*:1–3, 1889. See also Lancet *1*:436; 553, 1889.

Popp, W. C., and Olds, J. W.: Roentgen treatment of plantar warts. Radiology *31*:218–219, 1938.

Poulet, A.: De l'ostéopériostite rhumastismale des métatarsients au 3e régiment de Zouaves. Arch. Méd. Pharm. Mil. *12*:245–258, 1888.

Powers, H.: Dupuytren's contracture one hundred years after Dupuytren: its interpretation. J. Nerv. Ment. Dis. *80*:386–409, 1934.

Randell, Henry Kemp: *Elements of Osteology;* or the minute anatomy of the bones, intended for the use of students. London, S. Highley & Effingham Wilson, 1831, p. 206.

Reeves, H. A.: Remarks on the contraction of the palmar and plantar fasciae. Brit. M. J. *2*:1049, 1881.

Reeves, R. J., and Jackson, M. T.: Roentgen therapy of plantar warts. Am. J. Roentgenol. *76*: 977–978, 1956.

Ringertz, N., and Unander-Scharin, L.: Morton's disease—a clinical and patho-anatomical study. Acta Orthop. Scandinav. *19*:327–348, 1950.

Robinson, D. W.: Treatment of complications of plantar warts. Arch. Surg. *66*:434–439, 1953.

Roughton, E.: "Anterior metatarsalgia": its nature and treatment. Lancet *1*:553, 1889.

Rouillard, J., and Schwob, R. A.: Rétraction des aponévroses palmaires et plantaires; coexistence de gros troubles sensitifs du type syringomyélique. Bull. Mém. Soc. Méd. Hôp. Paris *55:*712–717, 1931.

Roux, C.: Aux pieds sensibles. Rev. Méd. Suisse Rom. *40:*62–83, 1920.

Rutledge, B. A., and Green, A. L.: Surgical treatment of plantar corns. U.S. Armed Forces M. J. *8:*219–221, 1957.

Schreiner, B. F., and Wehr, W. H.: Primary malignant tumors of the foot—a report of thirty-seven cases. Radiology *21:*513–521, 1933.

Schroeder, J. H.: Sarcoma (?) of thigh, with secondary sarcoma (?) of inguinal region, liver and lungs; recovery after intensive deep roentgen irradiation. J.A.M.A. *120:*23–25, 1923.

Schulte: Die sogennante Fussgeschwulst. Arch. Klin. Chir. *55:*872–892, 1897.

Shaw, M. H.: Treatment of chronic ulceration after irradiation of plantar wart. Brit. M. J. *1:*11, 1948.

Sirbu, A. B., and Palmar, A. M.: March fracture—a report of fifteen cases. Calif. West. Med. *57:* 123–127, 1942.

Skillern, P. G., Jr.: Eggshell fracture of head of metatarsal. Ann. Surg. *61:*371–372, 1915.

Skoog, T.: Dupuytren's contraction, with special reference to aetiology and improved surgical treatment; its occurrence in epileptics; note on knuckle-pads. Acta Chir. Scand. *96:*1–190, 1948.

Sloane, D., and Sloane, M. F.: March foot. Am. J. Surg. *31:*167–169, 1936.

Smillie, I. S.: Freiberg's infraction (Koehler's second disease). J. Bone Joint Surg. *37:*580, 1955.

Souza-Leite: Rétraction de l'aponévrose palmaire; —de l'aponévrose plantaire. —Rhumatisme articulaire aigu. —Affection cardiaque. Progr. Méd. *4:*816–818, 1886.

Specklin, P., and Stoeber, R.: Rétraction des aponévroses palmaires et plantaires avec névralgies; guérison par les radiations. Presse Méd. *30:*743–745, 1922.

Speed, J. S., and Blake, T. H.: March foot. J. Bone Joint Surg. *15:*372–382, 1933.

Stechow: Fussoeden und Roentgenstrahlen. Deutsche Mil.-Ärztl. Ztschr. *16:*465–471, 1897.

Stern, W. F.: Morton's painful disease of the toes. Amer. Med. *7:*221–225. 1904.

Straus, F. H.: Marching fractures of metatarsal bones—with a report of the pathology. Surg. Gynec. Obst. *54:*581–584, 1932 .

Strauss, M. J., Bunting, H., and Melnick, J. L.: Preliminary and short reports—eosinophilic inclusion bodies and cytoplasmic masses in verrucae. J. Invest. Dermat. *17:*209–211, 1951.

Sulkin, S. E., and Harford, C. G.: The laboratory diagnosis of virus diseases. J.A.M.A. *122:*646, 1943.

Thiele: Ueber Frakturen der Metatarsal-knochen durch indirekte Gewalt (die Ursache der sogenannten Fussgeschwulst). Deutsche Med. Wchnschr. *15:*158–161, 1899.

Trethowan, W. H.: Simple fractures of the upper and lower limbs. *In* Jones, R. (ed.): *Orthopaedic Surgery of Injuries.* 1921, Vol. I, pp. 88–89.

Tubby, A. H.: *Deformities Including Diseases of the Bones and Joints.* London, MacMillan & Co., 1912, p. 725.

Van Demark, R. E., and McCarthy, P. V.: March fracture. Radiology *46:*496–501, 1946.

Venturi, R.: Metatarsalgia di Morton. Chir. Org. Mov. *49:*327–339, 1960.

Wagner, A.: Isolated aseptic necrosis in the epiphysis of the first metatarsal bone. Acta Radiol. *11:*80–87, 1930.

Watson-Jones, R.: *Fractures and other Bone and Joints Injuries.* Baltimore, Williams & Wilkins Co., 1941, pp. 163–165 and 635–636.

Watson-Jones, R.: *Fractures and Joint Injuries.* Baltimore, Williams & Wilkins Co., 1951, Vol. 1, pp. 343–350.

Weisbach: Die sogenannte Fussgeschwulst (Syndesmitis metatarsea) des Infanteristen. Deutsche Mil.-Ärztl. Ztschr. *6:*551, 1877.

Whitfield, A.: On development of callosities, corns and warts. Brit. J. Derm. *44:*580–585, 1932.

Whitman, R.: Observations on Morton's painful affection of the fourth metatarso-phalangeal articulation and similar affections of the metatarsal region that may be included with it under the term anterior metatarsalgia. Trans. Amer. Orthop. Assoc., *11:*34–53, 1898.

Whitman, R.: *A Treatise on Orthopedic Surgery.* Philadelphia, Lea Brothers & Co., 1907, pp. 721–730.

Wile, U. J., and Kingery, L. B.: The etiology of common warts. J.A.M.A. *73:*970–973, 1919.

Winkler, H., Feltner, J. B., and Kimmelstiel, P.: Morton metatarsalgia. J. Bone Joint Surg. *30:*496–500, 1948.

Woodruff, C. E.: Incomplete luxations of the metatarsophalangeal articulations. Med. Rec. *1:*61–62, 1890.

Zarzecki, C. A.: Fibrosarcoma of the extremities—a review of thirty-eight cases. North Carolina M. J. *10:*605–607, 1949.

Zeitlin, A.: Some reflections on the etiology of Koehler's disease. Radiology *24:*360–363, 1935.

Zeitlin, A. A., and Odessky, I. N.: Zur Differential diagnose Metatarsafraktur oder morbus Deutschlaender. Arch. Orthop. u. Unfall-Chir. *34:*653–656, 1934.

Zwick, K. G.: Hygionesis of warts disappearing without topical medication. Arch. Derm. Syph. *25:*508–521, 1932.

Chapter Seventeen

SURGICAL COMPLICATIONS

In the present chapter if we seem to overstress hazards connected with hallux valgus surgery and say very little about those that accompany operations for other derangements of the forefoot, it is because attempts to correct the deformity of the great toe have been far more frequent and have entailed numerous complications, some of which have found their way into the literature. Published accounts of mishaps occurring in connection with the surgical treatment of hammered and clawed toes, plantar incarceration of the metatarsal heads, and corns or calluses have been extremely scarce. This does not mean they do not occur. They do. It is only that they have not been reported—not as often as complications of hallux valgus surgery.

Riedel (1886) started a healthy movement in recording a disabling type of metatarsalgia that followed Heuter resection of the first metatarsal head; he also registered his misgivings about the procedure he subsequently improvised, which we now call Keller resection. With the passing of years, the tradition of honest appraisal of one's results appears to have vanished. Surgeons of more recent vintage tend to minimize complications following their operations and criticize methods other than the one they favor. Not long ago a surgeon, whose name is identified with one of the operations for hallux valgus, was asked if he had ever performed Keller resection, which he so severely criticized. The answer was negative. The reason given was that it was "unphysiological"—a favored word of condemnation that has never been fully explained.

In an earlier chapter we said that preoperative treatment began while the operation was being performed. We may add that complications that manifest themselves after the operation have their inception earlier—during surgery or even before, when the patient is first examined. Judicious assessment of the patient, adequate preoperative preparation, selection of suitable procedure, and proper execution go long ways in preventing postoperative complications and some catastrophies.

Circulatory hazards. In cases of infected bunions, Aston Key (1836) warned against "opening the abscess, and discharging its contents. . . . I have known," he wrote, "gangrene of the foot, and death, ensue from opening an inflamed suppurating bunion; and in three cases, exfoliation of bones, with a most tedious and painful suppuration of the surrounding structure." Blodgett (1880) reported a case of gangrene of the foot following decapitation of the first metatarsal for hallux valgus. The patient was a 75 year old man. An Esmarch constrictor had been used during surgery. Gangrene of the foot and the leg followed, and the patient died 11 days after the operation. The surgeon who had operated this case ascribed the disaster to the use of a tourniquet. No mention was made of the fact that the patient might have had arteriosclerosis, diabetes, or arthritis that had not been detected before the operation.

A few years back we were called to see a young woman who was afflicted with advanced rheumatoid arthritis. She had undergone surgery for correction of bilateral hallux valgus and clawtoes. The operation, we were told, consisted of the following: bilateral osteotomy of the first metatarsal bones, Keller resection on both great toes, bilateral partial proximal phalangectomy of the lesser toes, manual correction of knuckled interphalangeal joints, and medullary pin fixation of all toes. Postoperatively the feet had been encased in circular casts. When the surgeon removed the casts he found both great toes and the third digit on one foot gangrenous. A pneumatic tourniquet had been used during surgery, which may have contributed to the mishap. But in this age group, in the absence of arteriosclerosis, one can hardly blame temporary constriction. A more plausible explanation would be that the vessels of the great toes and their metatarsals were damaged in the course of dissection and retraction necessitated by the extensive surgery. Vigorous manual correction of the knuckled, mummified lesser toe—which also became gangrenous —may have injured its vessels (Fig. 17–1).

In longstanding rheumatoid arthritis with severe deformity and stiffness of the toes, one must suppose that plantar digital vessels have undergone adaptive shortening. One also anticipates some shrinkage or constriction of these vessels due to the fibrosis of the surrounding tissues and immobility of the toe. Contracted, scarbound small digital vessels cannot tolerate stretching. One may draw an analogy between the type of deformed toe described and a knee that has been acutely flexed and has remained fixed in that position for a number of years. Many of us remember the days when such a knee was forcibly extended at the risk of rupturing the popliteal artery.

In fixed digital deformities due to inveterate rheumatoid disease, one should avoid overzealous correction of deformed toes either manually or surgically. It is best not to tamper with the knuckled interphalangeal joint of the toe and obtain a measure of flexibility at the metatarsophalangeal articulation by resecting the distal third of the corresponding metatarsal bone. Hallux valgus of rheumatoid arthritis is also treated better by decapitation of the first metatarsal than by operations that require extensive dissection and retraction. No muscles insert into the first metatarsal head; one can resect this portion of the bone with minimum dissection and retraction. The same holds true of the distal extremities of the lateral metatarsal bones.

A tourniquet should not be used on patients who are known to be diabetic, arteriosclerotic, or are too old. Not long ago, almost three quarters of a century after Blodgett's (1880) report, we were told of an elderly man who had both his feet operated on for hallux valgus. During surgery, a tourniquet had been applied on one leg only. On the side that had not been subjected to constriction, the surgical wound healed with primary intention. The skin flap on the other side sloughed, and infection intervened and involved the first metatarsal bone. Even disarticulation of the great toe at the tarsometatarsal junction did not avail; the limb had to be amputated at a higher level—through the leg (Fig. 17–2).

Skin slough. Necrosis of the skin is perhaps the most common complication of hallux valgus surgery. It is the main cause of delayed wound healing and infection. The earlier semilunar incisions of Weir (1897), Mayo (1908), or Silver (1923) necessitated extensive undermining. The skin at the highest point of the curve became blue and then black. Before the advent of toe extension and wire fixation, the hallux receded after Keller resection; the skin over the medial side of the joint puckered into a deep dorsoplantar fold and eventually sloughed. Postoperative splinting with a tongue depressor has also caused an untold number of skin necroses.

McBride (1935) recorded three cases of skin slough after his operations; all three patients were past 60 years of age; they had been operated on with the aid of local anesthesia. McBride considered the mishap as a "circulatory complication." Bade (1940) blamed infiltration anesthesia as a cause of skin slough and delayed wound healing. Local infiltration, Bade contended, compromised the viability of the skin over the first metatarsophalangeal joint and predisposed to infection. He argued that the skin over this joint was poorly nourished and local infiltration depressed its viability even more.

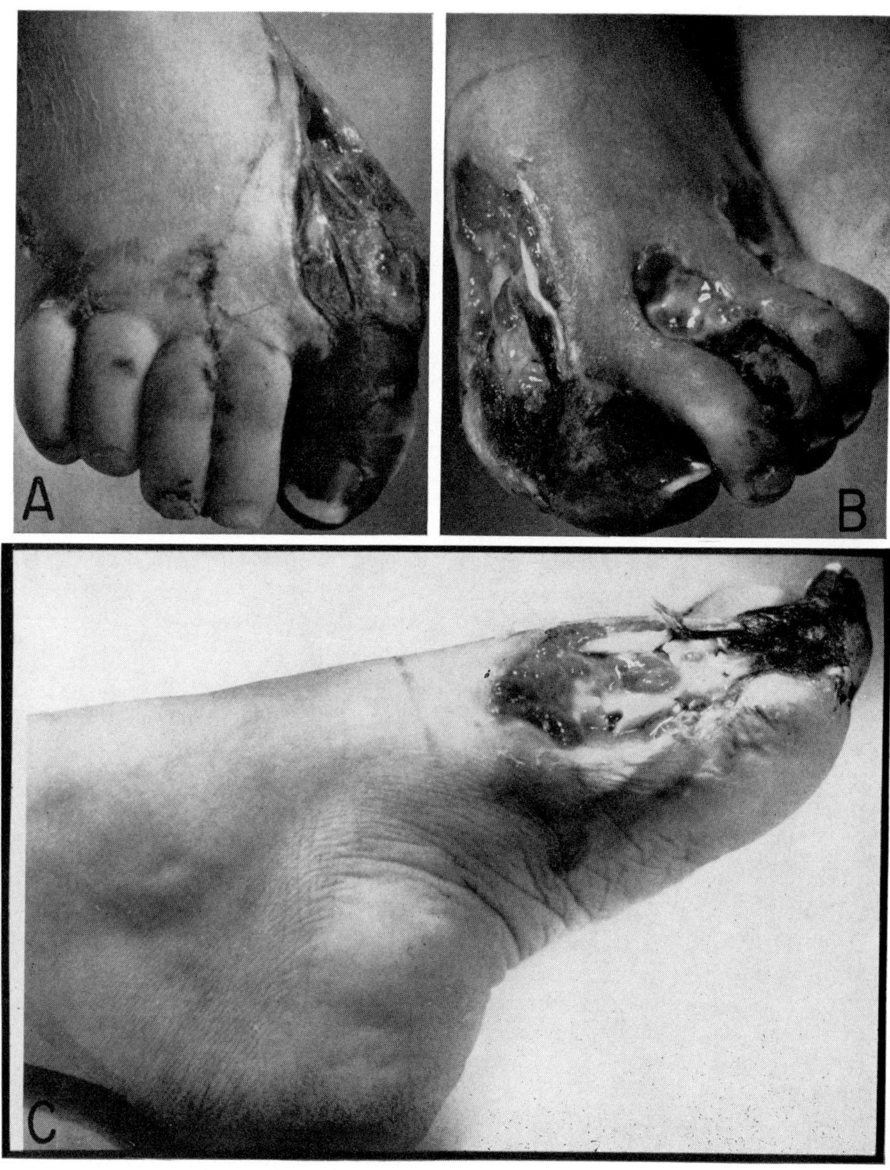

Figure 17–1. Gangrene of the toes following surgery in a case of advanced rheumatoid arthritis. *A,* Dorsal view of the right forefoot. *B,* Dorsal view of the left forefoot. *C,* Left foot seen from the medial aspect. Note the line of osteotomy of the first metatarsal.

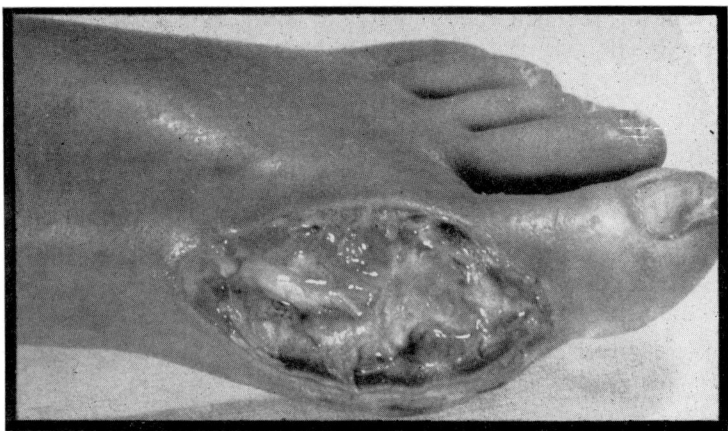

Figure 17–2. Necrosis of the skin following surgery for correction of hallux valgus.

Lapidus (1960) reported skin slough following his modification of Silver's operation. "In two cases," Lapidus wrote, "there was pressure necrosis of soft tissues over the bunion; in one of these . . . a satisfactory result and complete healing were obtained four months after the operation. The second case subsequently developed involvement of the bone of the base of the proximal phalanx of one big toe that later required resection of the Keller-Brandes type. The postoperative disability lasted on and off for about 1 year, and the final result after the Keller-Brandes operation on one foot was considered to be unsatisfactory by our standards."

Infiltration anesthesia may at times be indicated in forefoot surgery. It should be avoided when there is any question of sluggish circulation. The risk of circulatory embarrassment of the toes is greater if epinephrine has been added to procaine. In older individuals, curved incisions and extensive undermining or attenuation of the skin should also be avoided. If the integument over the medial aspect of the first metatarsophalangeal joint appears parchment-thin —precarious—one should approach this articulation through an incision between the bases of the two medial toes, where there is better circulation.

In most instances the area of skin necrosis after reconstructive surgery of the forefoot is small. Weekly application of Unna's paste boot will usually help denuded areas to epithelialize. One may have to undermine the skin edges and approximate them by secondary sutures. Larger defects may require grafting. Deeper wounds usually lead to involvement of the underlying skeletal elements, in which instance the infected bone has to be resected.

Infections. Skin slough invariably leads to infection. Severe infections after forefoot surgery are comparatively rare these days; they have been recorded in the past. Zacharie (1860) condemned the use of a penknife in paring corns and spoke of "the most appalling spasms, convulsions, and lockjaw. . . ." Both Reverdin (1881) and Riedel (1886) reported suppuration after hallux valgus surgery, but did not say what caused it. There have been sporadic remarks about rough handling of tissues, the use of coarse suture materials, in particular chromicized catgut, and constricting stitches. More often the blame is placed on: laked blood, an infected bursa, a devitalized fascial flap, and foreign body inserts.

Laked blood. As a cause of infection, laked blood has long been recognized. When a pneumatic tourniquet is used for hemostasis, it is good practice to reduce pressure completely at the completion of the main reconstructive work and ligate or cauterize the bleeders before closing the skin. Too much reliance is being placed on pressure bandages to control postoperative bleeding. Hematoma not only invites infection but also causes tension, pain, and skin slough.

Infected bursa. The bursa on the

medial aspect of the first metatarsophalangeal joint has often been blamed for infection following hallux valgus surgery. Payr (1894) promulgated the concept that, in about 10 per cent of cases, the bursa communicated with the joint cavity. Subsequently it was deemed dangerous to open the bursa for fear of introducing infection into the articular cavity. Robert Jones (1924) wrote: "We not uncommonly find suppurating joints due entirely to the fact that the surgeon has attempted a reconstructive operation during the inflammatory stage of the bursa. This condition is very apt to occur, and it is essential to allow an interval of a few weeks to pass between the recovery of the bursa and the operative attack."

We learn from Bade (1940) that the question of the bursa as a source of infection was debated in Germany. On the contention by Weimer that wound infections after surgery for hallux valgus were caused by bacteria contained in the inflamed bursa, Pick had cultured the fluid from clinically inflamed—swollen, red, tender— bursae. Pick obtained no growth, except in three cases that showed a few cocci; he ascribed these to secondary contamination. After surveying Weimer's and Pick's findings, Bade commented: "We are of the opinion that the surgeon is to be blamed for poor healing after hallux valgus operations and not the bursa which supposedly contains bacteria—obviously there are bacteria in the bursa if there is suppuration. In such a case one must not operate. But if the skin is intact, then the bursa is sterile. . . ."

The devitalized fascial flap. As a cause of infection resulting in persistent drainage after hallux valgus surgery, the devitalized fascial flap has not been sufficiently emphasized. The capsulobursal flap of Mayo (1908), or Silver's (1923) triangular flap, was detached proximally where most arterial twigs penetrated it and run toward the tip of the great toe. The flap was left attached distally to the base of the proximal phalanx, from which site it could hardly be expected to receive adequate nutrient supply. To make matters worse, in these operations the distally pedicled flap was sutured over or imbricated.

Foreign material inserts. As causes of infection, foreign material inserts have also been recorded. Infection at times follows pin tracks, which have come into practice of late in connection with Keller's operation and osteotomy of the first metatarsals. Screws, staples, or compression clamps utilized for arthrodesis of the first metatarsophalangeal joint may at times be responsible for infection. Seiffert (1953) described a method of arthroplasty of the first metatarsophalangeal joint, covering the end of the bones with nylon. In a number of cases, 6 to 8 weeks after surgery, infection became manifest, necessitating secondary operation removal of the interposed nylon.

Joint stiffness. Infection often leads to stiffness of the joints. One of the four patients Riedel (1886) operated on, resecting the medial eminence and the base of the proximal phalanx, became infected and ended with a completely stiff first metatarsophalangeal joint. The arthroplastic resections of Mayo (1908), Singley (1913), and others have also been followed by this complication. Joint stiffness is more likely to occur when the base of the proximal phalanx or the head of the first metatarsal is resected through cancellous bone, which has great proliferative power, especially in young people. Operations that require opening of the joint are more likely to be followed by joint stiffness than extra-articular procedures.

Occasionally the infected joint goes into solid ankylosis, with the toe in functional position, as in the case reported by McKeever (1952), in which instance it should be regarded as a salutary event. More commonly, fusion is incomplete and painful or the toe has become fixed in a position incompatible with walking or wearing shoes. Fixed plantar incarceration of the metatarsal heads and loss of resilience at the metatarsophalangeal joints are also known to occur incident to prolonged immobilization necessitated by delayed osteosynthesis following osteotomy of the first metatarsal or attempted fusion of the

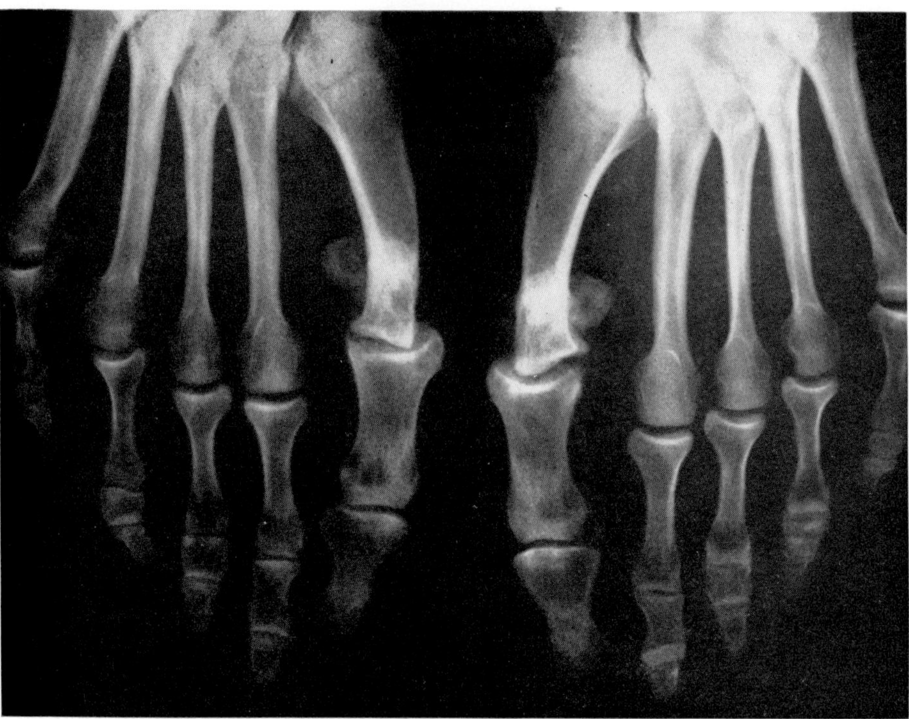

Figure 17–3. Roentgenograms of forefeet that had been operated on employing decapitation of the first metatarsals. Note the incongruity of the articular surface of first metatarsal stumps.

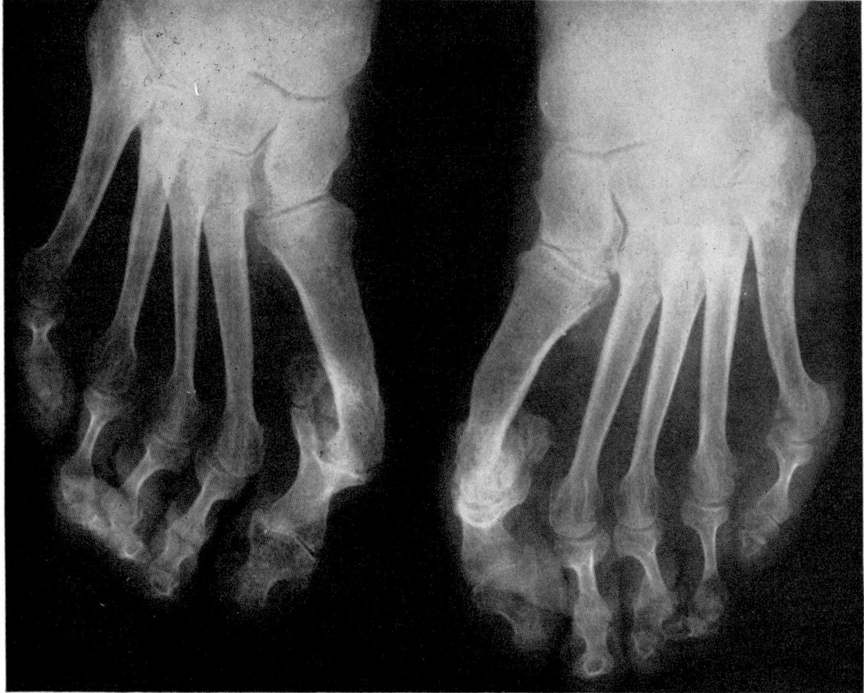

Figure 17–4. Bony proliferation after Keller's resection. The proximal phalanx of each great toe had obviously been resected through the cancellous base instead of the less reactive tubular shaft.

innermost cuneometatarsal articulation.

Painful stiffness of the first metatarsophalangeal joint is best treated by Keller's resection or fusion. The choice depends on the presence or absence of metatarsalgia. Fusion of the first metatarsophalangeal joint is preferred when metatarsalgia is unbearable. Rigidly incarcerated distal extremities of the outer metatarsal bones are resected and each

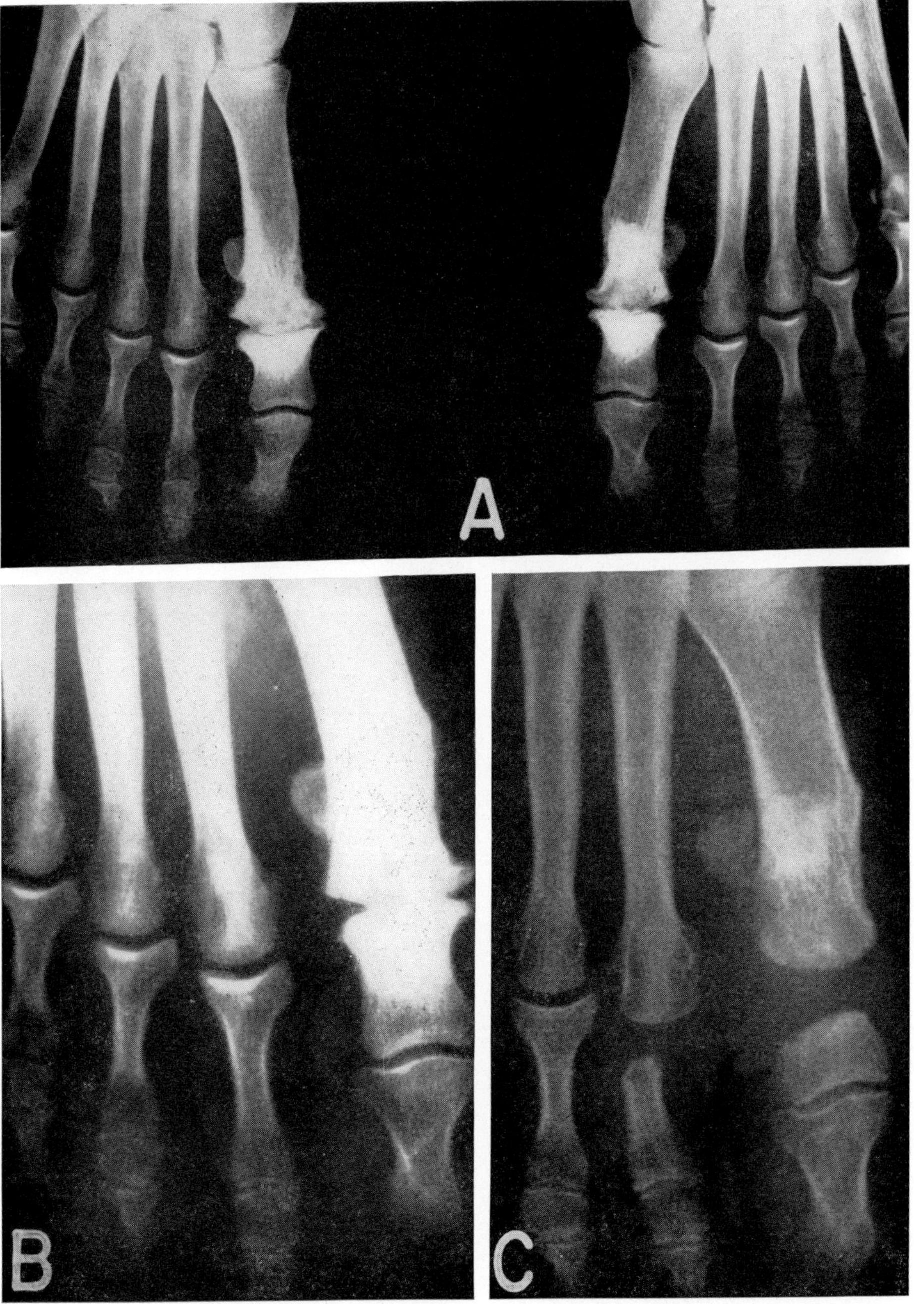

Figure 17–5. Woman, 47 years of age, with stiff great toes and inability to wear shoes even with Cuban heels. Previous surgery: bilateral Keller resection. Secondary surgery: resection of more bone from the remaining stumps of the proximal phalanges of the great toe, partial proximal phalangectomy of the second toe, and syndactylia of the second and third toes. *A,* Roentgenogram of both feet when first seen. *B,* Left foot, before resection of more bone from the remainder of the proximal phalanx. *C,* The same after resection.

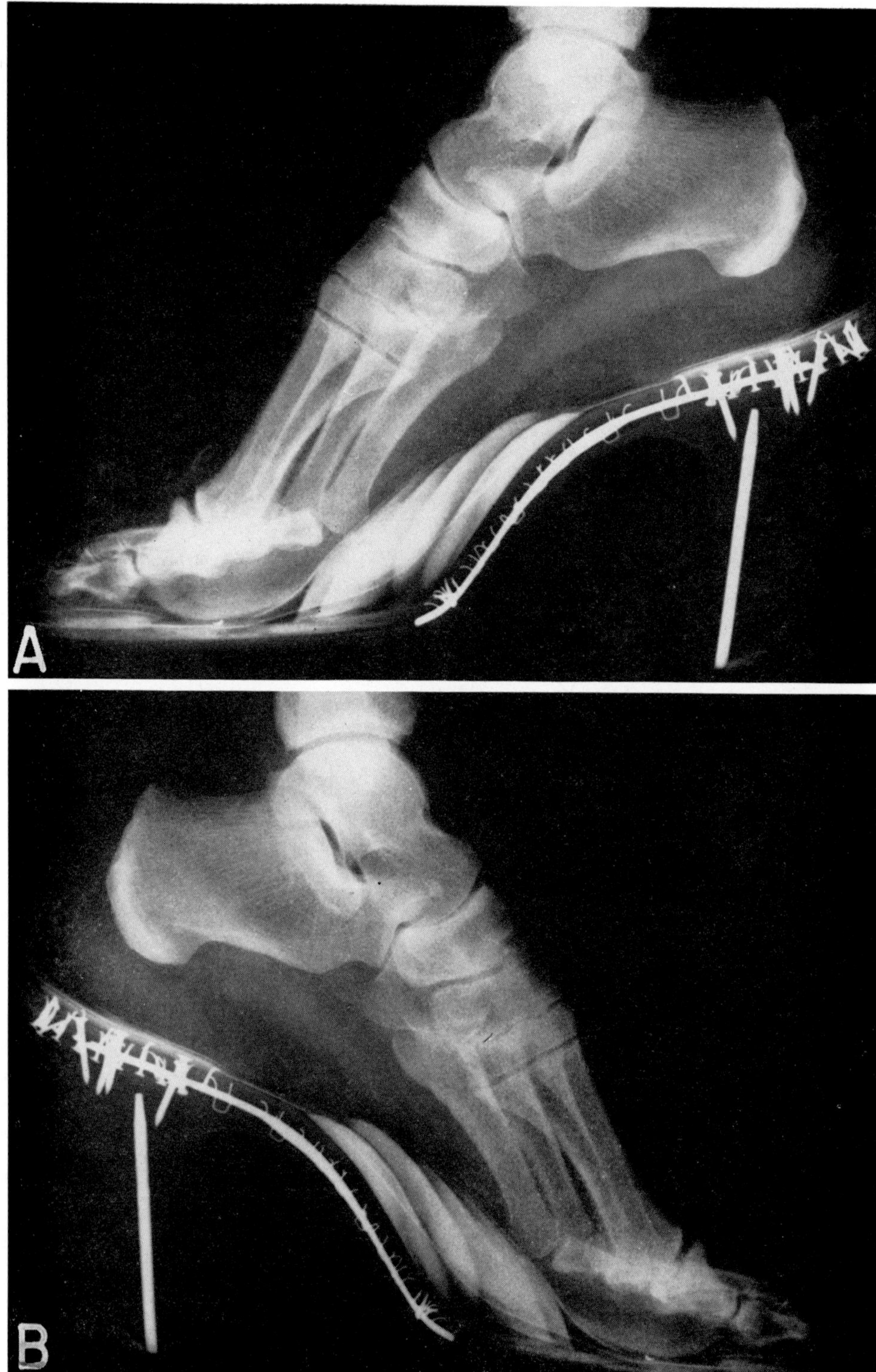

Figure 17–6. The same case as in Figure 17–5. Patient is wearing high-heeled shoes. *A,* Right foot. *B,* Left foot.

pair of adjacent toes syndactylized. In the absence of metatarsalgia, stiffness following Keller's resection is treated by resecting more bone from the stump of the proximal phalanx of the great toe (Figs. 17–3 to 17–13).

Weakened propulsive power of the great toe. Rogers and Joplin (1947) stated that after Keller's resection the propulsive power of the great toe was diminished. Writing alone, Joplin (1950) had this to say: "The reconstructive push-off mechanism either appeared weaker after operation than before, or was unchanged in eighty-nine percent of the cases; this condition is due to weakness of the flexor mechanism of the great toe. . . ."

The fallacy of such criticism lies in the fact that an operation that is—or should be—reserved for older patients is judged by standards of muscle power and function of young robust individuals or of unshod natives. In civilized adults, accustomed to wearing prefabricated footwear with unyielding material and walking on smooth hard surfaces, the "flexor mechanism of the great toe" hardly matters. Moreover, the age group subjected to Keller's resection—mainly because of arthritis of the first metatarsophalangeal joint—have long lost their

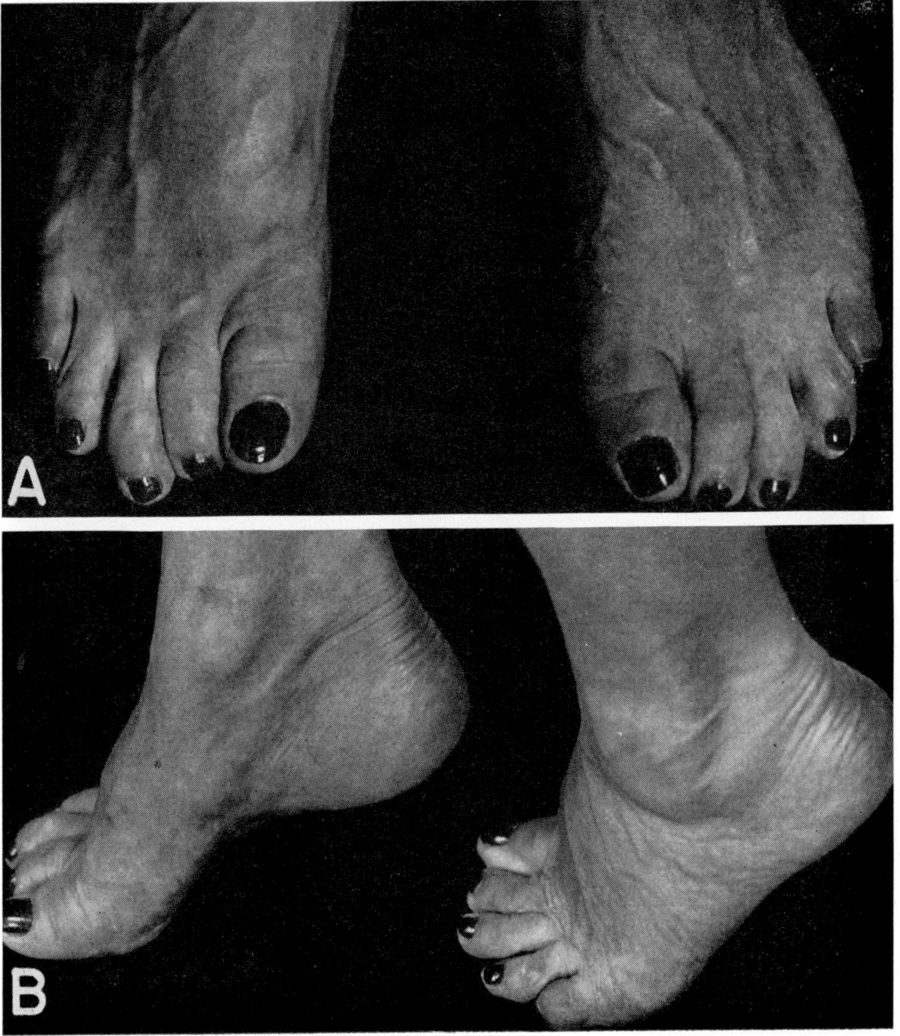

Figure 17–7. Same case. *A,* Dorsal view several months after surgery. *B,* Patient rising on her toes. She was extremely satisfied.

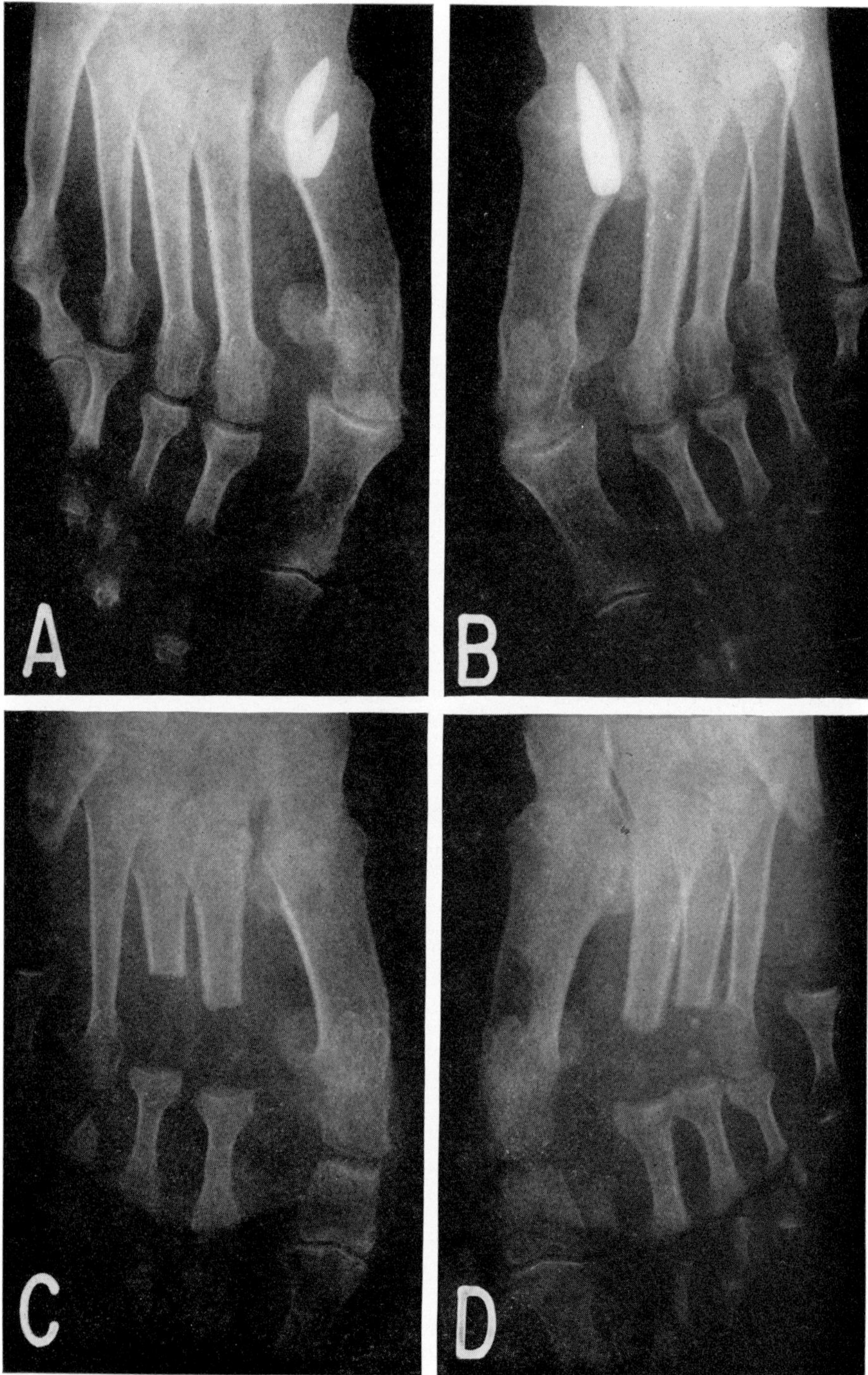

Figure 17–8. Woman, 48 years of age, with stiff great toes, metatarsalgia under the second and third metatarsal heads, and digitus quintus varus on one side. Previous surgery: bilateral Lapidus procedure with the use of staples plus Silver's operation. Secondary surgery: removal of staples, bilateral Keller resection, resection of distal thirds of second, third and fifth metatarsals, and surgical syndactylia of each pair of lesser toes. *A* and *B,* Roentgenogram before surgery. *C* and *D,* Roentgenogram after surgery.

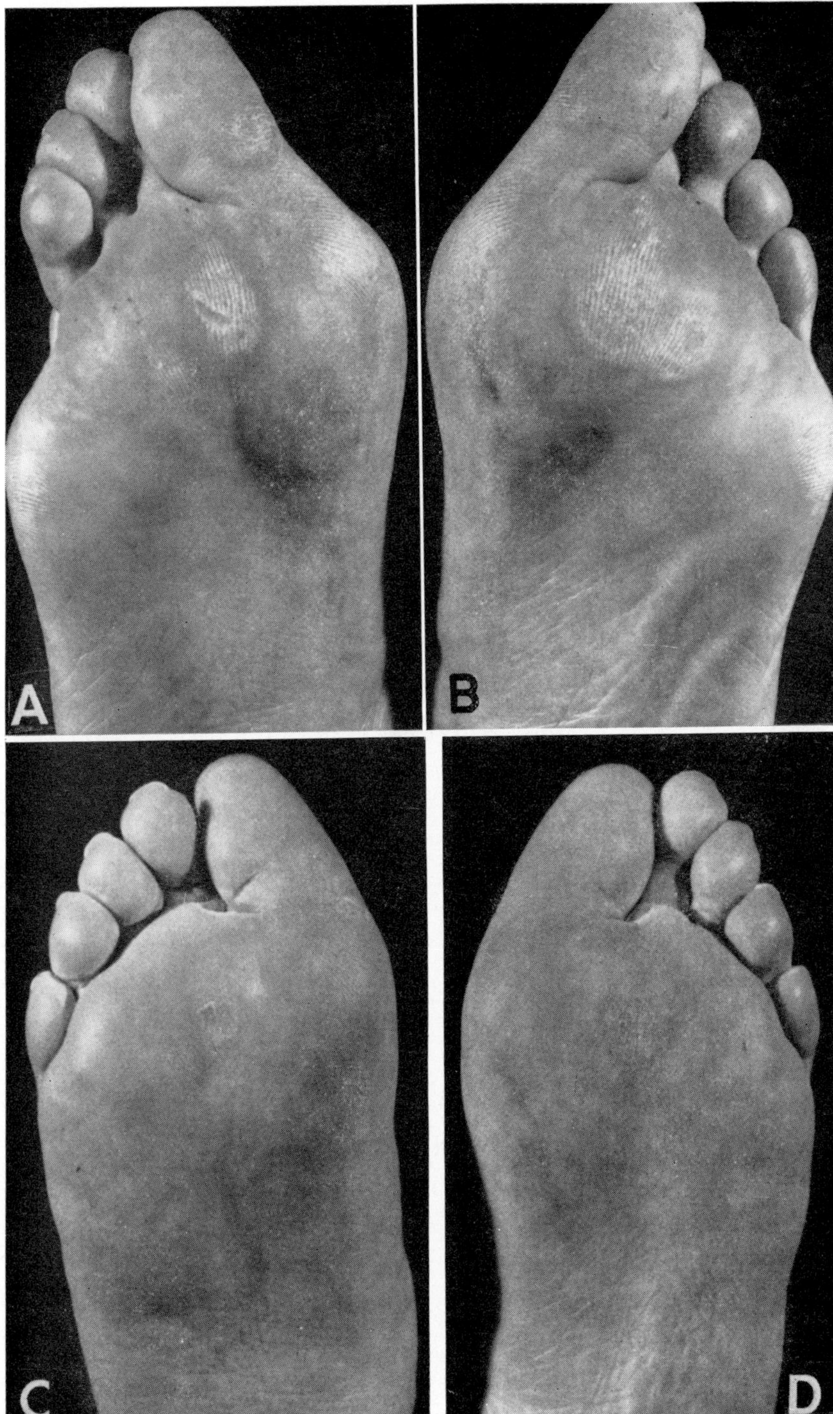

Figure 17–9. The same case as in Figure 17–8. *A* and *B*, Plantar view before surgery. *C* and *D*. The same after surgery.

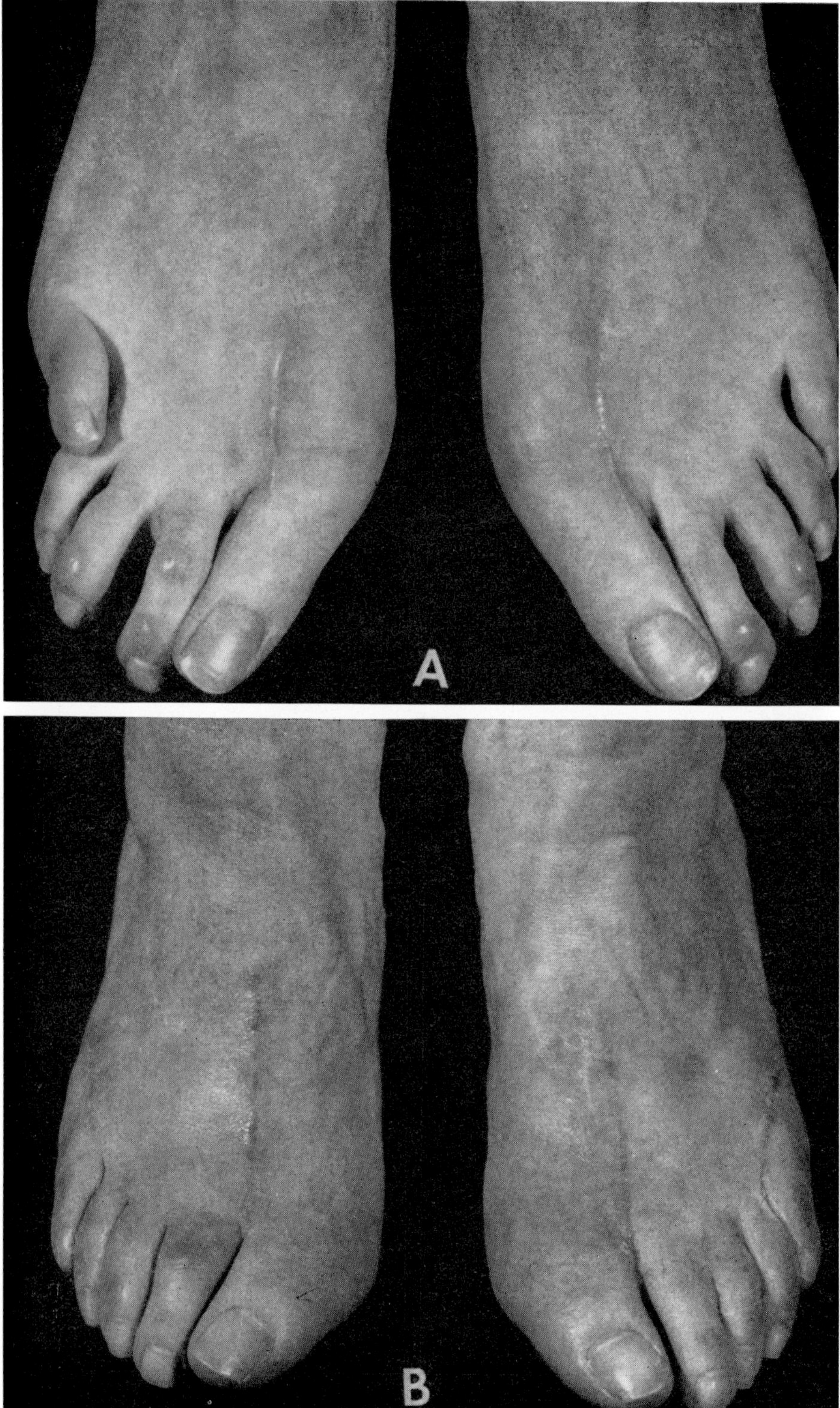

Figure 17–10. The same case as in Figures 17–8 and 17–9. *A,* Dorsal view before operation. *B,* Dorsal view after surgery. Patient was satisfied.

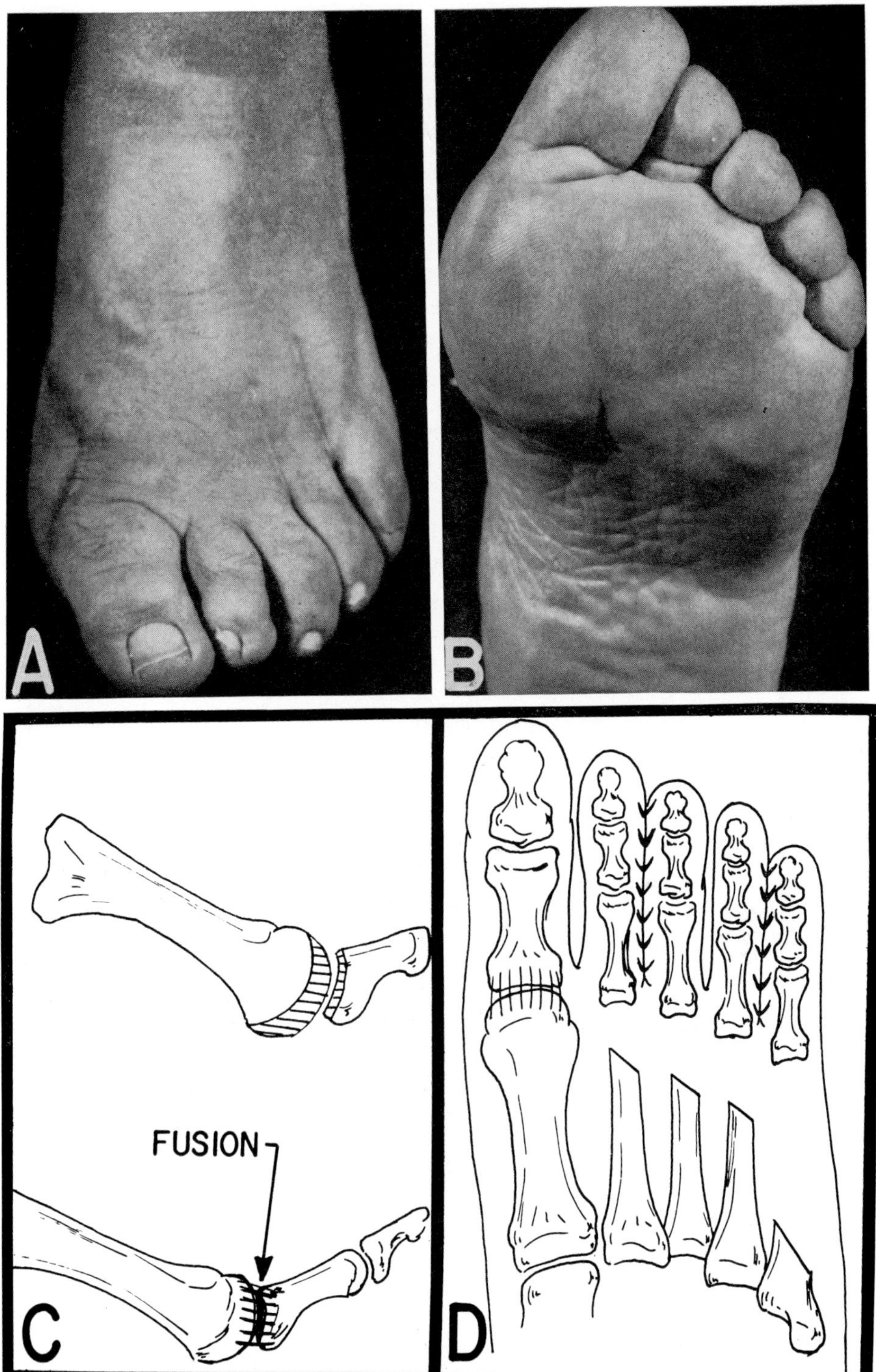

Figure 17–11. Woman, 51 years of age, obese, with stiff great toe and intractable metatarsalgia. Previous surgery: Silver's procedure and neurectomy of the third and fourth digital nerves. Secondary surgery: fusion of the first metatarsophalangeal joint, resection of incarcerated distal segments of the middle metatarsals, and syndactylia of each pair of lesser digits. *A,* Dorsal view when patient was first seen. *B,* Plantar view. *C* and *D,* Interpretative diagrams.

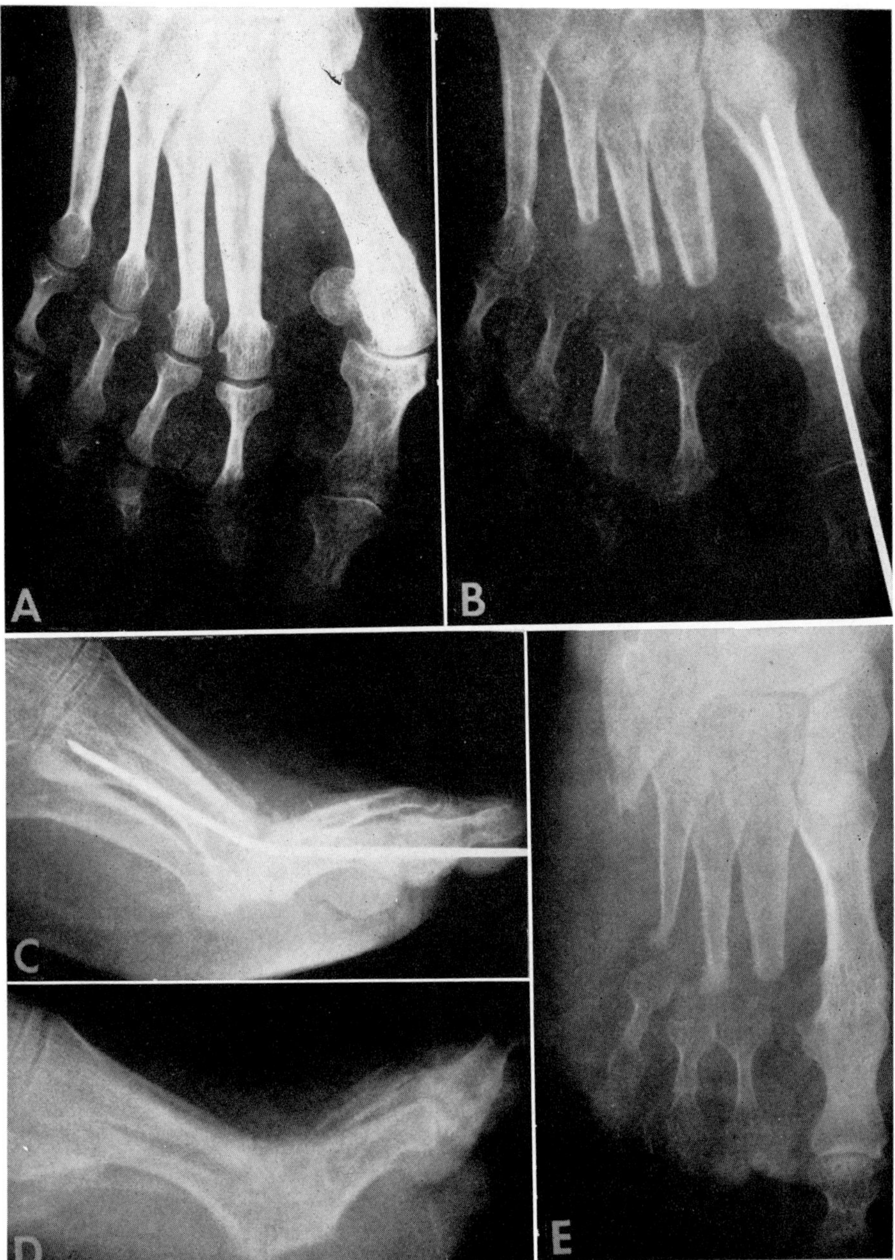

Figure 17–12. The same case as in Figure 7–11. *A,* Roentgenogram when patient was first seen. Note the metatarsus primus varus. *B,* Roentgenogram soon after secondary surgery. Subsequently, the distal three-fourths of the fifth metatarsal had to be resected. *C, D,* and *E,* Progress of fusion of the first metatarsophalangeal joint.

push-off power. In such a case it is questionable if any operation, including Joplin's, can ever restore this power.

There is something to be said in favor of the statement made by Thompson and McElvenny (1940) that "the propulsive action of the great toe is not essential for the normal gait"—anyway, not in the age group seeking advice for longstanding hallux valgus with degenerative arthritis of the first metatarsophalangeal joint, and surely not in modern women who no longer lift the heel first and rise on their toes in walking, but contact the ground simultaneously with both points. Joplin's criticism would be valid if Keller's resection were carried out on a young patient or on one who is athletically inclined. Push-off mechanism is important in athletes and dancers, who should not be subjected to Keller's resection.

Recurrence of the deformity. Weir (1897), Porter (1909), Fuld (1916), Silver (1923), Payr (1925), F. Schede (1927), McBride (1928), and Stein (1938) have reported reappearance of hallux valgus after so-called conservative operations. Occasionally infection will disrupt the plastic repair of the medial capsule and cause hallux valgus to recur. In some instances the adductor tension on the lateral side of the joint has not been adequately released. A more common cause of recurrence is the failure to have recognized and corrected the metatarsus primus varus. If recurrence is due to this cause, the first metatarsal should be osteotomized and the distal fragment shifted laterally. Failure to recognize hypermobile first metatarsal should also be considered. If recurrence can be definitely ascribed to this last cause and the innermost cuneometatarsal joint is painful or shows arthritic changes, it should be fused. Not uncommonly this joint has been tampered with for the purpose of removing the dorsal prominence–the *overbone.* It is not realized that this overgrowth is due to hypermobile first metatarsal and secondary arthritis; it usually recurs after resection (Figs. 17–14 and 17–15).

Reversal of the deformity. Hallux varus was reported by Silver (1923) in two patients operated on by his method –"persisting in one for several weeks and in the other for several months." McBride (1935) wrote: "In two of my cases the forces of abduction seemed to gain too great an advantage, and as weight was born the toe spread out in a most undesirable varus. Both patients were under 25 years of age. . . . The complication was well overcome in both cases by lengthening the abductor tendon and by reinforcing the fascia and the tendinous tissue at the outer side of the base of the proximal phalanx." It was not clear what McBride meant by the last part of this statement, since in his operation the tendinous tissue or the conjoined tendon is severed from the outer side of the base of the proximal phalanx and sutured to the back of the first metatarsal head. Campbell's (1963)

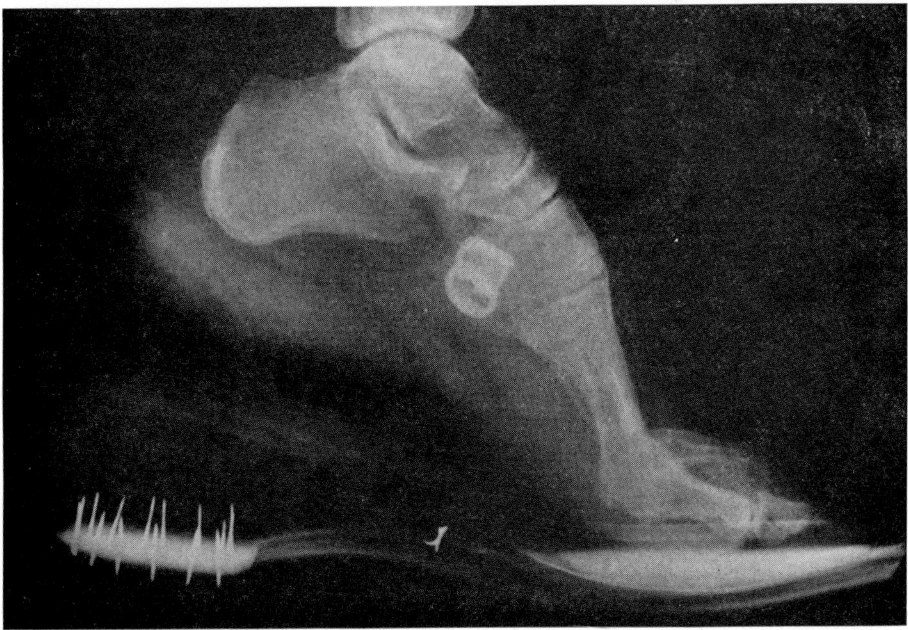

Figure 17–13. The same case as in Figures 7–11 and 7–12. The patient, wearing high-heeled shoes was satisfied.

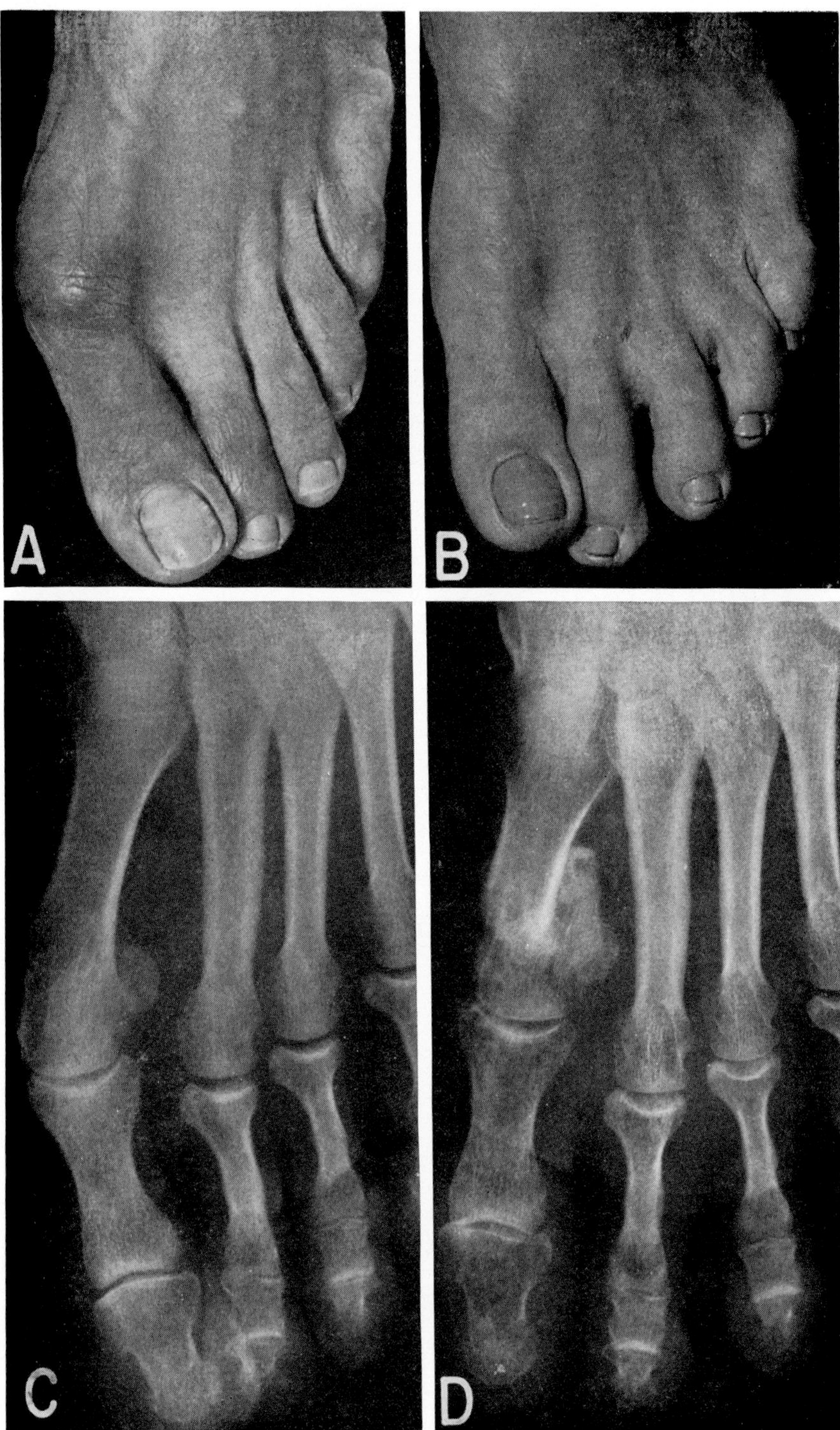

Figure 17–14. Woman, 42 years of age. Previous surgery: Silver's operation. Complaint: recurrence of deformity and pain over the dorsum of the first metatarsal. Secondary surgery: lateral displacement osteotomy of the distal end of first metatarsal. *A,* Photograph when patient was first seen. *B,* After osteotomy. *C,* Roentgenogram before osteotomy. Note the metatarsus primus varus. *D,* Roentgenogram after osteotomy. Patient was satisfied.

Operative Orthopaedics featured the photograph of a foot with hallux varus following McBride's operation. After hallux valgus surgery, overcorrection should be avoided. As a complication of his sling procedure, Joplin (1964) reported "medial subluxation of the sesamoids with hallux varus" in eight feet.

Postoperative hallux varus of some months standing is usually accompanied with stiffness of the first metatarsophalangeal joint. We have remedied these cases by Keller's resection and surgical syndactylia of the hallux with the second toe. Rarely, the long extensor tendon needs to be lengthened. If flexibility of one of the lateral metatarsophalangeal joints is impaired, the basal portions of the proximal phalanx of the involved toe is resected and this digit is syndactylized with its neighbors (Figs. 17–16 and 17–17).

Metatarsalgia. Pain under the ball of the forefoot, often present as a part of the symptom complex of hallux valgus, should not be confused with metatar-

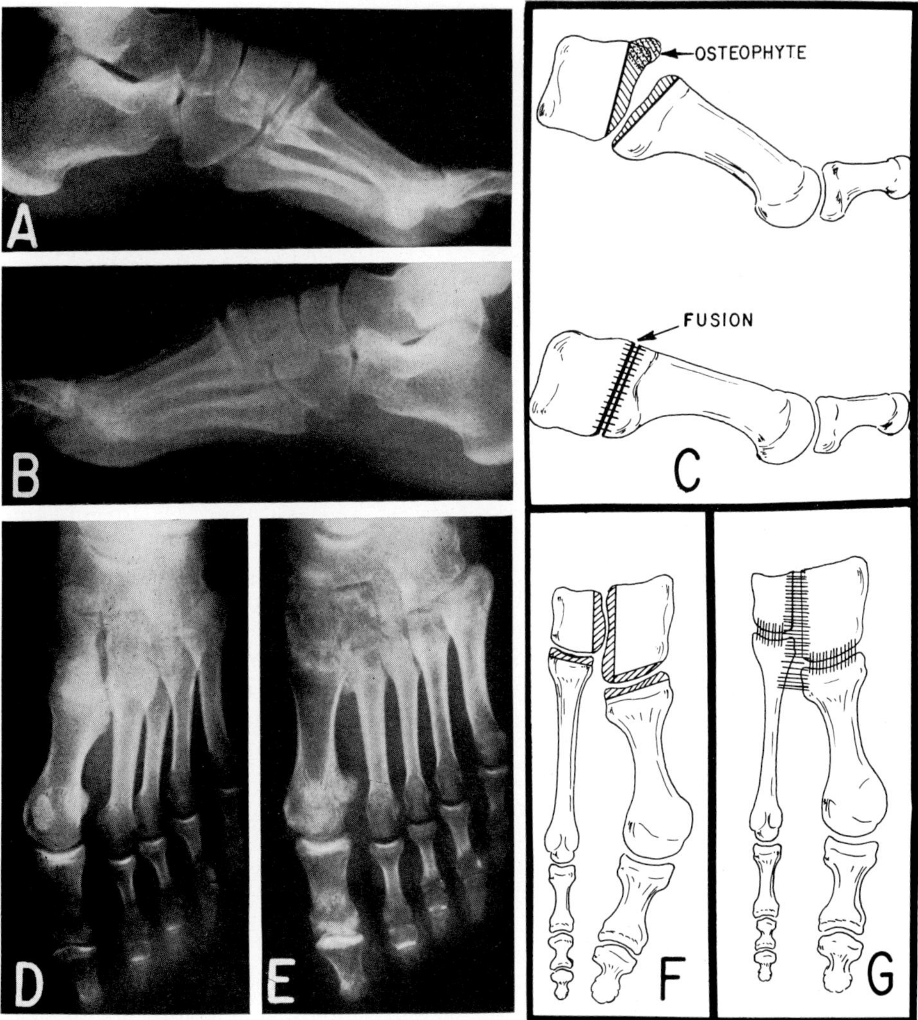

Figure 17–15. Girl, 17 years of age, who has had *overbones* removed from the dorsal aspect of the innermost cuneiform bone of both feet. Complaint: recurrence of osteophytes and pain. Secondary surgery: fusion of the innermost cuneometatarsal joint, fusion of the bases of first and second metatarsals, and fusion of medial and middle cuneiform bones. *A* and *B,* Side views of feet when patient was first seen. *C,* Interpretative diagram to show the overbone and plantarflexed first metatarsal. *D,* Left foot before secondary surgery. *E,* Left foot after surgery. *F* and *G,* Interpretative diagrams. The patient complains of slight pain in the right foot, but is otherwise satisfied.

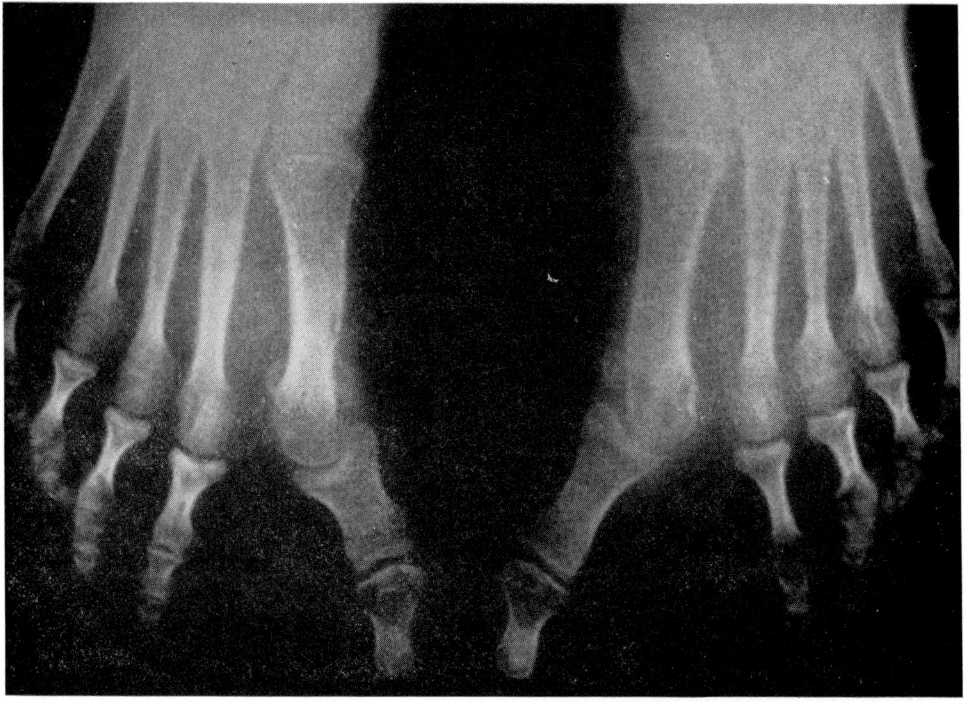

Figure 17–16. Bilateral hallux varus following Silver's procedure.

salgia following surgery. The procedures that are said to commonly aggravate pre-existing metatarsalgia or initiate a new one are: decapitation of the first metatarsal; osteotomy of the first metatarsal, followed by dorsal tilt of the distal fragment; resection of the proximal portion of the basal phalanx of the great toe; proximal phalangectomy of the lesser toes; inadequate resection of metatarsal heads for relief of pressure keratoses; and stress fractures of the lateral metatarsals, known to occur after some forefoot operations.

Metatarsalgia following decapitation of the first metatarsal bone. Metatarsalgia of this nature was first reported by Riedel (1886). He pointed out that resection of the first metatarsal head deprived the foot of an important weight-sustaining pillar and caused pain in the planta pedis. It was reasoned by Hoffa (1894) and others that when the first metatarsal was shortened, its allotted share of the weight was relegated to the outer heads, forcing these bones to dig their way toward the sole. The corresponding digits became displaced dorsally, the retracted toes failed to touch the ground and relieve the metatarsal heads of the excessive load, and the stress was concentrated on the central metatarsal heads and caused pain. Following a similar rationalization, Massart (1934) and Morton (1952) condemned decapitation of the first metatarsal. Becker (1952) evoked corroborating evidence by pointing out that after the Hueter-Mayo operation the second metatarsal became thick in response to the excessive stress thrown on it. Hypertrophy of the proximal phalanx of the great toe is also known to occur following decapitation of the first metatarsal early in life (Fig. 17–18).

Dorsal tilt of the distal fragment. This is recognized, following osteotomy of the first metatarsal, as a definite cause of metatarsalgia. After osteotomy through the neck of the first metatarsal, Hohmann (1951) considered the dorsal displacement of the capital fragment undesirable. Mitchell and his associates (1958) also viewed this complication with dismay. Theoretically, the first metatarsal head, which has tilted up, will have an effect as though it were removed by resection: it will not sustain its share

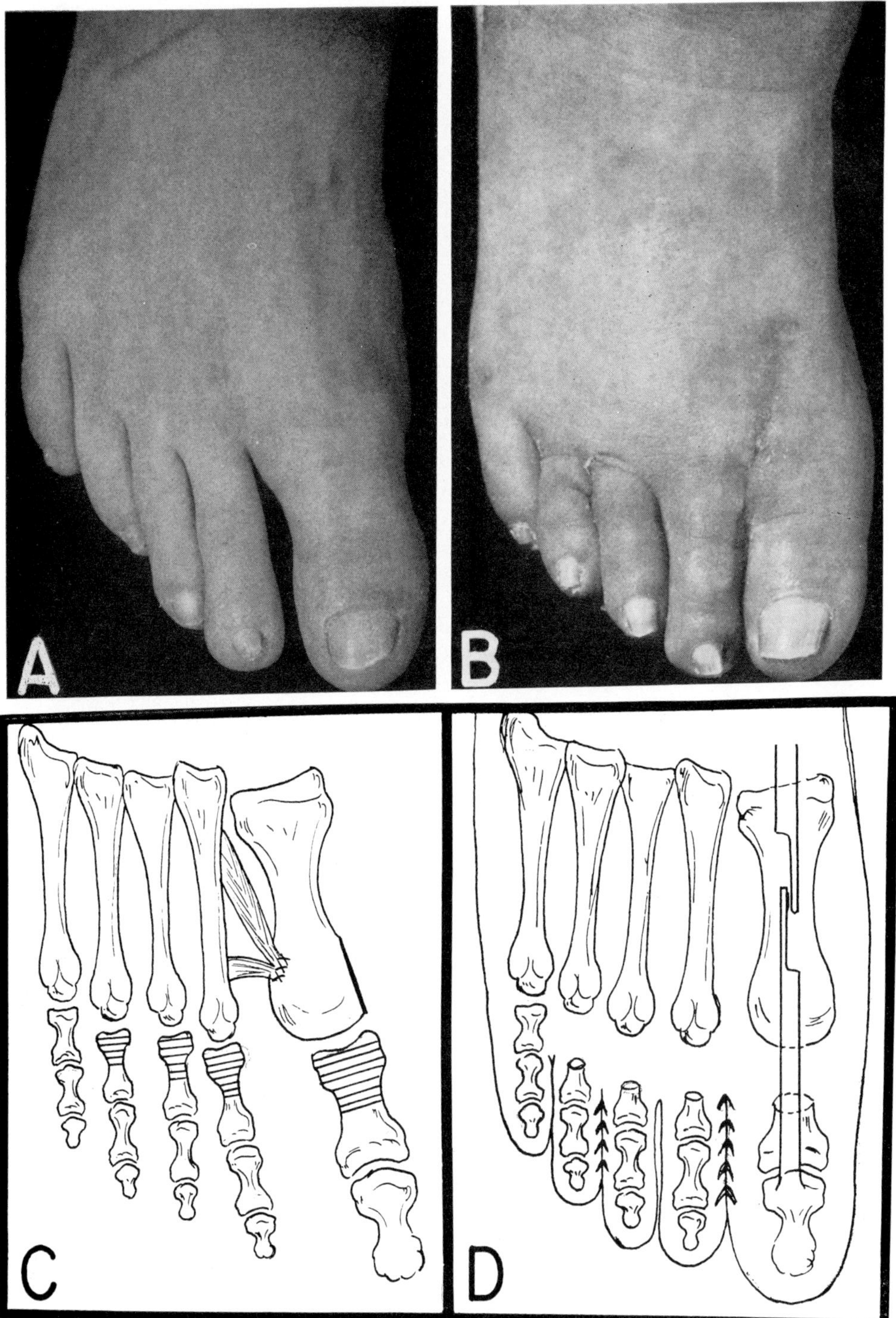

Figure 17–17. Woman, around 45 years of age, with medially deflected hallux and stiff first metatarsophalangeal joint. Previous operation: resection of the medial eminence through interdigital approach. Secondary surgery: Keller's resection, lengthening of the long extensor tendon, partial proximal phalangectomy of the three middle toes, and surgical syndactylia of the first with the second, and third with the fourth toes. *A,* Photograph when patient was first seen. *B,* After secondary operation. *C* and *D,* Interpretative diagrams. The condition was improved but the patient was not completely satisfied.

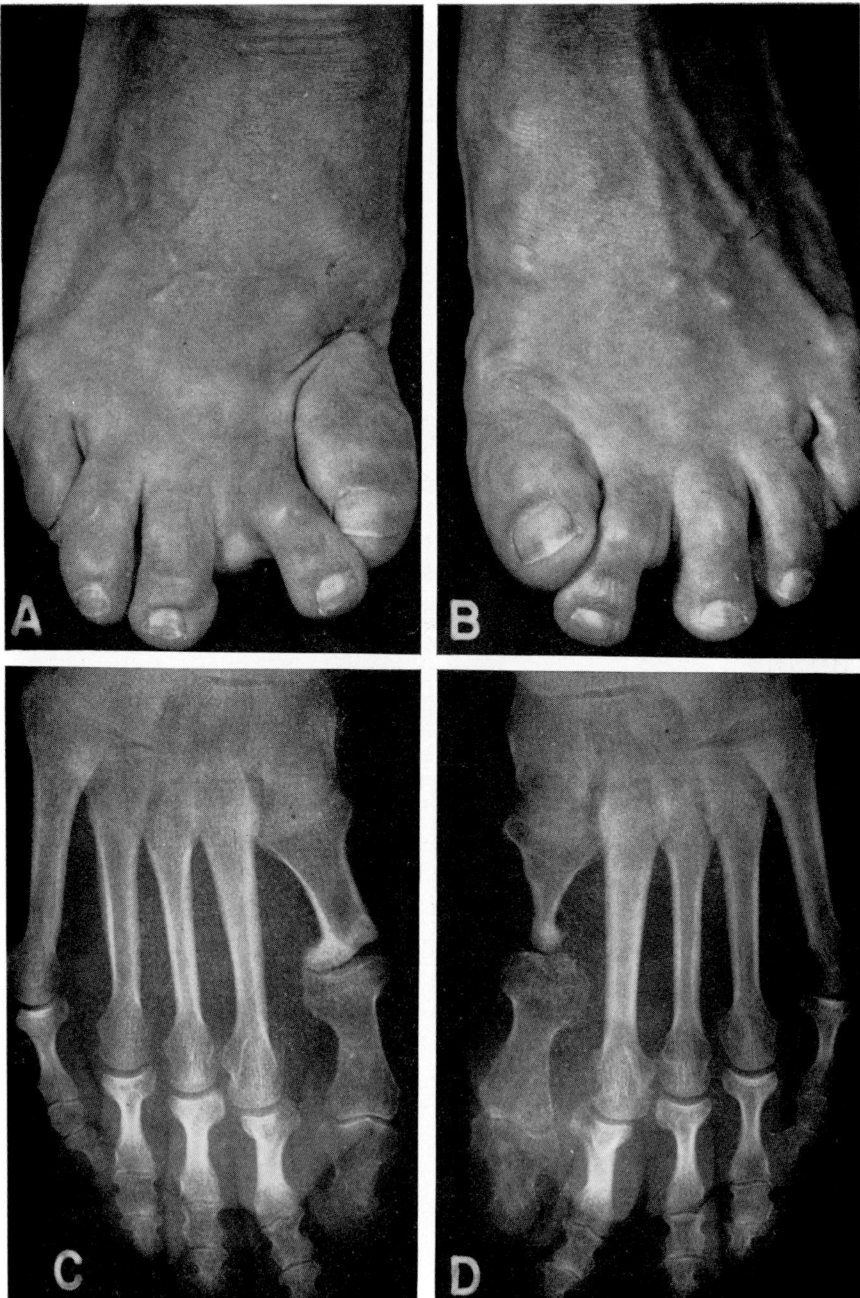

Figure 17–18. Woman, around 40. In childhood she had had decapitation of the first metatarsals of both feet. There was not much complaint at the time the photographs were taken. Note the hypertrophied proximal phalanges in *C* and *D*.

of weight, and the adjacent bones will be subjected to excessive stress (Fig. 17–19).

Metatarsalgia following Keller's operation. This type of metatarsalgia was ascribed by Morton (1952) to the retraction of the short flexor of the great toe and rearward shift of the sesamoids. "The resulting pain and callus formation are similar to those of a short first metatarsal bone," Morton wrote. A more common criticism leveled against Keller's operation is that, when the base of the proximal phalanx is removed, intrinsic mus-

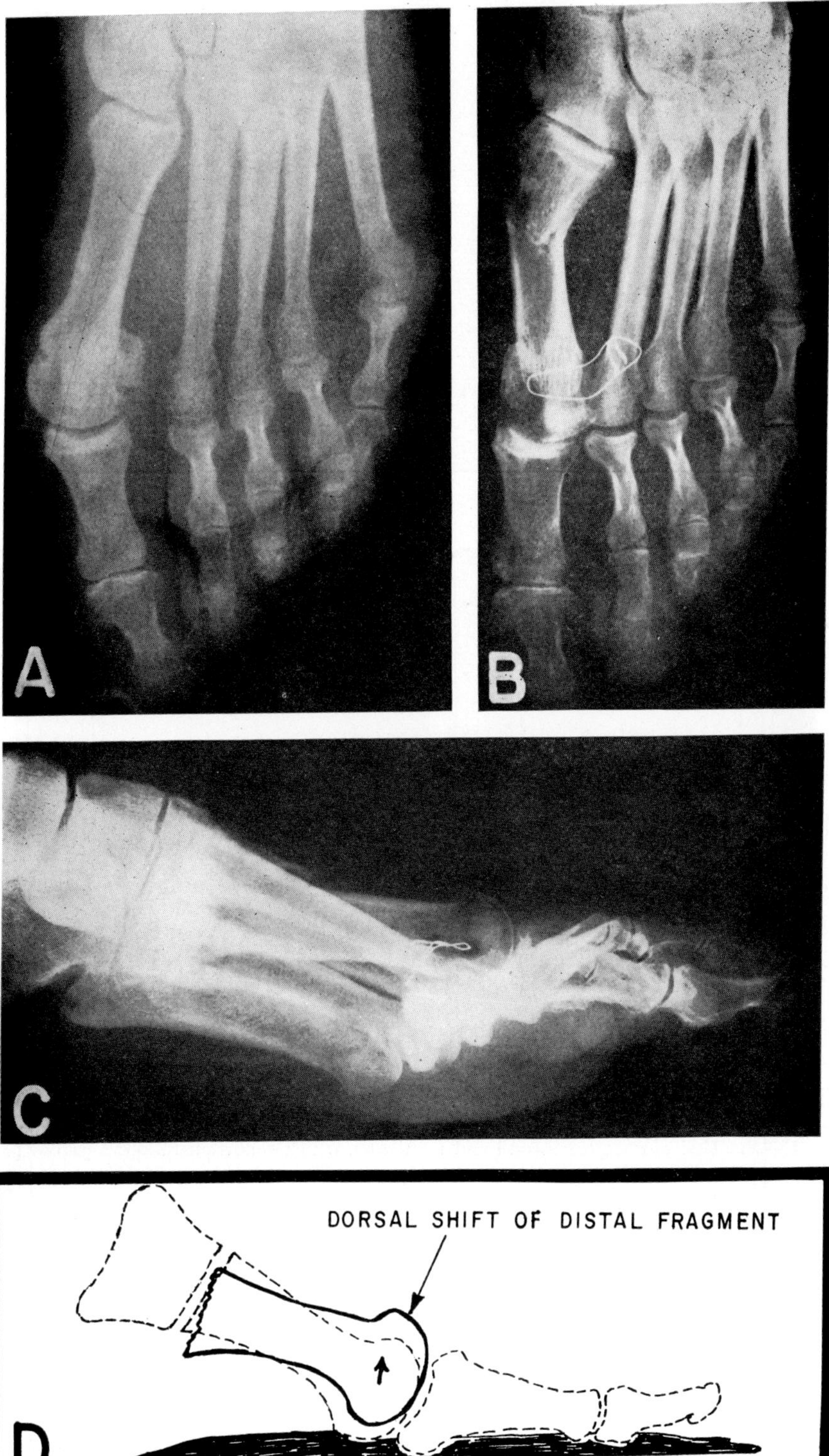

Figure 17–19. Woman, around 45. She had had osteotomy of first metatarsal. *A* and *B*, Dorsoplantar view roentgenograms. *C*, Lateral view showing dorsal tilt of the distal fragment. *D*, Interpretative diagram. Complaint: metatarsalgia.

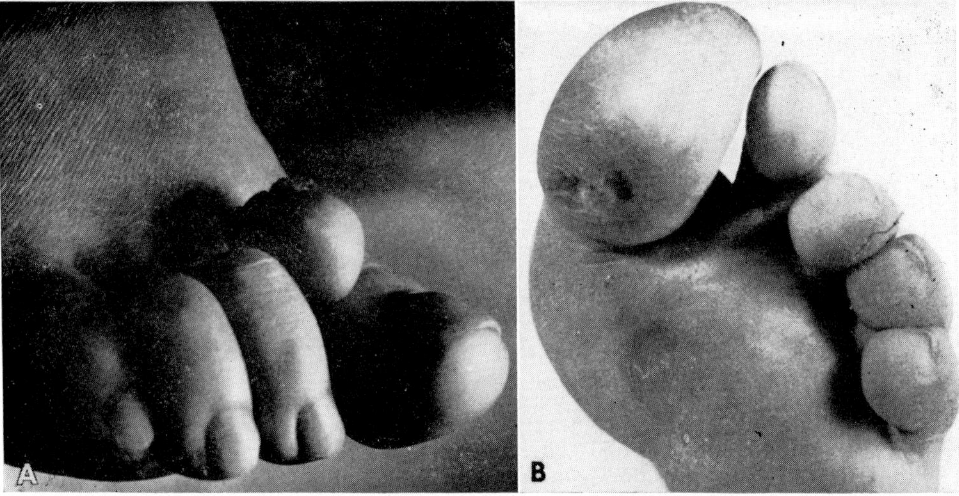

Figure 17–20. Retracted second toes that had been subjected to partial proximal phalangectomy.

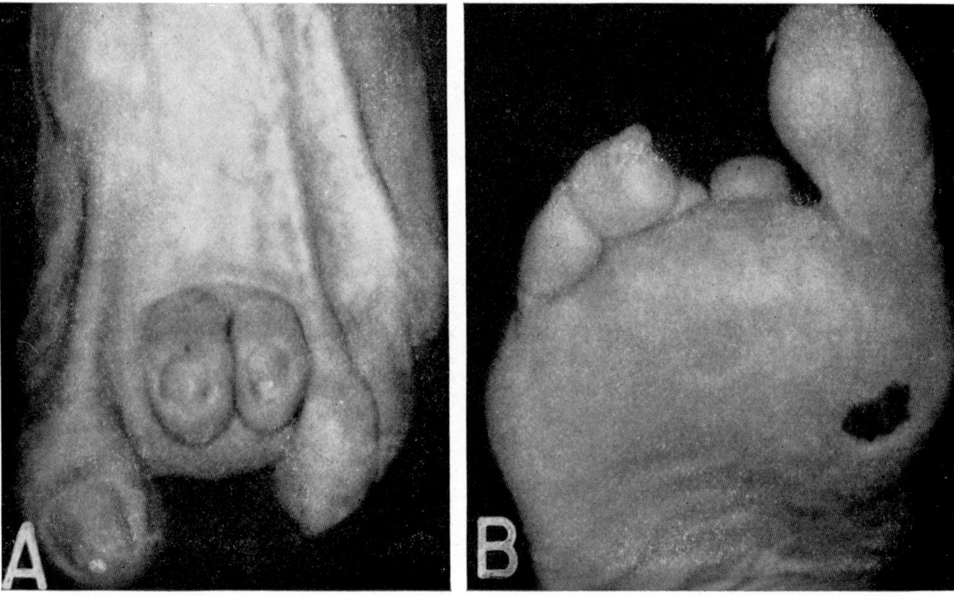

Figure 17–21. Useless retracted second and third toes, which condition followed partial proximal phalangectomy.

cles of the hallux lose their anchorage and cannot contribute to the pressing-down action of the great toe. The hallux becomes weaker, and its area of contact with the ground is curtailed. The great toe cannot effectively press down, establish a broad base for the long flexor to pull from, lift the first metatarsal up, and thus save it from untimely wear. As we have noted, Keller's resection should not be performed in the young and robust with as yet active intrinsic muscles, nor in the old with pre-existing metatarsalgia of some severity.

Metatarsalgia following proximal phalangectomy of the lesser toes. Metatarsalgia from this procedure has been explained by a similar reasoning. Toes that have lost their bases dangle and become retracted; they fail to touch the proffered surface, press upon it and broaden the tread, and relieve the corresponding metatarsal heads of the excessive load. This hazard may be ob-

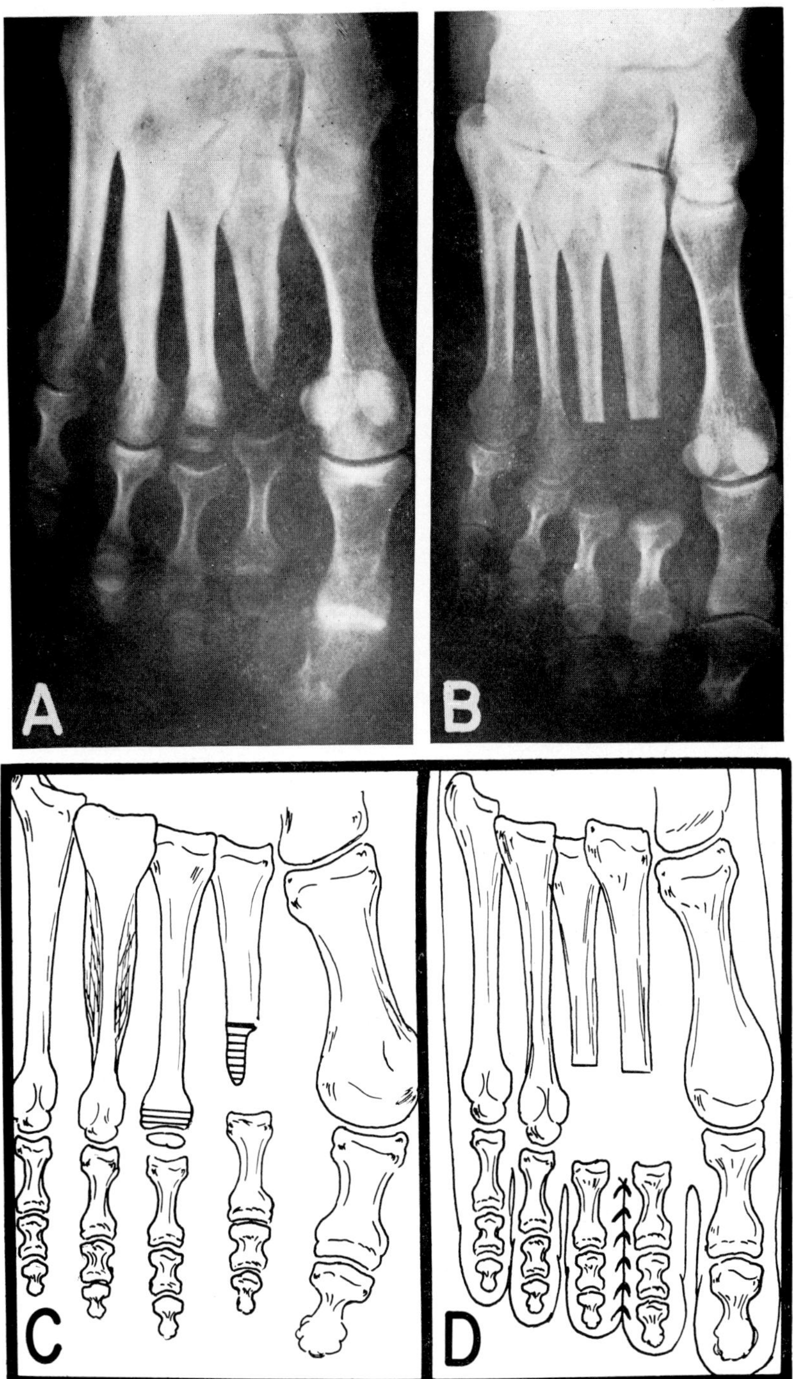

Figure 17–22. *A,* Roentgenogram showing inadequate resection of the distal ends of the second and third metatarsals. Note the recession of the second toe and stress hypertrophy of the fourth metatarsal shaft. *B,* Roentgenogram showing adequate resection of the distal segments of the second and third metatarsals. Note that the proximal phalanges of the second and third toes have not receded. This hazard was obviated by surgical syndactylia of the involved toes. *C,* Diagram interpreting *A*. *D*. Diagram interpreting *B*.

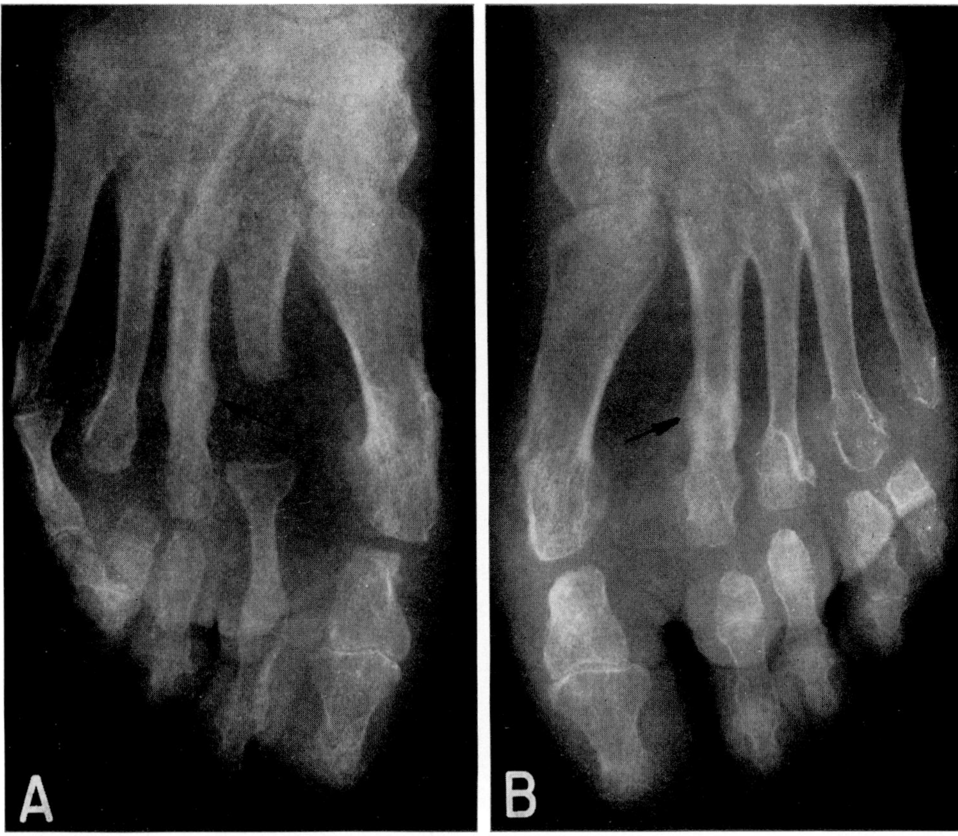

Figure 17–23. Woman, 65 years of age, with postoperative stress fracture of the metatarsal bones. See the text for explanation. *A,* Roentgenogram of right foot. *B,* Left foot.

viated if, after proximal phalangectomy, the two adjacent toes are syndactylized (Fig. 17–20 and 17–21).

Inadequate resection of incarcerated metatarsal heads. Insufficient resection is often followed by recurrence of pressure keratosis and aggravation of the pre-existing metatarsalgia. In fixed incarceration of the central heads, the distal third of the involved metatarsal should be resected and the adjacent toes syndactylized (Fig. 17–22).

Stress fractures of the lateral metatarsal bones. Meyerding and Pollock (1938) mentioned a patient who had "undergone excision of the first metatarsal head" and developed march fracture of the neighboring metatarsal. Stress fractures of the outer metatarsals were recorded by Cleveland and Winant (1950) in two cases—the first, two and one-half; the second, six months—after Keller's resection. There was no history of injury in either instance. The fractures were not suspected, but because of constant complaints by the patients, roentgenograms were taken, which revealed a fracture of the second metatarsal in one case, and of the third metatarsal in the other. In addition to hallux valgus, the latter patient also had Freiberg's infraction of the second metatarsal head, which had been treated surgically.

"Not uncommonly," Watson-Jones (1957) wrote, "fatigue fracture of the second metatarsal occurs several weeks after operative correction of hallux valgus deformity." He gave the following explanation: "With hallux valgus there is already splaying of the metatarsals and transverse flatfoot, and the muscle control is impaired still more by the immobility that follows the operation." Watson-Jones considered "early exercises for the transverse arch with sustained active flexion of all toes . . . an important measure in after-treatment." He said that following surgery for hallux valgus, these "exercises should be practiced regularly before weight-bearing is resumed."

The present writer operated on a patient of bilateral hallux valgus with metatarsalgia and hammered toes. Keller's procedure was carried out on both great toes. In addition, on the right side the incarcerated distal portion of the second metatarsal was resected and the proximal phalanges of the third and fourth toes were partially excised. On the left side the basal halves of the proximal phalanges of all the toes were removed. Six months after surgery the patient came back complaining of metatarsalgia on the left side. Roentgenography revealed a fracture of the shaft of the second metatarsal. Routine roentgenograms of the right foot showed a typical march fracture of the third metatarsal with exuberant callus formation. The patient had no complaint referable to the right foot. The left foot was enclosed in a short leg cast with a rubber heel. Six weeks later the cast was removed and an elastic stocking was prescribed. Metatarsalgia disappeared (Fig. 17–23).

Miscellaneous mishaps. Lloyd (1935) reported alteration of the gait following resection of the first metatarsal head or the proximal portion of the basal phalanx of the great toe. Postoperatively, he noted "a great tendency for patients to try to spare the inner border of the foot by walking on its outer edge, and this," Lloyd said, "is the commonest cause of failure after operation. Every patient should be told that he *must* bear weight on the inner border of the foot, lest he gives himself a secondary metatarsalgia. A. Blundell Bankart has advised an *outside* wedge of 1/4 inch after operation, and this should be a standard postoperative precaution."

Flail hallux. This is known to occur after resection of the articular ends of the main bones entering into the formation of the first metatarsophalangeal joint. In older individuals "dangle toe" may be left alone. In the young an attempt should be made to stabilize the toe. The alternatives are fusion or surgical syndactylia of the hallux with the second toe.

Hallux extensus. Dorsal retraction of the great toe is also known to occur following Keller's resection, perhaps owing to injury to the flexor mechanism or failure to procure an anchorage to the detached intrinsic muscles. Hallux extensus due to taut long extensor tendon is often accompanied with hallux varus. Differentiation between this type of varus and that caused by the contracted medial capsule may be made by pushing the toe laterally. In varus deformity due to taut extensor tendon the toe can be pushed with ease; in varus due to a contracted medial capsule this attempt will meet with some resistance.

Malleus deformity. Hammered deformity of the great toe at times follows Keller's resection. The hallux knuckles at the interphalangeal joint, and there is a painful callus on its dorsal aspect. The condition is best remedied by

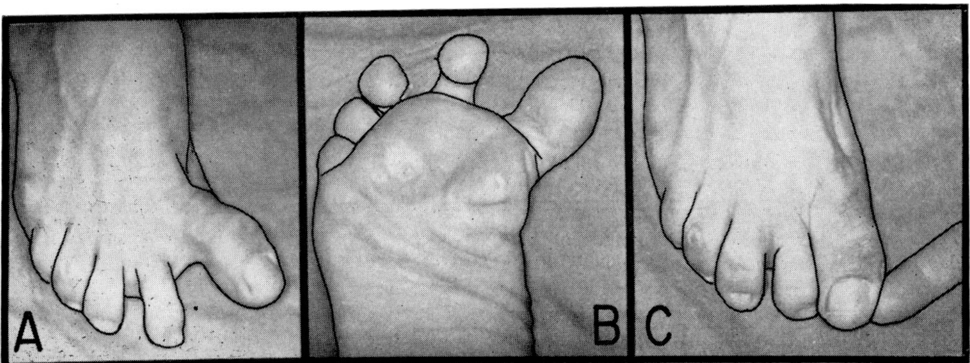

Figure 17–24. Postoperative hallux varus extensus due to taut medially displaced long extensor tendon of the great toe. *A,* Dorsal view. *B,* Plantar view. *C,* Reduced by gentle push, meeting no resistance.

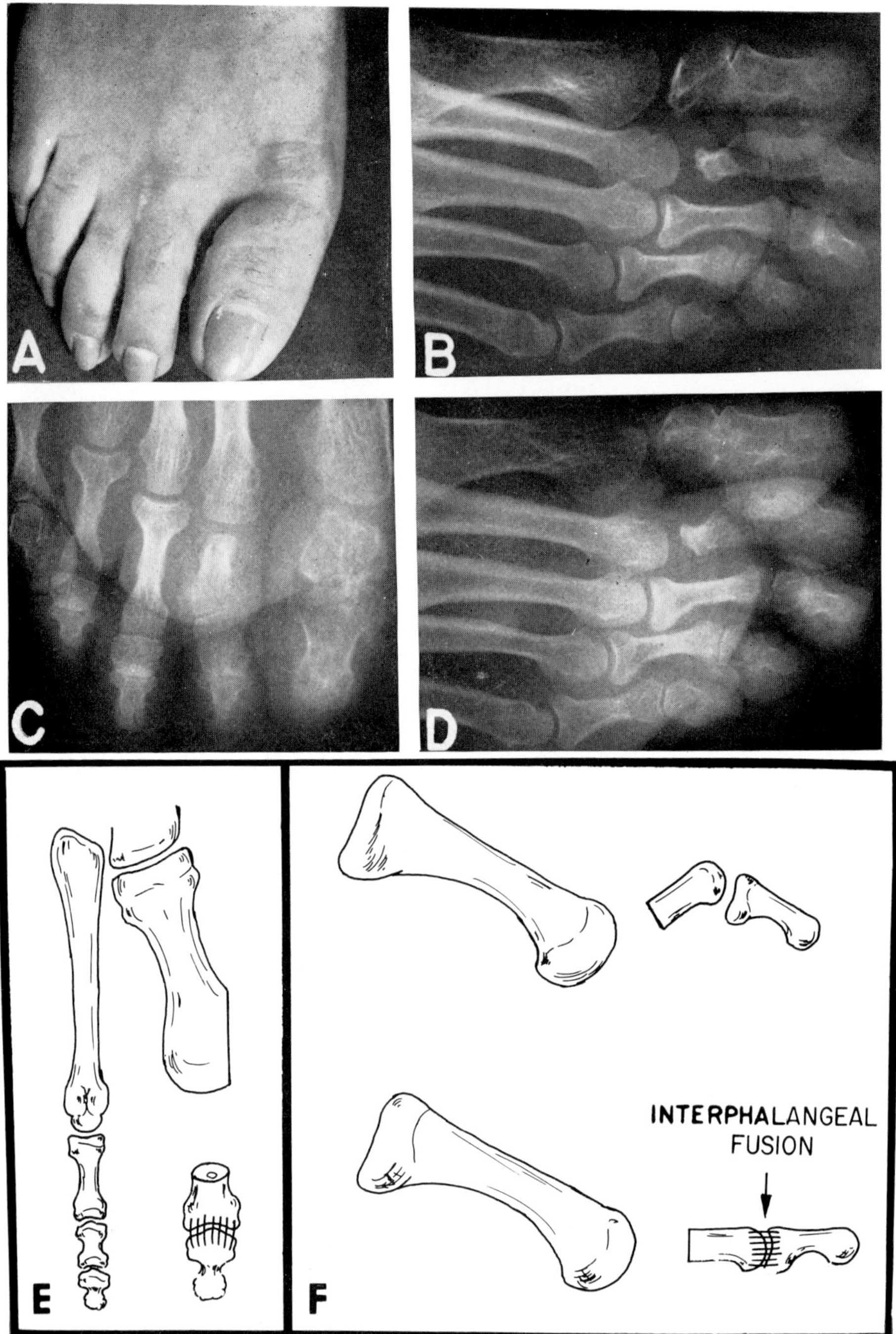

Figure 17–25. Woman, 30 years of age, with right side developed malleus of the great toe and pain over the dorsal aspect of the interphalangeal joint of the great toe. Previous surgery by the author: bilateral Keller resection, resection of proximal phalanges of second toes, and syndactylia of second toe with third toe on both sides. Secondary operation: resection of more bone from the remaining stump of the proximal phalanx of the great toe, interphalangeal fusion, and syndactylia of first and second toes. *A,* Before secondary surgery. *B,* Dorsoplantar view roentgenogram before secondary surgery. *C,* Dorsoplantar view roentgenogram after fusion of the interphalangeal joint of the great toe. *D,* Oblique view of the same. *E* and *F,* Interpretative diagrams.

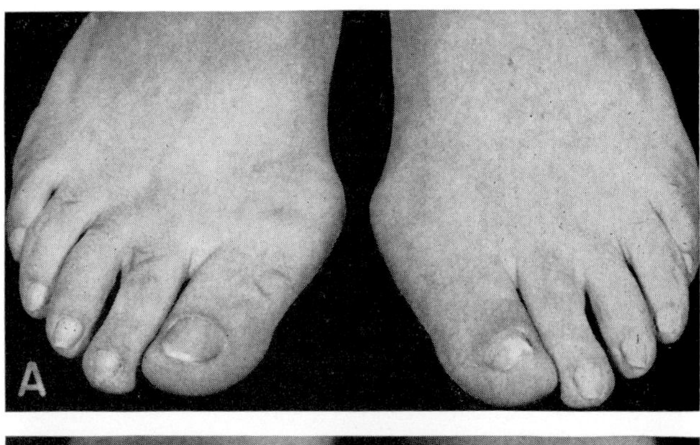

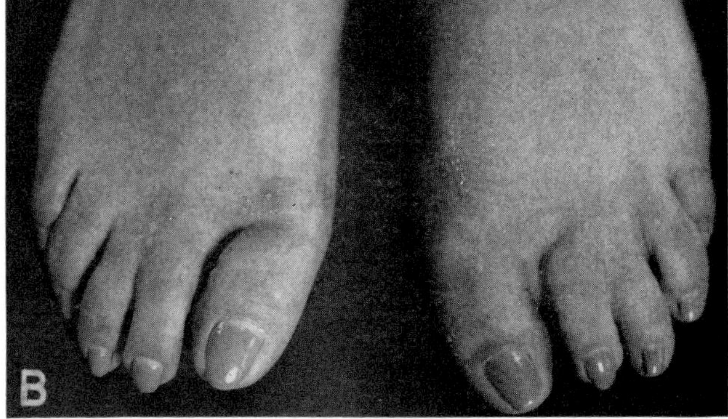

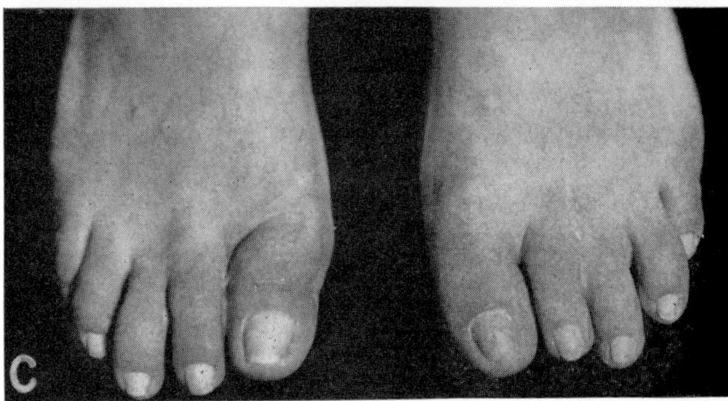

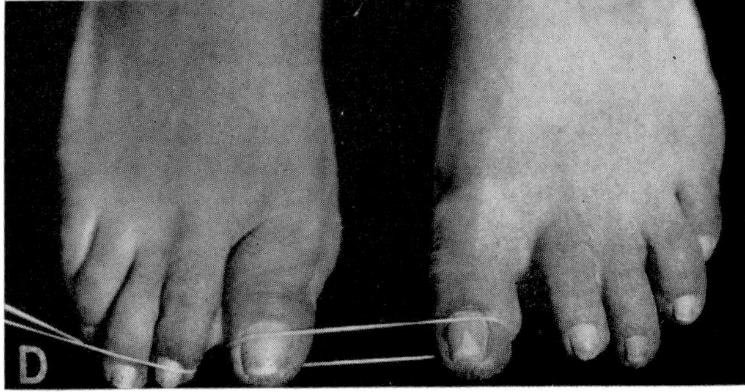

Figure 17–26. The same case as in Figure 17–25. *A,* Before the first operation. *B,* After the first operation. *C,* After the second operation. *D,* The surgical syndactylia of the first and second toes on the right side. The patient was satisfied.

tenotomy of the long extensor and fusion of the interphalangeal joint. After tenotomy and attempted fusion, the hallux is stabilized by surgical syndactylia with the second toe.

Discrepancy in the lengths of the two great toes. Another complication that follows forefoot surgery is discrepancy in the lengths of the two great toes, or of the first and second toes. When only one foot is subjected to Keller's resection, the patient will sometimes complain of having to wear shoes of unequal sizes.

Hammered deformity of the second toe. This often occurs when the hallux is inordinately shortened by decapitation of the first metatarsal or resection of the proximal two thirds of the basal phalanx. Following these procedures, the second toe gains in relative length; it juts far in advance of the great toe and eventually knuckles into a typical hammered deformity. After operations that cause abbreviation of the length of the great toe, we prophylactically shorten the second digit, subjecting it to proximal phalangectomy and surgical syndactylia with its partner on one or the other side. We also shorten the second toe when the tip of the hallux is amputated for relief of ingrown or deformed toe nail (Figs. 17–24 to 17–30).

Subluxation of the smaller digits at the metatarsophalangeal joint. Watson-Jones (1957) dramatized the plight of a surgeon who had operated on a "bunion" without recognizing the "spontaneous dislocation" of the second toe. The surgeon was threatened by medicolegal proceedings, because the patient had

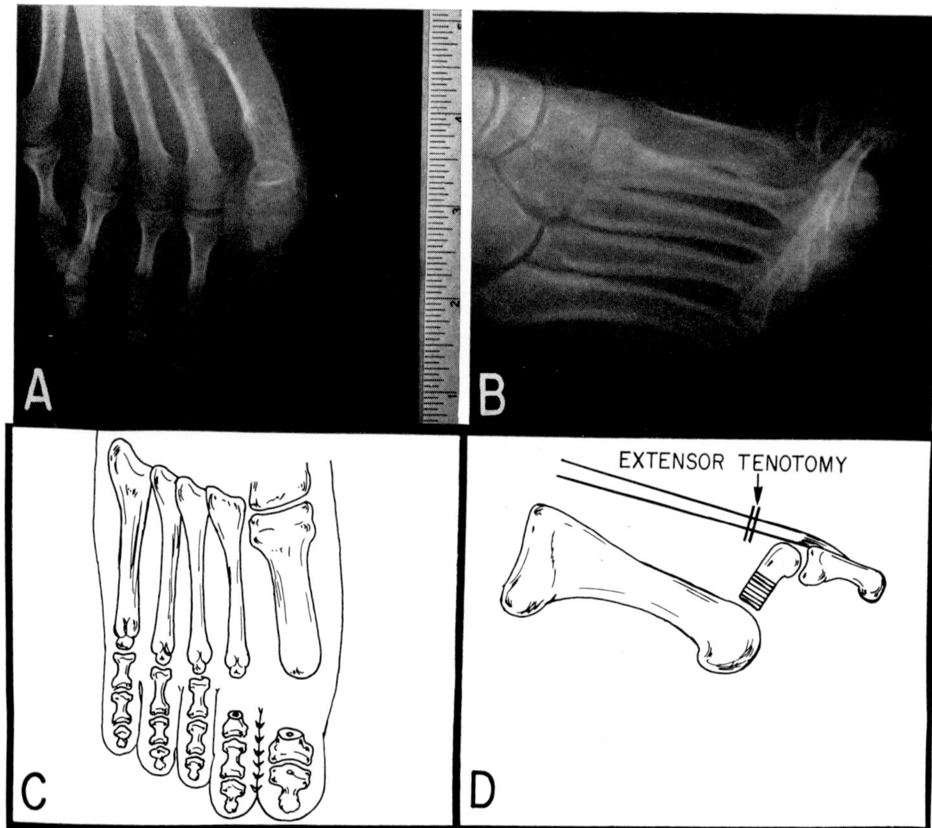

Figure 17–27. Woman, 34 years of age, with stiff painful great toe and inability to wear shoes. Two previous operations had been performed elsewhere, the last one apparently a Keller resection. Secondary surgery: extensor tenotomy, resection of more bone from the stump of the proximal phalanx of the great toe, partial proximal phalangectomy of the second toe, and surgical syndactylia of the first and second toes. *A,* Dorsoplantar roentgenogram when the patient was first seen. *B,* Oblique view of same. *C* and *D,* Interpretative diagrams.

known of no injury and blamed him for the dislocation. The implication was that spontaneous dislocation may occur coincidentally with hallux valgus, which is true enough, but not following surgery. We have seen subluxation of the toe occurring at the fourth metatarsophalangeal joint after correction of hallux valgus and resection of distal portions of the second, third, and fifth metatarsal bones.

Other mishaps. Massart (1934) spoke of *painful adherent scars* after hallux valgus surgery. *Pseudoarthrosis* has been reported both after attempted fusion of the first metatarsophalangeal joint and following osteotomies. Nonunion was reported by Mygind (1953) after Thomasen's *peg-and-hole* osteotomy. Gibson Piggott (1962) also reported a case of nonunion after a *spike-and-hole* type of subcapital osteotomy. This case was subsequently treated by bone graft; it resulted in painful hallux rigidus. Mitchell and his associates (1958), and Hammond, who discussed their paper, spoke of *aseptic necrosis* of the osteotomized head.

Some patients complain of persisting *insensibility* of the toe, undoubtedly due to nerve injury; others speak of *sensitive scars* and prolonged pain. To alleviate *persistent postoperative* pain, Bloomberg (1940) recommended crushing of the sensory nerves that supply the basal articulation of the great toe. With the aid of local infiltration of 0.5 per cent procaine, using a curved dorsomedian incision, Bloomberg exposed the medial

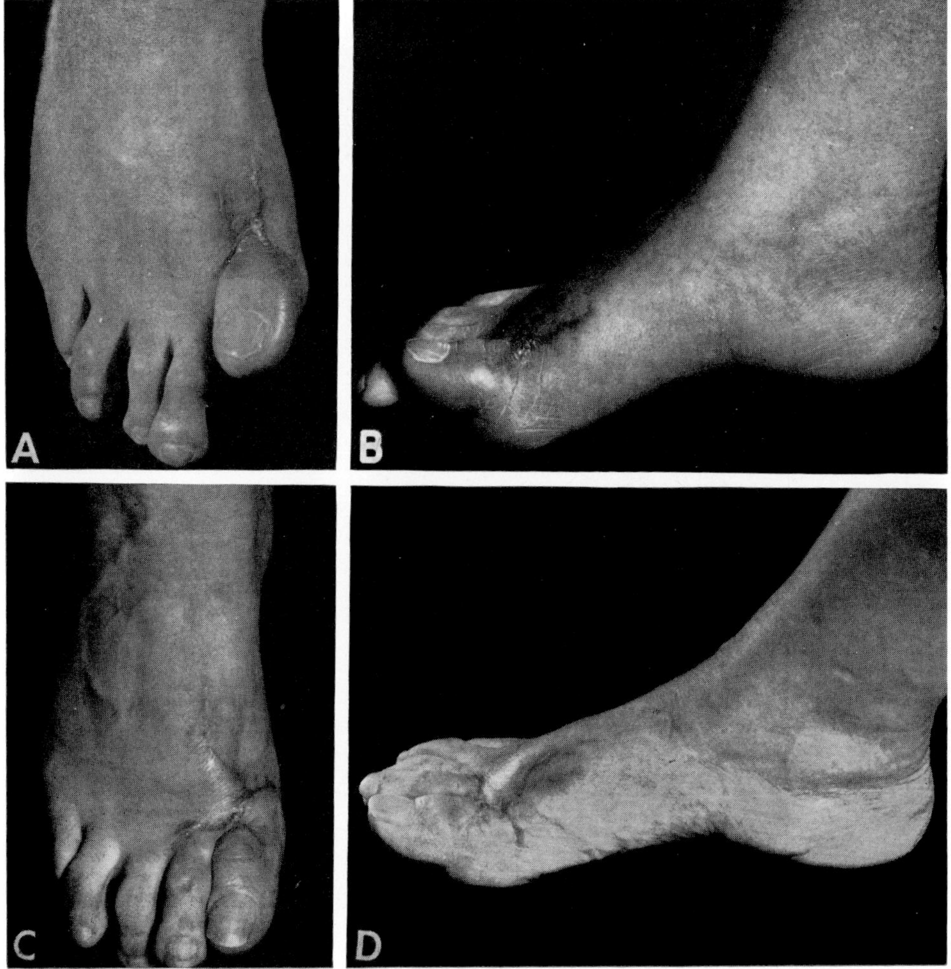

Figure 17–28. Same case as in Figure 17–27. *A* and *B*, Photographs when patient was first seen. *C* and *D*, After secondary surgery. Patient was satisfied.

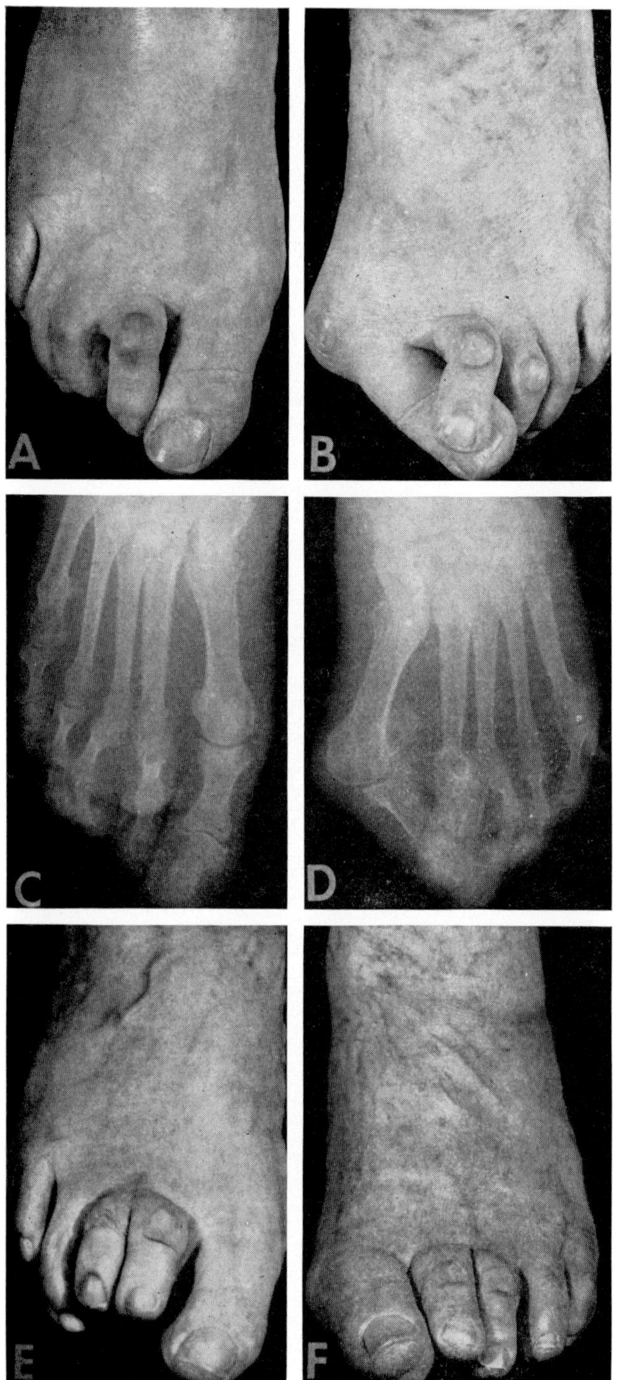

Figure 17–29. Woman, about 50 years of age, operated on by the author, was unable to wear shoes of equal sizes because of Keller resection on one side (left), which considerably shortened the foot. *A* and *B,* Before surgery. *C* and *D,* Roentgenograms before surgery. *E* and *F,* After surgery—partial proximal phalangectomy and surgical syndactylia of the hammered second and third toes on the right side, Keller resection of the great toe, and partial proximal phalangectomy of the lateral toes followed by surgical syndactylia of each pair. Patient was dissatisfied.

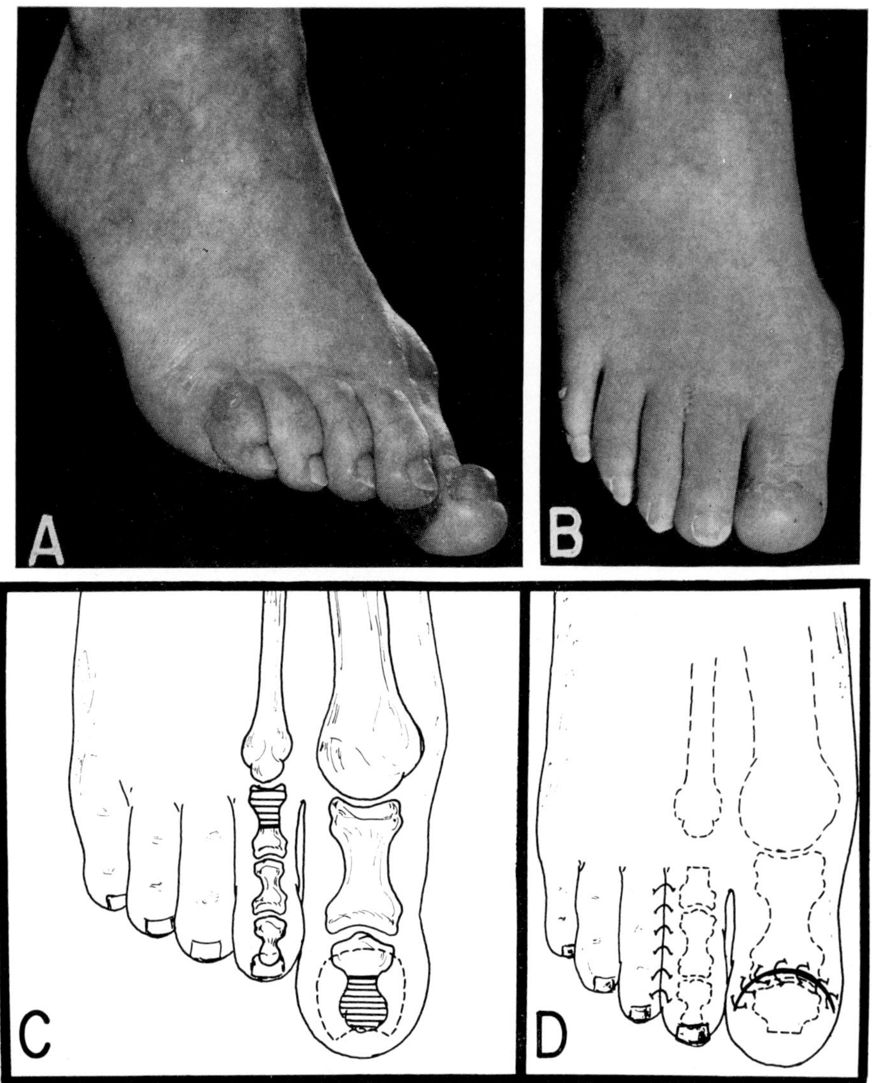

Figure 17–30. Woman, about 30 with onychogryposis that necessitated partial amputation of the terminal phalanx of the great toe. To obviate hammered deformity, the second toe was subjected to partial proximal phalangectomy and syndactylized with the third toe. Patient was satisfied.

and lateral dorsal digital nerves of the great toe and crushed them for a distance of 1 cm. with a hemostat. Joplin (1964) resected "the medial proper digital nerve" to procure smoother convalescence. We rely on periodic injections of procaine and cortisone to allay severe postoperative pain.

REFERENCES

Bade, P.: *Der Hallux valgus.* Ztschr. Orthop. Grenzbt., Stuttgart, F. Enke, 1940, pp. 1–84.

Becker, A.: Ist die Operation nach Hueter-Mayo eine brauchbare Methode in der Behandlung des Hallux valgus? Verh. Deut. Orthop. Ges. *81*:248–251, 1952.

Blodgett, A. N.: Hallux valgus, with a report of two successful cases. Med. Rec. New York *18:* 34–37, 1880.

Bloomberg, M.: A method for the control of postoperative pain in hallux valgus operations. Am. J. Surg. *48*:412–413, 1940.

Campbell's *Operative Orthopaedics* (A. H. Crenshaw, ed.). 4th Ed. St. Louis, C. V. Mosby Co., 1963, Vol. 2, p. 1603 (Fig. 1390).

Cleveland, M., and Winant, E. M.: An end-result of the Keller operation. J. Bone Joint Surg. *32*:163–175, 1950.

Fuld, J. E.: Transplantation of the abductor hallucis tendon in the surgical treatment of hallux valgus. Surg. Gyn. Obst. *23*:626–628, 1916.

Gibson, J., and Piggott, H.: Osteotomy of the neck of the first metatarsal in the treatment of hallux valgus. J. Bone Joint Surg. *44*:349–355, 1962.

Hoffa, A.: *Lehrbuch der Orthopaedischen Chirurgie*. Stuttgart, F. Enke, 1894, pp. 739–744.

Hohmann, G.: *Fuss und Bein*. Munich, J. F. Bergmann, 1951, pp. 145–192.

Jones, R.: Discussion on the treatment of hallux valgus and rigidus. Brit. Med. J. *2*:651–656, 1924.

Joplin, R. J.: Sling procedure for correction of splay-foot, metatarsus primus varus, and hallux valgus. J. Bone Joint Surg. *32*:779–785, 1950.

Joplin, R. J.: Sling procedure for correction of splay-foot, metatarsus primus varus, and hallux valgus. J. Bone Joint Surg. *46*:690–693, 1964.

Key, A.: Some observations on the nature and treatment of ganglion, bunion, etc. Guy's Hosp. Rep. *1*:415–428, 1836.

Lapidus, P. W.: Author's bunion operation from 1931 to 1959. Clin. Orthoped. *16*:119–135, 1960.

Lloyd, E. J.: Prognosis of hallux valgus and hallux rigidus. Lancet *2*:263, 1935.

McBride, E. D.: A conservative operation for bunion. J. Bone Joint Surg. *10*:735–739, 1928.

McBride, E. D.: The conservative operation for "bunions". J.A.M.A. *105*:1164–1168, 1935.

McKeever, D. C.: Arthrodesis of the first metatarsophalangeal joint for hallux valgus, hallux rigidus, and metatarsus primus varus. J. Bone Joint Surg. *34*:129–134, 1952.

Massart, R.: Les résultats déplorables des opérations d'hallux valgus. Bull. Mém. Soc. Chir. *26*:669–674, 1934.

Mayo, C. H.: The surgical treatment of bunions. Ann. Surg. *48*:300–302, 1908.

Mitchell, C. L., Fleming, J. L., Allen, R., Glenney, C., and Sanford, G. A.: Osteotomy-bunionectomy for hallux valgus. J. Bone Joint Surg. *40*:41–60, 1958.

Meyerding, H. W., and Pollock, G. A.: March fracture. Surg. Gyn. Obst. *67*:234–242, 1938.

Morton, D. J.: *Human Locomotion and Body Form*. Baltimore, Williams & Wilkins Co., 1952, pp. 104–106.

Mygind, H. B.: Some views on the surgical treatment of hallux valgus. Acta Orthop. Scand. *23*:152–158, 1953.

Payr, E.: *Pathologie und Therapie des Hallux valgus*. Vienna and Leipzig, W. Braumueller, 1894, pp. 1–77.

Payr, E.: Zur Hallux-valgus-Operation; Kapselbandexzision an der lateralen Seite des Gelenkes. Zbl. Chir. *52*:2292–2296, 1925.

Porter, J. L.: Why operations for bunions fail with a description of one which does not. Surg. Gyn. Obst. *8*:89–90, 1909.

Reverdin, J.: De la déviation en dehors du gros orteil (hallux valgus, vulg. "oignon", "bunions", "Ballen") et de son traitement chirurgical. Trans. Intern. Med. Congr. *2*:408–412, 1881.

Riedel: Zur operativen Behandlung des Hallux valgus. Cbl. (later became Zbl.) Chir. *44*:753–755, 1886.

Rogers, W. A., and Joplin, R. J.: Hallux valgus, weak foot and the Keller operation: an end-result study. Surg. Clin. N. Amer. *27*:1295–1302, 1947.

Schede, F.: Hallux valgus, Hallux flexus und Fussenkung. Ztschr. Orthop. Chir. *48*:569–571, 1927.

Seiffert, J.: Nylon als Knorpelersatz bei der Hallux-valgus-Operation. Dtsch. Med. J. *4*:414–415, 1953.

Silver, D.: The operative treatment of hallux valgus. J. Bone Joint Surg. *5*:225–232, 1923.

Singley, J. D.: The operative treatment of hallux valgus and bunion. J.A.M.A. *61*:1871–1872, 1913.

Stein, H. C.: Hallux valgus. Surg. Gyn. Obst. *66*: 889–898, 1938.

Thompson, F. R., and McElvenny, R. T.: Arthrodesis of the first metatarsophalangeal joint. J. Bone Joint Surg. *22*:555–558, 1940.

Watson-Jones, R.: *Fractures and Joint Injuries*. 4th Ed., Baltimore, Williams & Wilkins Co., 1957, Vol. 1, pp. 345–347.

Weir, Robert F.: The operative treatment of hallux valgus. Ann. Surg. *25*:444–453, 1897. See also the discussion on pp. 480–485, 1897.

Zacharie, T.: *Surgical and Practical Observations on the Diseases of the Human Foot*. New York, C. B. Norton, 1860, pp. 36–46.

Chapter Eighteen

SUMMARY AND SUGGESTIONS

When we decided to write this book, we set as our aim clarification of the current confusion about hallux valgus, related deformities of the forefoot, and metatarsalgia. We hoped we would establish an accord between our own and the recorded experience of others. Ideas emanate from experience. We soon discovered that, on several points, our views clashed with those expressed in some books and articles. Clash tends to be more impressive than harmony. It may have passed unnoticed that—as regards to basic principles of anatomy, interpretation of structural changes, and surgery—we endorsed, in some instances reflected, the concepts expressed by most of our predecessors—by Camper (1781), Durlacher (1845), Broca (1852), Volkmann (1856), Henry Morris (1879), Lane (1887), Ellis (1890), Hilton (1891), Anderson (1897) Ewald (1912), Silver (1923), Wood Jones (1949), and Hohmann (1951), to mention some of the classic and a few of the recent authors.

In the introduction of this book we said it has become fashionable to overlook the obvious—shoes as the most common cause of forefoot deformity. Another obvious fact that seems to have been overlooked or forgotten pertains to the interdependence of various parts of the forefoot. Too often the deformities of the toes and disorders of the metatarsal segment are regarded as isolated, independent entities. It is not realized—not often enough—that these parts are organically and functionally related and the disorder of one will have its inevitable effect on the other.

The forefoot, moreover, is an integral part of the body, heir to all its ailments, and shares or reflects some of its pains. What sets the forefoot apart and makes it seem unique is the discrepancy between its construction and the dual duties it is asked to perform—support the body weight and at the same time impart a measure of springiness to the gait. Support presupposes stability. The hindfoot is well suited for this function. It consists of solid blocks of bones that are bound together firmly by strong ligaments and braced by stout tendons. Its joints yield only slightly to the forces from above or below. The bones of the forefoot on the other hand are long and narrow; its ligaments are weak and it has no tendinous brace. Its joints yield to pressure from above, from below, form behind, and from in front—at the tip of the toes. The subsidiary function of the forefoot—which we said is to impart resilience to the gait—requires that it should allow considerable movement. The joints of the forefoot that permit the greatest range of motion are placed near where most of the body weight is born, which makes the metatarsophalangeal junction vulnerable to distorting forces. In almost every type of deformity of the toes, one may suspect a derangement at the corresponding metatarsophalangeal joint—subluxation, erosion of the hyaline surface, or both. By failing to contact the proffered surface and thus to enlarge the tread, stiff distorted toes in their turn fail to relieve the metatarsal heads of the excessive stress and aggravate the pain under them, or even cause it.

In Chapter 17, on surgical complications, we mentioned some of the reasons for allotting more space to the discussion of hallux valgus than to other deformities of the forefoot. We said that hallux valgus has evoked extensive discussions and attempts to correct it have been numerous, and we may add, diversified. The multiplicity of methods suggests that no single procedure has been entirely satisfactory or without some objectionable feature—hence, the need for modification or even innovation. Careful analysis of unsatisfactory results will show that, in most instances, not enough attention has been paid to disorders of the metatarsal segment or deformities of the lesser toes. But even with adequate care of all these derangements, one must not expect the impossible—a forefoot that after surgery is completely painless, functions well, and is shapely.

The results of surgical correction of hallux valgus and related forefoot deformities are at best relative. We deal with a combination of deformities that may have been reversible at the start but in time become fixed. There is also the fact that this part of the anatomy is subjected to the repeated injury of weight-bearing and walking; it cannot easily cast off the added insult of surgical trauma. Moreover, the toes are far away from the central circulation and their recuperative power is comparatively meager; their wounds—surgical or otherwise—heal sluggishly. But with commensurate care they do, in time.

Many a surgeon of undeniable integrity has developed his own method of coping with the problems of forefoot surgery and has eventually obtained gratifying results. There is perhaps something to the saying that it is not so much what is done as how well it is done that counts. A surgeon can better execute the operation he has performed most often or knows how to do well. On the other hand, however skillful, if the surgeon applies the same set of steps to one and all varieties of deformity, he is likely to spawn more than his share of deplorable results.

Surgeons in the past usually favored one procedure and reported glowing results. They used the word "cure" indiscriminately and did not always state what was cured. Writing about the operative treatment of "bunion," Parker Syms (1897) stated: "A thorough removal of the inner condyle will cure the majority of cases." Augustus Wilson (1906) said that his personal experience with 53 cases warranted him to advocate "excision for the internal aspect of the distal extremity of the first metatarsal in all cases." John L. Porter (1909) claimed his method of sagittal resection of the medial two-thirds of the first metatarsal head never failed. Bromeis (1931) from Kirschner's clinic contended that "thorough smooth chiseling" of the medial eminence was not likely to be followed by failure.

We now know that, however generous, sagittal resection of the medial eminence of the first metatarsal head does not correct the outward deviation or axial rotation of the great toe; it merely reduces the swelling along the tibial border of the forefoot and relieves the discomfort due to chafing by the shoe. Both these benefits are transient, temporary. Even when supplemented with release of adductor tension on the lateral aspect of the first metatarsphalangeal joint and reinforcement of the capsule on the other side, sagittal resection of the medial eminence is often followed by recurrence. All the same, it is perhaps the best method for hallux valgus in the aged, who want a measure of comfort when wearing shoes and are not interested in the correction of the outward deviation of the great toe.

Syms, Wilson, and Porter were Americans; Bromeis was German. But overconfidence was not endemic in America alone or in Germany. Speaking at a meeting in the Royal National Hospital, London, Jackson Clarke (1913) said he had resected the first metatarsal head "in about a thousand successive cases without a mishap. . . ." George Perkins (1927) wrote: "The operation of excision of the head of the metatarsal can be relied on always and completely to cure symptoms due to hallux valgus and to hallux rigidus." As a young surgeon, Blandell Bankart (1913) penned a cautious article on hallux valgus and took pains to prove that the operation of excision of the head of the first metatarsal was a "bad one," because it "permanently" destroyed the arch and "greatly" impaired the usefulness of the foot. Years later, as a mature surgeon, Bankart (1935) wrote: . . . "excision of the head of the first metatarsal, which has stood the test of time and is unquestionably in my opinion the best treatment." Granted, age and experience engender confidence. Do they also qualify one to pontificate positive statements?

In America, Cleveland (1927) reviewed the results of 200 operations for correction of hallux valgus in 108 patients subjected to one of the following operations: decapitation of the first metatarsal; sagittal resection of the medial eminence, Keller's resection, exostectomy and capsulorrhaphy, and cuneiform osteotomy of the first metatarsal or of the basal phalanx of the great toe. "In this series," Cleveland wrote, "the most satisfactory operation for correction of hallux valgus was resection of the metatarsal head, together with removal of exostosis." A quarter of a century later, Cleveland and his associate (1950) arrived at the following conclusion: "Arthroplasty of the metatarsophalangeal joint of the great toe by the Keller procedure gave good or excellent results in 93 per cent of 193 operations. . . ."

Time changes. Techniques improve. Criteria as to what constitutes a good result vary. Cleveland (1927) made the distinction between cosmetic and functional results; he stressed the greater importance of the latter. According to him, the functional result expressed the mobility of the great toe, the amount of control that the patient had over it, and its general efficiency in the propulsion of the body in walking. He considered the presence or absence of pain also an important factor in determining the end result. Perkins (1927) admitted that the procedure he praised—excision of the metatarsal head—did not relieve metatarsalgia. Mitchell and associates (1958) wrote: "relief of pre-existing metatarsalgia cannot be considered a prerequisite of a satisfactory result." In view of what has been said about the interrelation of deformed toes and metatarsalgia, no result of hallux valgus surgery can be considered satisfactory if afterwards the pain under the ball of the forefoot persists.

As years go by, techniques multiply. When Syms (1897) wrote about the surgical treatment of hallux valgus, he had at most five methods to choose from. Even though he favored sagittal resection of the medial eminence, he advised employing "different operative procedures according to the degree and character of the deformity." A quarter century later Olivecrona (1924) could select from two dozen surgical methods, yet he wrote: "There is no single operative procedure which is uniformly successful. It is further evident that each operation has its special indications and limitations and that the results may be improved if the same operation is not made routine in every case but the type of operation is selected according to the condition prevailing in each case." Harding (1927) implied the same in an article entitled, "Bunions: Different Types, Different Treatment." Stamm (1957) wrote: "The surgical treatment of hallux valgus . . . exemplifies to perfection the fact that surgery is an art, for each case presents a different problem which is capable of solution in a number of different ways, success depending upon the most careful assessment of all the factors involved as well as upon the technical skill and meticulous attention to detail."

It can now be said that perhaps in no endeavor to solve a surgical problem has human ingenuity devised so many diversified methods as for the surgical treatment of hallux valgus and related forefoot deformities. At this writing there are over a hundred operations on record for the correction of hallux valgus alone. The author of this book has tried to mention most of them and has perhaps overlooked a few. It should have been evident that he does not approve of many and sanctions some with reservation.

He considers the following as valuable steps for the correction of uncomplicated hallux valgus in comparatively young individuals: effacement of the medial eminence, release of the adductor tension on the lateral aspect of the first metatarsophalangeal articulation, and reinforcement of the medial capsule by transposition of the abductor hallucis to a more dorsal plane on the side of the joint—in other words *Silver's* procedure or some modification of it. This is an intra-articular operation. Following surgery, the joint stiffens some. It is important that the patient can beforehand actively extend the great toe and that pushing the hallux in dorsal direction does not cause pain.

When hallux valgus is accompanied by more than 15 degrees of varus of the first metatarsal, this bone should be osteotomized. If the basal joint of the great toe does not require redressement, the first metatarsal is sectioned across its distal extremity. When one also has to carry out resection of the medial eminence and release the lateral capsule, the site of the osteotomy is shifted toward the proximal end of the bone. Of the distal osteotomies, *Thomasen's peg-and-hole method* is preferred because it is the most stable. The author's choice for proximal osteotomy is a modified form of *Kutzenberger's* **V** cut. Prerequisite for osteotomy of the first metatarsal is that there should be no interlocking type of arthritis at the joint or that the great toe possesses a measure of unimpeded painless motion. When hallux valgus is complicated by a painfully stiff first metatarsophalangeal joint, one has two choices—Keller's resection or fusion. In the presence of severe metatarsalgia, fusion is to be preferred, especially when the patient is relatively young and has an occupation that necessitates long hours of standing or walking. Unfortunately, most patients do not easily accept the idea of going through life with ankylosed great toes.

The author does not wish to convey the impression that he is against other procedures, some of which may beneficially be utilized when indicated. He definitely disapproves of the practice of recommending the same set of surgical steps for any and all types of deformities. It is important that one knows what Schede, Keller, or Silver did in the past. With the accumulated knowledge since their time and with more modern tools and technical facilities, the surgeon must improve on the methods of his predecessors. He must feel free to delete a step or add another to the historically sanctioned surgical procedures. If necessary, he must deviate and design his own pattern to meet the requirements of the case under his care. The operation must suit the condition and not the other way around.

The word *condition* is used here in a broad sense. It does not merely refer to the deformity of the toes, the forefoot, or the foot; but it takes into account the patient's general health, his emotional make-up, occupation, and the number of weeks he can afford to be out of work. Osteotomy and fusion necessitate wearing casts for 6 weeks or more; they require an extended period of convelescence. The surgeon may decide in favor of Thomasen's osteotomy, but the patient cannot afford the time necessary for consolidation of the surgical fracture. In such an instance a compromise has to be made in favor of another procedure—perhaps Silver's. By the same token, the surgeon may think that fusion of the first metatarsophalangeal joint would be more appropriate, but the time element may induce him to perform the next best operation—Keller's resection.

In planning a suitable procedure for

a case, the surgeon must consider the following local factors: the circulatory state of the foot, the location of metatarsalgia and of tender points, the splaying of the forefoot under body weight and its compressibility, the degree of metatarus primus varus and of metatarsus quintus valgus, the extent of plantar bulge of central metatarsal heads and if they do or do not yield to upward thrust, the flexibility of metatarsophalangeal joints, the degree of outward deviation of the great toe and its axial rotation, the presence of interlocking arthritis of the first metatarsophalangeal joint as determined by push-down and push-up tests, and the deformities of the lesser toes and the mobility of their joints. It is important that one ascertain the duration of the discomfort or deform-

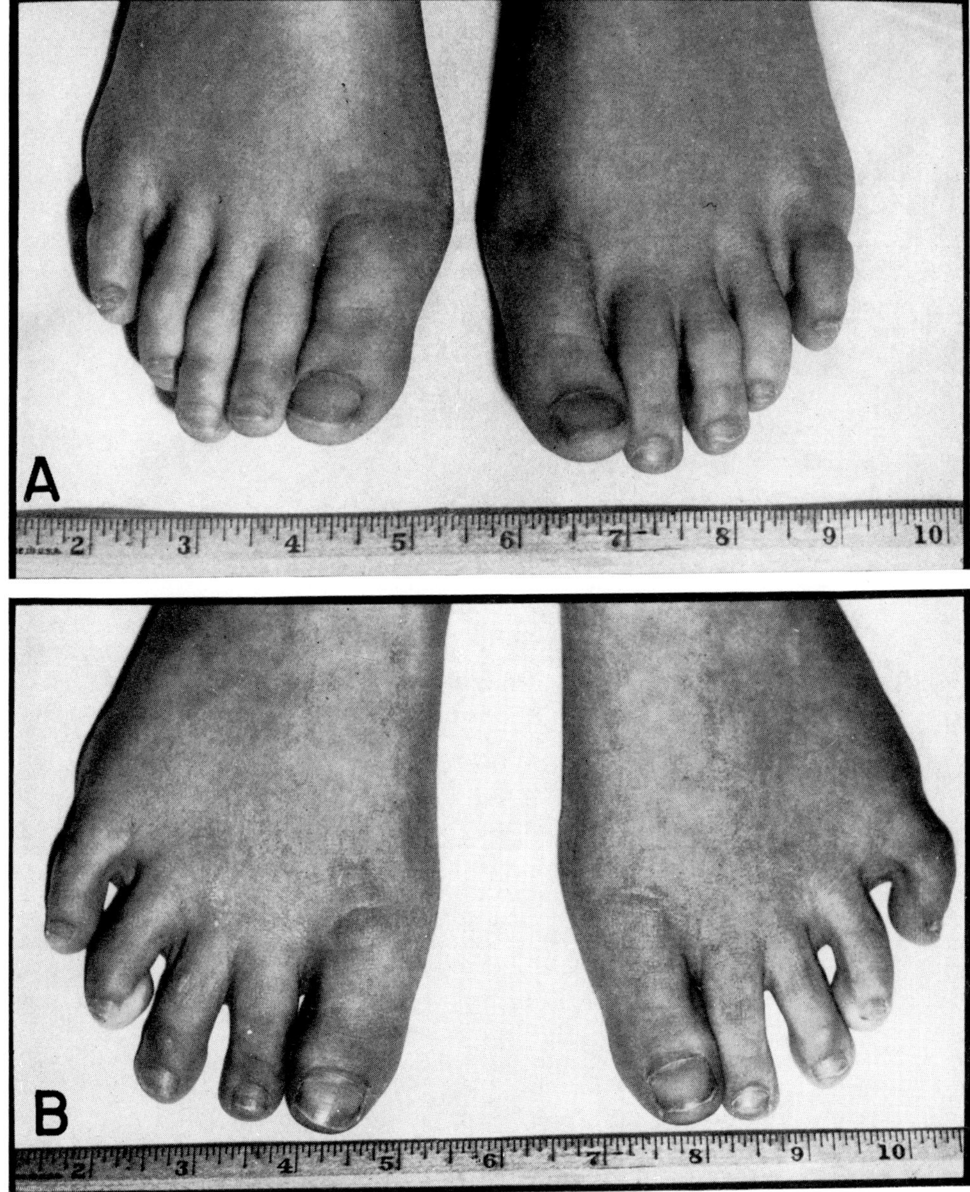

Figure 18–1. Widening of the forefeet under body weight. *A,* Photograph when no weight is borne. *B,* When weight is born. Note the widening of the forefoot. This was a case of early dynamic splaying of the forefoot in a 14 year old girl. It was symptomatic.

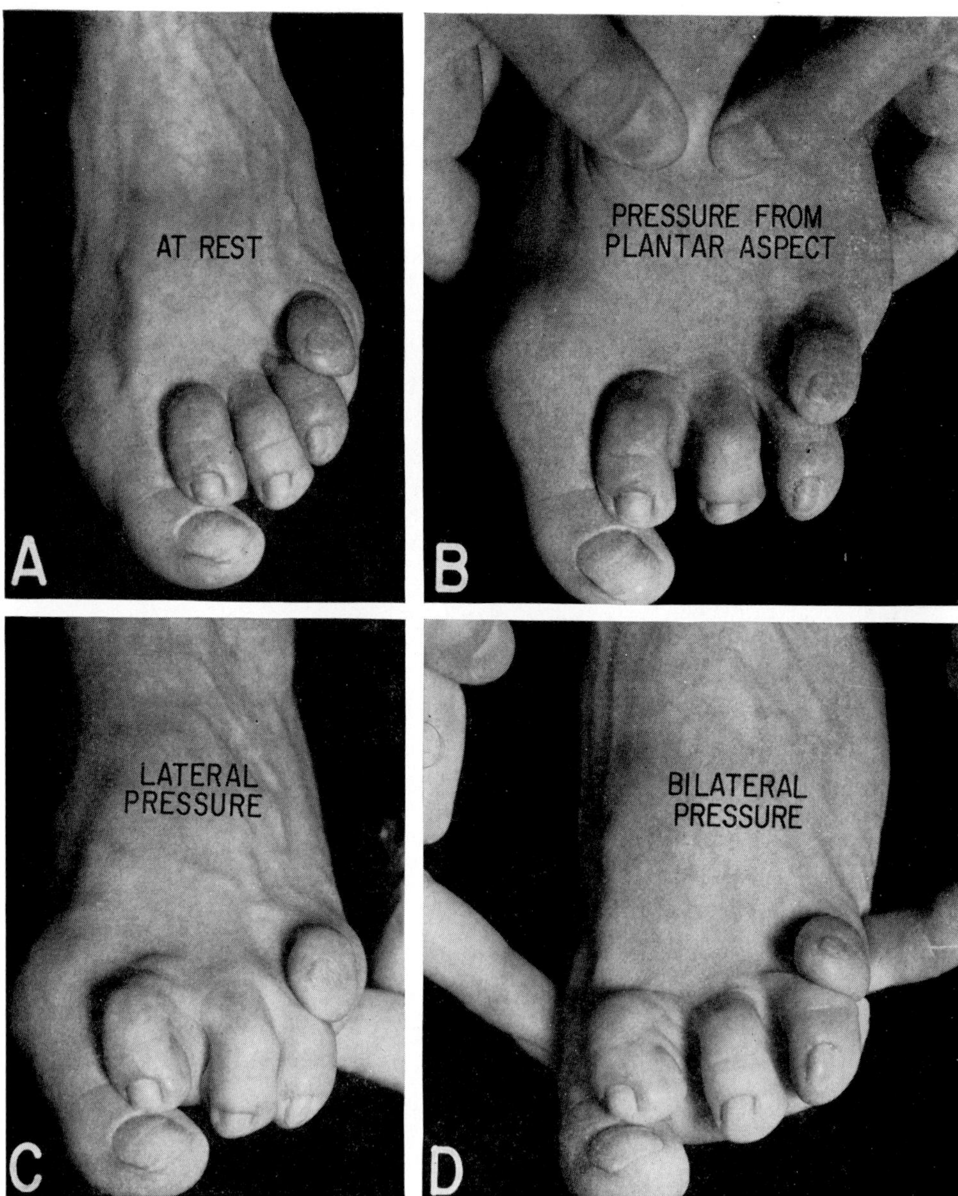

Figure 18–2. Compressibility of the forefoot. *A,* Photograph when no weight is borne on the forefoot. *B,* With pressure from the plantar aspect. Note the forefoot spread. *C,* Pressure on the head of fifth metatarsal narrows the forefoot. *D,* Pressure on the sides of marginal metatarsals reduces the transmetatarsal span considerably. This was a case of dynamic splaying of the forefoot in a woman around 60. It was also symptomatic. The deformed toes are considered to result from the late effects of splaying.

ity and its connection to trauma and shoe changes. One also looks for insignia of neurofibromatosis, contractures, and arthritis elsewhere in the body. A pigmented patch of skin in some other part may supply a clue for the obscure pain in the forefoot. When fibromatosis involves the palmar and plantar aponeuroses of the same patient, one may see the nodular thickening in the hand but not in the foot. Seeing the former makes one search for the latter carefully. Perhaps more important—at least more common—is the simultaneous involvement of the hands and feet in osteo- and rheumatoid arthritis. (Figs. 18–1 to 18–6).

The age of the patient needs to be considered in some instances. We know when a child reaches puberty and an adolescent evolves into adulthood. But when does an adult stop being young and merge into senescence? Shouldn't the surgeon be more concerned with the sluggishness of the patient's circulation and the stiffness of his joints than by his actual age? Judged by their arteries, their joints, and general tissue turgor, some patients are old at 40 or even before; others at 70 are young. In children, adolescents, and teenagers, cir-

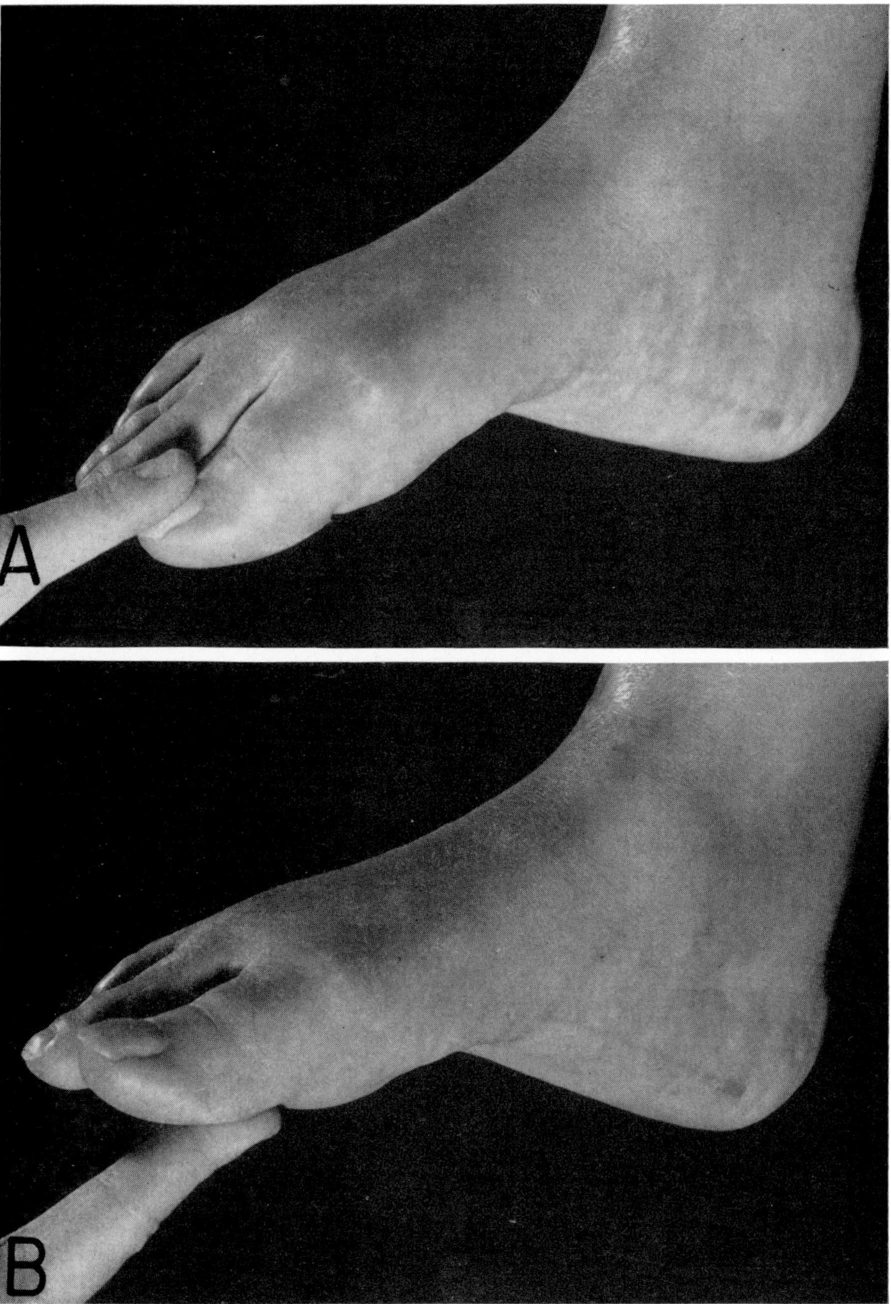

Figure 18–3. The limitation of motion of the first metatarsophalangeal joint. *A,* Push-down test. *B,* Push-up test. Note that there is almost no passive yield in dorsal direction. This was a young woman, 32 years of age, with no evidence of arthritis elsewhere.

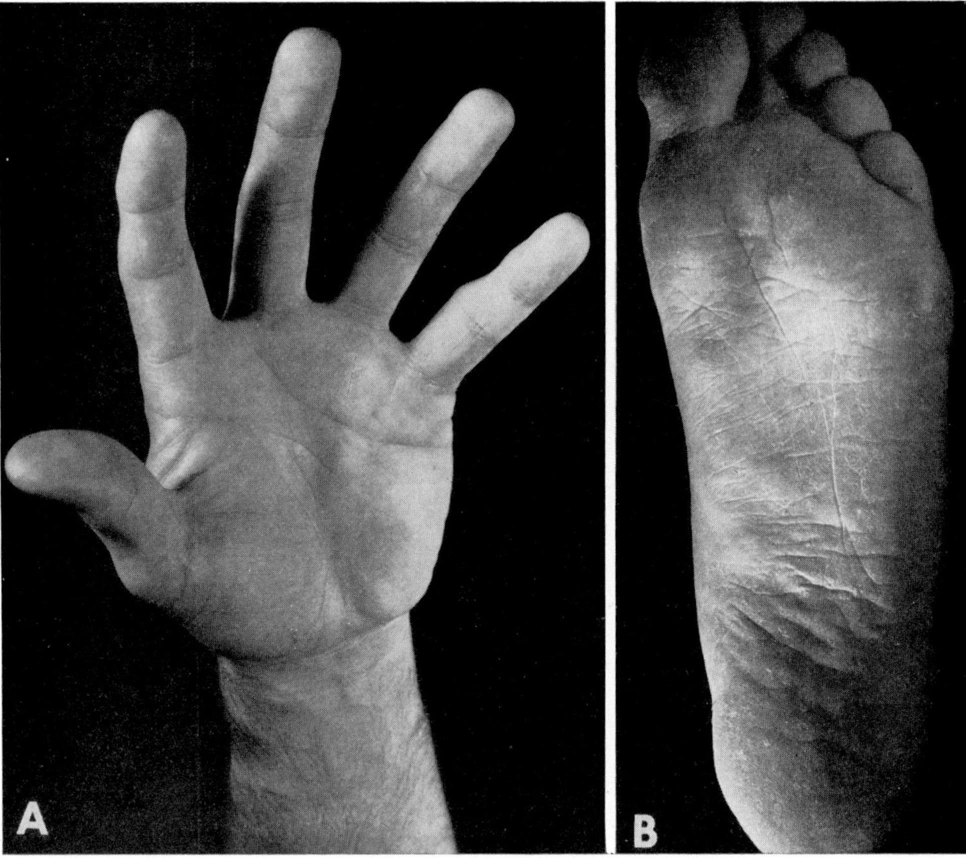

Figure 18–4. *A,* Visible nodule on the ulnar aspect of the palm of a man who had fibromatosis of both palmar and plantar aponeuroses on both right and left sides. *B,* Barely visible but palpable nodules along the medial border of the sole.

culatory disturbances of the foot seldom become a matter of concern, and the joints of the toes are rarely interlocked. In this age group one has to think mainly of the following factors: the stage of epiphysial growth, in particular of the proximal phalanx of the great toe; the propensity of young bones to throw exuberant callus; and hypermobility of marginal metatarsals. Keller's resection is avoided before epiphysial maturation; it would mean resection of the only growth center of the proximal phalanx of the great toe. Moreover, the remaining bone will in time proliferate profusely, encroach on the metatarsal head, and cause stiffness and pain. In the very young, sagittal resection of the medial or lateral eminence is likely to be followed with recurrence due to the hypermobility of the first or fifth metatarsals.

By far the majority of deformities in infants and growing children are congenital in origin: supernumerary digits, absent toes, microdactylia, digital gigantism, curling, overriding toes, and so on. The following present special problems of treatment: hallux valgus interphalangeus, hallux varus, metatarsus primus varus, and metatarsus multiplex varus. Hallux valgus interphalangeus is treated by cuneiform osteotomy through the shaft of the proximal phalanx of the great toe with the base of the resected wedge of bone lying medially. Seldom at birth does the great toe turn toward the midline of the body from the metatarsophalangeal junction. More commonly, congenital hallux varus is secondary to metatarsus primus varus—after wearing shoes for several years, the patient's great toe, which seems to have been deflected medially, will begin to turn in a lateral direction and simulate

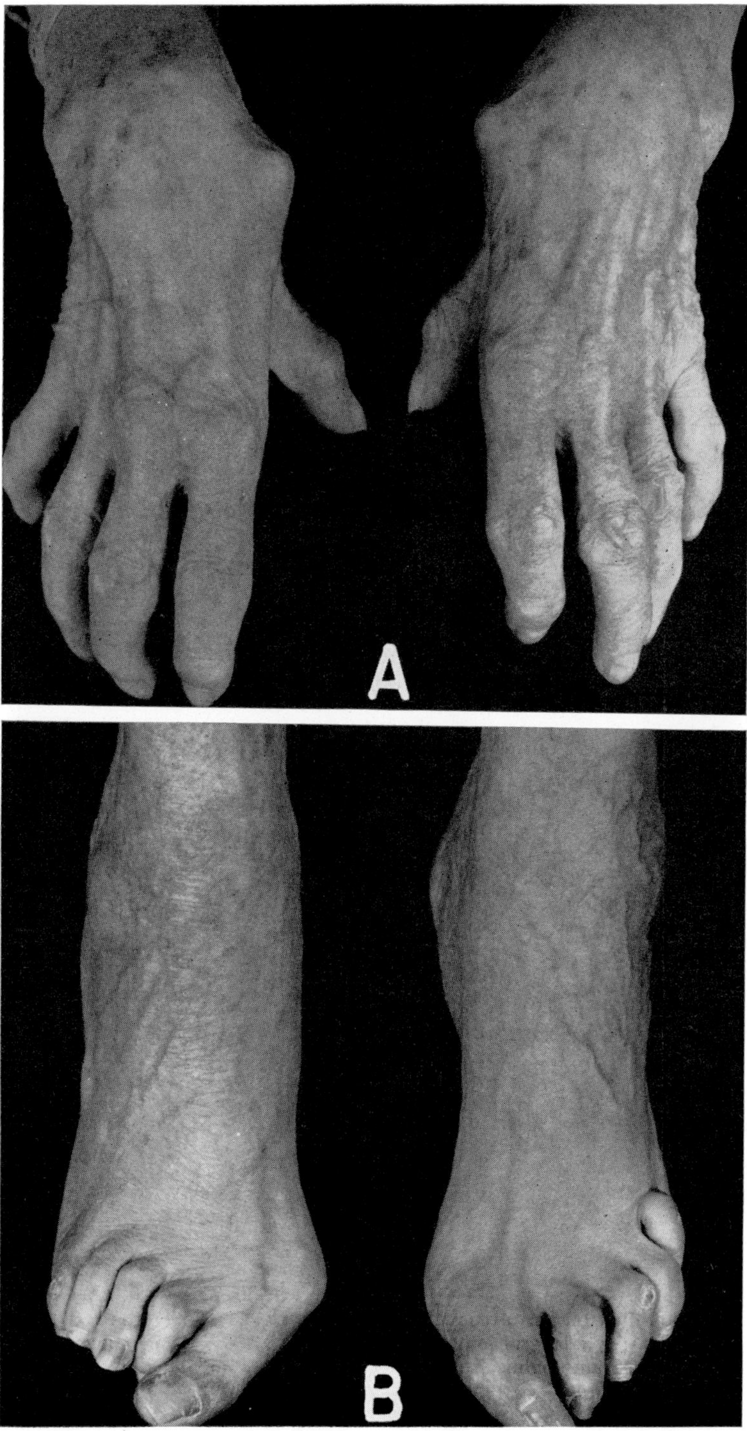

Figure 18–5. Simultaneous involvement of the hands and feet by osteo- or degenerative arthritis. Note the lack of swelling of the metacarpophalangeal joints (*A*) and the knuckling of the interphalangeal joints (*B*). Osteoarthritis appears to favor the distal digital joints of both the hand and the foot.

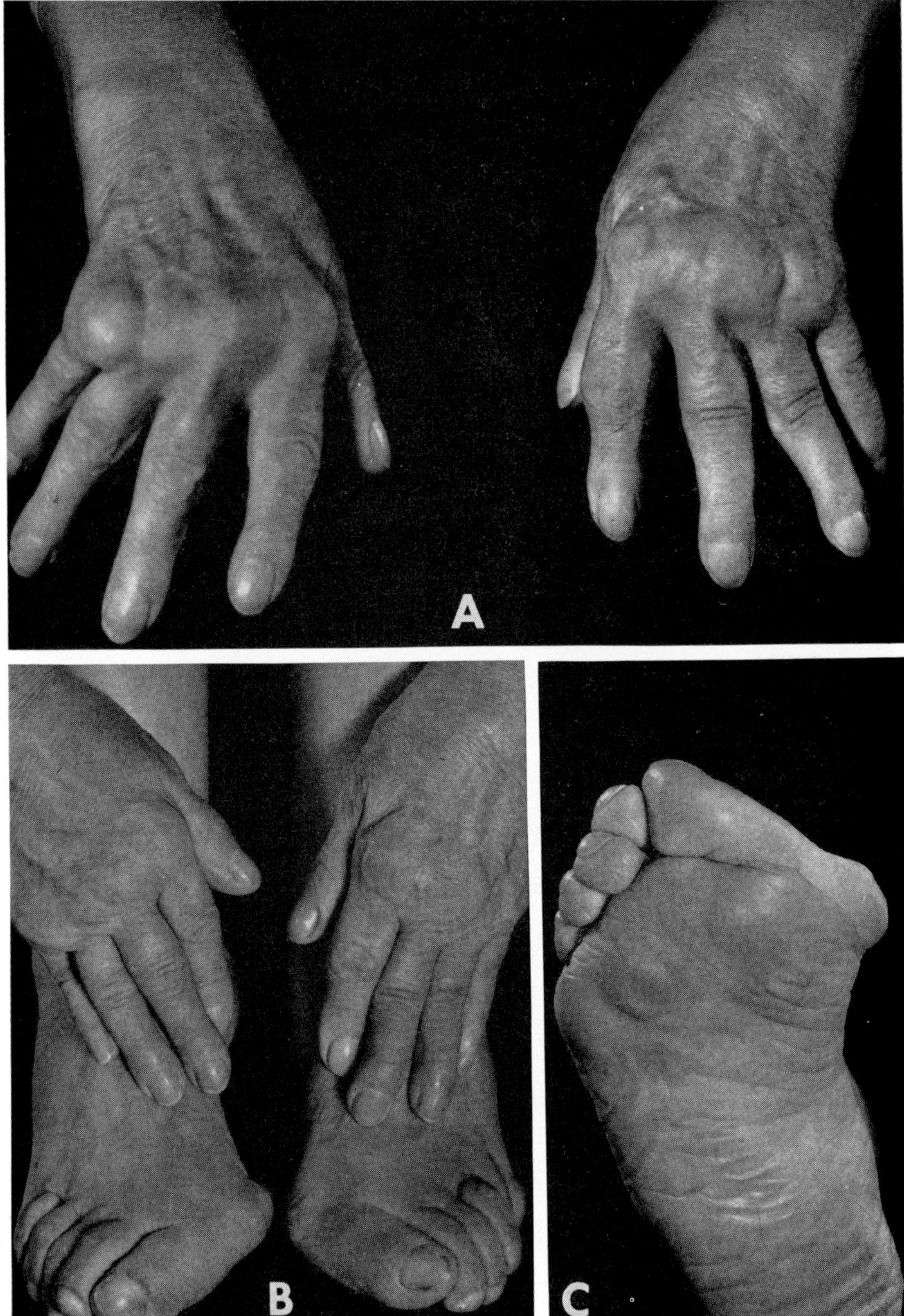

Figure 18–6. Simultaneous involvement of the hands and feet in rheumatoid arthritis. *A,* Note that mainly the metacarpophalangeal joints are involved. *B,* The hand in juxtaposition with the feet. Note that the toes also deviate mainly from the metatarsophalangeal junction. *C,* Plantar view of one foot.

hallux valgus. The rare primary hallux varus of congenital origin is treated by surgical syndactylia of the first and second toes. The more common secondary hallux varus is remedied by V osteotomy of the shaft of the first metatarsal, angulating the distal fragment laterally. In case the great toe has already begun to deviate toward the outer border of the foot, osteotomy of the first metatarsal is combined with release of adductor tension on the lateral side of the first metatarsophalangeal joint. The multiple variety of metatarsus varus depends on inversion of the heel. The first metatarsal bone is not only deflected medially but also plantarflexed, giving the impression of a cavus foot. The varus of the heel is corrected by Dwyer's osteotomy of the os calcis. The forefoot

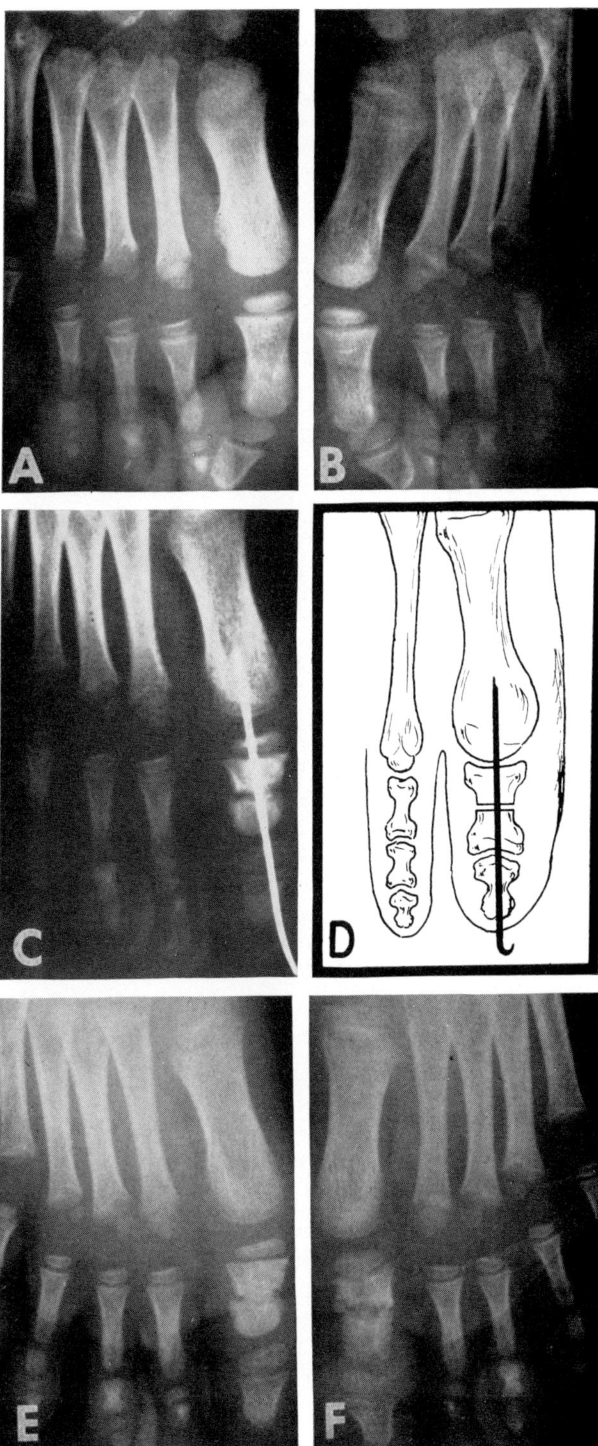

Figure 18–7. Boy, 2 years old, with bilateral congenital hallux valgus interphalangeus Mother's complaint: the second toes became blistered with the wearing of shoes. Surgery consisted of cuneiform osteotomy of the proximal phalanx of the great toe, the base of the resected wedge of bone lying medially; and fixation of the fragments by intramedullary wire. *A* and *B*, Preoperative roentgenograms of both feet. *C*, Right foot soon after surgery. *D*, Interpretative diagram. *E* and *F*, Postrecovery roentgenograms of both feet.

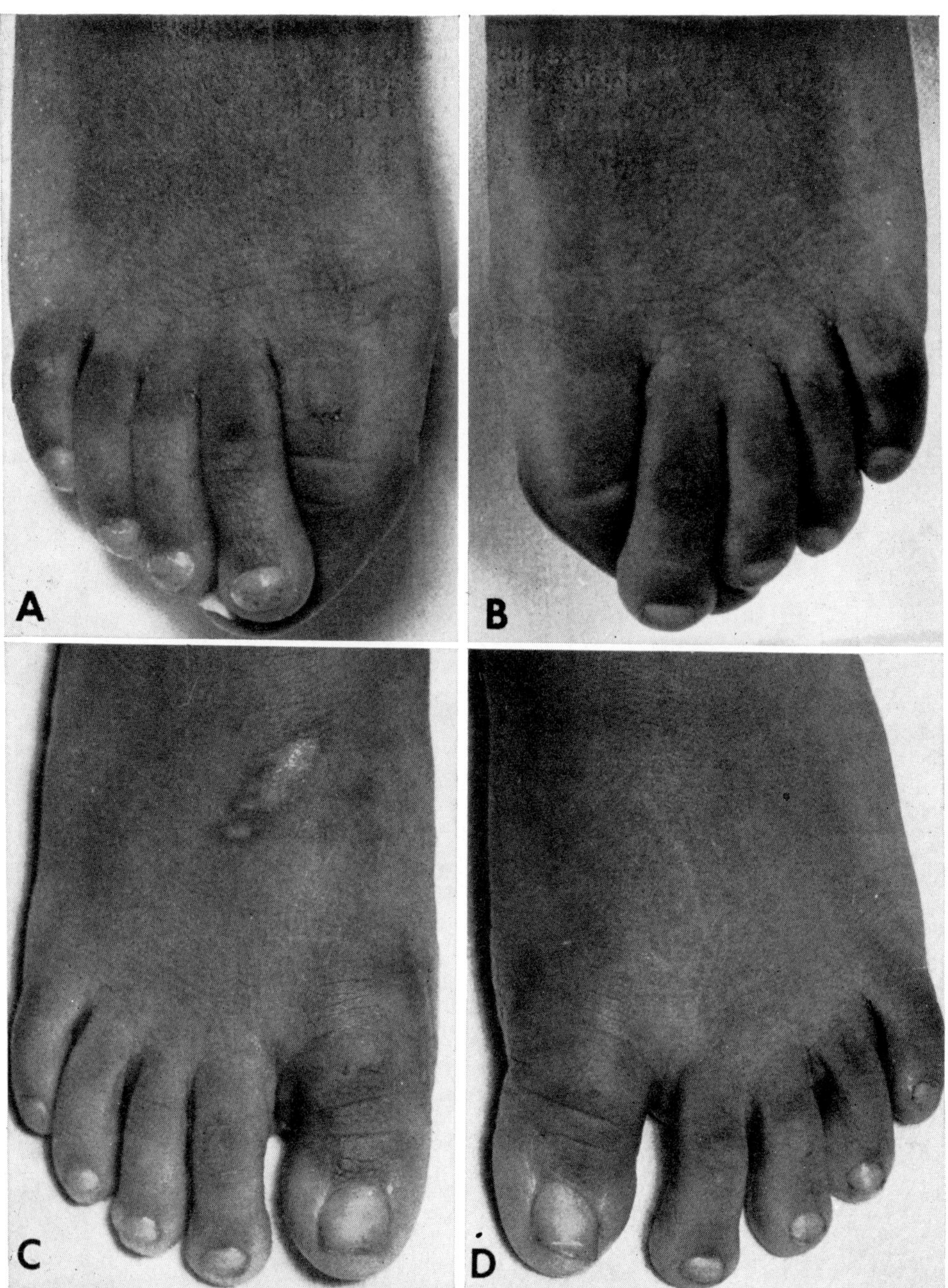

Figure 18–8. The same case as in Figure 18–7. *A* and *B,* Preoperative photographs of both feet. *C* and *D,* Postrecovery photographs. The child wears shoes in comfort. The second toes no longer become blistered.

deformity is remedied by transfer of the anterior tibial insertion to the lateral cuneiform. A plantarflexed and medially inclined first metatarsal is dealt with by osteotomy, tilting the distal fragment up and outward (Figs. 18–7 to 18–12).

Between the time of epiphysial maturation and the twentieth year, symptoms referable to Freiberg's infraction may become manifest. It is generally agreed that aseptic necrosis of one of the lateral metatarsal heads usually has its inception before epiphysial closure but remains asymptomatic until arthritic changes take place. Metatarsus primus varus and hypermobile first metatarsal are also carried over, from earlier to later years. A characteristic complaint by girls around the age of 14 to 18 is pain on the sides of the first and fifth metatarsal heads due to dynamic splaying of the forefoot. The marginal metatarsals spread sideways on weight-bearing; the forefoot overflows as it were, beyond the confines of the shoe; the heads of the first and fifth metatarsals bulge out and are chafed by the shoe. The girl complains of considerable discomfort on wearing shoes and cannot tolerate them. In some instances there is already established hallux valgus. If symptomatic, the widened forefoot of teenagers is narrowed by the following procedures: V osteotomy at the proximal shaft of first metatarsal, angulating the distal fragment laterally; oblique resection of the distal third of the fifth metatarsal; and surgical syndactylia of the fourth

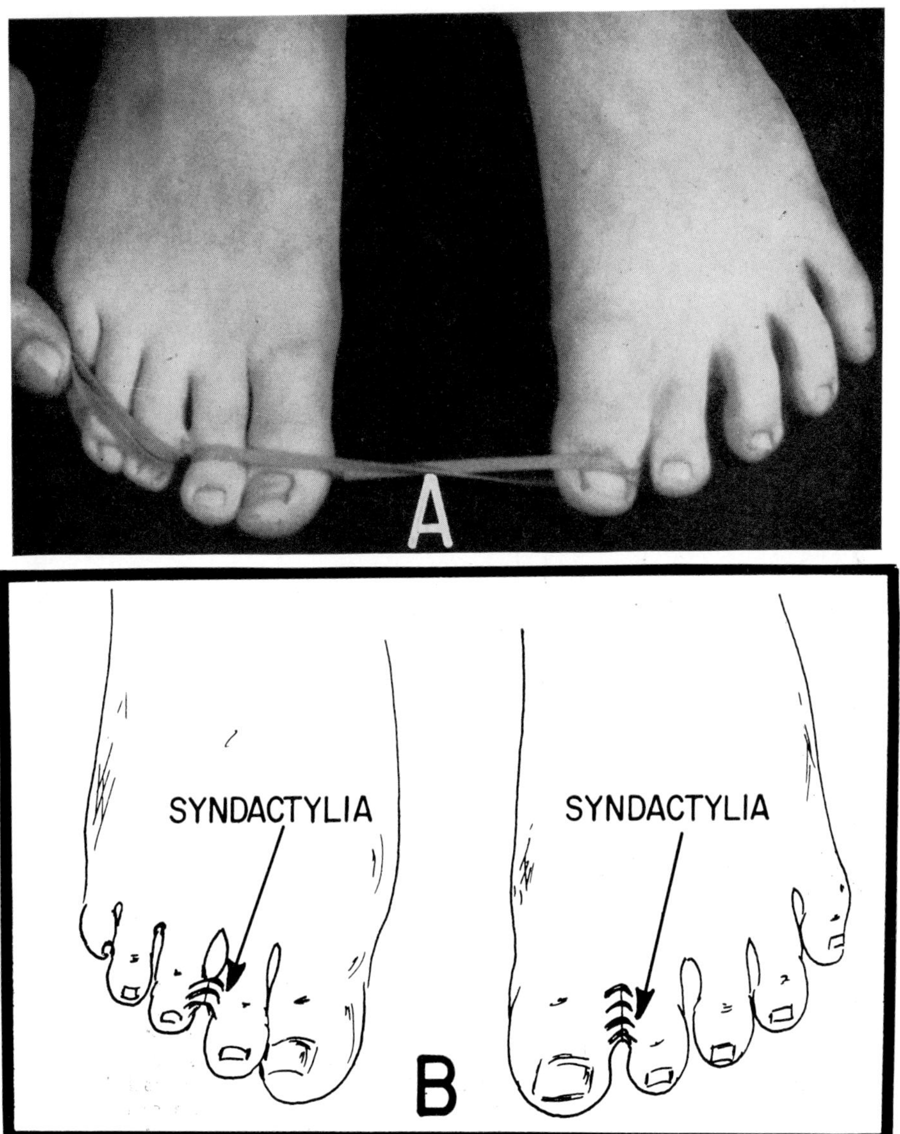

Figure 18–9. Boy, 3 years old, with curling third toe on the right side and "pigeontoe" on the left. The latter was primary congenital hallux varus without metatarsus primus varus. Surgery on the right foot consisted of partial surgical syndactylia between the second and third toes; on the left foot subtotal syndactylia of first and second toes was employed. The hallux is pulled medially to show the extent of anastomosis. *C,* Interpretative diagram. The parents were satisfied.

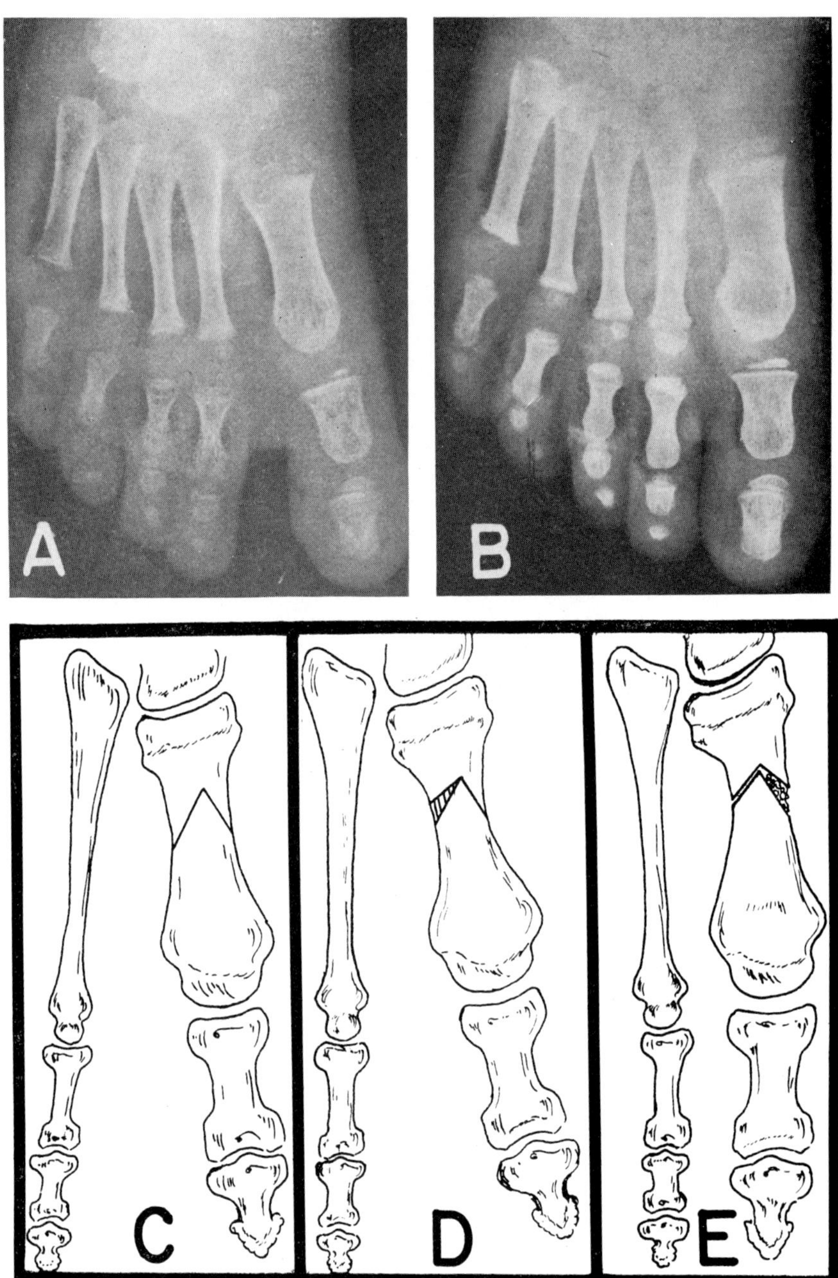

Figure 18–10. Boy, 3 years of age, with persisting "pigeontoes." This was secondary hallux varus due to metatarsus primus varus. Surgery consisted of V osteotomy of first metatarsal shaft, angulating the distal fragment laterally. *A,* Roentgenogram before osteotomy. *B,* After recovery. *C, D,* and *E,* Interpretative diagrams. Patient now wears ordinary shoes in comfort and parents are satisfied.

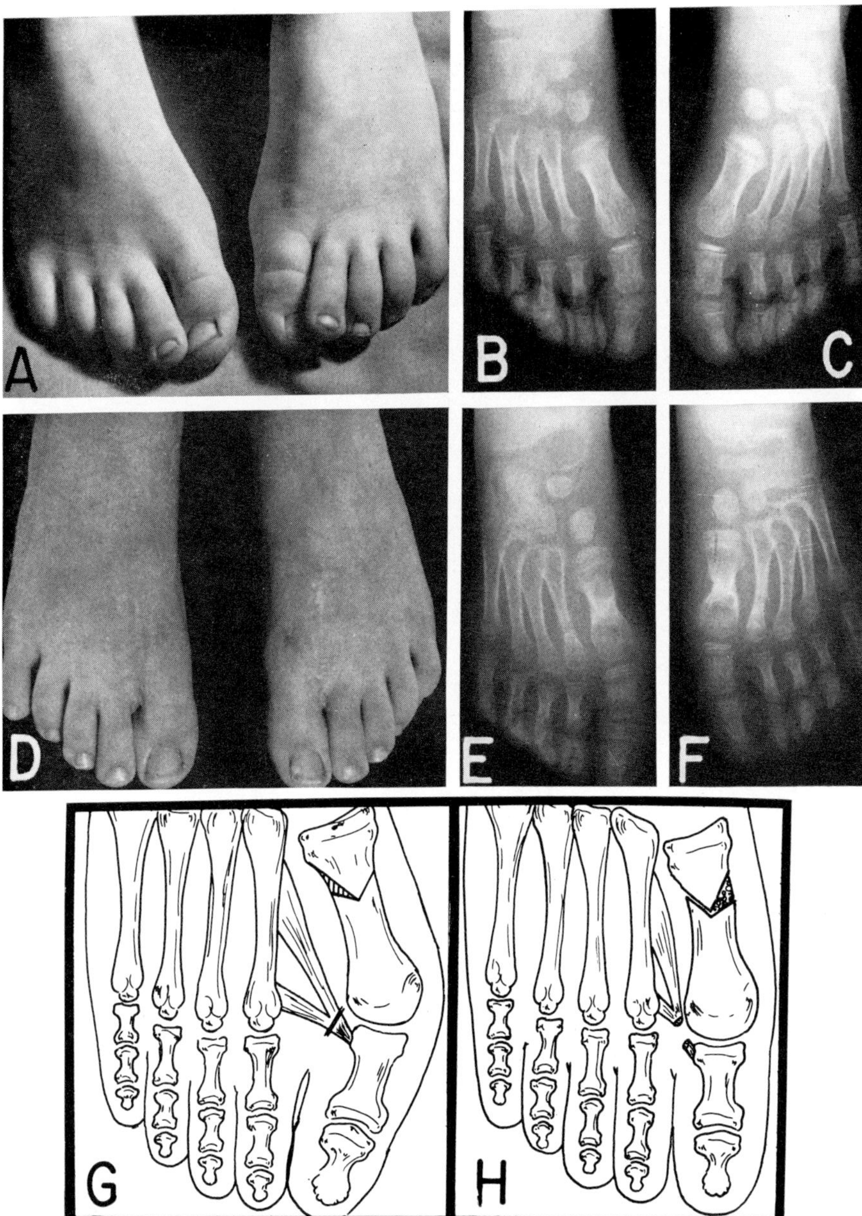

Figure 18–11. Girl, 4 years of age. Mother's complaint: "crooked big toes." This was a case of bilateral metatarsus primus varus and beginning hallux valgus on both sides. Surgery consisted of angulation osteotomy of first metatarsal and release of adductor tension on the lateral side of the first metatarsophalangeal joint. *A,* Before surgery. *B* and *C,* Roentgenograms before surgery. *D,* After recovery. *E* and *F,* Roentgenograms after recovery. *G* and *H,* Interpretative diagrams illustrating surgery on the right foot. Left foot was similarly operated on. Patient wears ordinary shoes in comfort and mother is satisfied.

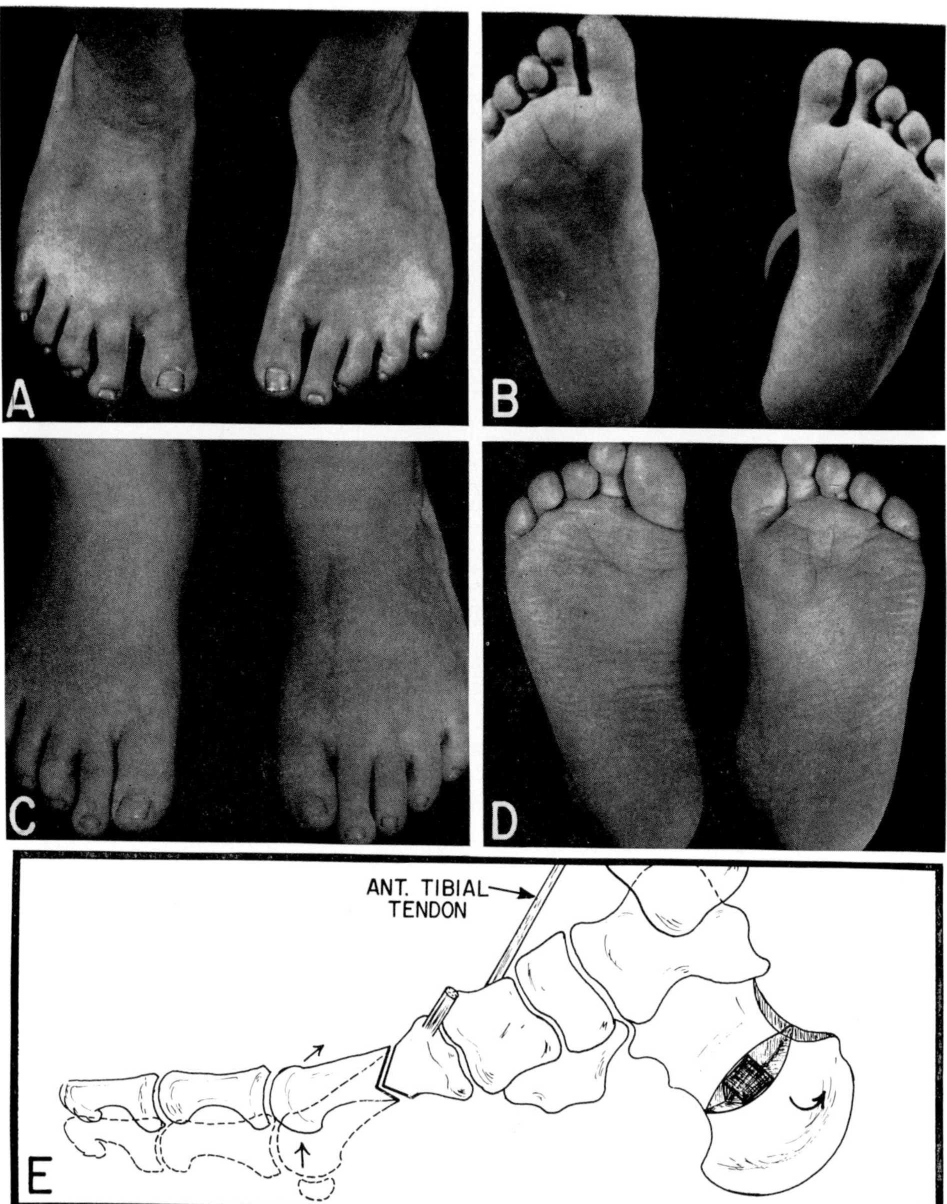

Figure 18–12. Boy, 4 years of age, with short left foot and blisters on the outer border of the sole. Diagnosis: forefoot varus, inversion of the entire foot and pes cavus. Surgery consisted of modified Dwyer osteotomy of os calcis; transfer of the anterior tibial insertion into the lateral cuneiform; and V osteotomy of the first metatarsal shaft, angulating the distal fragment dorsally and laterally. *A,* Dorsal view of both feet. *B,* Plantar view. Note that left foot is shorter and that there is a pressure keratosis under the base of the fifth metatarsal. *C,* Dorsal view 2 years after surgery. *D,* Plantar view. Note that the left foot is catching up in length and that the pressure keratosis has disappeared. *E,* Interpretative diagram of surgery. Patient now wears ordinary shoes in comfort and parents are satisfied.

and fifth toes. When there is established hallux valgus, the osteotomy side is shifted closer to the head of the first metatarsal (Figs. 18–13 to 18–17).

Freiberg's infraction may have remained dormant and unnoticed until after the twentieth year of life, when symptoms due to degenerative arthritis of the involved metatarsophalangeal joint arouse suspicion. Stress fractures of the metatarsals occur after this age. After the age of 20 or 30, acquired deformities prevail and begin to get complicated. The great toe not only deviates in a lateral direction, but it also rotates around it axis, and mounts over or slips under its neighbor. The lesser toes are hammered, clawed, crowded together, or sometimes diverge from one another. As time goes on, marginal metatarsals may lose some of their mobility and central heads bulge prominently under the plantar aspect of the forefoot and may even become fixed in that location, or

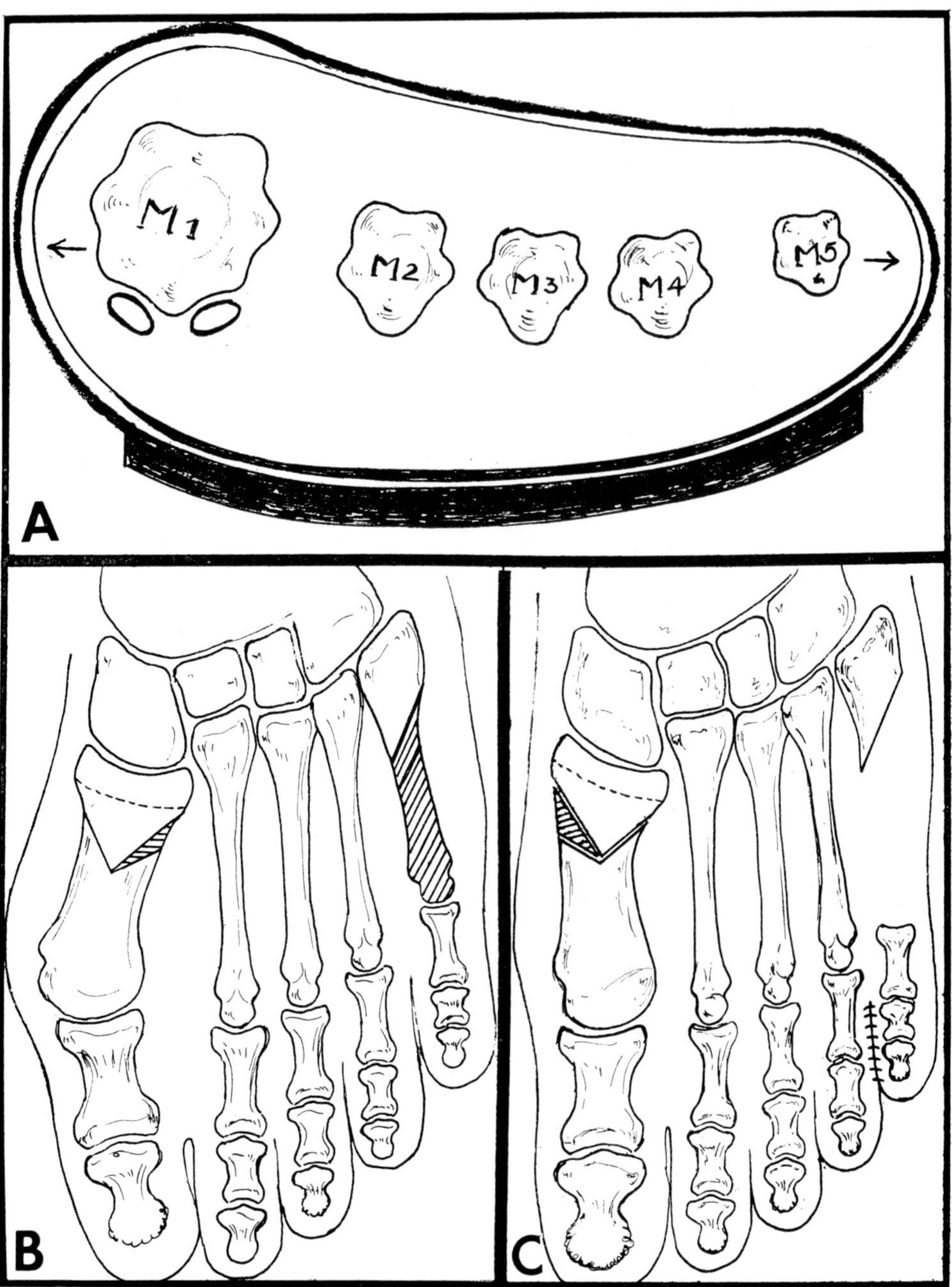

Figure 18–13. *A,* Diagram of forefoot "overflow" beyond the bounds of the shoe sole. *B* and *C,* The surgical procedures utilized for the correction of dynamic splaying of the forefoot: V osteotomy of the first metatarsal followed by angulation of the distal fragment laterally, and resection of distal two-thirds of the fifth metatarsal followed by surgical syndactylia of fourth and fifth toes.

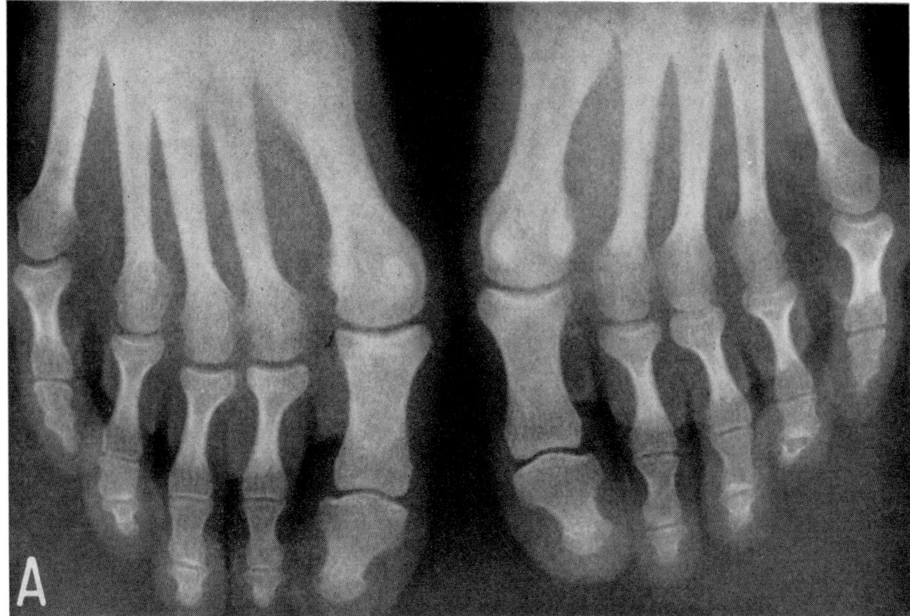

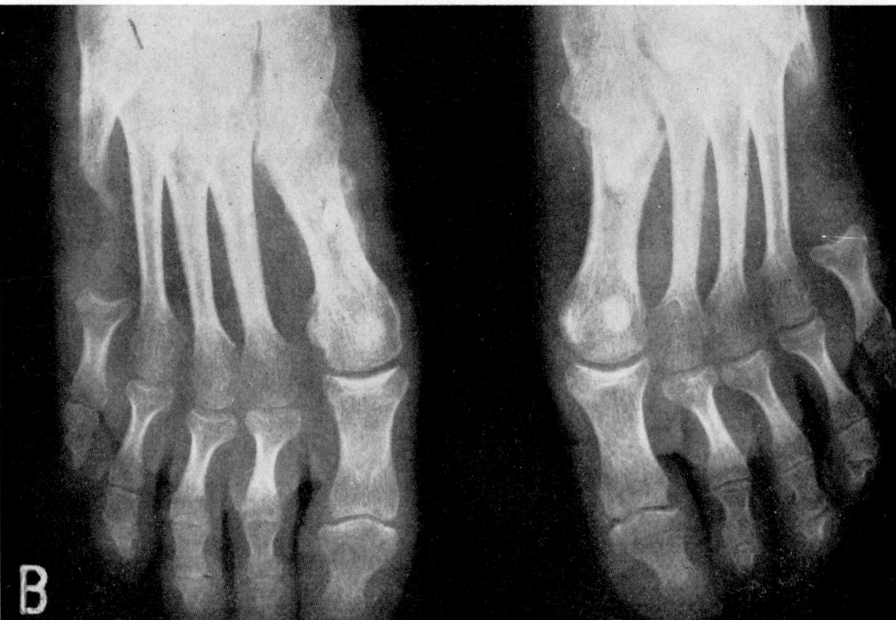

Figure 18–14. Girl, 14 years of age, unable to wear closed-toe shoes because of pain on the sides of first and fifth metatarsal heads. Diagnosis: dynamic splaying of forefoot. Surgery consisted of lateral angulation osteotomy of the first metatarsal, resection of distal two-thirds of fifth metatarsal, and surgical syndactylia of fourth and fifth toes. *A,* Roentgenogram of both feet before surgery. *B,* After recovery.

incarcerated. The metatarsophalangeal joints stiffen and the forefoot as a whole loses its resilience.

In the absence of arthritis, metatarsus primus varus, or hypermobile first metatarsal, hallux valgus in comparatively young adults may be treated by Silver's operation or some modification of it. When there is definite axial rotation of the hallux, metatarsus primus varus, or hypermobile first metatarsal, we prefer Thomasen's operation—peg-and-hole osteotomy of the distal end of the first metatarsal. In the absence of metatarsalgia, the capital fragment is displaced laterally, closer to the second metatarsal; if there is also metatarsalgia, the distal fragment is in addition depressed plantarward. In axial rotation of the great toe, after invaginating the spiked end of the proximal fragment into the capital piece, the hallux is derotated until its nail assumes a horizontal position. Hammertoes are corrected by partial phalangectomy and surgical syndactylia. Persistent dynamic splaying of the fifth metatarsal is remedied by resection of the distal half, or more, of this bone and by surgical syndactylia of the fifth toe with the fourth. Incarcerated central meta-

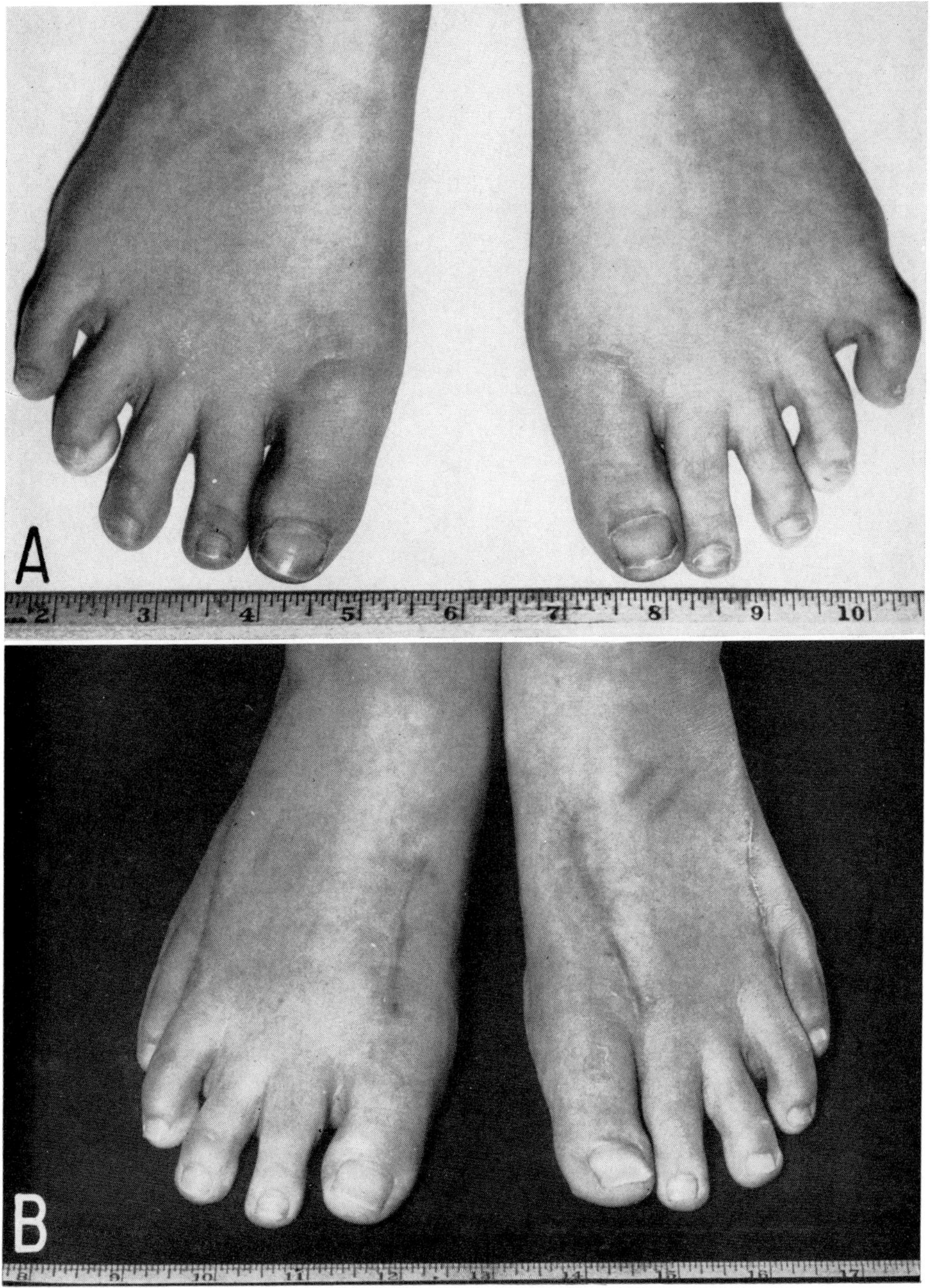

Figure 18–15. The same case as in Figure 18–14. *A,* Before surgery. *B,* After recovery. She wears closed-toe shoes in comfort and is happy with narrowed forefeet.

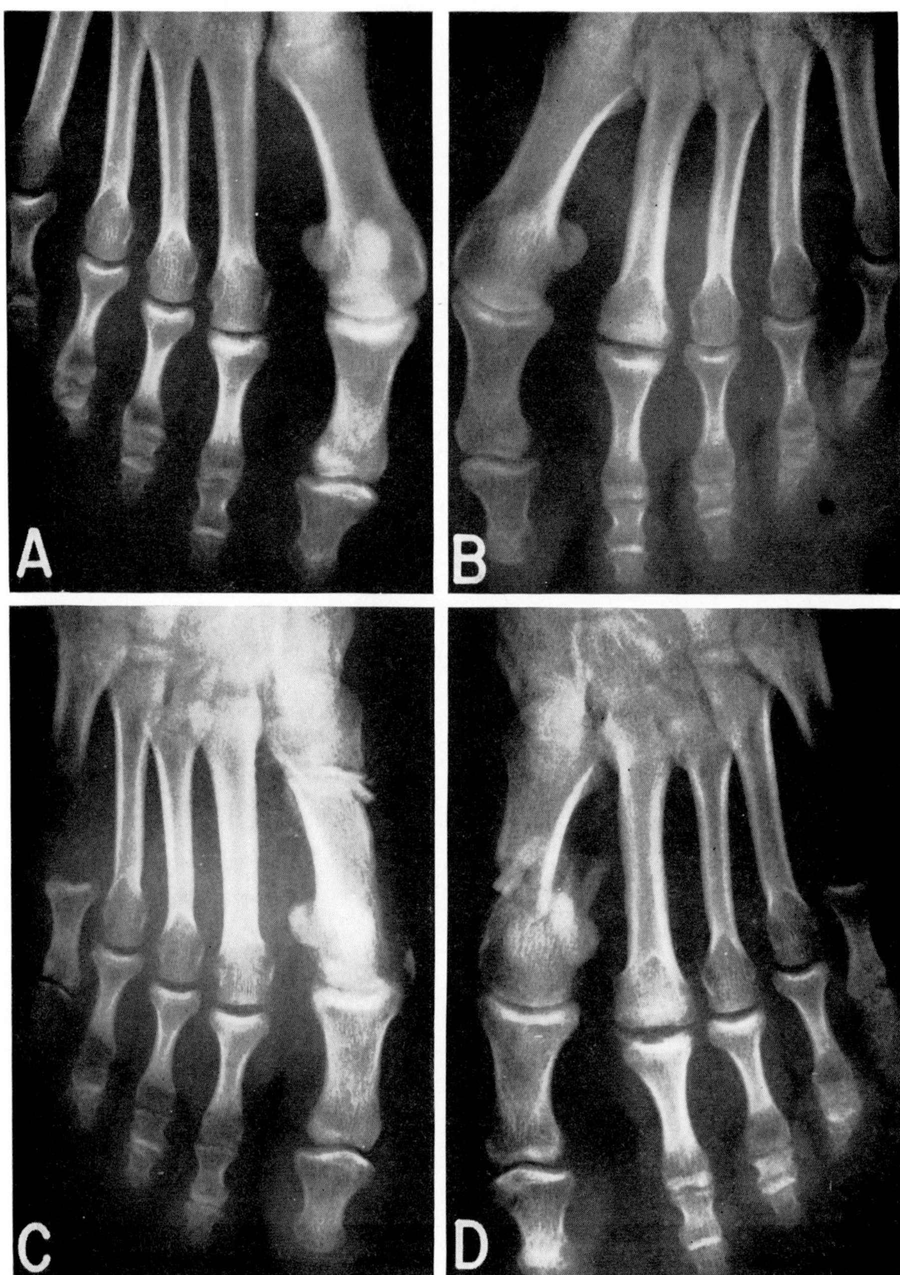

Figure 18–16. Girl, 18 years of age, with pain along the borders of the forefeet and "bunions." Diagnosis: bilateral dynamic splaying of forefeet and hallux valgus. Surgery on right foot consisted of V osteotomy of first metatarsal base and sagittal resection of medial eminence; on left foot, lateral displacement osteotomy of the distal end of the first metatarsal was employed. On both sides, resection of distal half of the fifth metatarsal, and surgical syndactylia of fourth and fifth toes were performed. *A* and *B,* Preoperative roentgenograms. Note the flattening of the second metatarsal head in *B. C* and *D,* Roentgenograms after recovery.

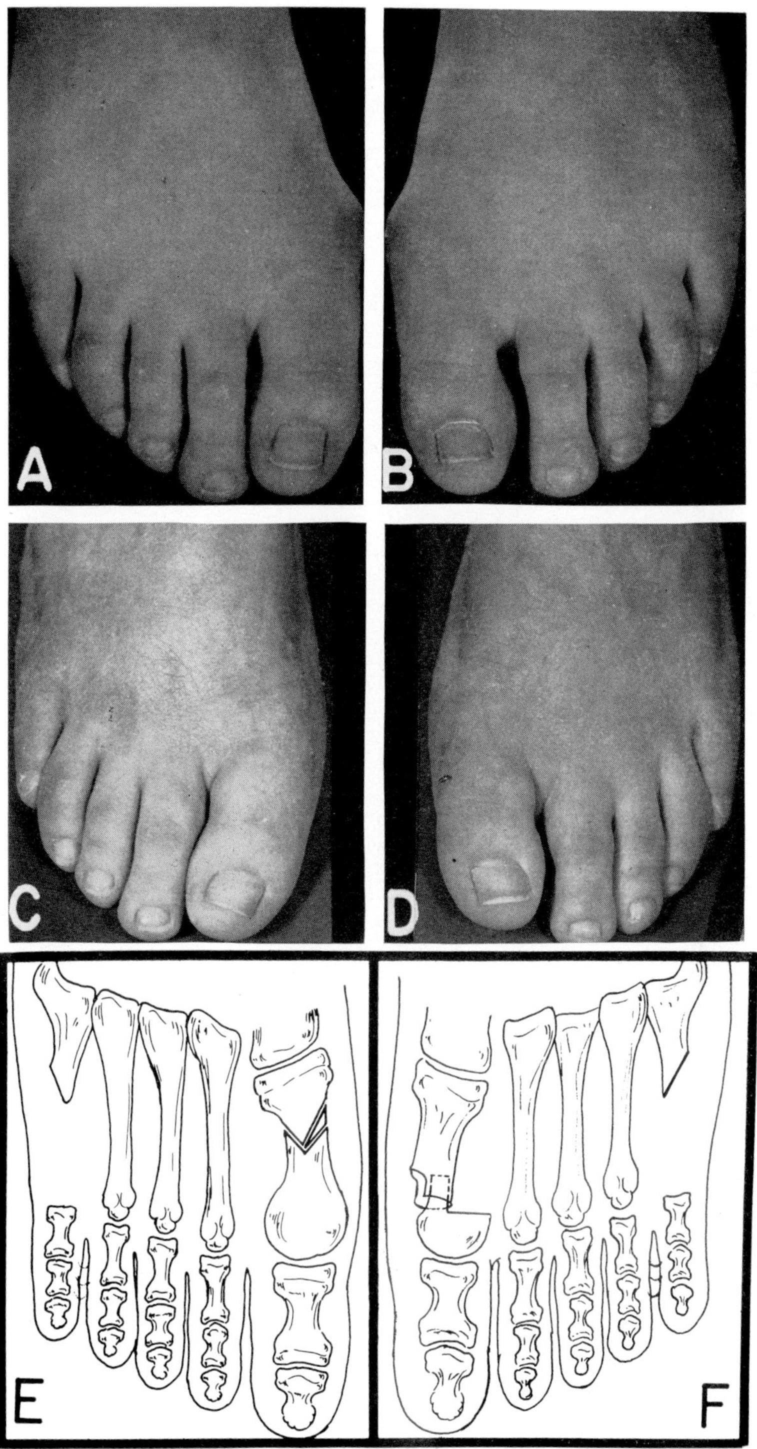

Figure 18–17. The same case as in Figure 18–16. *A* and *B,* Before surgery. *C* and *D,* After recovery. *E* and *F,* Interpretative diagrams. Patient is satisfied with narrowed feet, but complains of some pain over first metatarsophalangeal joints.

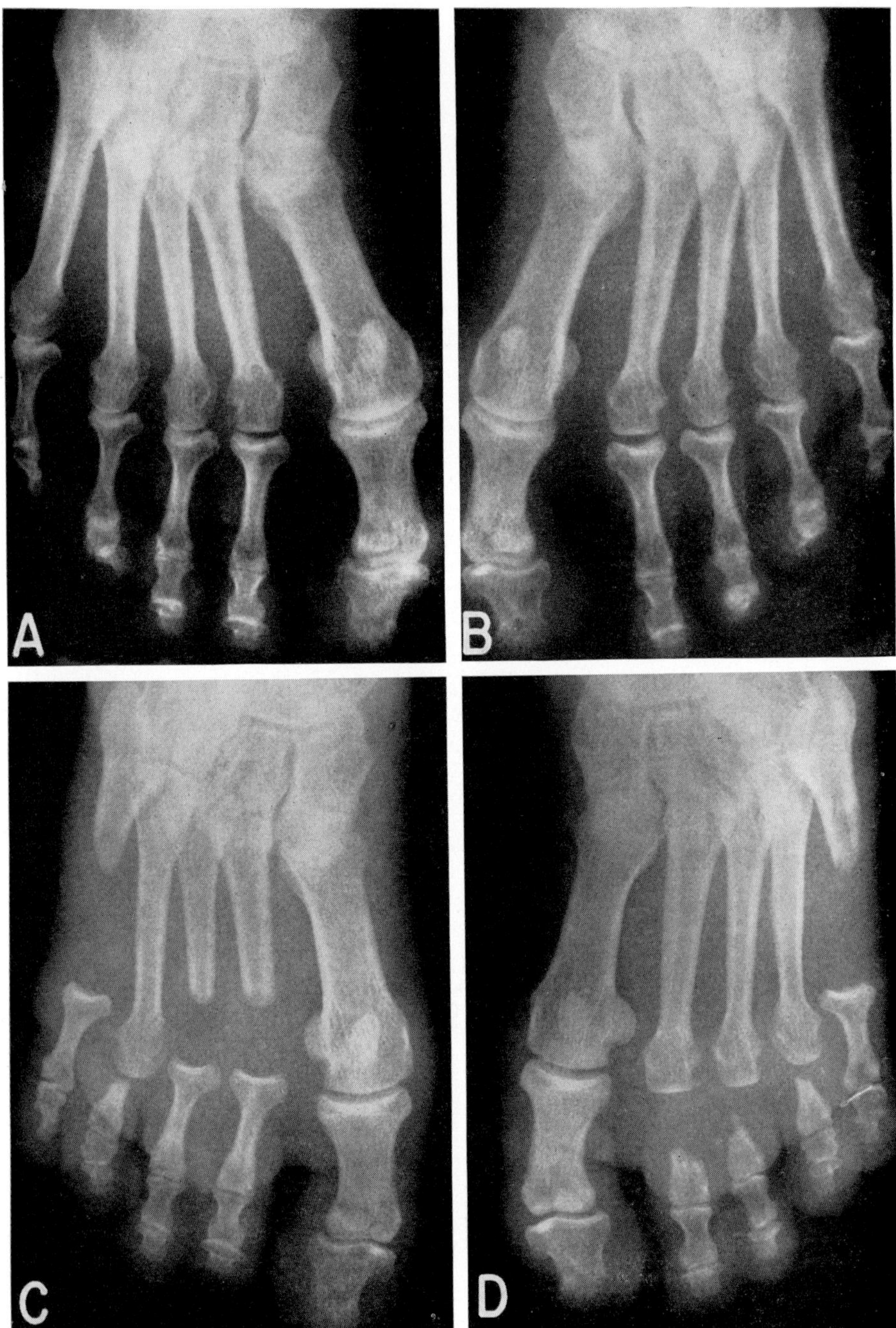

Figure 18–18. Woman, 38 years of age, with pain over the heads of both fifth metatarsals and pain under second and third metatarsal heads of right foot. Diagnosis: on the right side, dynamic splaying of the fifth metatarsal and fixed incarceration of second and third metatarsal heads; on the left side, dynamic splaying of the fifth metatarsal and resilient plantar bulge of the central metatarsal heads. Surgery on the right side consisted of resection of distal ends of second and third metatarsals and surgical syndactylia of second and third toes, and resection of distal two-thirds of the fifth metatarsal and surgical syndactylia of fourth and fifth toes; on the left side, partial proximal phalangectomy of the three middle toes, resection of distal two-thirds of fifth metatarsal, and syndactylia of second with third and fourth with fifth toes were performed. *A* and *B,* Preoperative roentgenograms. *C* and *D,* Roentgenograms after recovery.

tarsal heads may also need excision, in which instance the corresponding toes are stabilized by surgical syndactylia. Occasionally, one sees patients past the age of 60 or 70 with symptomatic hallux valgus and metatarsus primus varus and no sign of arthritis of the first metatarsophalangeal joint. If the circulation of the foot is unimpaired, the deformity of the great toe and its metatarsal should be corrected by osteotomy, as in young individuals (Figs. 18–18 to 18–25).

Hallux valgus with a stiff first metatarsophalangeal joint is treated by Keller's resection. Keller's resection is also preferred when the hallux rides over or has slipped under the second toe, in which case the operation is carried out by an interdigital approach and the first and second toes are syn-

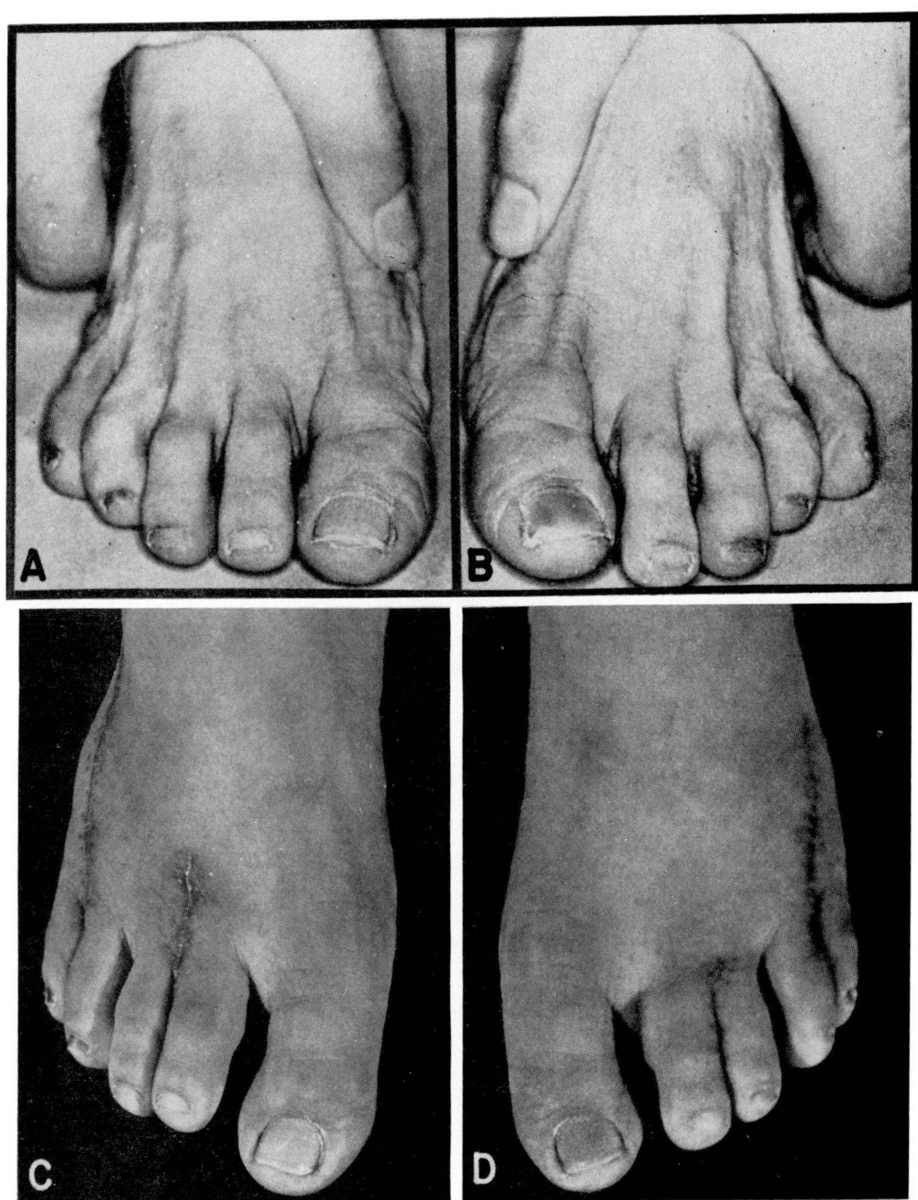

Figure 18–19. The same case as in Figure 18–18. *A* and *B,* Preoperative photographs. The forefeet are being compressed. *C* and *D,* After recovery. Patient is very happy with her narrowed feet and experiences no discomfort.

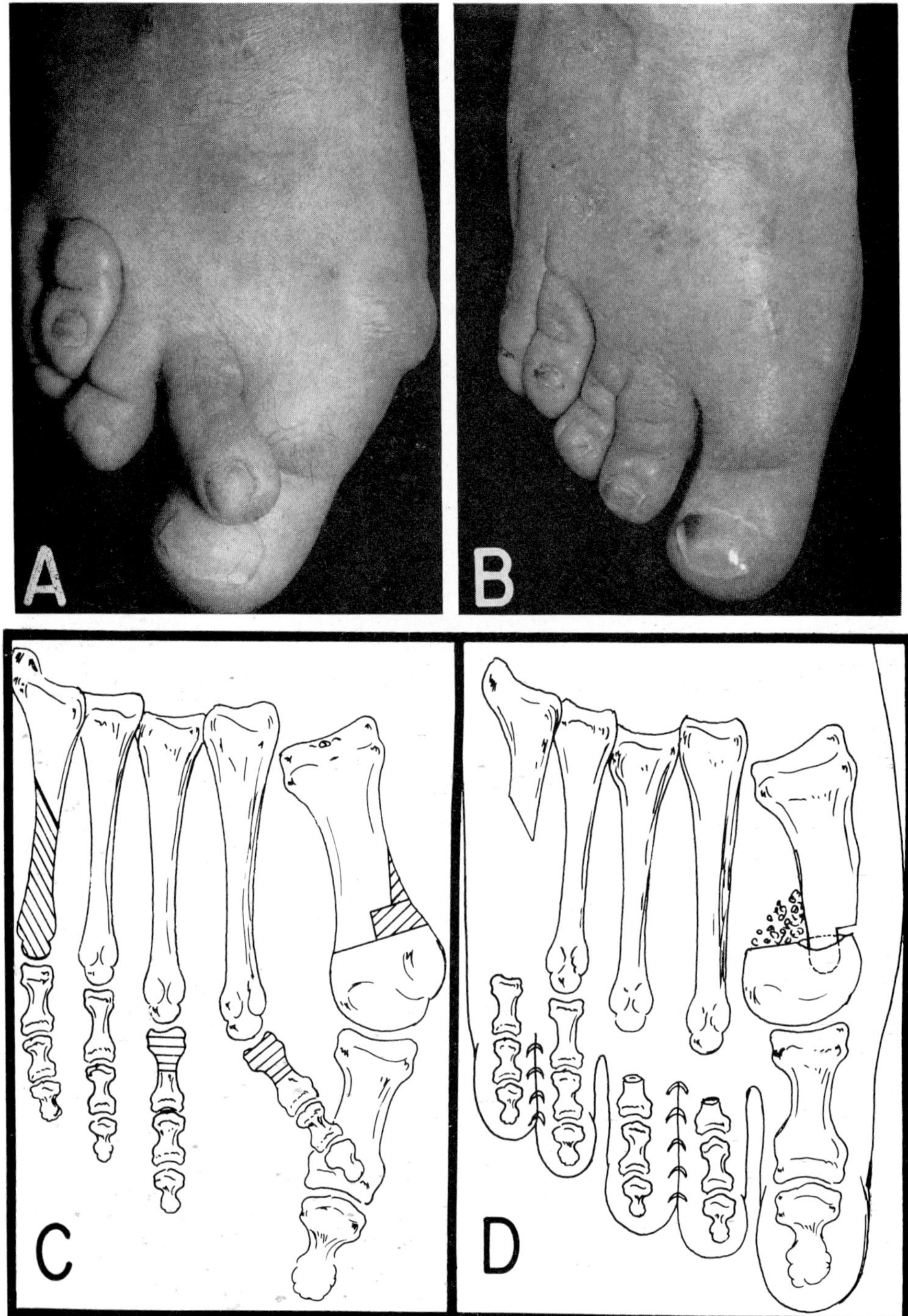

Figure 18–20. Woman, 33 years of age, with malformed toes and pain on the borders of her forefoot when wearing shoes. Diagnosis: dynamic splaying of the forefoot, hammered and overriding toes, and hallux valgus. Surgery consisted of lateral displacement osteotomy of the distal extremity of the first metatarsal, partial proximal phalangectomy of the second and third toes, resection of the distal two-thirds of the fifth metatarsal, and surgical syndactylia of second toe with the third and fourth toe with the fifth. *A,* Preoperative photograph. *B,* Postrecovery photograph. *C* and *D,* Interpretative diagrams. Patient was very satisfied.

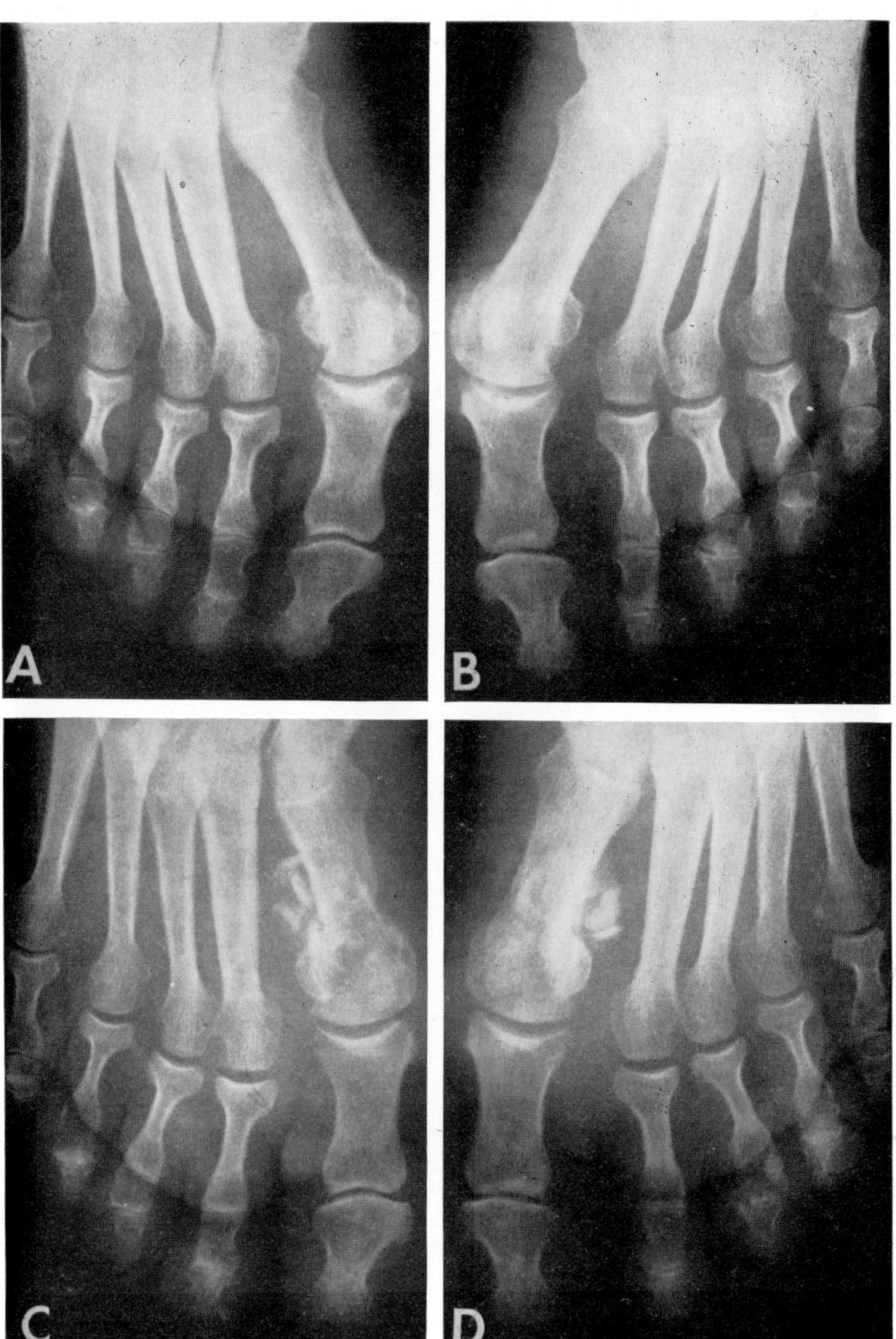

Figure 18–21. Woman, 64 years of age, with deformed great toes and pain on the medial aspects of the first metatarsophalangeal joints. Diagnosis: bilateral hallux valgus with metatarsus primus varus in a woman who, in spite of her age, was considered young and treated as such. Surgery consisted of distal osteotomy with lateral and plantar displacement of capital fragment. *A* and *B*, Preoperative roentgenograms. *C* and *D*, Postrecovery roentgenograms.

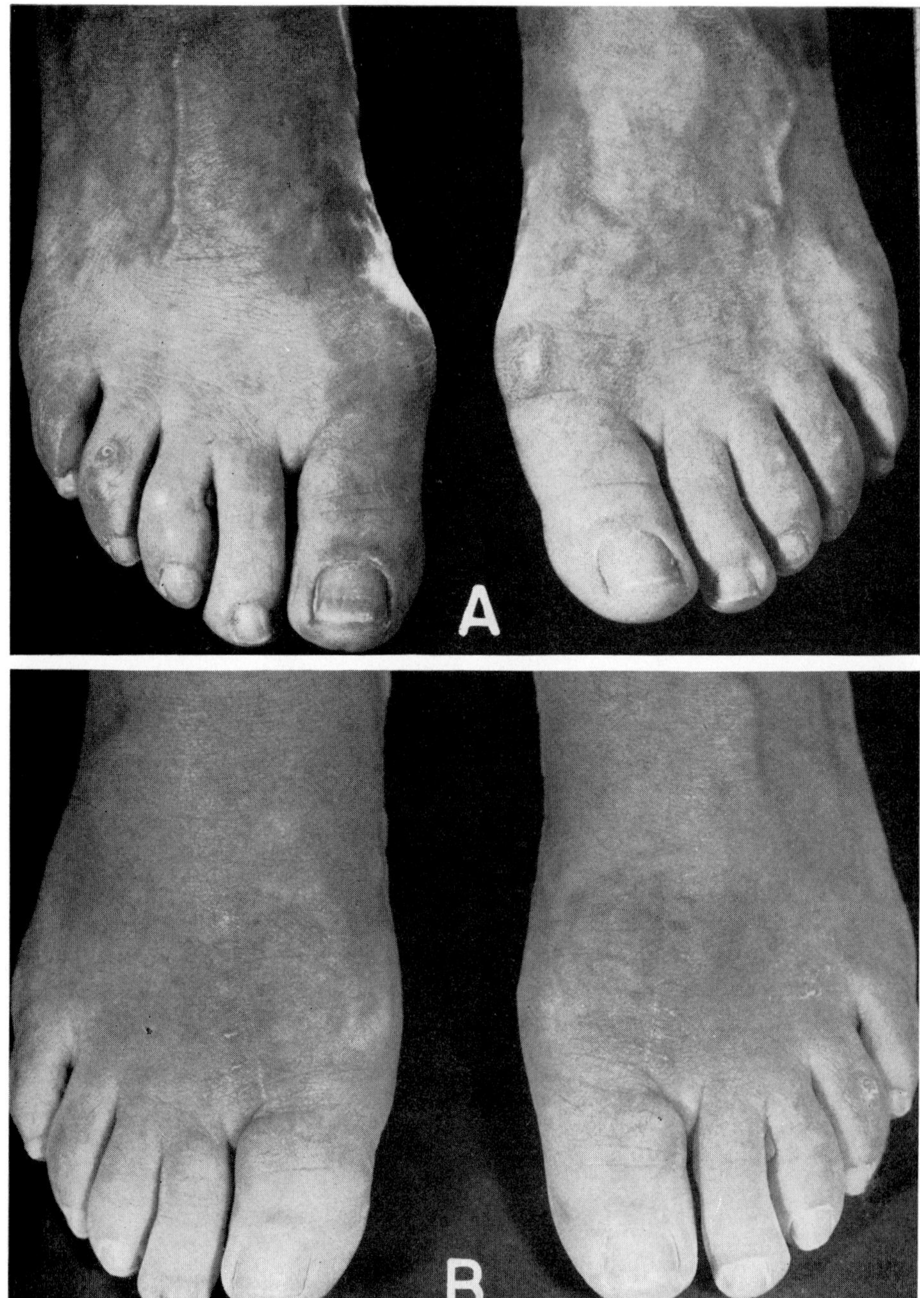

Figure 18–22. The same case as in Figure 18–21. *A,* Before surgery. *B,* After recovery. Patient is satisfied.

dactylized together. This approach is also preferred when the skin over the medial aspect of the first metatarsophalangeal joint appears precarious. In some cases the first metatarsophalangeal joint of one foot is arthritic, while articulation on the opposite side is free of degenerative changes. The deformity on the arthritic side is corrected by Keller's resection; that on the other side is remedied by Thomasen's osteotomy. The great toes are shortened equally. Occasionally, hallux valgus, degenerative arthritis of the first metatarsal joint, and metatarsus primus varus coexist. In such a case the first metatarsal is osteotomized at or near its base to correct its varus, and Keller's resection is

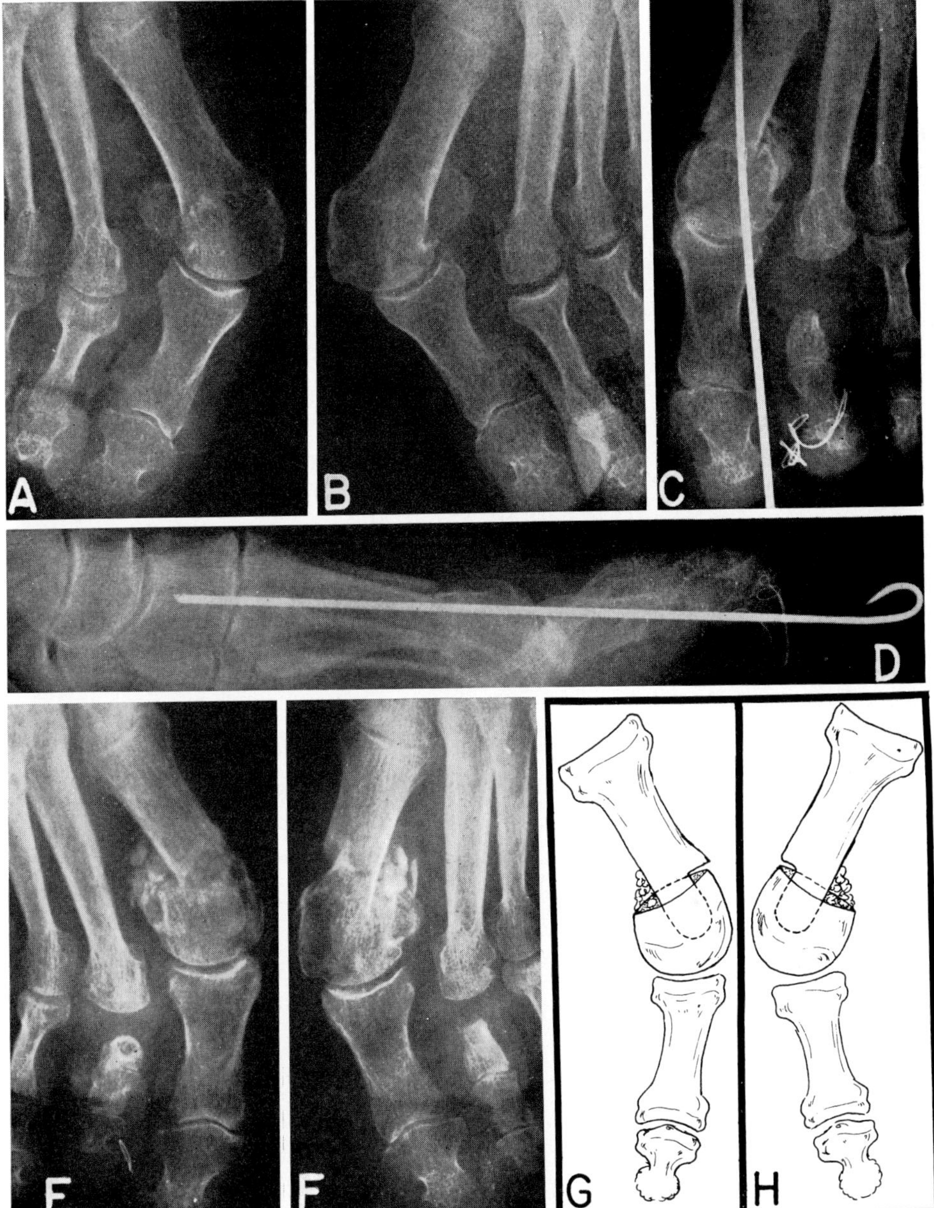

Figure 18–23. Woman, 75 years of age, with bilateral "bunions," hammertoes, and pain around the big toe joints but with no stiffness. Notwithstanding her advanced years, she had resilient feet. Her chief complaint was that she walked on the nail of the right second toe and experienced metatarsalgia proximal to this. Diagnosis: bilateral hallux valgus with axial rotation, fixed metatarsus primus varus, resilient plantar bulge of the second metatarsal head, and hammered second toe. Surgery consisted of distal osteotomy of the first metatarsal with lateral displacement and plantar depression of the distal fragment on each foot, and partial proximal phalangectomy of second toes and syndactylia each with the hallux. *A* and *B,* Preoperative roentgenograms. *C,* Postoperative roentgenogram of left foot showing intramedullary fixation by Kirschner wire. *D,* The same seen from the lateral side. Note the plantar shift of the capital fragment. *E* and *F,* Postrecovery roentgenograms. *G* and *H,* Diagrams demonstrating peg-and-hole invagination.

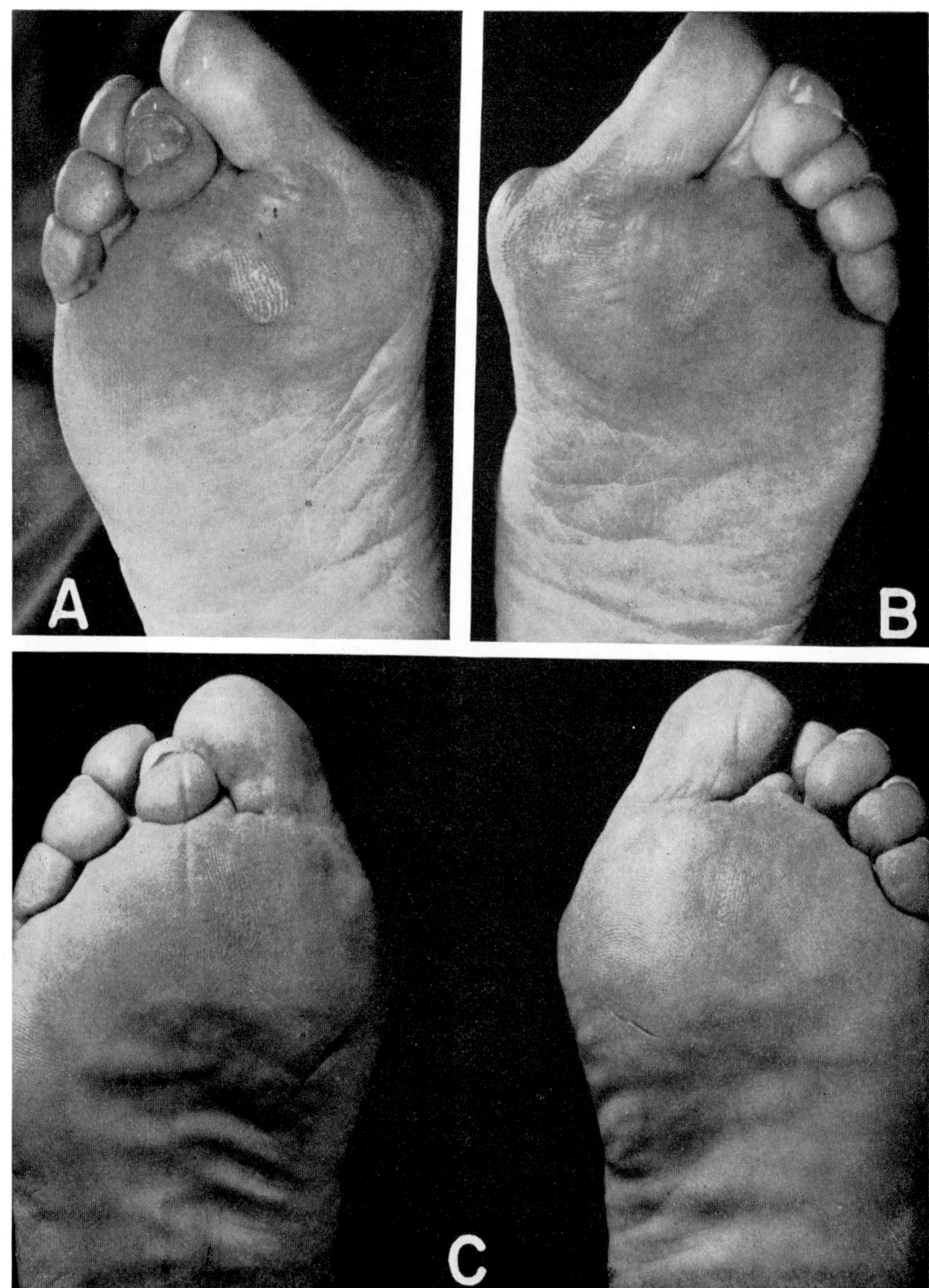

Figure 18–24. The same case as in Figure 18–23. Preoperative (*A*) and (*B*) postoperative (*C*) plantar views of both feet.

utilized for the correction of hallux valgus with degenerative joint changes (Figs. 18–26 to 18–32).

The author of this book is aware that he has said almost nothing about deformities of the forefoot caused by gout, diabetic neuropathy, upper and lower motor neuron lesions, and so on. A surgical pattern that has been utilized for disabilities from one cause may—with some modification—be advantageously used to remedy disorders from another source.

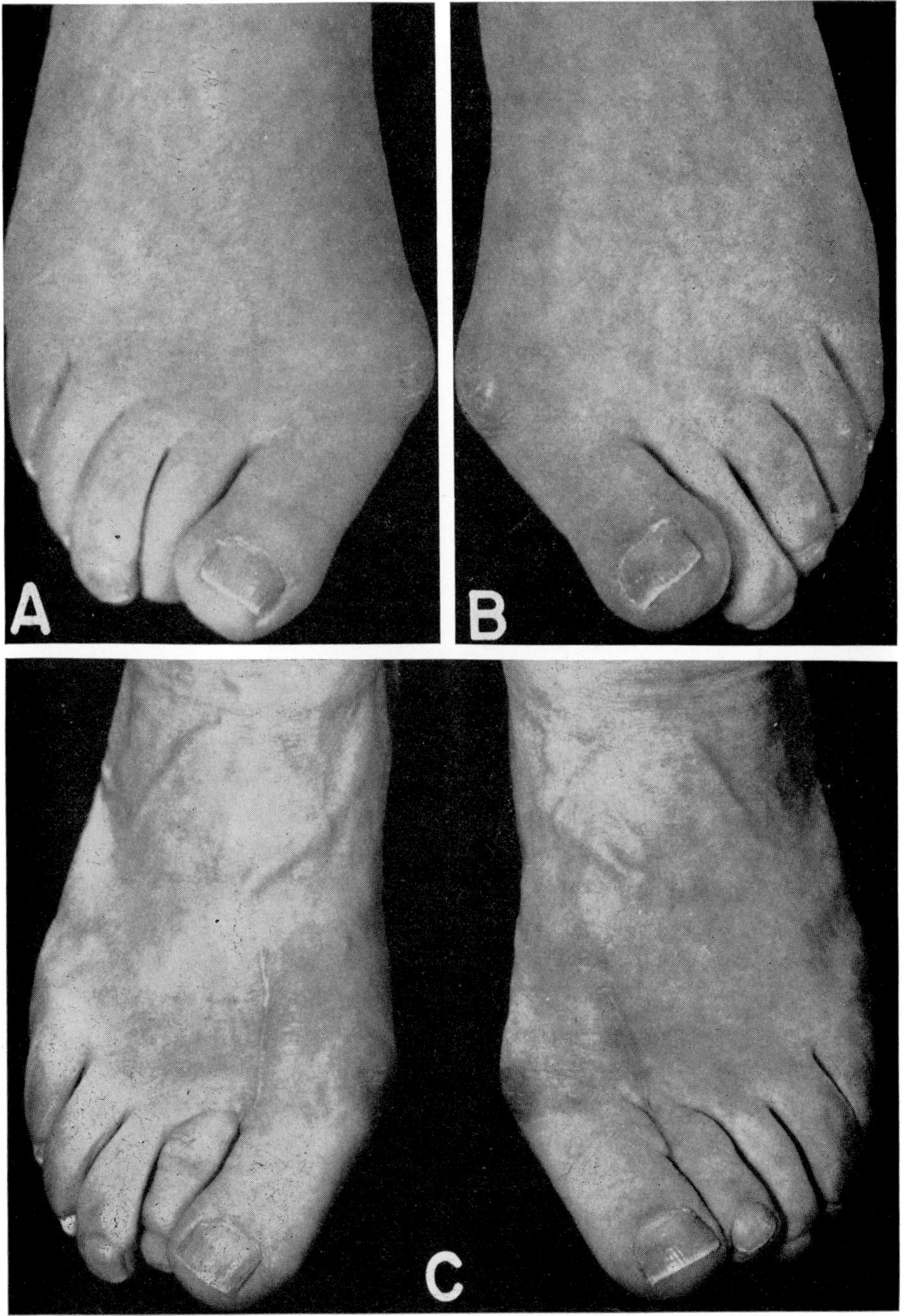

Figure 18–25. Same case. *A* and *B*, Preoperative dorsal view photograph. *C*, Postoperative dorsal view. Patient completely happy with the results.

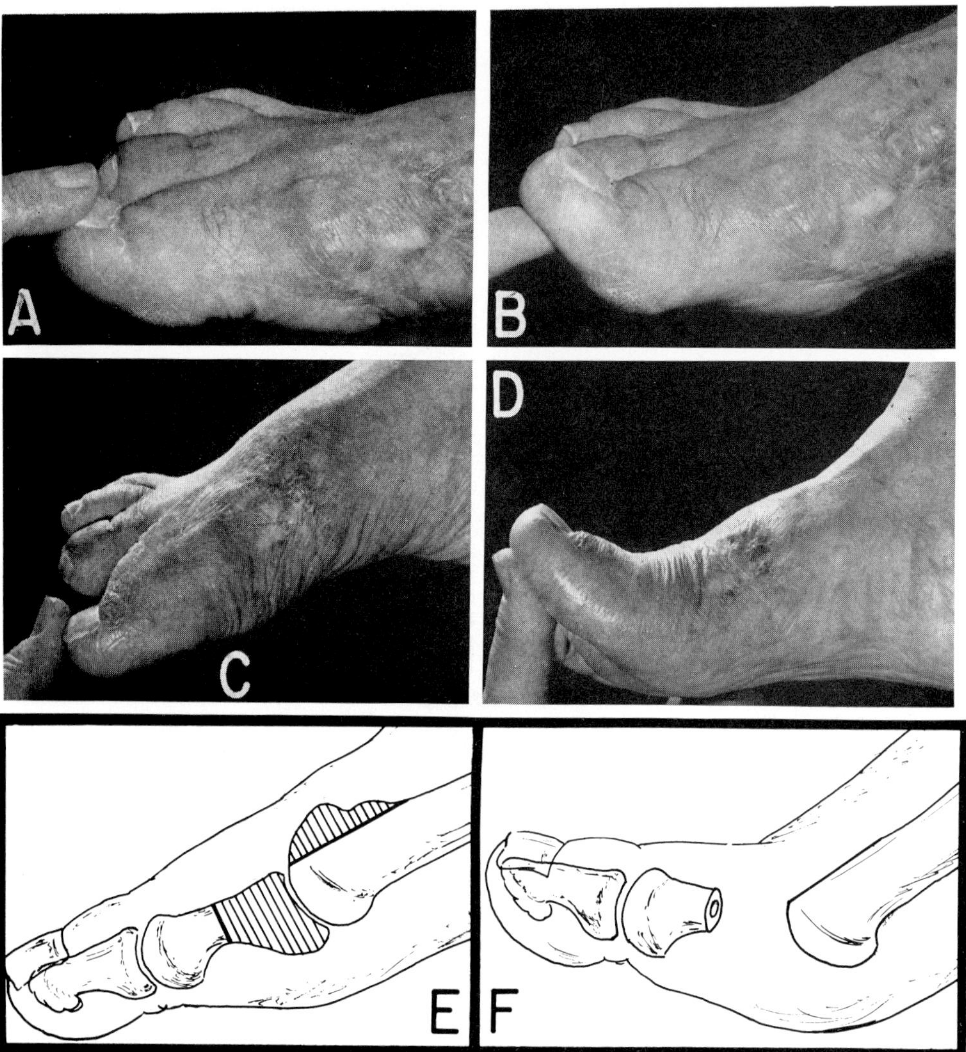

Figure 18–26. Woman, around 45, with stiff and painful great toe and "dorsal bunion." Diagnosis: hallux rigidus. Surgery consisted of resection of the proximal half of the first phalanx of the great toe and effacement of dorsal osteophyte. *A,* Preoperative push-down test showing the great toe barely flexing at the metatarsophalangeal joint. *B,* Preoperative push-up test—the hallux extends at the interphalangeal but not at the metatarsophalangeal joint. *C* and *D,* Postrecovery tests. *E* and *F,* Interpretative diagrams. Patient was satisfied.

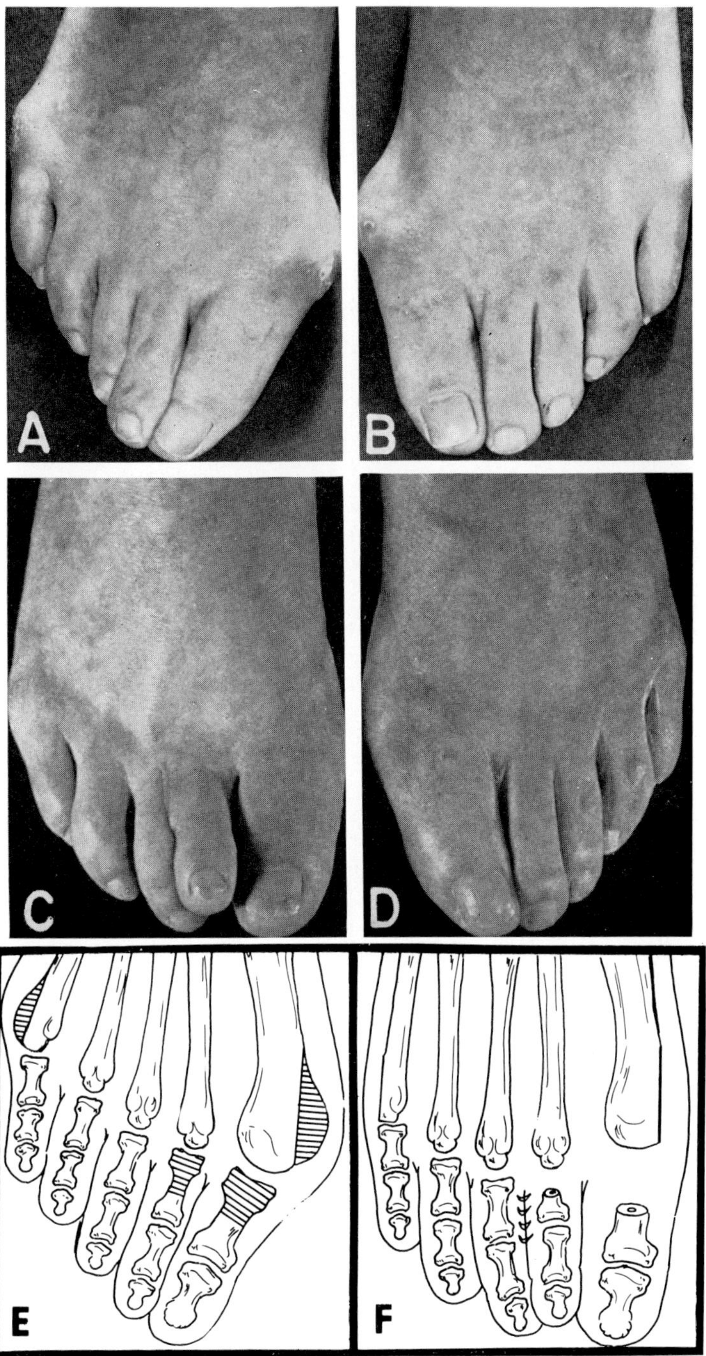

Figure 18–27. Woman, 55 years of age, with pain on the sides of the first and fifth metatarsophalangeal joint. Diagnosis: bilateral valgus, corn on the third right toe, and bunionette due to fixed metatarsus quintus valgus. Surgery consisted of a Keller resection, partial proximal phalangectomy and syndactylia of the second and third toes, and sagittal resection of the lateral eminence of the fifth metatarsal head. *A* and *B*, Before surgery. *C* and *D*, After recovery. *E* and *F*, Interpretative diagrams. The patient was satisfied, notwithstanding the overriding right second toe due to inadequate surgical syndactylia.

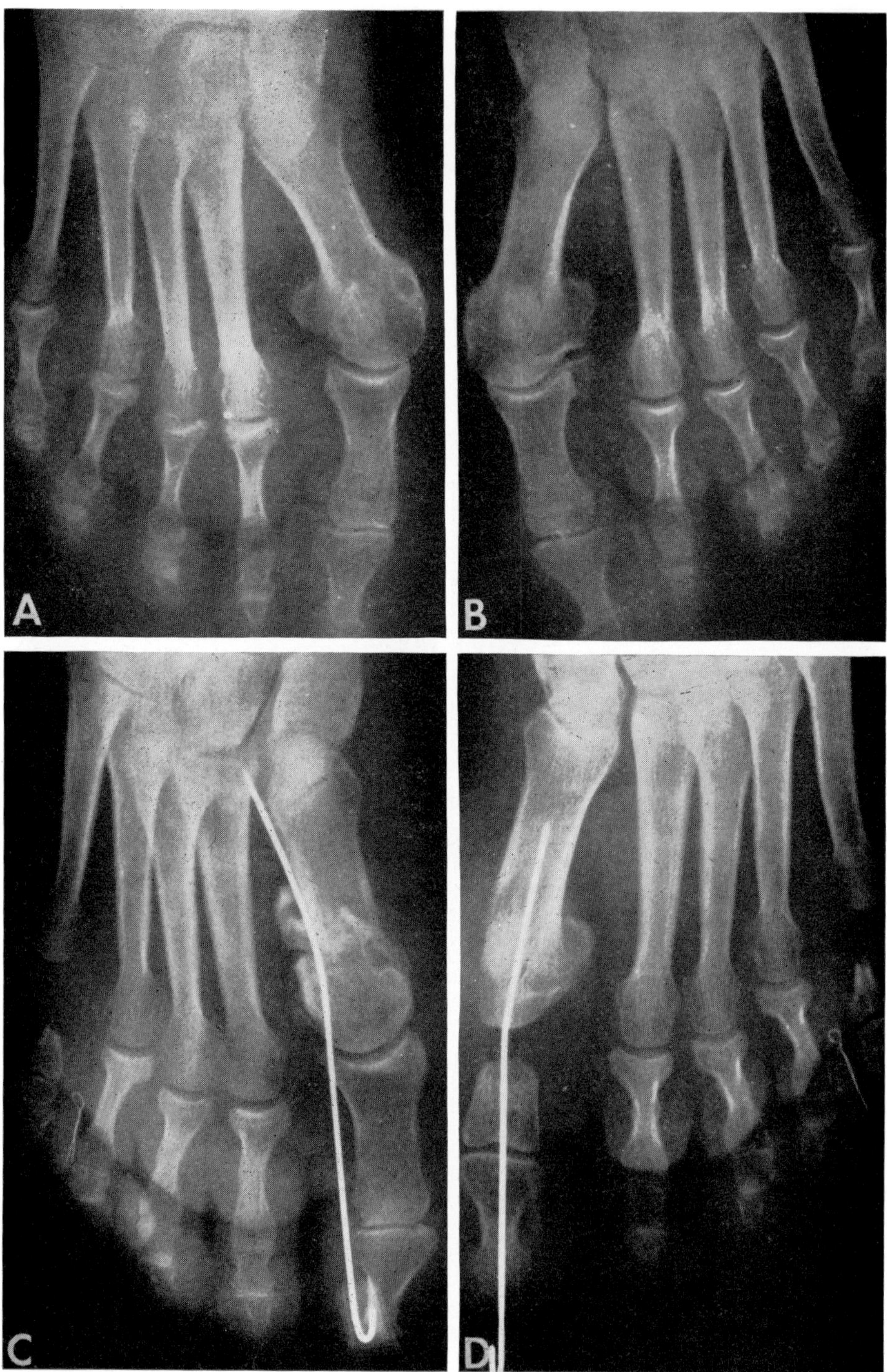

Figure 18–28. Woman, 53 years of age, with right side "bunion," a stiff painful big toe on the left side, and hammered small toes on both feet. Diagnosis: bilateral metatarsus primus varus, bilateral hallux valgus, bilateral fixed metatarsus quintus valgus, and bilateral contracted small toes. Surgery consisted of lateral displacement osteotomy of the distal extremity of the first metatarsal on the right side, a Keller resection on the left side, and partial proximal phalangectomy of the fifth toe and syndactylia of this digit with its neighbor on both sides. *A* and *B,* Preoperative roentgenograms. *C* and *D,* Immediate postoperative roentgenograms. Note fixation wires.

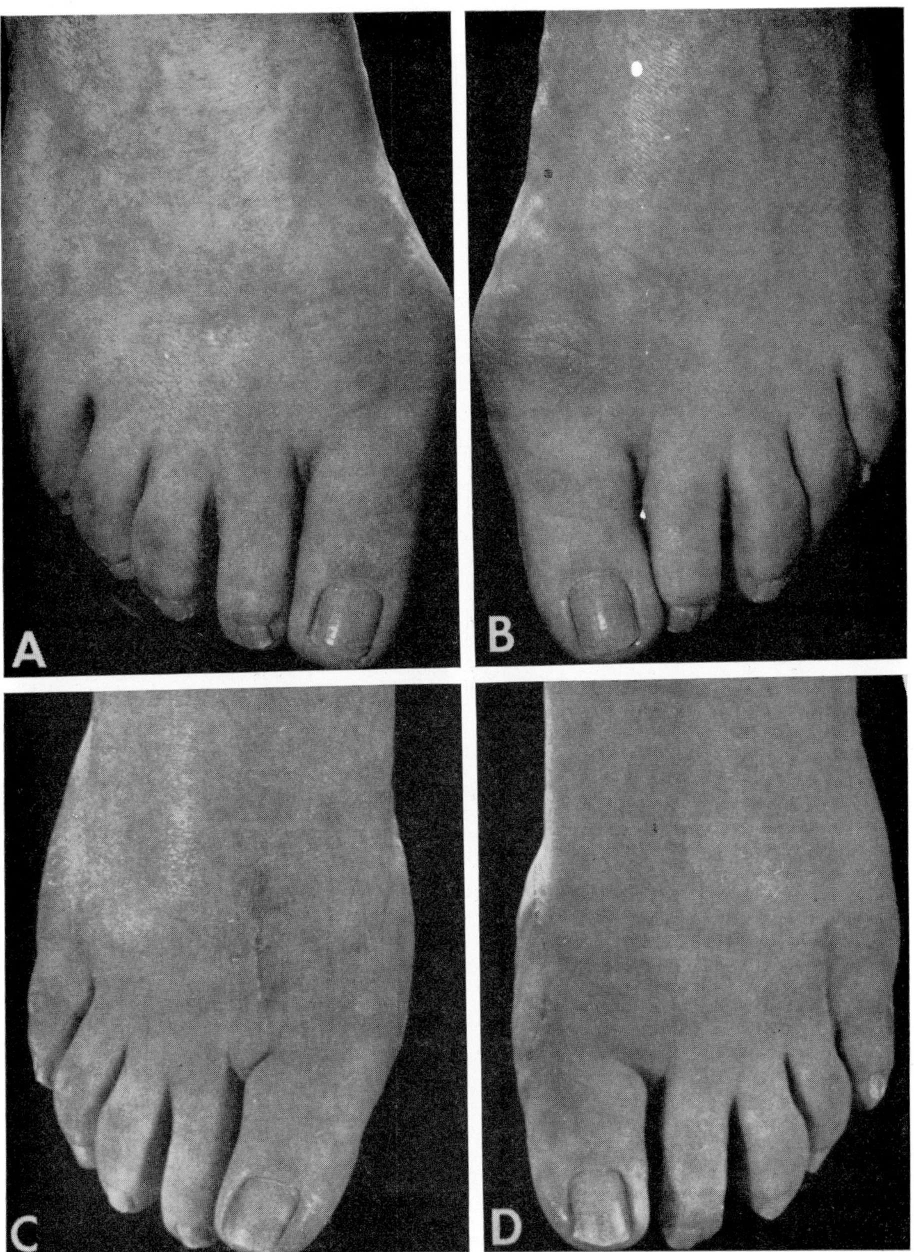

Figure 18–29. The same case as in Figure 18–28. *A* and *B,* Preoperative photographs. *C* and *D,* Postrecovery photographs. The patient is satisfied and works 8 hours a day as a saleslady.

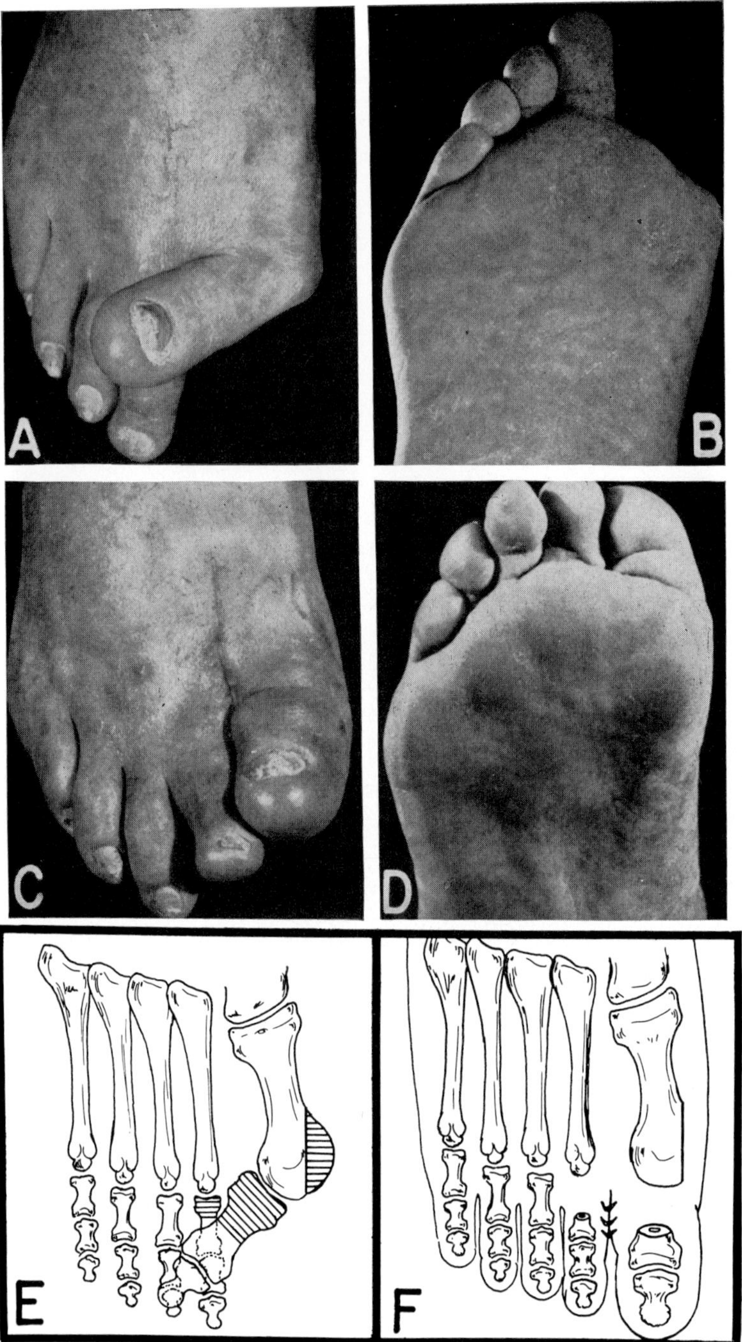

Figure 18–30. Man, near 80, cannot wear shoe because of "crooked" big toe. Diagnosis: outwardly deviated, axially rotated, overriding hallux, thin skin over the medial aspect of the first metatarsophalangeal joint and precarious circulation. Surgery consisted of a Keller resection through interdigital approach, and surgical syndactylia of first and second toe; no tourniquet was used. *A,* Dorsal view before surgery. *B,* Preoperative plantar view. *C,* Postrecovery dorsal view. *D,* Postrecovery plantar view. *E* and *F,* Interpretative diagrams. The syndactylia did not hold near the tip of the toes. Patient can now wear shoes in comfort.

The pattern offered may be as simple as that employed for the eradication of a clavus or as complicated as those utilized for correction of clawtoes, loose-jointed or contracted forefeet, and for the extremely disabling fixed plantar incarceration of the metatarsal heads due to rheumatoid arthritis (Figs. 18–33 to 18–40).

The author has consciously avoided statistical documentation of surgical results. Almost all statistics about the surgical treatment of hallux valgus and related deformities of the forefoot leave out an important factor: the surgeon. By this is not merely meant the man who operates with variable degree of dexterity, but he who also knows what to do and when, and is prepared to vary his technique to meet the needs of the patient. The imaginative surgeon does not cling to any stereotyped procedure, even if he feels attached to it for his having played a part in its invention.

As it should have been evident, the author believes that hallux valgus, hammer- or clawtoes, dynamic or fixed splaying of marginal metatarsals, and plantar prominence of the central heads are complex deformities in themselves. In varying combinations they create complicated problems. To cope with these problems one needs to combine many steps and improvise an operation that would meet all the needs of the case under consideration. Obviously such "tailored" operations cannot be categorized, labeled, "pigeonholed." Nor can the results obtained be fitted into a stereotype scale.

Instead of interpolating a statistical tabulation of results, the author has presented a number of representative cases, shown in the illustrations accompanying the text. Photographs before and after surgery should supply the necessary information concerning the cosmetic outcome. Unfortunately, cosmetic and functional results do not always go hand in hand. A shapely foot can sometimes be excruciatingly painful; conversely, a deformed foot may cause no discomfort and serve its possessor well. Paraphrased testimonies by the patients or—in case of

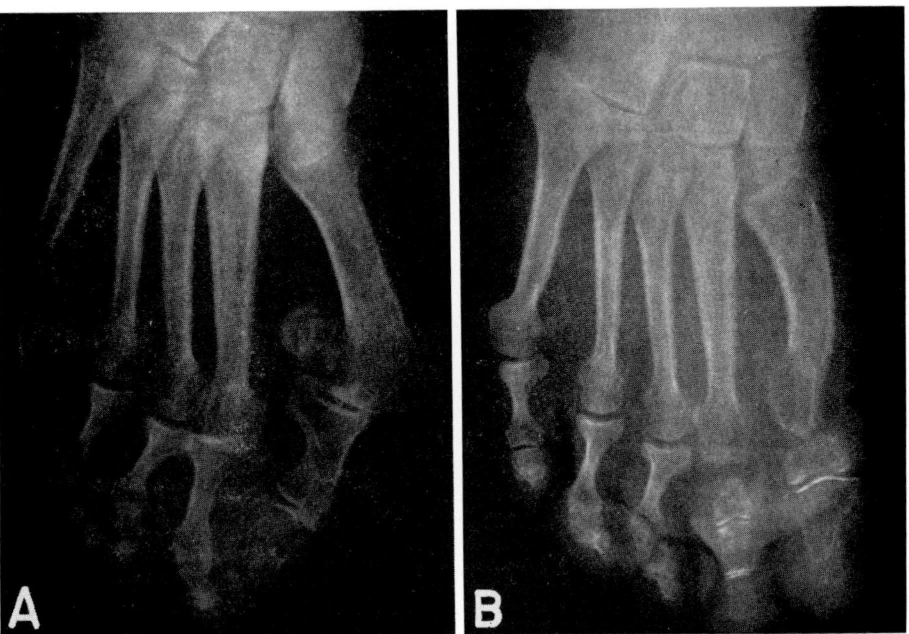

Figure 18–31. Woman, 55 years of age, with painful, stiff overriding and twisted great toe and spread out forefoot, and pain under the ball of the great toe. Diagnosis: hallux valgus and rigidus with fixed axial rotation of the great toe and metatarsus primus varus. Surgery consisted of V osteotomy of the base of the first metatarsal followed by angulation of the distal fragment laterally, Keller resection, sesamoidectomy, prophylactic shortening of the second toe, and surgical syndactylia of the first with the second toe. *A,* Roentgenogram before surgery. *B,* Roentgenogram after recovery.

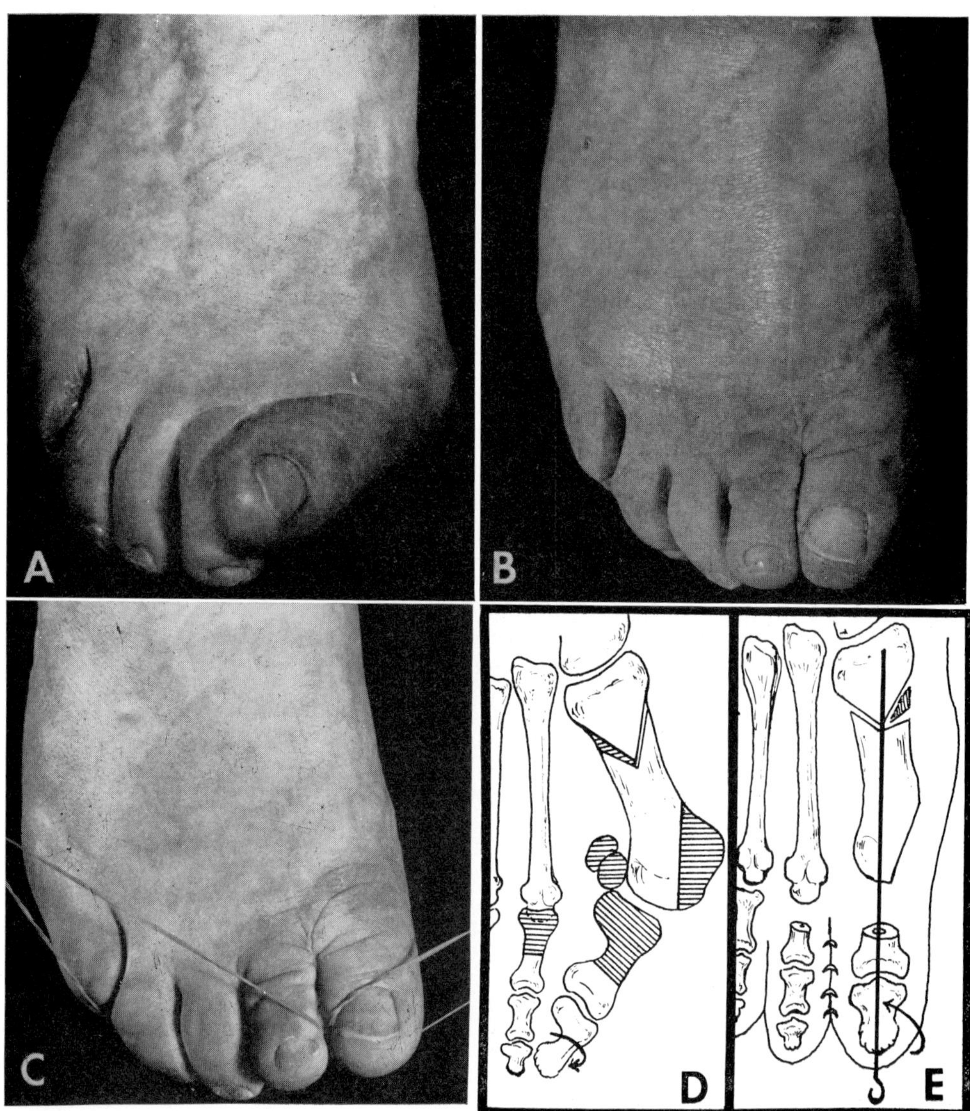

Figure 18–32. The same case as in Figure 18–31. *A,* Before surgery. *B,* After recovery. *C,* First and second toes are pulled apart to show the advanced web between them. *D* and *E,* Interpretative diagrams. Patient is completely satisfied.

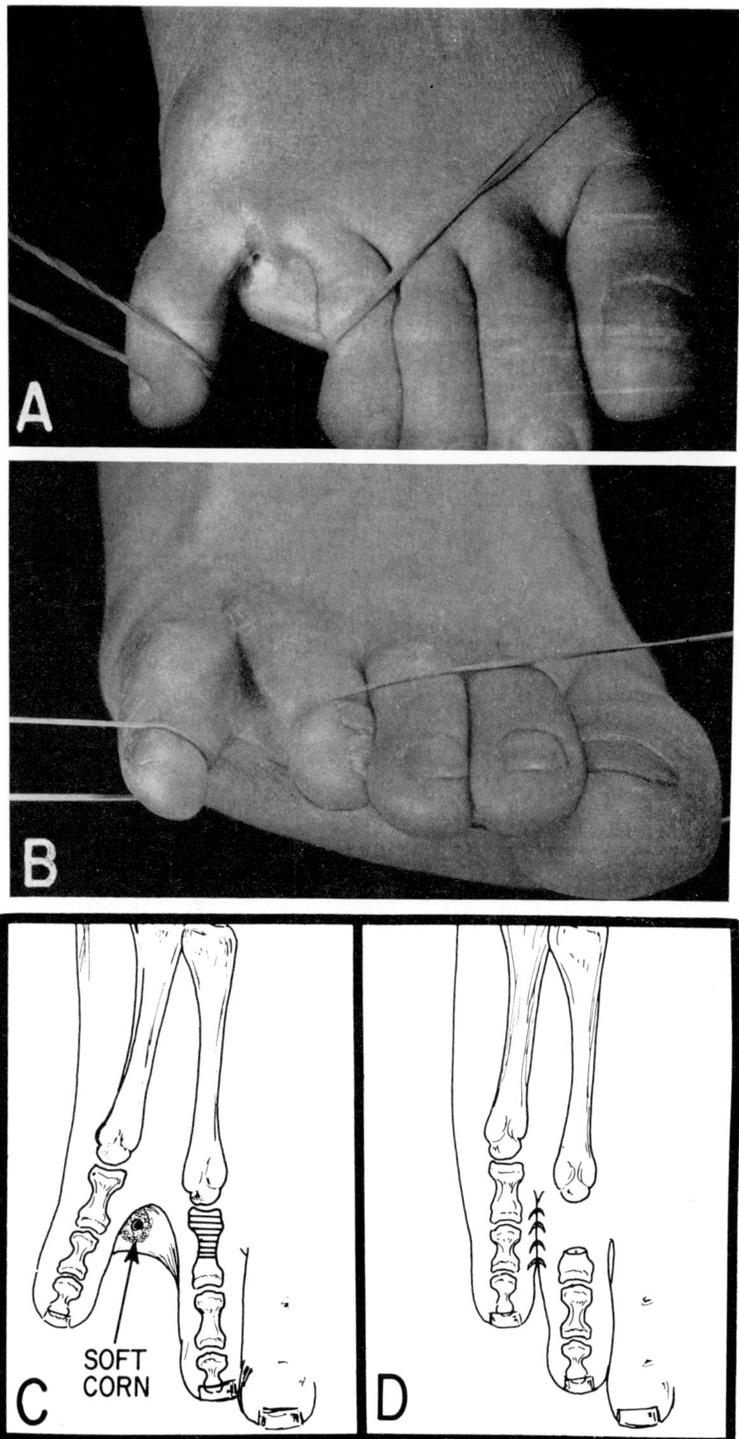

Figure 18–33. Woman, 30 years of age, with painful, soft corn. Diagnosis: interdigital clavus. Surgery consisted of resection of clavus, partial proximal phalangectomy of fourth toe, and surgical syndactylia of fourth and fifth toes. *A,* Preoperative photograph. *B,* Postrecovery photograph. Toes have been pulled apart by rubber bands to show the extent of syndactylia. *C* and *D,* Interpretative diagrams. There has been no recurrence.

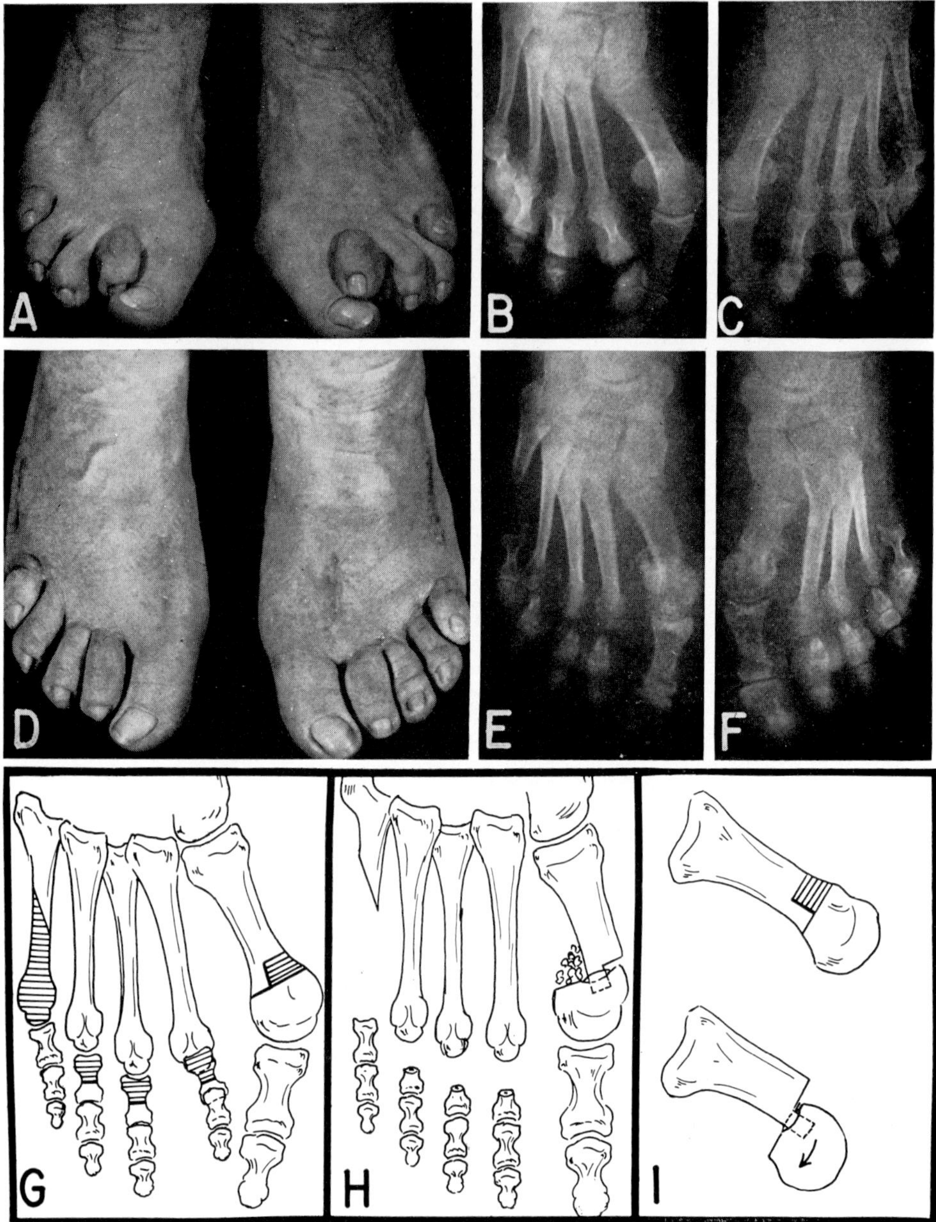

Figure 18–34. Woman, in her 60's, with metatarsalgia, spread out forefeet, and deformed toes. Diagnosis: bilateral hallux valgus, hammered overriding toes, hypermobile marginal metatarsals, and extremely loose-jointed, compressible feet. Surgery consisted of distal osteotomy of the first metatarsal, displacing the capital fragment laterally and plantarward; partial proximal phalangectomy of the middle toes; resection of the distal two-thirds of the fifth metatarsal; and surgical syndactylia of each pair of lesser toes. *A,* Preoperative photograph. *B* and *C,* Preoperative roentgenograms. *D,* Postrecovery photograph. *E* and *F,* Postrecovery roentgenograms. *G, H,* and *I,* Interpretative diagrams. Patient was elated with the outcome.

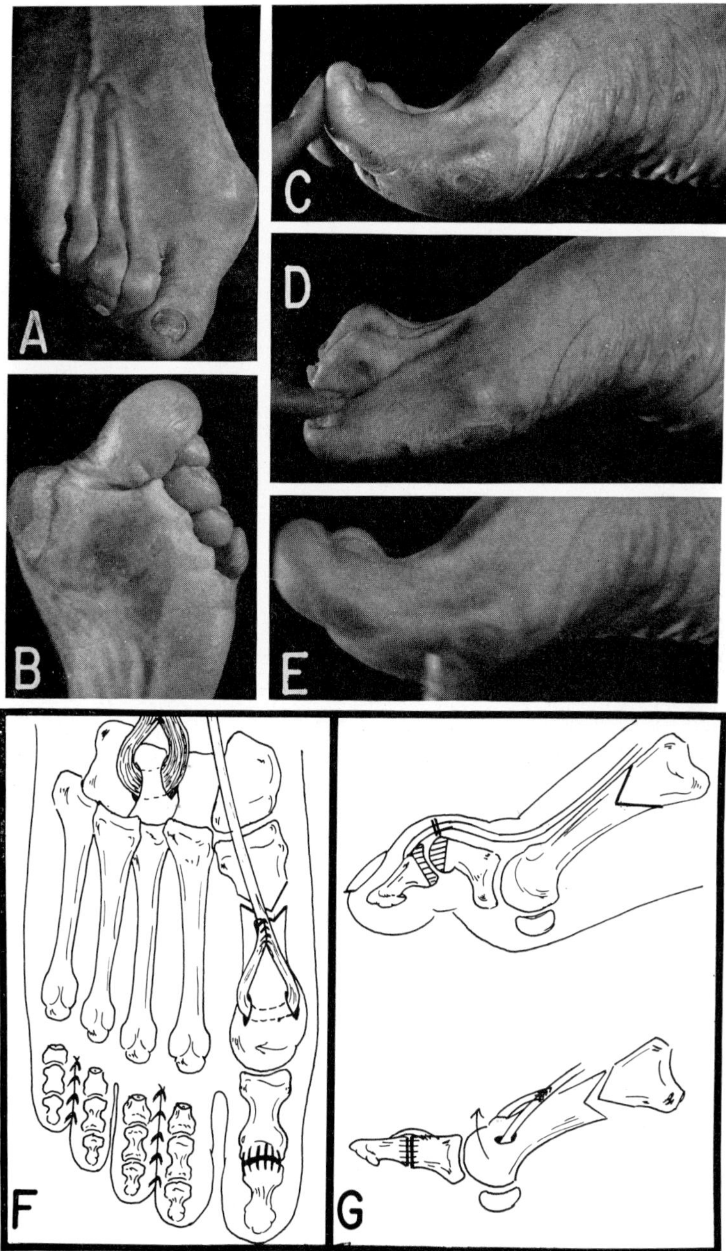

Figure 18–35. Man, around 40 years of age, with bilateral hallux valgus, clawtoes, plantarflexed first metatarsal, fixed plantar incarceration of the middle metatarsal heads, and taut digital extensors. Charcot-Marie-Tooth disease was a concomitant condition. Patient complained of inability to wear shoes with comfort. Surgery consisted of osteotomy of first metatarsal near its base—the distal fragment was pushed laterally, lifted up, and suspended by the long extensor of the great toe; fusion of interphalangeal joint of great toe; transfer of extensor tendons of lesser toes to the lateral cuneiform; and partial proximal phalangectomy of lesser toes and surgical syndactylia of each pair. *A,* Dorsal view of right foot showing hallux valgus deformity, clawed lesser toes, and taut extensor tendons. *B,* Plantar view. *C,* The great toe could be pushed up. *D,* The hallux could not be pushed plantarward because of taut long extensor. *E,* Pressure on the ball of the foot failed to bring the toes down. *F* and *G,* Diagrams illustrating the main step of surgical procedure used on the right foot. The left foot was similarly operated on.

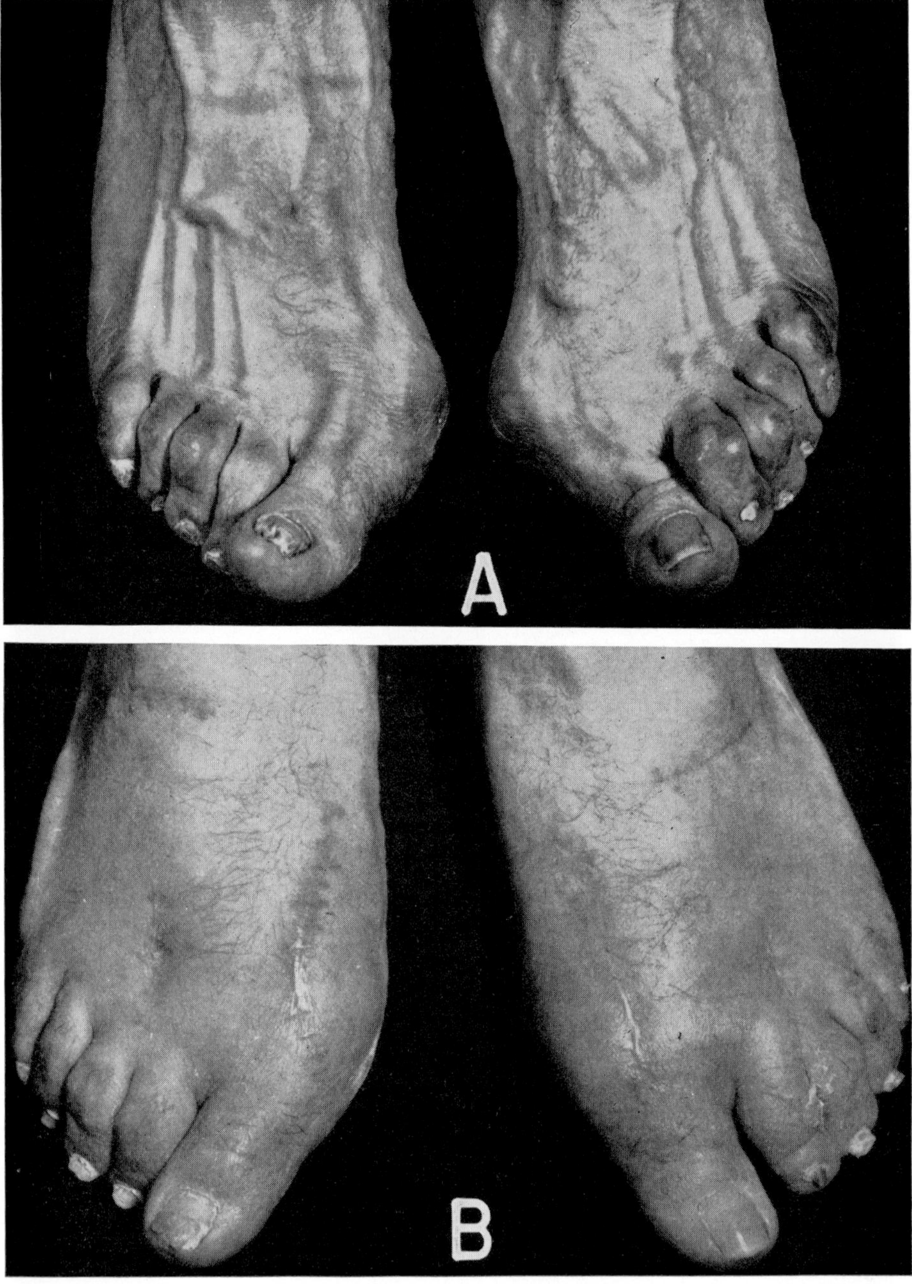

Figure 18–36. The same case as in Figure 18–35. *A,* Preoperative dorsal view. Note the split nail of the second toe and pressure keratosis on the right side. *B,* Postoperative dorsal view.

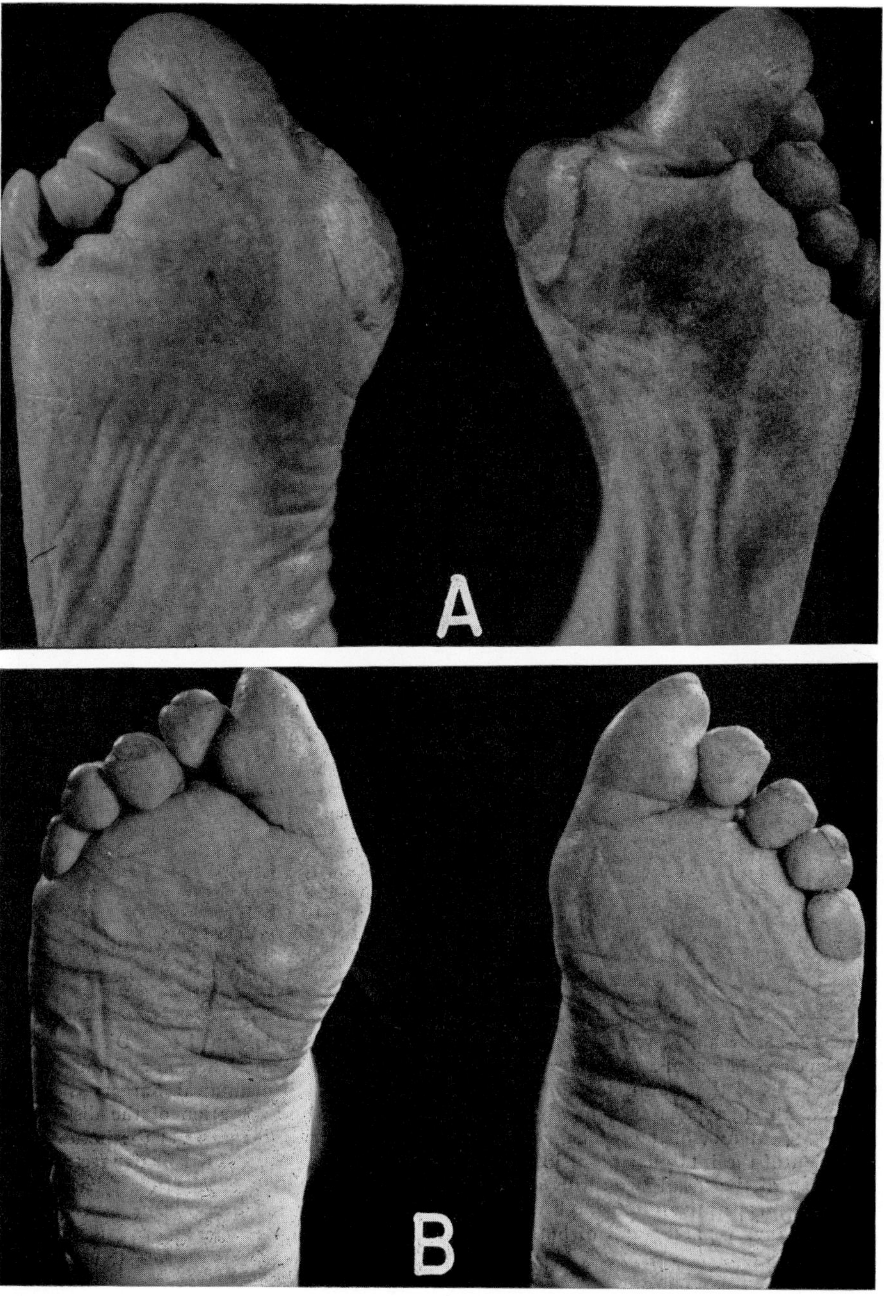

Figure 18–37. The same case as in Figures 18–35 and 18–36. Preoperative (*A*) and postoperative (*B*) plantar views. Patient is happy he can now wear shoes in comfort.

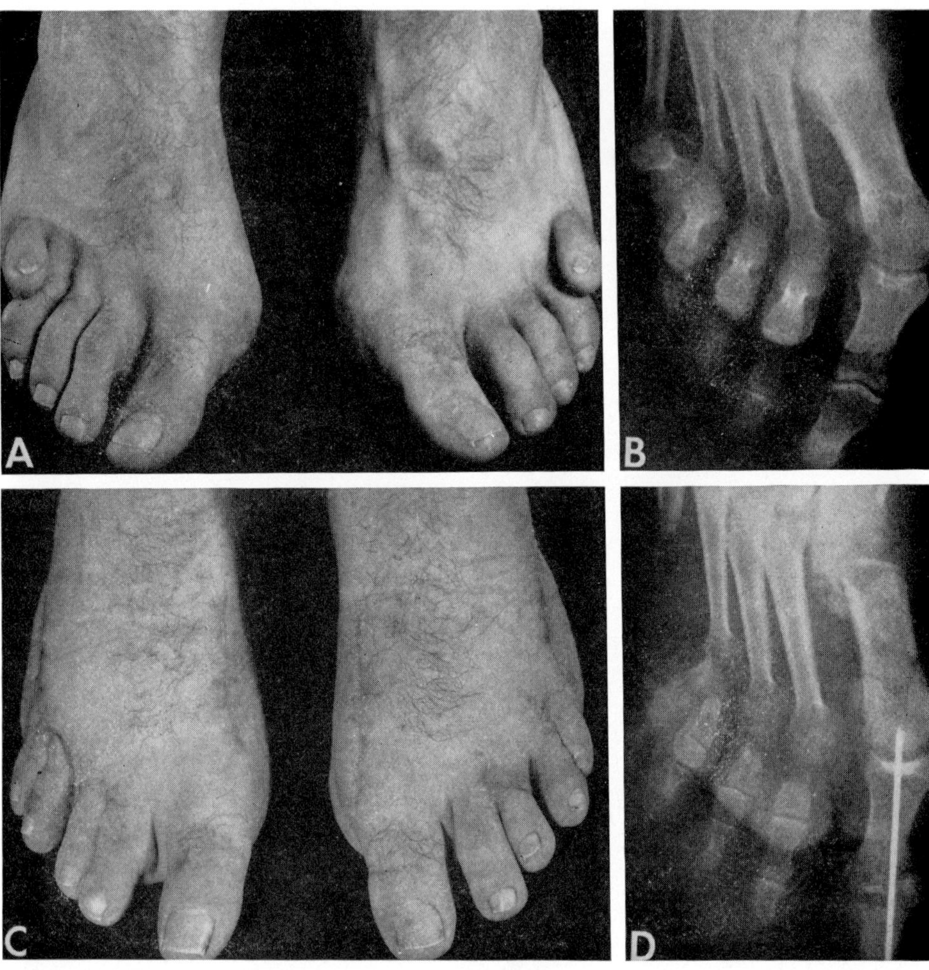

Figure 18–38. Man, 32 years of age, with painful forefeet and deformed toes. Diagnosis: bilateral hallux valgus and hammered middle toes, digitus minimus varus, plantar flexion and varus of the first metatarsal, varus of the middle metatarsals, and hypermobile fifth metatarsal. Surgery consisted of V osteotomy of the first metatarsal base with lateral angulation and elevation of the distal fragment, using the long extensor of the great toe for suspension as shown in diagrams at the bottom of Figure 18–35; fusion of the interphalangeal joint of the great toe; partial proximal phalangectomy of lesser toes; resection of the distal two-thirds of the fifth metatarsal; and surgical syndactylia each pair of lesser toes. *A,* Preoperative photograph of both forefeet. *B,* Preoperative roentgenogram of right forefoot. *C,* Postrecovery photograph of both forefeet. *D,* Postoperative roentgenogram of right forefoot. Patient was satisfied.

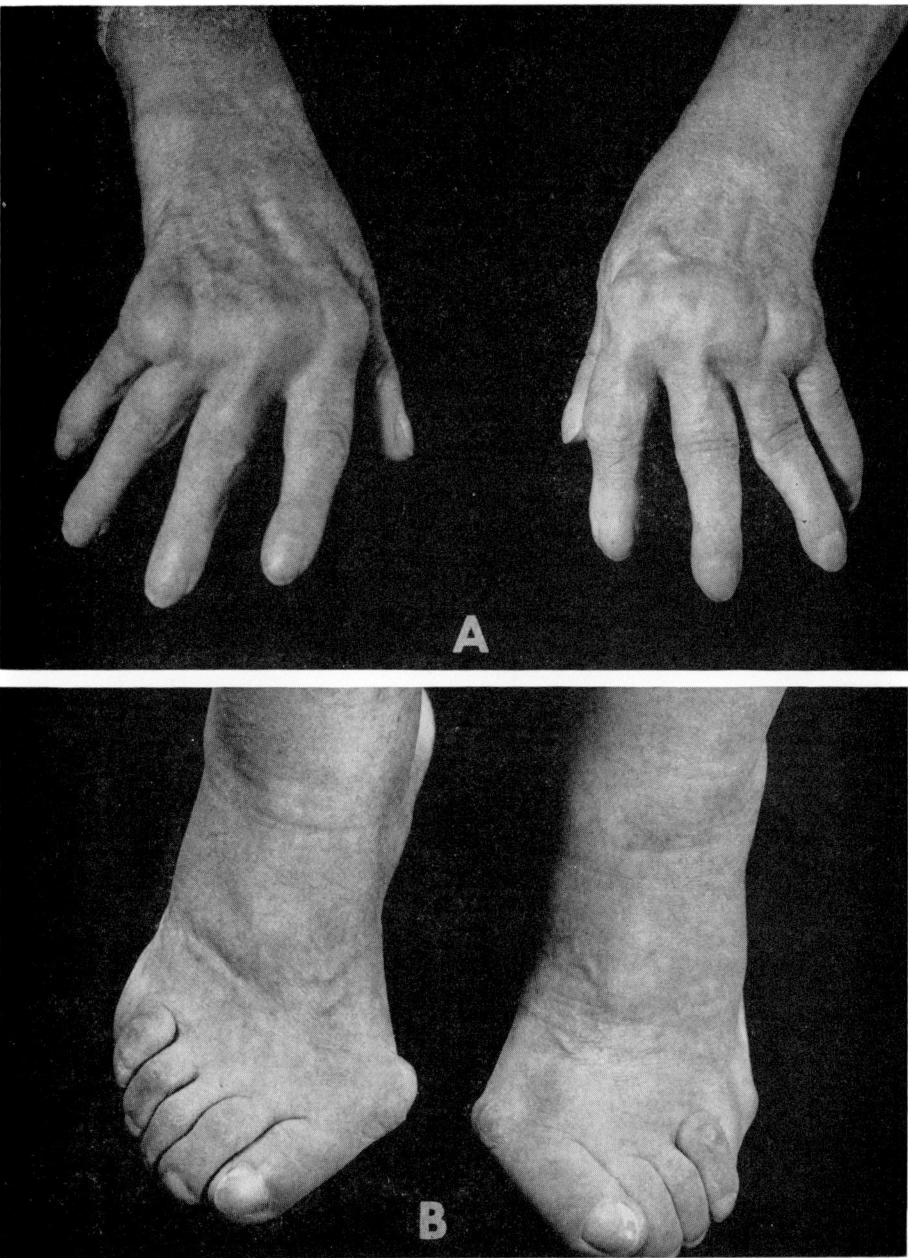

Figure 18–39. Woman, in her 50's, with painful clawtoes. Diagnosis: clawtoes with fixed plantar incarceration of the metatarsal heads due to rheumatoid arthritis. Surgery consisted of resection of the heads and part of adjacent shaft of all metatarsals, and surgical syndactylia of the first with the second and the third with the fourth toes. *A*, Photograph of the hands. *B*, Photograph of the feet.

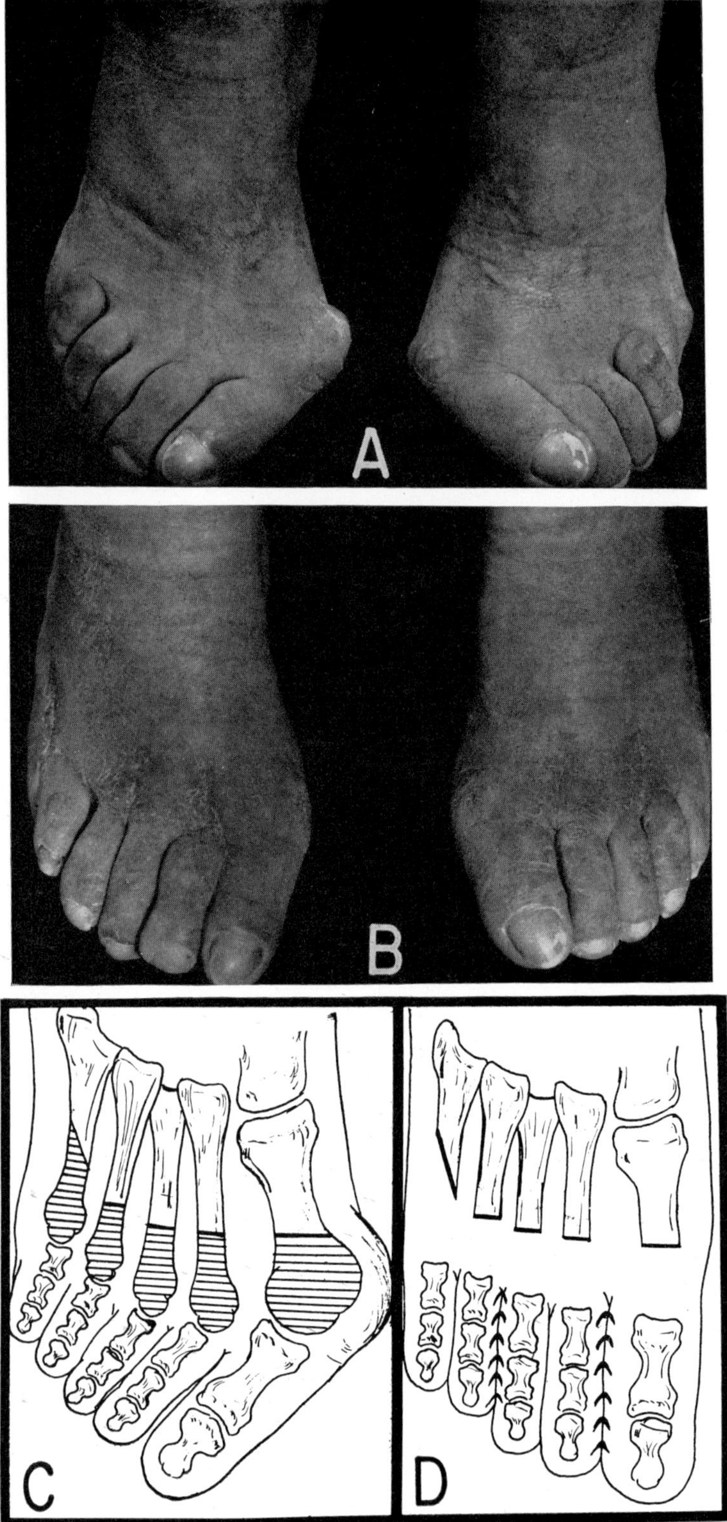

Figure 18–40. The same case as in Figure 18–39. *A,* Feet before surgery. *B,* Postrecovery photograph. *C* and *D,* Interpretative diagrams. Patient was satisfied.

children—by their parents should suggest the degree of comfort and functional usefulness secured by surgery.

REFERENCES

Anderson, W.: *The Deformities of the Fingers and Toes.* London, J. & A. Churchill, 1897.

Bankart, A. S. B.: Pathology and treatment of hallux valgus. Med. Press Circ. *96*:33–35, 1913.

Bankart, A. S. B.: The treatment of minor maladies of the foot. Lancet *1*:249–252, 1935.

Broca, P.: Des deformités de la partie anterieure du pied produite par l'action de la chaussure. Bull. Soc. Anat. *27*:60–67, 1852.

Bromeis, H.: Unsere Erfahrungen mit der Hallux valgus—Operation nach M. Schede. Chirurg *3*:465–471, 1931.

Camper, P.: *On the Best Form of Shoe,* published with Dowie's treatise, *The Foot and Its Covering.* London, R. Hardwicke, pp. 1–44, 1861. The French version, called *Dissertation sur le Meilleur Forme des Souliers,* appeared in Paris, 1781.

Clarke, J. J.: Operation for painful affection of the great toe joints. Med. Press Circ. *95*: 284–285, 1913.

Cleveland, M.: Hallux valgus—final results of two hundred operations. Arch Surg. *14*:1123–1135, 1927.

Cleveland, M., and Winant, E. M.: An end-result of the Keller operation. J. Bone Joint Surg. *32*:163–175, 1950.

Durlacher, L.: *A Treatise on Corns, Bunions, Disease of the Nails and the General Management of the Feet.* London, Simkin, Marshall & Co., 1845.

Ellis, T. S.: *The Human Foot.* New York, W. Wood Co., 1890.

Ewald, P.: Die Aetologie des Hallux Valgus. Dtsch. Ztschr. Chir. *114*:90–103, 1912.

Harding, M. C.: Bunions: different types, different treatment. Southw. Med. *11*:360–362, 1927.

Hilton, J.: *Rest and Pain.* Reprinted from the last London edition. Cincinnati and Cleveland, P. W. Garfield, 1891.

Hohmann, G.: *Fuss Und Bein.* Munich, J. Bergmann, 1951.

Jones, F. W.: *Structure and Function as Seen in the Foot.* 2nd Ed. London, Bailliere, Tindall & Cox, 1949.

Lane, A.: The causation, pathology and physiology of the deformities which develop during young life. Guy's Hosp. Rep. *44*:307–317, 1887.

Mitchell, C. L., Fleming, J. L., Allen R., Glenney, C., and Sanford, G. A.: Osteotomy—bunionectomy for hallux valgus. J. Bone Joint Surg. *40*:41–60, 1958.

Morris, H.: *Anatomy of the Joints.* London, J. & A. Churchill, 1879.

Olivecrona, H.: An operation for certain cases of hallux valgus. Acta. Chir. Scand. *57*:396–402, 1924.

Perkins, G.: Removal of the metatarsal head for hallux valgus and hallux rigidus. Lancet *1*: 540–541, 1927.

Porter, J. L.: Why operations for bunions fail with a description of one which does not. Surg. Gynec. Obst. *8*:89–90, 1909.

Silver, D.: The operative treatment of hallux valgus. J. Bone Joint Surg. *5*:225–232, 1923.

Stamm, T. T.: The surgical treatment of hallux valgus. Guy's Hosp. Rep. *106*:273–279, 1957.

Syms, P.: Bunion: its aetiology, anatomy and operative treatment. New York J. Med. *66*:448–451, 1897.

Volkmann, R.: Ueber die sogenannte Exostose der grossen zehe. Virchows Arch. Path. Anat. Physiol. *10*:297–306, 1856.

Wilson, H. A.: An analysis of 152 cases of hallux valgus in 77 patients with a report upon an operation for relief. Am. J. Orthop. Surg. *3*: 214–230, 1906.

Index

Page numbers in **bold face** indicate illustrations.